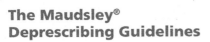

The Maudsley®
Deprescribing Guidelines

T0131356

The Maudsley Guidelines

Other books in the *Maudsley Prescribing Guidelines* series include:

The Maudsley® Deprescribing Guidelines

Antidepressants, Benzodiazepines, Gabapentinoids and Z-drugs

Mark Horowitz, BA, BSc(Med), MBBS(Hons), MSc, GDipPsych, PhD

Clinical Research Fellow in Psychiatry and Co-lead clinician in the Psychotropic Deprescribing Clinic
North East London NHS Foundation Trust, Ilford, UK
Honorary Clinical Research Fellow, Department of Psychiatry, University College London, London, UK

David Taylor, PhD, FFRPS, FRPharmS, FRCPEdin, FRCPsych(Hon)

Director of Pharmacy and Pathology
South London and Maudsley NHS Foundation Trust
Professor of Psychopharmacology, King's College London, London, UK

WILEY Blackwell

This edition first published 2024
© 2024 John Wiley & Sons Ltd

The right of Mark Horowitz and David Taylor to be identified as the authors of this work has been asserted in accordance with law.

Registered Offices
John Wiley & Sons, Inc., 111 River Street, Hoboken, NJ 07030, USA
John Wiley & Sons Ltd, The Atrium, Southern Gate, Chichester, West Sussex, PO19 8SQ, UK

For details of our global editorial offices, customer services, and more information about Wiley products visit us at www.wiley.com.

Wiley also publishes its books in a variety of electronic formats and by print-on-demand. Some content that appears in standard print versions of this book may not be available in other formats.

Limit of Liability/Disclaimer of Warranty
The contents of this work are intended to further general scientific research, understanding, and discussion only and are not intended and should not be relied upon as recommending or promoting scientific method, diagnosis, or treatment by physicians for any particular patient. In view of ongoing research, equipment modifications, changes in governmental regulations, and the constant flow of information relating to the use of medicines, equipment, and devices, the reader is urged to review and evaluate the information provided in the package insert or instructions for each medicine, equipment, or device for, among other things, any changes in the instructions or indication of usage and for added warnings and precautions. While the publisher and authors have used their best efforts in preparing this work, they make no representations or warranties with respect to the accuracy or completeness of the contents of this work and specifically disclaim all warranties, including without limitation any implied warranties of merchantability or fitness for a particular purpose. No warranty may be created or extended by sales representatives, written sales materials or promotional statements for this work. This work is sold with the understanding that the publisher is not engaged in rendering professional services. The advice and strategies contained herein may not be suitable for your situation. You should consult with a specialist where appropriate. The fact that an organization, website, or product is referred to in this work as a citation and/or potential source of further information does not mean that the publisher and authors endorse the information or services the organization, website, or product may provide or recommendations it may make. Further, readers should be aware that websites listed in this work may have changed or disappeared between when this work was written and when it is read. Neither the publisher nor authors shall be liable for any loss of profit or any other commercial damages, including but not limited to special, incidental, consequential, or other damages.

Library of Congress Cataloging-in-Publication Data Applied for
ISBN: 9781119822981 (Paperback); 9781119823018 (Adobe PDF); 9781119823025 (EPub)

Cover design: Wiley

Set in 10/12pt Sabon by Straive, Pondicherry, India

SKY10066215_013024

Contents

Preface

'It is an art of no little importance to administer medicines properly; but it is an art of much greater and more difficult acquisition to know when to suspend or altogether omit them.'

Philippe Pinel 1745–1826

This is not a book that questions the validity or effectiveness of medicines used for mental health conditions. It is a guide to the deprescribing of psychotropic medication in situations where deprescribing is, on balance, agreed to be a better option than continued prescribing. The agreement here is between prescriber and patient. The core tenet of this text is that decisions are made jointly in the patient's best interest.

Patients have expressed dissatisfaction – and sometimes outrage – with available medical assistance for stopping psychiatric medications. This has led to many tens of thousands of patients seeking advice from online peer-support forums. When surveyed, these patients report that their doctors were often unhelpful either because they recommended tapering too quickly or because they were not familiar enough with withdrawal effects to provide helpful advice.[1] Some doctors are apparently still suggesting that antidepressants do not cause withdrawal symptoms. The main requests from these patients are that health professionals are sufficiently well informed to provide personalised, flexible reduction plans and that access is provided to smaller doses to facilitate tapering (either liquid versions of medication, or specially compounded smaller dose tablets or capsules).[1] We hope this textbook will contribute to a broader understanding of these issues, a greater expertise in helping patients and a better outcome for all.

In writing this textbook we took on what some might consider an impossible task. Safely stopping psychiatric medications is not simply a matter of outlining a regimen of reducing doses for patients to follow. There are too many aspects of the drug, the individual and their lives that come into play such that adjustments inevitably need to be made, often involving a certain amount of trial and error. Yet the most common request we receive from patients and clinicians is to provide tapering schedules to guide reductions. It can be daunting to begin a journey without a map to follow. So in this book we have tried to balance specific guidance with flexibility, offering different routes to reducing doses, whilst trying to accommodate the complexity required for adjusting the course for an individual. We have also tried to acknowledge the tenets of other guidance in this field. The advice given here is, for example, largely consistent with the UK NICE guidelines on this topic, but we aimed to provide greater detail on how to implement the broad principles outlined.

Balancing competing priorities has proved difficult. On the one hand, patients often report that they are tapered off psychiatric drugs too quickly, and on the other, patients should not be exposed for an unnecessarily long time to a drug that could be stopped more quickly. Added to this is the awareness that there is great variation from one person to another – and that we have little to guide us in predicting how an individual will react. We have therefore attempted to accommodate a wide variety of circumstances with further instructions on how to make changes from the suggested regimens.

We wrote this book partly because of our own difficulties in coming off various psychiatric drugs. Our main motivation has been that, by clarifying what is known about safe deprescribing and applying that to practice, we will spare others some of the difficult experiences we have endured. It is perhaps the book that we wished our prescribers had possessed.

It is sobering to consider that had we not experienced stopping medication first-hand we would have found it hard to believe the accounts of patients, which can seem almost fantastical in the variety and severity of symptoms (what one experienced practitioner in this field has called 'the unbelievability factor'[2]). We hope this book will help clinicians develop a greater appreciation for the difficulties some patients experience when trying to stop psychotropic medication.

We recognise that much of the guidance included in this book requires confirmation and clarification from further research but we also appreciate that people are already reducing and stopping their medication and that we should not let the perfect be the enemy of the good. The main messages of the textbook could be summed up in a few words: go slowly, at a rate the patient can tolerate and proceed even more cautiously for the last few milligrams, which are often the hardest to stop.

One major barrier for prescribers we have observed is a reluctance to prescribe liquid versions of drugs, compounded medication or other unlicensed (but widely used) methods to make up the smaller doses of medication necessary for optimal tapering. Often this is for good reasons like cost and complexity. However, minute doses are likely to be required for a substantial proportion of long-term users if they are to stop their medication safely. Many patients report that once a clinician has traversed this psychological moat the process of tapering off their medication becomes substantially easier.

We have also sought to empower patients in the process of coming off their drugs. Patient autonomy is increasingly highlighted in medicine (and psychiatry more widely), but in the area of deprescribing where relatively little is known and where patient experience is so central, it is even more important. We have observed that patients soon become the experts in understanding what rate they can tolerate in reducing their medications and we hope that clinicians will support patients in this process. An old adage from another area of medicine – 'Pain is what the patient says it is' – might be borrowed here. Withdrawal is what the patient says it is.

On this topic, we have also included in this textbook the voices of patient experts and advocates who have been instrumental in drawing attention to the problems many patients face in withdrawal, and in working out innovative approaches to minimise risks. Some of these patient experts have medical training, and some have published research in academic journals. Their experience of being both patients and, in some cases, clinicians brings unique insight into the process.

When discussing withdrawal syndromes from psychiatric drugs, the concepts of addiction or misuse and abuse often arise. However, we have emphasised throughout this textbook that physical dependence is a predictable physiological response to chronic use of psychotropic medication. This inevitably and predictably leads to a withdrawal syndrome on stopping or reducing the dose and does not indicate addiction, misuse or abuse.

This book has been written so that it may be read from cover to cover but it is also designed to be sampled as needed by the busy clinician. To this end, there are 'quick start' guides for tapering specific drugs that are designed to be intelligible largely independent of the rest of the book. The chapters on individual drug classes outline the issues specific to each class but also to tapering in general, given some commonalities. This deliberate design has necessitated some degree of repetition, the reasons for which we hope the reader will understand.

We would like to pay special tribute to Adele Framer for sharing the wisdom gained from years of supporting patients to safely stop antidepressants and other psychiatric drugs in peer-led forums, combining lived experience with academic knowledge. Also, Nicole Lamberson and Christy Huff, medical professionals with lived experience, for contributing their long experience in helping people to safely stop benzodiazepines via peer-led forums. We would also like to thank Bryan Shapiro for his help putting together the section on gabapentinoids, and Andrea Atri Mizrahi and Ivana Clark for their tireless efforts in assembling and checking for accuracy substantial parts of the drug-specific guidance. Lastly we would like to record our appreciation for the support of Robin Murray in our work in the field of deprescribing.

Mark Horowitz
David Taylor
London
November 2023

References

1. Read J, Moncrieff J, Horowitz MA. Designing withdrawal support services for antidepressant users: patients' views on existing services and what they really need. *Journal of Psychiatric Research* 2023. https://www.sciencedirect.com/science/article/pii/S0022395623001309.
2. Frederick B. *Recovery and Renewal: Your Essential Guide to Overcoming Dependency and Withdrawal from Sleeping Pills, Other 'Benzo' Tranquilisers and Antidepressants*, rev. edn. London: RRW Publishing, 2017.

Acknowledgements

We thank the following for their contributions to *The Maudsley® Deprescribing Guidelines*

Adele Framer
Alex Macaulay
Andrea Atri Mizrahi
Anna Lembke
Britain Baker
Bryan Shapiro
Christian Müller
Christy Huff
Constantin Volkmann
Daniel Cohrs
Ivana Clark
James Richard O'Neill
Jessica Overton
Laura Nininger Devlin
Louise Bundock
Mary Ita Butler
Michael O'Connor
Nicole Lamberson
Robin Murray
Samuel Bruneau-Dubuc
Tom Stockmann

Notes on using The Maudsley® Deprescribing Guidelines

The main aim of *The Guidelines* is to provide clinicians with practically useful advice on the deprescribing of psychotropic agents in commonly encountered clinical situations. The advice contained in this handbook is based on a combination of literature review, clinical experience and expert contribution, including from patient experts and advocates. We do not claim that this advice is necessarily 'correct' or that it deserves greater prominence than the guidance provided by other professional bodies or special interest groups. We hope, however, to have provided guidance that helps to assure the safe, effective and economical use of medicines in psychiatry, including when they are no longer required.

We hope also to have made clear precisely the sources of information used to inform the guidance given. Please note that some of the recommendations provided here involve the use of unlicensed formulations of some drugs in order to facilitate tapering. Note also that, while we have endeavoured to make sure all quoted doses are correct, clinicians should always consult statutory texts before prescribing. Users of *The Deprescribing Guidelines* should also bear in mind that the contents of this handbook are based on information available to us in November 2023. Much of the advice contained here will become out-dated as more research is conducted and published.

No liability is accepted for any injury, loss or damage, however caused.

Notes on inclusion of drugs

The Deprescribing Guidelines originate in the UK but are intended for use in other countries outside the UK. With this in mind, we have included in this edition those drugs in widespread use throughout the Western world in November 2023. These include drugs not marketed in the UK, such as desvenlafaxine, vilazodone, amongst several others. Many older drugs or those not widely available are either only briefly mentioned or not included on the basis that these drugs were not in widespread use at the time of writing. This book was written to have worldwide utility, although it retains a mild emphasis on UK practice and drugs.

Contributors' Conflict of Interest

Most of the contributors to *The Deprescribing Guidelines* have not received funding from pharmaceutical manufacturers for research, consultancy or lectures, although some have. Readers should be aware that these relationships inevitably colour opinions on such matters as drug selection or preference. However, in the case of a textbook that advises on stopping psychiatric drugs, and that generally recommends not using medications to treat withdrawal from another, such conflicts may be less pertinent than in other circumstances. As regards direct influence, no pharmaceutical company has been allowed to view or comment on any drafts or proofs of *The Deprescribing Guidelines*, and none has made any request for the inclusion or omission of any topic, advice or guidance. To this extent, *The Deprescribing Guidelines* have been written independent of the pharmaceutical industry.

Abbreviations List

% CI	percentage confidence interval	DSM-III-R	Diagnostic and Statistical Manual of Mental Disorders 3rd revised edition
ADHD	attention deficit hyperactivity disorder		
AMPA	α-amino-3-hydroxy-5-methyl-4-isoxazolepropionic acid	DSM-V	Diagnostic and Statistical Manual of Mental Disorders 5th revised edition
APA	American Psychiatric Association		
BDD	body dysmorphic disorder		
BIND	benzodiazepine-induced neurological dysfunction	EMA	European Medicines Agency
BNF	British National Formulary	EMPOWER	Eliminating Medications Through Patient Ownership of End Results
BZD	benzodiazepine		
BzRAs	benzodiazepine receptor agonists	ER	extended release
CABG	coronary artery bypass graft	FDA	US Food and Drugs Administration
CANMAT	Canadian Network for Mood and Anxiety Treatments	FND	functional neurological disorder
CBT	cognitive behavioural therapy	GABA	gamma-aminobutyric acid
		$GABA_A$	gamma-aminobutyric acid type A receptor
CBT-I	cognitive behavioural therapy for insomnia	GAD	generalised anxiety disorder
CFS	chronic fatigue syndrome	GMC	General Medical Council
CNS	central nervous system	GP	general practitioner
COPD	chronic obstructive pulmonary disease	HAM-A	Hamilton Anxiety Rating Scale
CR	controlled release	HAM-D	Hamilton Depression Rating Scale
CSM	Committee on the Safety of Medicines	HPA	hypothalamic-pituitary-adrenal
DAT	dopamine transporter	IBS	irritable bowel syndrome
DAWSS	Discriminatory Antidepressant Withdrawal Symptom Scale	ICD-10-CM	The International Classification of Diseases, 10th Revision, Clinical Modification
DESS	discontinuation-emergent signs and symptoms		

IR	immediate-release	PPWS	persistent post-withdrawal syndrome
LGIB	lower gastrointestinal bleeds		
MADRS	Montgomery-Åsberg Depression Rating Scale	PSSD	post-SSRI sexual dysfunction
		PTSD	post-traumatic stress disorder
MAO	monoamine oxidase	PWS	persistent withdrawal symptoms
MAOI	monoamine oxidase inhibitor		
MB-CT	mindfulness based cognitive therapy	RCPsych	Royal College of Psychiatrists
MDD	major depressive disorder	RCT	randomised controlled trial
MDMA	3,4-methylenedioxymethamphetamine	RIMA	reversible inhibitor of monoamine oxidase A
MHRA	Medicines and Healthcare Products Regulatory Agency	RLS	restless leg syndrome
		RO	receptor occupancy
MMSE	Mini Mental State Examination	RPS	Royal Pharmaceutical Society
MUS	medically unexplained symptoms	SAD	social anxiety disorder
		SARI	serotonin antagonist and reuptake inhibitors
NaSSAs	noradrenaline and specific serotonergic antidepressants		
		SERT	serotonin transporter
NET	noradrenaline transporter	SIADH	syndrome of inappropriate secretion of antidiuretic hormone
NEWT	North East Wales NHS Trust		
NGO	non-governmental organisation		
		SMD	standardised mean difference
NHS	National Health Service	SmPC	summary of product characteristics
NICE	National Institute for Health and Care Excellence		
		SNRI	serotonin and norepinephrine reuptake inhibitor
NIDA	National Institute on Drug Abuse		
		SR	sustained-release
NMDA	N-methyl-D-aspartate	SSRI	selective serotonin reuptake inhibitor
NNT	number needed to treat		
NPS	National Prescribing Service	STOPP	Screening Tool of Older Persons' Prescriptions
OCD	obsessive compulsive disorder		
ODV	O-desmethylvenlafaxine	TCAs	tricyclic antidepressants
ONS	Office of National Statistics	TI	The Therapeutics Initiative
OR	odds ratio	TIA	transient ischaemic attack
PAWS	post-acute withdrawal syndrome	UGIB	upper gastrointestinal bleeds
		WHO	World Health Organization
PD	panic disorder	XR or XL	extended-release
PET	positron-emission tomography	Z-drugs	nonbenzodiazepine sedative-hypnotics
PIL	patient information leaflet		

Chapter 1

Introduction to Deprescribing Psychiatric Medications

Deprescribing as an Intervention

Deprescribing is the planned and supervised process of reducing or stopping medication for which existing or potential harms outweigh existing or potential benefits.[1] The term 'deprescribing' originates from geriatric medicine where polypharmacy in frail patients can cause more harm than benefit.[1] Deprescribing is increasingly recognised to be a key component of good prescribing – reducing doses when they are too high, and stopping medications when they are no longer needed.[2] This process cannot occur in a vacuum of theoretical concerns but should take into account the patient's health, current level of functioning and, importantly, their values and preferences.[1] Deprescribing seeks to apply best practice in prescribing to the process of stopping a medication. It requires the same skill and experience as for the process of prescribing from prescribers, as well as support from pharmacists and other healthcare staff to obtain the best results. Importantly, it should place patients at the centre of the process to ensure medicines optimisation.[3]

There has historically been little attention paid to deprescribing in psychiatry. There is a dearth of research into a structured approach to stopping psychiatric medication, with the exception of some early studies examining stopping benzodiazepines[1] and in some specific populations, like people with learning disabilities. The focus of research efforts has been predominantly the prescribing of psychiatric medications – for example, there are estimated to be about 1,000 (published and unpublished) studies on starting antidepressants and only 20 on stopping them.[4] Concern about this imbalance is not specific to psychiatry with other medical specialties, such as cardiology, also engaging in a re-appraisal of long-term medication continuation, with support for developing strategies for repeated risk–benefit analyses over time.[5]

The Maudsley® Deprescribing Guidelines: Antidepressants, Benzodiazepines, Gabapentinoids and Z-drugs, First Edition. Mark Horowitz and David Taylor.
© 2024 John Wiley & Sons Ltd. Published 2024 by John Wiley & Sons Ltd.

The context for deprescribing

Over-prescription in psychiatry

Despite evidence of benefit for psychiatric drug treatment, there have been concerns raised regarding over-prescription. 1 in 6 people in western countries are prescribed an antidepressant in any given year, with rates rising a few per cent each year.[4,6] These increasing prescription numbers are mostly caused by longer periods of prescribing – the median duration of use of antidepressants is now more than 2 years in the UK and more than 5 years in the USA.[6] Some commentators have suggested that the increasing duration of prescriptions in part reflect the difficulty people have in stopping these medications due to withdrawal effects.[7] In practice, 30–50% of patients do not have evidence-based reasons for the continued prescription of antidepressants,[8–10] prompting calls to action to reduce associated risks.[6,11] There have been similar concerns about the high rates of antipsychotic use in conditions other than serious mental illness,[12] as well as a reconsideration of their open-ended use in psychotic conditions for all patients.[13,14] There are long-standing worries about levels of benzodiazepine and z-drug prescribing,[15,16] and more recent concerns about gabapentinoid prescribing.[17]

High rates of medication prescribing has also gained governmental attention in the UK,[17] with a particular focus on psychiatric drugs. A government report has noted that 1 in 4 adults in the UK are prescribed at least one dependence forming medication each year, with some patients having difficulties stopping these medications.[18] One central concern is that short-term symptom control might be prioritised over long-term functional outcomes, especially as most studies guiding treatment protocols measure symptomatic outcomes over short time periods rather than functional outcomes (or other outcomes often valued by patients) over longer time periods.[13,19,20]

Alongside this disquiet regarding over-prescription there has been renewed scrutiny of the effectiveness of some psychiatric medications. There is some consensus in the UK and Europe that benzodiazepines and z-drugs have limited effectiveness in the long term, with guidance recommending against long-term treatment for anxiety and insomnia,[21] matched by guidance in the USA from some health management organisations.[15] Preliminary studies have recently found similar outcomes in the treatment of selected patients with first-episode psychosis with or without antipsychotics in the context of comprehensive psychosocial support,[22,23] and non-drug treatment for serious mental illness has attracted increasing interest, including a large randomised controlled trial (RCT).[24] There have been calls from clinicians and patients for 'minimal medication' options for the treatment of psychotic conditions, such as have been established in Norway and parts of the USA.[25] There has continued to be debate regarding the efficacy of antidepressants[26,27] with arguments being made for their use in selected populations.[28] Concerns have emerged regarding the efficacy and safety of gabapentinoids.[17] In some countries there has been a shift away from a drug-centric approach in some patient groups – for example, in England and Wales the National Institute for Health and Care Excellence (NICE) now recommends that mild depression should not be treated with antidepressants as a first-line treatment, and suggests eight equally effective (and cost-effective) non-pharmacological treatment options for severe depression, alongside medication options.[29]

In addition to the above, there has also been significant critical attention directed towards the relapse prevention properties of psychiatric drugs.[30,31] All psychiatric drug classes are recognised to cause withdrawal effects when stopped that may be misinterpreted as relapse of the initial condition necessitating treatment.[32] These withdrawal symptoms are often ignored in discontinuation studies examining relapse prevention properties.[30,33,34] As a result there have been questions raised as to whether the relapse prevention properties of psychiatric drugs have been over-stated by mis-classification of withdrawal effects as relapse,[30,33,34] indicating we should be cautious in our interpretation of these studies.

Research and guideline establishment in deprescribing

In recent years interest in psychiatric deprescribing has increased exponentially. Numerous studies have been conducted or are ongoing exploring reducing and stopping antipsychotics in first and multi-episode psychotic conditions, in Taiwan, France, Denmark, the Netherlands, England, Australia and Germany, including the establishment of an international research consortium.[14] Some of these studies are examining gradual reductions, or hyperbolic dose reductions specifically.[14,35] Alongside this there are studies looking at how to help patients stop antidepressants – in the UK,[36] the Netherlands[37] and in Australia[38] – as well as several published studies looking at substitutions for antidepressant treatment like preventative cognitive therapy or mindfulness-based cognitive therapy.[39–41]

There has been increasing interest in the process of stopping medication based on the pharmacological properties of the drugs,[42–45] as well as in the practical means for making gradual dose reduction (for example, using compounded tablets in very small doses).[46–48] There has also been increased focus on the non-pharmacological aspects of reducing and stopping medication – the positive and negative impact on people's lives, as well as the barriers and the facilitators.[1,49–52]

In parallel, there has been increasing institutional interest in deprescribing in some countries. In the UK, in recent years, there has been guidance issued by the Royal College of Psychiatrists on how to safely stop antidepressants,[53] as well as guidance from NICE on how to stop antidepressants, benzodiazepines, z-drugs, opioids and gabapentinoids.[54] Similar guidance on how to stop antipsychotics has been called for.[55] In England, the National Health Service (NHS) has introduced structured medication reviews to reduce the use of unnecessary medication, including some psychiatric drugs,[56] and the Department of Health and Social Care has been tasked with upscaling deprescribing capacity in the NHS.[18]

Many clinicians report an interest in deprescribing and in receiving training for its practice. In total, 75% of UK clinicians working in first-episode psychosis services thought that early discontinuation of antipsychotic medication was beneficial for most patients.[57] In patients with multiple psychotic episodes English psychiatrists reported that they would feel comfortable supporting about 20% of their patients to discontinue their antipsychotics, with a minority of psychiatrists comfortable to support greater proportions.[58] In a survey 68% of GPs expressed a desire for more training on the withdrawal effects of antidepressants.[59] As mentioned, in Norway, government directives have led to the establishment of 'drug-free' wards, in which deprescribing is a central activity.[25] There are several dedicated psychiatric drug deprescribing services established around the world situated either in public or private healthcare settings or run by

NGOs partnered with health systems.[60] Indeed, several academics and psychiatrists have written about their own experience stopping psychiatric medication, often with the theme that this process was far more difficult than the published literature or their training had intimated.[61–63]

Patient knowledge and advocacy

This rise in academic, professional and institutional interest in psychiatric drug deprescribing has lagged behind decades of interest in the topic by patient groups who have sought ways to rationalise (and generally reduce) their medication in the relative absence of professional help. This movement seems driven by the subjectively unpleasant effects and physical health consequences from being on such medications.[64–67] It is noteworthy that much of the academic work now being conducted in deprescribing borrows from the expertise developed by patient groups.[44,48,62,66] Groups of patients (often supported by clinicians) have created guidance and advice on the topic of deprescribing in various guides and websites.[64,66,68] Manuals like *The Ashton Manual* (written by the clinical pharmacologist Professor Heather Ashton) are widely used in peer-led withdrawal communities,[69] and this manual has influenced NICE guidance on withdrawing from benzodiazepines.[70] Alongside this there has been substantial patient advocacy for more clinical services for deprescribing, which has been part of the driving force in the shift of interest to this topic,[64,71–73] as well as increasing media attention to the issue of how to safely stop psychiatric medications and the adverse consequences of stopping too rapidly.[74–78]

References

1. Gupta S, Cahill JD. A Prescription for 'Deprescribing' in Psychiatry. *Psychiatric Services* 2016; 67: 904–7.
2. Farrell B, Mangin D. Deprescribing is an essential part of good prescribing. *Am Fam Physician* 2019; 99: 7–9.
3. Department of Health and Social Care. Good for you, good for us, good for everybody: a plan to reduce overprescribing to make care better and safer, support the NHS, and reduce carbon emissions. 2022.
4. Davies J, Read J. A systematic review into the incidence, severity and duration of antidepressant withdrawal effects: are guidelines evidence-based? *Addict Behav* 2019; 97: 111–21.
5. Rossello X, Pocock SJ, Julian DG. Long-term use of cardiovascular drugs: challenges for research and for patient care. *J Am Coll Cardiol* 2015; 66: 1273–85.
6. Kendrick T. Strategies to reduce use of antidepressants. *Br J Clin Pharmacol* 2021; 87: 23–33.
7. Healy D, Aldred G. Antidepressant drug use and the risk of suicide. *Int Rev Psychiatry* 2005; 17: 163–72.
8. Cruickshank G, MacGillivray S, Bruce D, Mather A, Matthews K, Williams B. Cross-sectional survey of patients in receipt of long-term repeat prescriptions for antidepressant drugs in primary care. *Ment Health Fam Med* 2008; 5: 105–9.
9. Ambresin G, Palmer V, Densley K, Dowrick C, Gilchrist G, Gunn JM. What factors influence long-term antidepressant use in primary care? Findings from the Australian diamond cohort study. *J Affect Disord* 2015; 176: 125–32.
10. Eveleigh R, Grutters J, Muskens E, et al. Cost-utility analysis of a treatment advice to discontinue inappropriate long-term antidepressant use in primary care. *Fam Pract* 2014; 31: 578–84.
11. Wallis KA, Donald M, Moncrieff J. Antidepressant prescribing in general practice: a call to action. *Aust J Gen Pract* 2021; 50: 954–6.
12. Byng R. Should we, can we, halt the rise in prescribing for pain and distress? *Br J Gen Pract* 2020; 70: 432–3.
13. Murray RM, Quattrone D, et al. Should psychiatrists be more cautious about the long-term prophylactic use of antipsychotics? *Br J Psychiatr* 2016; 209: 361–5.
14. Sommer IEC, Horowitz M, Allott K, Speyer H, Begemann MJH. Antipsychotic maintenance treatment versus dose reduction: how the story continues. *Lancet Psychiatry* 2022; 9: 602–3.
15. Kaiser Permanente. Benzodiazepine and z-drug safety guideline expectations for Kaiser Foundation Health Plan of Washington Providers. 2019. https://wa.kaiserpermanente.org/static/pdf/public/guidelines/benzo-zdrug.pdf (accessed 19 October 2022).
16. Davies J, Rae TC, Montagu L. Long-term benzodiazepine and z-drugs use in the UK: a survey of general practice. *Br J Gen Pract* 2017; doi:10.3399/bjgp17X691865.

17. Horowitz MA, Kelleher M, Taylor D. Should gabapentinoids be prescribed long-term for anxiety and other mental health conditions? *Addict Behav* 2021; 119: 106943.

18. Public Health England. Dependence and withdrawal associated with some prescribed medicines. An evidence review. 2019. www.gov.uk/government/publications/prescribed-medicines-review-report (accessed 25 May 2021).

19. Wunderink L, Nieboer RM, Wiersma D, Sytema S, Nienhuis FJ. Recovery in remitted first-episode psychosis at 7 years of follow-up of an early dose reduction/discontinuation or maintenance treatment strategy long-term follow-up of a 2-year randomized clinical trial. *JAMA Psychiatry* 2013; 70: 913–20.

20. Moncrieff J. Antipsychotic maintenance treatment: time to rethink? *PLoS Med* 2015; 12: 1–7.

21. National Institute for Health and Care Excellence (NICE). Generalised anxiety disorder and panic disorder in adults: management. *NICE clinical guideline CG113* 2011. www.nice.org.uk/guidance/cg113/chapter/2-Research-recommendations#the-effectiveness-of-physical-activity-compared-with-waiting-list-control-for-the-treatment-of-gad (accessed 19 October 2022).

22. Morrison AP, Pyle M, Maughan D, et al. Antipsychotic medication versus psychological intervention versus a combination of both in adolescents with first-episode psychosis (MAPS): a multicentre, three-arm, randomised controlled pilot and feasibility study. *Lancet Psychiatry* 2020; published online 23 July. doi:10.1016/S2215-0366(20)30248-0.

23. Francey SM, O'Donoghue B, Nelson B, et al. Psychosocial intervention with or without antipsychotic medication for first-episode psychosis: a randomized noninferiority clinical trial. *Schizophr Bull Open* 2020; 1. doi:10.1093/schizbullopen/sgaa015.

24. Pilling S, Clarke K, Parker G, et al. Open dialogue compared to treatment as usual for adults experiencing a mental health crisis: protocol for the ODDESSI multi-site cluster randomised controlled trial. *Contemp Clin Trials* 2022; 113: 106664.

25. Cooper RE, Mason JP, Calton T, Richardson J, Moncrieff J. Opinion piece: the case for establishing a minimal medication alternative for psychosis and schizophrenia. *Psychosis* 2021; 13: 276–85.

26. Horowitz M, Wilcock M. Newer generation antidepressants and withdrawal effects: reconsidering the role of antidepressants and helping patients to stop. *Drug Ther Bull* 2022; 60: 7–12.

27. Munkholm K, Paludan-Müller AS, Boesen K. Considering the methodological limitations in the evidence base of antidepressants for depression: a reanalysis of a network meta-analysis. *BMJ Open* 2019; 9: e024886.

28. Stone MB, Yaseen ZS, Miller BJ, Richardville K, Kalaria SN, Kirsch I. Response to acute monotherapy for major depressive disorder in randomized, placebo controlled trials submitted to the US Food and Drug Administration: individual participant data analysis. *BMJ* 2022; 378: e067606.

29. National Institute for Health and Care Excellence (NICE). Depression in adults: treatment and management | Guidance | NICE. 2022; published online June. www.nice.org.uk/guidance/ng222 (accessed 16 July 2022).

30. Récalt AM, Cohen D. Withdrawal confounding in randomized controlled trials of antipsychotic, antidepressant, and stimulant Drugs, 2000–2017. *Psychother Psychosom* 2019; 88: 105–13.

31. Cohen D, Récalt A. Discontinuing psychotropic drugs from participants in randomized controlled trials: a systematic review. *Psychother Psychosom* 2019; 88: 96–104.

32. Cosci F, Chouinard G. Acute and persistent withdrawal syndromes following discontinuation of psychotropic medications. *Psychother Psychosom* 2020; 89: 283–306.

33. Hengartner MP. How effective are antidepressants for depression over the long term? A critical review of relapse prevention trials and the issue of withdrawal confounding. *Ther Adv Psychopharmacol* 2020; 10: 2045125320921694.

34. Horowitz MA, Taylor D. Distinguishing relapse from antidepressant withdrawal: clinical practice and antidepressant discontinuation studies. *BJPsych Advances* 2022; 28: 297–311.

35. Moncrieff J, Lewis G, Freemantle N, et al. Randomised controlled trial of gradual antipsychotic reduction and discontinuation in people with schizophrenia and related disorders: the RADAR trial (Research into Antipsychotic Discontinuation and Reduction). *BMJ Open* 2019; 9: e030912.

36. Kendrick T, Geraghty AWA, Bowers H, et al. REDUCE (Reviewing long-term antidepressant use by careful monitoring in everyday practice) internet and telephone support to people coming off long-term antidepressants: protocol for a randomised controlled trial. *Trials* 2020; 21: 419.

37. Vinkers CH, Ruhé HG, Penninx BW. Antidepressant discontinuation: in need of scientific evidence. *J Clin Psychopharmacol* 2021; 41: 512–5.

38. RELEASE: REdressing Long-tErm Antidepressant uSE in general practice. 2021; published online 4 September. https://medical-school.uq.edu.au/release (accessed 3 October 2022).

39. Breedvelt JJF, Warren FC, Segal Z, Kuyken W, Bockting CL. Continuation of antidepressants vs sequential psychological interventions to prevent relapse in depression: an individual participant data meta-analysis. *JAMA Psychiatry* 2021; 78: 868–75.

40. Huijbers MJ, Wentink C, Simons E, Spijker J, Speckens A. Discontinuing antidepressant medication after mindfulness-based cognitive therapy: a mixed-methods study exploring predictors and outcomes of different discontinuation trajectories, and its facilitators and barriers. *BMJ Open* 2020; 10: e039053.

41. Kuyken W, Hayes R, Barrett B, et al. Effectiveness and cost-effectiveness of mindfulness-based cognitive therapy compared with maintenance antidepressant treatment in the prevention of depressive relapse or recurrence (PREVENT): a randomised controlled trial. *Lancet* 2015; 386: 63–73.

42. Horowitz MA, Jauhar S, Natesan S, Murray RM, Taylor DM. A method for tapering antipsychotic treatment that may minimize the risk of relapse. *Schizophr Bull* 2021; 47: 1116–29.

43. Horowitz MA, Taylor D. How to reduce and stop psychiatric medication. *Eur Neuropsychopharmacol* 2021; 55: 4–7.

44. Horowitz MA, Taylor D. Tapering of SSRI treatment to mitigate withdrawal symptoms. *Lancet Psychiatry* 2019; 6: 538–46.

45. Horowitz MA, Moncrieff J, de Haan L, et al. Tapering antipsychotic medication: practical considerations. *Psychol Med* 2021; 1–4.

CHAPTER 1

46. Groot PC, van Os J. Successful use of tapering strips for hyperbolic reduction of antidepressant dose: a cohort study. *Ther Adv Psychopharmacol* 2021; 11: 20451253211039330.

47. Groot PC, van Os J. Outcome of antidepressant drug discontinuation with taperingstrips after 1–5 years. *Ther Adv Psychopharmacol* 2020; 10: 204512532095460.

48. Groot PC, van Os J. How user knowledge of psychotropic drug withdrawal resulted in the development of person-specific tapering medication. *Ther Adv Psychopharmacol* 2020; 10: 204512532093245.

49. Maund E, Dewar-Haggart R, Williams S, et al. Barriers and facilitators to discontinuing antidepressant use: a systematic review and thematic synthesis. *J Affect Disord* 2019; 245: 38–62.

50. Moncrieff J, Gupta S, Horowitz MA. Barriers to stopping neuroleptic (antipsychotic) treatment in people with schizophrenia, psychosis or bipolar disorder. *Ther Adv Psychopharmacol* 2020; 10: 2045125320937910.

51. Gupta S, Cahill JD, Miller R. Deprescribing antipsychotics: a guide for clinicians. *BJPsych Advances* 2018; 24: 295–302.

52. Karter JM. Conversations with clients about antidepressant withdrawal and discontinuation. *Ther Adv Psychopharmacol* 2020; 10: 2045125320922738.

53. Burn W, Horowitz M, Roycroft G, Taylor D. Stopping antidepressants. *Stopping Antidepressants*. 2020. www.rcpsych.ac.uk/mental-health/treatments-and-wellbeing/stopping-antidepressants (accessed 19 October 2022).

54. National Institute for Health and Care Excellence (NICE). Medicines associated with dependence or withdrawal symptoms: safe prescribing and withdrawal management for adults | Guidance | NICE. www.nice.org.uk/guidance/ng215/chapter/Recommendations (accessed 27 June 2022).

55. Cooper RE, Grünwald LM, Horowitz M. The case for including antipsychotics in the UK NICE guideline: 'Medicines associated with dependence or withdrawal symptoms: safe prescribing and withdrawal management for adults.' *Psychosis* 2020; 12: 89–93.

56. National Health Service. Network contract directed enhanced service: structured medication reviews and medicines optimisation: guidance. 2022.

57. Thompson A, Singh S, Birchwood M. Views of early psychosis clinicians on discontinuation of antipsychotic medication following symptom remission in first episode psychosis. *Early Interv Psychiatry* 2016; 10: 355–61.

58. Long M, Stansfeld J, Kikkert M, et al. Views and practice of antipsychotic discontinuation among 241 UK psychiatrists: a survey. (in preparation).

59. Read J, Renton J, Harrop C, Geekie J, Dowrick C. A survey of UK general practitioners about depression, antidepressants and withdrawal: implementing the 2019 Public Health England report. *Ther Adv Psychopharmacol* 2020; 10: 204512532095012.

60. Cooper RE, Ashman M, Lomani J, Moncrieff J, Guy A. "Stabilise-reduce, stabilise-reduce": A survey of the common practices of deprescribing services and recommendations for future services. PLoS One. 2023. Available: https://journals.plos.org/plosone/article?id=10.1371/journal.pone.0282988

61. Stockmann T. What it was like to stop an antidepressant. *Ther Adv Psychopharmacol* 2019; 9: 2045125319884834.

62. Horowitz M. Stopping antidepressants: what is the best way to come off them? Evidently Cochrane. 2021; published online 4 June. www.evidentlycochrane.net/stopping-antidepressants-what-is-the-best-way-to-come-off-them/ (accessed 3 October 2022).

63. Taylor D. Truth withdrawal. *Open Mind*. 1999; September/October.

64. Inner Compass Initiative. The Withdrawal Project. 2021. https://withdrawal.theinnercompass.org/ (accessed 19 October 2022).

65. White E, Read J, Julo S. The role of Facebook groups in the management and raising of awareness of antidepressant withdrawal: is social media filling the void left by health services? *Ther Adv Psychopharmacol* 2021; 11: 2045125320981174.

66. Framer A. What I have learnt from helping thousands of people taper off psychotropic medications. *Ther Adv Psychopharmacol* 2021; 11: 204512532199127.

67. Witt-Doerring J, Shorter, K. Online communities for drug withdrawal: what can we learn? *Psychiatr Times* https://cdn.sanity.io/files/0vv8moc6/psychtimes/a601f0899ba233e43e83ac7a649028b77df79749.pdf/PSY0418_PDF%20w%20Classifieds.pdf (accessed 19 October 2022).

68. Hall W. Harm reduction guide to coming off psychiatric drugs and withdrawal. The Icarus Project and Freedom Center, 2012.

69. Ashton H. Benzodiazepines: How They Work & How to Withdraw, The Ashton Manual. 2002. Available: http://www.benzo.org.uk/manual/bzcha01.htm (accessed 7 October 2022)

70. Scenario: Benzodiazepine and z-drug withdrawal. https://cks.nice.org.uk/topics/benzodiazepine-z-drug-withdrawal/management/benzodiazepine-z-drug-withdrawal/ (accessed 7 October 2022).

71. Akathisia Alliance for Education and Research. https://akathisiaalliance.org/about-akathisia/ (accessed 17 September 2022).

72. International Institute for Psychiatric Drug Withdrawal. https://iipdw.org/ (accessed October 7, 2022).

73. APPG for Prescribed Drug Dependence. http://prescribeddrug.org/ (accessed 7 October 2022).

74. Carey B. How to quit antidepressants: very slowly, doctors say. *The New York Times*. 2019; published online 6 March. www.nytimes.com/2019/03/05/health/depression-withdrawal-drugs.html (accessed 7 October 2022).

75. Carey B, Gebeloff R. Many people taking antidepressants discover they cannot quit. *The New York Times*. 2018; published online 7 April. www.nytimes.com/2018/04/07/health/antidepressants-withdrawal-prozac-cymbalta.html (accessed 7 October 2022).

76. Boseley S. Antidepressants: is there a better way to quit them? *The Guardian*. 2019; published online 22 April. www.theguardian.com/lifeandstyle/2019/apr/22/antidepressants-is-there-a-better-way-to-quit-them (accessed 7 October, 2022).

77. Aviv R. The Challenge of Going Off Psychiatric Drugs. The New Yorker. 2019; published online March 29. www.newyorker.com/magazine/2019/04/08/the-challenge-of-going-off-psychiatric-drugs (accessed 7 October 2022).

78. Piore A. Antidepressants work better than sugar pills only 15 percent of the time. Newsweek. 2022; published online 21 September. www.newsweek.com/2022/09/30/antidepressants-work-better-sugar-pills-only-15-percent-time-1744656.html (accessed 7 October 2022).

Why deprescribe?

A variety of clinical scenarios may warrant deprescribing. These include:

- high-dose prescribing,
- polypharmacy (drug-drug interactions, effects on adherence, and medical risk in vulnerable populations).
- inappropriate prescribing (wrong drug, dose or duration),
- patient preference,
- harms outweighing benefits,
- condition improved, resolution of stressors or alternative coping strategies developed.

High-dose prescribing, polypharmacy, inappropriate prescribing

It is widely agreed that high-dose prescribing and polypharmacy can, in many instances, produce more harm than benefit.[1] For many psychiatric conditions, including major depressive disorder, there is no clear advantage to high-dose pharmacotherapy, although the risks of adverse effects can increase as a function of dose.[2] The lower range of licensed doses is thought to achieve an optimal balance between efficacy, tolerability and acceptability in acute treatment.[2] The potential harms of high-dose antipsychotic prescribing and psychiatric drug polypharmacy are also well recognised.[1] Additionally, potentially inappropriate prescribing of psychiatric medication occurs commonly – including chronic polypharmacy for patients with personality disorders, in which guidance generally recommends avoiding pharmacological treatment or employing it for short-term use.[3] Deprescribing may be warranted for long-term benzodiazepine and z-drug use, which is generally officially frowned upon,[4] and in the substantial proportion of patients on antidepressants with no evidence-based reason for ongoing treatment (for example, the antidepressant may have had no beneficial effect or it might have been effective but has been continued for too long).[5]

Patient preference

In an era in which medical treatment in general is moving towards patient-centred treatment and away from paternalism, patient preference should be a central consideration, unless a patient is legally required to comply with treatment via a community treatment order.[6,7] Many patients report that their clinicians decline to help them reduce or stop their medication.[8] In some cases this can lead to patients following more risky options like stopping abruptly, the technique most likely to lead to aversive outcomes. Many people feel compelled to seek advice from online peer-support communities instead of their clinicians because of their clinicians' reluctance to support deprescribing, or lack of knowledge of how to do so.[8,9] Clinicians and patients may have different priorities with clinicians concerned with risk of relapse, symptom control and potential legal consequence for aversive outcomes, while patients may prioritise fulfilling social roles or quality of life, over being symptom free (although there is wide variation on this matter).[10] Negotiating a balance between differing priorities amongst patients and clinicians may be beneficial for outcomes, including treatment alliance and adherence to treatment recommendations in general.[7]

Harms outweigh benefits

For a portion of patients the benefits of medication will be outweighed by adverse effects.

Limited benefits

In some people the medication may never have been particularly effective but has continued because of inertia, a lack of attention to deprescribing or a desire not to 'rock the boat'.[11,12] Even in short-term trials the number needed to treat (NNT) for many forms of psychiatric medication is 6–10 or more meaning many patients are not helped by a specific effect of the medication to an appreciable degree. For some patients the medication may have been initially helpful, but through the development of tolerance to the drug this benefit has diminished.[13,14] This is well recognised for benzodiazepines and z-drugs, is also an issue for gabapentinoids,[15] and has also been somewhat controversially implicated in the long-term use of antidepressants,[16,17] and antipsychotics.[18,19]

Many medications are continued after initial symptoms have resolved with the intention of preventing future relapse. However, as above, there are significant concerns about the certainty of the evidence for the prophylactic properties for psychiatric drugs.[20-23] These discontinuation studies often stop psychiatric drugs abruptly or rapidly, do not take into account withdrawal effects, which are likely to be mis-classified as relapse in the discontinuation arms of these trials.[20-23] This phenomenon would provide an exaggerated estimation of the relapse prevention properties of psychiatric drugs,[20-23] and should lead us to be more cautious in interpreting the extent of the relapse prevention properties of some long-term psychiatric medications.

Adverse effects

The myriad adverse effects from psychiatric drugs range from weight gain and other metabolic consequences, particularly noted for atypical antipsychotics, to more subtle effects such as impaired capacity for feeling, memory or concentration caused by many psychiatric drug classes. Sexual side effects are very common, especially with selective serotonin reuptake inhibitors (SSRIs), where they occur in half or more of patients[24,25] and other adverse effects often thought to be short term have been found to persist.[26] There are also risks of long-term use such as possible cortical loss with antipsychotic treatment,[19,27] increased risk of dementia for some medications,[28,29] as well as falls and increased mortality, especially as people age.[30,31] Extra-pyramidal side effects from first-generation antipsychotics and tremor from lithium can be aversive.[1] When substantial benefits to a patient are provided by psychiatric drugs, these risks may be acceptable, but in other cases the balance of harms and benefits may not be favourable. As patients age the risks may increase owing to impaired metabolism of drugs and greater frailty, while the benefits may decrease, due to tolerance and perhaps the improvement of their condition over time.[7] Lastly, withdrawal effects are particularly associated with increased duration of medication use; one reason to stop medication earlier rather than later.[32,33]

Mental health condition improved or alternative coping

For some patients the original condition for which they were prescribed medication will have resolved or improved over time. The most obvious example is the circumstance in which a stressor that precipitated depression or anxiety has resolved, with a corresponding improvement in the patient's condition. Even conditions often considered life-long such as psychotic conditions or affective disorders can improve with time – as reported in several cohorts of patients,[19,34,35] with up to 40% of people with psychotic conditions being well and on no or little medication years after first diagnosis.[19,36] The behaviours diagnosed as personality disorders generally improve over time;[37] patients may have found more stable personal or professional circumstances and maturity may limit emotional instability. For some patients, especially those who are stable, medication may have less benefit than during more active periods of their condition. Or patients may have developed or be interested in pursuing alternative approaches to managing their mental health conditions. As one example, NICE has identified a dozen treatments that are as effective (and cost-effective) as antidepressants in the treatment of depression.[38]

References

1. Taylor D, Barnes T, Young A. *The Maudsley Prescribing Guidelines in Psychiatry*, 114th edn. Hoboken, NJ: Wiley-Blackwell; 2021.
2. Furukawa TA, Cipriani A, Cowen PJ, Leucht S, Egger M, Salanti G. Optimal dose of selective serotonin reuptake inhibitors, venlafaxine, and mirtazapine in major depression: a systematic review and dose-response meta-analysis. *Lancet Psychiatry* 2019; 6. 601–9.
3. National Institute for Health and Care Excellence (NICE). Borderline personality disorder: recognition and management. *Cg78* 2009; 1–40.
4. Byng R. Should we, can we, halt the rise in prescribing for pain and distress? *Br J Gen Pract* 2020; 70: 432–3.
5. Kendrick T. Strategies to reduce use of antidepressants. *Br J Clin Pharmacol* 2021; 87: 23–33.
6. Gupta S, Cahill JD, Miller R. Deprescribing antipsychotics: a guide for clinicians. *BJPsych Advances* 2018; 24: 295–302.
7. Gupta S, Cahill JD. A prescription for 'Deprescribing' in Psychiatry. *Psychiatric Services* 2016; 67: 904–7.
8. White E, Read J, Julo S. The role of Facebook groups in the management and raising of awareness of antidepressant withdrawal: is social media filling the void left by health services? *Ther Adv Psychopharmacol* 2021; 11: 2045125320981174.
9. Framer A. What I have learnt from helping thousands of people taper off psychotropic medications. *Ther Adv Psychopharmacol* 2021; 11: 204512532199127.
10. Crellin NE, Priebe S, Morant N, et al. An analysis of views about supported reduction or discontinuation of antipsychotic treatment among people with schizophrenia and other psychotic disorders. *BMC Psychiatry* 2022; 22: 185.
11. Gupta S, Cahill J, Miller R. *Deprescribing in Psychiatry* 2019; 1–16.
12. Maund E, Dewar-Haggart R, Williams S, et al. Barriers and facilitators to discontinuing antidepressant use: a systematic review and thematic synthesis. *J Affect Disord* 2019; 245: 38–62.
13. Peper A. A theory of drug tolerance and dependence I: a conceptual analysis. *J Theor Biol* 2004; 229: 477–90.
14. Baldessarini RJ, Ghaemi SN, Viguera AC. Tolerance in antidepressant treatment. *Psychother Psychosom* 2002; 71: 177–9.
15. Horowitz MA, Kelleher M, Taylor D. Should gabapentinoids be prescribed long-term for anxiety and other mental health conditions? *Addict Behav* 2021; 119: 106943.
16. Kinrys G, Gold AK, Pisano VD, et al. Tachyphylaxis in major depressive disorder: a review of the current state of research. *J Affect Disord* 2019; 245: 488–97.
17. Fava GA. May antidepressant drugs worsen the conditions they are supposed to treat? The clinical foundations of the oppositional model of tolerance. *Ther Adv Psychopharmacol* 2020; 10: 2045125320970325.
18. Chouinard G, Samaha AN, Chouinard VA, et al. Antipsychotic-induced dopamine supersensitivity psychosis: pharmacology, criteria, and therapy. *Psychother Psychosom* 2017; 86: 189–219.
19. Murray RM, Quattrone D, et al. Should psychiatrists be more cautious about the long-term prophylactic use of antipsychotics. *British Journal of Psychiatry* 2016; 209: 361–5.
20. Récalt AM, Cohen D. Withdrawal confounding in randomized controlled trials of antipsychotic, antidepressant, and stimulant drugs, 2000–2017. *Psychother Psychosom* 2019; 88: 105–13.
21. Cohen D, Récalt A. Discontinuing psychotropic drugs from participants in randomized controlled trials: A systematic review. *Psychother Psychosom* 2019; 88: 96–104.
22. Hengartner MP. How effective are antidepressants for depression over the long term? A critical review of relapse prevention trials and the issue of withdrawal confounding. *Ther Adv Psychopharmacol* 2020; 10: 2045125320921694.
23. Baldessarini RJ, Tondo L. Effects of treatment discontinuation in clinical psychopharmacology. *Psychother Psychosom* 2019; 88: 65–70.
24. Higgins A, Nash M, Lynch AM. Antidepressant-associated sexual dysfunction: impact, effects, and treatment. *Drug Healthc Patient Saf* 2010; 2: 141–50.
25. Serretti A, Chiesa A. Treatment-emergent sexual dysfunction related to antidepressants: a meta-analysis. *J Clin Psychopharmacol* 2009; 29: 259–66.
26. Bet PM, Hugtenburg JG, Penninx BWJH, Hoogendijk WJG. Side effects of antidepressants during long-term use in a naturalistic setting. *Eur Neuropsychopharmacol* 2013; 23: 1443–51.

27. Voineskos AN, Mulsant BH, Dickie EW, et al. Effects of antipsychotic medication on brain structure in patients with major depressive disorder and psychotic features: neuroimaging findings in the context of a randomized placebo-controlled clinical trial. *JAMA Psychiatry* 2020; published online 26 February. doi:10.1001/jamapsychiatry.2020.0036.

28. Coupland CAC, Hill T, Dening T, Morriss R, Moore M, Hippisley-Cox J. Anticholinergic drug exposure and the risk of dementia: a nested case-control study. *JAMA Intern Med* 2019; 179: 1084–93.

29. Richardson K, Fox C, Maidment I, et al. Anticholinergic drugs and risk of dementia: case-control study. *BMJ* 2018; 361: k1315.

30. Coupland C, Dhiman P, Morriss R, Arthur A, Barton G, Hippisley-Cox J. Antidepressant use and risk of adverse outcomes in older people: population based cohort study. *BMJ* 2011; 343: d4551.

31. Guina J, Merrill B. Benzodiazepines I: upping the care on downers: the evidence of risks, benefits and alternatives. *J Clin Med Res* 2018; 7: 17.

32. National Institute for Health and Care Excellence (NICE). Medicines associated with dependence or withdrawal symptoms: safe prescribing and withdrawal management for adults I Guidance I NICE. www.nice.org.uk/guidance/ng215/chapter/Recommendations (accessed 27 June 2022).

33. Horowitz MA, Framer A, Hengartner MP, Sørensen A, Taylor D. Estimating risk of antidepressant withdrawal from a review of published data. CNS Drugs 2023; 37: 143–57.

34. Morgan C, Lappin J, Heslin M, et al. Reappraising the long-term course and outcome of psychotic disorders: the AESOP-10 study. *Psychol Med* 2014; 44: 2713–26.

35. Larsen-Barr M, Seymour F, Read J, Gibson K. Attempting to discontinue antipsychotic medication: withdrawal methods, relapse and success. *Psychiatry Res* 2018; 270: 365–74.

36. McGorry P, Alvarez-Jimenez M, Killackey E. Antipsychotic medication during the critical period following remission from first-episode psychosis. *JAMA Psychiatry* 2013; 70: 898.

37. Paris J. Personality disorders over time: precursors, course and outcome. *J Pers Disord* 2003; 17: 479–88.

38. National Institute for Health and Care Excellence (NICE). Depression in adults: treatment and management I Guidance I NICE. 2022; published online June. www.nice.org.uk/guidance/ng222 (accessed 16 July 2022).

Barriers and facilitators to deprescribing

There are numerous factors that can facilitate or hinder deprescribing. A narrative review outlined these factors with regard to stopping antidepressants, many of which are applicable to a variety of drug classes (Table 1.1).[1] Some of these factors can be addressed through education and support, as discussed in subsequent chapters. Additionally, there are many institutional factors that act as barriers to deprescribing: while deprescribing can produce benefits for patient health and well-being, as well as health services (e.g. reduced adverse effect burden) in the long term, in the short term it often involves greater resources (e.g. increased contact, monitoring and support), which can act as a deterrent.[2]

Importantly, previous experience of stopping medication – either planned or, more usually, spontaneously by the patient, often abruptly or rapidly – with negative consequences can deter patients and clinicians from wishing to trial this process again.[2] The sometimes alarming presentations with severe symptoms after drug cessation that have generally been interpreted as relapse can strongly re-enforce the impression of a need for medication. However, there is some evidence now that these presentations – even when they are delayed for some time after drug cessation – may in fact represent withdrawal effects or the consequence of withdrawal effects, sometimes called withdrawal-associated relapse (e.g. genuine relapse as a consequence of withdrawal effects such as insomnia).[3,4] There is further evidence, presented in subsequent chapters, that in at least some of these cases a more gradual, structured and pharmacologically informed approach to reduction may minimise or avoid some of the more negative aspects of this process.[2]

Table 1.1 Barriers and facilitators for patients to stop psychiatric medications. Adapted from [1] (2019).

Domain	Barriers	Facilitators
Psychological and physiological factors	▪ Stressful life circumstances ▪ Aversive experience of discontinuation in past leading to deterioration (withdrawal effects or relapse) ▪ Lack of effective coping strategies ▪ Physical dependence on psychiatric medications (leading to withdrawal effects)	▪ Confidence in ability to discontinue ▪ Life circumstances stable ▪ Well-informed about approach to tapering
Perceived cause of mental health condition	▪ Long-term (perhaps life-long) condition requiring long-term treatment ▪ Primarily biochemical (or other biological) cause	▪ Primarily life circumstances
Fears	▪ Fear of relapse ▪ Fear of withdrawal effects	▪ Fear of 'addiction', physical dependence ▪ Fear of adverse effects and long-term health complications
Personal goals/ motivations	▪ Self-identity as 'disabled' ▪ Stopping as threat to stability ▪ Benefit of continuing to others around them ▪ Cure is not possible, only management	▪ Self-identity as 'healthy' ▪ Desire to function without psychiatric medication ▪ Feeling better ▪ Dislike having to take a psychiatric medication

(Continued)

Table 1.1 (*Continued*)

Domain	Barriers	Facilitators
Perception of psychiatric medications	■ Positive effect ■ Natural or benign ■ Lack of concern over adverse/side effects	■ Ineffectual ■ Unacceptable adverse/side effects ■ Unnatural ■ Unhappy about long-term use
Information about the discontinuation process	■ Inadequate information about the discontinuation process, and risks and benefits of this	■ Information on how to safely discontinue and what to expect
Support network (friends, family, professionals)	■ Pressure to stay on medication	■ Support to come off medication

References

1. Maund E, Dewar-Haggart R, Williams S, et al. Barriers and facilitators to discontinuing antidepressant use: a systematic review and thematic synthesis. *J Affect Disord* 2019; 245: 38–62.
2. Moncrieff J, Gupta S, Horowitz MA. Barriers to stopping neuroleptic (antipsychotic) treatment in people with schizophrenia, psychosis or bipolar disorder. *Ther Adv Psychopharmacol* 2020; 10. doi: 10.1177/2045125320937910.
3. Horowitz MA, Jauhar S, Natesan S, Murray RM, Taylor DM. A method for tapering antipsychotic treatment that may minimize the risk of relapse. *Schizophr Bull* 2021; 47: 1116–29.
4. Framer A. What I have learnt from helping thousands of people taper off psychotropic medications. *Ther Adv Psychopharmacol* 2021; 11. doi: 10.1177/2045125321991274.

Withdrawal Effects from Psychiatric Medications

The two major negative consequences of reducing and stopping psychiatric medication are relapse and withdrawal. The risks of relapse are well known and explored extensively elsewhere so we will focus on the less-commonly addressed issue of withdrawal effects. All classes of psychiatric drugs can cause withdrawal effects.[1,2] These include benzodiazepines, z-drugs, gabapentinoids, mood stabilisers, stimulants, antipsychotics and antidepressants.[1,2] There is a great degree of overlap in the withdrawal symptoms from different drug classes, including symptoms such as dizziness, nausea, anxiety, impaired concentration, irritability, agitation, headache, tremor, sleep disturbances, depressed mood and fatigue.[1] There are also withdrawal symptoms more typical of specific classes of drug that may reflect effects on particular receptor targets and downstream processes – for example, brain zaps, myoclonus, depersonalisation and derealisation in SSRI and serotonin and norepinephrine reuptake inhibitor (SNRI) withdrawal, and derealisation/depersonalisation and delirium in benzodiazepine withdrawal.[2]

Withdrawal effects have not been systematically evaluated for all classes of psychiatric medication but they are common – about 50% of patients who stop antidepressants[3] will experience withdrawal effects, and 32%–42% of people taking benzodiazepines will be unable to stop their drug because of withdrawal effects.[4] The other commonality across drug classes are that withdrawal effects can manifest in psychological symptoms,[1,2] likely due to effects on the central nervous system.[1] Psychological withdrawal symptoms can include low mood, anxiety, insomnia, panic attacks, obsessive thinking, suicidality and there are reported cases of psychotic symptoms due to withdrawal from antidepressants,[1] benzodiazepines[2] and antipsychotics.[5]

Mis-diagnosis of withdrawal effects as relapse

The presence of withdrawal symptoms that manifest psychologically makes it easy to mistake these symptoms for relapse of an underlying condition by both patients and clinicians.[6-8] Patients commonly report that their withdrawal symptoms are mis-diagnosed as relapse of the condition for which their drug was originally prescribed, or as a new-onset mental health disorder.[6-8] Such mis-diagnosis is understandable, given the limited awareness of withdrawal symptoms from psychiatric drugs, including their severity and duration and because they have often been downplayed as 'discontinuation' symptoms, or characterised as 'mild and brief' based on short-term industry trials.[9] The waters have also been muddied by commentators claiming that some psychiatric drugs can not cause withdrawal effects because they are not addictive[10,11] – whereas adaptation to a drug over time (often called 'physical dependence') is all that is required for withdrawal symptoms to emerge when reducing or stopping the drug, without the need for addiction (which involves psychological dependence as well, characterised by craving, compulsion, etc).[12,13]

On the other hand, physicians are well practised at detecting relapse: when patients present with mood or anxiety symptoms, other psychiatric symptoms or disordered behaviour, especially when such symptoms are severe and long lasting, relapse is often higher on a list of differentials than withdrawal.[6,8] However, over the past few years there has been increasing recognition that withdrawal effects from psychiatric drugs can cause severe symptoms, which can themselves be long-lasting and in some instances appear similar to the presentation of other mental health conditions.

Physical dependence vs addiction

The term 'dependence' has come to be used interchangeably with 'addiction' (to mean uncontrolled drug-seeking behaviour).[12] Inevitably this has led to some unfortunate confusion.[12] This choice of language was made in DSM-III-R because the term 'addiction' was thought to be pejorative whilst the word 'dependence' was thought more neutral.[12] However, the original usage of the word 'dependence' referred to 'physiological adaptation that occurs when medications acting on the central nervous system are ingested with rebound when the medication is abruptly discontinued'.[12] The National Institute on Drug Abuse (NIDA) in the USA states 'Dependence means that when a person stops using a drug, their body goes through "withdrawal": a group of physical and mental symptoms that can range from mild (if the drug is caffeine) to life-threatening ... Many people who take a prescription medicine every day over a long period of time can become dependent; when they go off the drug, they need to do it gradually, to avoid withdrawal discomfort. But people who are dependent on a drug or medicine aren't necessarily addicted.'[13] In addition, Goodman and Gilman's textbook of pharmacology points out 'The appearance of a withdrawal syndrome when administration of the drug is terminated is the only actual evidence of physical dependence.'[14]

All major classes of psychiatric drugs can be associated with withdrawal symptoms on cessation or dose reduction. These symptoms occur in a substantial proportion of patients, as a result of physical dependence (a normal neurobiological response to drugs that act on the central nervous system).[2,12,15–18] Physical dependence to psychiatric drugs arises because the body and brain undergo adaptations to the presence of a drug, countering its effect in order to maintain homeostasis.[12,19,20] It is also clear that many psychiatric drugs – with the exception of benzodiazepines, stimulants and some antidepressants such as tranylcypromine and amineptine – do not cause addiction, as they do not induce compulsion, craving and other symptoms of addiction.[11,21] Sometimes misunderstanding that withdrawal symptoms arise merely from adaptation to psychiatric drugs after chronic use leads to misplaced accusations of addiction, misuse or abuse when patients report withdrawal symptoms on trying to stop.

Some patients may be less interested in academic distinctions between dependence and addiction and more interested in the reality that they cannot stop their psychiatric drugs because of unpleasant withdrawal effects. They may therefore describe them colloquially as 'addictive',[22,23] though most psychiatric drugs do not fit the strict definition of this property. Some patients may also not be happy being described as 'dependent' on psychiatric drugs (which they may still associate with the concept of addiction), and in this case, it may be better to talk in terms of 'neuroadaptation' or 'adaptation'.

Withdrawal symptoms vs discontinuation symptoms

The term 'discontinuation symptom' was promoted by drug manufacturers to minimise patient concerns regarding their product and to prevent an association with the idea of addiction.[9,24] There is now widespread recognition that this euphemism is misleading and that its use minimises the potentially adverse consequences of stopping psychiatric drugs; withdrawal symptoms do not imply addiction.[9,25,26] The more pharmacologically accurate term is 'withdrawal symptoms', now adopted by Royal College of Psychiatrists,[9,27] the British Medical Association[9] and NICE in the UK for antidepressants[28,29] and by academics for antipsychotics,[1,2,30] mood stabilisers,[2] and long used with regards benzodiazepines, stimulants and gabapentinoids.[2]

References

1. Cosci F, Chouinard G. Acute and Persistent withdrawal syndromes following discontinuation of psychotropic medications. *Psychother Psychosom* 2020; 89: 283–306.
2. Lerner A, Klein M. Dependence, withdrawal and rebound of CNS drugs: an update and regulatory considerations for new drugs development. *Brain Commun* 2019; 1: fcz025.
3. Davies J, Read J. A systematic review into the incidence, severity and duration of antidepressant withdrawal effects: Are guidelines evidence-based? *Addict Behav* 2019; 97: 111–21.
4. Schweizer E, Rickels K, Case WG, Greenblatt DJ. Long-term therapeutic use of benzodiazepines. II. Effects of gradual taper. *Arch Gen Psychiatry* 1990; 47: 908–15.
5. Horowitz MA, Jauhar S, Natesan S, Murray RM, Taylor DM. A method for tapering antipsychotic treatment that may minimize the risk of relapse. *Schizophr Bull* 2021; 47: 1116–29.
6. Framer A. What I have learnt from helping thousands of people taper off psychotropic medications. *Ther Adv Psychopharmacol* 2021; 11: 204512532199127.
7. White E, Read J, Julo S. The role of Facebook groups in the management and raising of awareness of antidepressant withdrawal: is social media filling the void left by health services? *Ther Adv Psychopharmacol* 2021; 11: 2045125320981174.
8. Horowitz MA, Taylor D. Distinguishing relapse from antidepressant withdrawal: clinical practice and antidepressant discontinuation studies. *BJPsych Advances* 2022; 28: 297–311.
9. Massabki I, Abi-Jaoude E. Selective serotonin reuptake inhibitor 'discontinuation syndrome' or withdrawal. *Br J Psychiatry* 2020; 1–4.
10. Haddad P, Anderson I. Antidepressants aren't addictive: clinicians have depended on them for years. *J Psychopharmacol* 1999; 13: 291–2.
11. Jauhar S, Hayes J, Goodwin GM, Baldwin DS, Cowen PJ, Nutt DJ. Antidepressants, withdrawal, and addiction; where are we now? *J Psychopharmacol* 2019; 33: 655–9.
12. O'Brien C. Addiction and dependence in DSM-V. *Addiction* 2011; 106: 866–7.
13. National Institute on Drug Abuse. Is there a difference between physical dependence and addiction? National Institute on Drug Abuse. https://nida.nih.gov/publications/principles-drug-addiction-treatment-research-based-guide-third-edition/frequently-asked-questions/there-difference-between-physical-dependence-addiction (accessed 31 May 2022).
14. Brunton LL, Chabner BA, Knollmann BC. *Goodman & Gilman's The Pharmacological Basis of Therapeutics*, 12e. McGraw-Hill Education, 2011.
15. Howland RH. Potential adverse effects of discontinuing psychotropic drugs: part 2: antidepressant drugs. *J Psychosoc Nurs Ment Health Serv* 2010; 48: 9–12.
16. Haddad PM, Anderson IM. Recognising and managing antidepressant discontinuation symptoms. *Adv Psychiatr Treat* 2007; 13: 447–57.
17. Public Health England. Dependence and withdrawal associated with some prescribed medicines. An evidence review. 2019. https://www.gov.uk/government/publications/prescribed-medicines-review-report (accessed 25 May 2021).
18. Taylor D, Stewart S, Connolly A. Antidepressant withdrawal symptoms – telephone calls to a national medication helpline. *J Affect Disord* 2006; 95: 129–33.
19. Turton S, Lingford-Hughes A. Neurobiology and principles of addiction and tolerance. *Medicine* 2016; 44: 693–6.
20. Hyman SE, Nestler EJ. Initiation and adaptation: a paradigm for understanding psychotropic drug action. *Am J Psychiatry* 1996; 153: 151–62.
21. Haddad P. Do antidepressants have any potential to cause addiction? *J Psychopharmacol* 1999; 13: 300–7.
22. Read J, Williams J. Adverse effects of antidepressants reported by a large international cohort: emotional blunting, suicidality, and withdrawal effects. *Curr Drug Saf* 2018; 13: 176–86.
23. Burn W, Horowitz M, Roycroft G, Taylor D. Stopping antidepressants. 2020. https://www.rcpsych.ac.uk/mental-health/treatments-and-wellbeing/stopping-antidepressants (accessed 4 July 2022).
24. Nielsen M, Hansen EH, Gotzsche PC. What is the difference between dependence and withdrawal reactions? A comparison of benzodiazepines and selective serotonin re-uptake inhibitors. *Addiction* 2012; 107: 900–8.
25. Lugg W. The case for discontinuation of the 'discontinuation syndrome'. *Aust N Z J Psychiatry* 2021; doi:10.1177/00048674211043443.
26. Fava GA, Gatti A, Belaise C, Guidi J, Offidani E. Withdrawal symptoms after selective serotonin reuptake inhibitor discontinuation: A systematic review. *Psychother Psychosom* 2015; 84: 72–81.
27. Royal College of Psychiatrists. Position statement on antidepressants and depression. 2019 https://www.rcpsych.ac.uk/docs/default-source/improving-care/better-mh-policy/position-statements/ps04_19---antidepressants-and-depression.pdf?sfvrsn=ddea9473_5 (accessed 4 July 2022).
28. National Institute for Health and Care Excellence (NICE). Depression in adults: recognition and management. (NICE Guideline 90). London: NICE, 2009.
29. Iacobucci G. NICE updates antidepressant guidelines to reflect severity and length of withdrawal symptoms. *BMJ* 2019; 367: l6103.
30. Brandt L, Bschor T, Henssler J, et al. Antipsychotic withdrawal symptoms: a systematic review and meta-analysis. *Front Psychiatry* 2020; 11: 569912.

Pathophysiology of psychiatric drug withdrawal symptoms

Drug withdrawal effects are effectively part of the pharmacology of any drug which the body eliminates faster than adaptations to the presence of the drug take to subside.[1] Based on this definition, any evidence of adaptation to a drug strongly suggests that withdrawal symptoms will occur when the drug is stopped.[1]

Homeostatic adaptation to psychiatric drugs

During ongoing administration of psychiatric drugs, as with other drugs acting on the central nervous system, neuroadaptation establishes a new homeostatic equilibrium, in which the system accommodates to alterations produced by the drug. When the medication is reduced or stopped, the new homeostatic set-point is perturbed, resulting in withdrawal symptoms.[1-3] Adaptations to the presence of the drug predict withdrawal effects because these adaptations do not resolve instantaneously upon stopping the drugs but will persist for some further period.

There are a variety of specific adaptations to each class of drug, explored in the relevant chapters. In general, because of a homeostatic drive towards equilibrium, the brain responds to antagonists by up-regulating the number or sensitivity of receptors to increase signal (e.g. dopaminergic hypersensitivity in response to long-term treatment with dopamine antagonists).[4] The brain responds to agonists or drugs that increase synaptic availability of transmitters by down-regulating the number or sensitivity of receptors to reduce the signal (e.g. reduced serotonergic receptor sensitivity in response to blockade of the serotonin transporter).[5] It is also likely that withdrawal symptoms are not mediated simply by changes to the receptors that are directly affected by medications, but also by the myriad transmitters and processes downstream or otherwise connected to these effects.[1,6]

Animal studies and some human studies show that these changes can persist after the drugs are removed from the body and can be long-lasting for months and years in some cases. This has been demonstrated in clinical studies of antidepressants[7] and suggested by long-lasting changes to some people who have taken antipsychotics manifesting in tardive dyskinesia,[8] and supported by animal studies.[9]

Homeostatic disruption on psychiatric medication discontinuation

When a psychiatric drug taken long-term is reduced in dose or stopped, the homeostatic equilibrium that had been established is perturbed. The difference between the 'expected' level of activity by the system and the actual 'input' by the drug is responsible for withdrawal symptoms (Figure 1.1).[1-3] Withdrawal symptoms will persist for the time taken for the brain to re-adapt to lower levels (or the absence) of the drug – that is, the time taken for a new homeostatic equilibrium to be established.

It is sometimes erroneously believed that withdrawal symptoms last for the time taken for the drug to be eliminated from the system.[6] This misunderstanding sometimes leads clinicians to tell patients that they could not be experiencing long-lasting withdrawal symptoms because 'the drug is out of their system' – however, as in Figure 1.1, it can be seen that while the onset of withdrawal symptoms is strongly determined by the elimination half-life of a drug (shorter half-life, quicker onset), the duration of

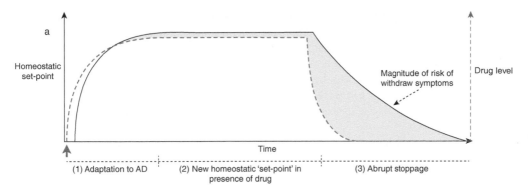

Figure 1.1 The neurobiology of psychiatric drug withdrawal. In this diagram, the homeostatic 'set-point' is shown in black and psychiatric drug levels are shown in purple dashed lines. Adapted from Horowitz and Taylor (2021).[10] (1) The system is at baseline. At the Solid purple arrow, a psychiatric mediation is administered; drug plasma levels increase. Physiological adaptations of the system to the presence of the drug begin. (2) At the plateau, drug plasma levels (and target receptor activation) have reached a steady state with a new homeostatic set-point of the system established. (3) The drug is abruptly ceased, and plasma drug levels drop to zero (exponentially, according to the elimination half-life of the drug). This difference between the homeostatic set-point (the 'expectations' of the system) and the level of drug in the system (dashed purple line) causes withdrawal symptoms. Hence, withdrawal symptoms may worsen or peak even long after the drug has been eliminated from the system. The shaded area under the curve, representing the difference between the homeostatic set-point and the level of the drug, indicates the degree of risk of withdrawal symptoms: the larger the area the greater the risk. With permission of Elsevier.

withdrawal is determined by the plasticity of the system in returning to a 'pre-drug' homeostatic equilibrium.[1,6]

An analogy might be made to the experience of walking out of a loud concert (more signal as with the increased synaptic neurotransmitter during agonist treatment) into a quiet street (physiological levels of transmitter after drug removal), where sounds appear muted. This experience of muted sounds arises because of reduced tympanic sensitivity (as for reduced receptor sensitivity) for a few minutes while your tympanic membrane re-accommodates to a lower average amount of sound (analogous to the delay for the system to re-adapt to less transmitter signal – although it takes much longer than a few minutes). The time for the sound to dissipate (or for synaptic transmitter levels to normalise on removal of the drug) is trivial; it is the time taken for tympanic re-accommodation that determines the duration of the withdrawal effects (as for re-accommodation of the processes affected by long-term psychiatric drug use – which can take months or years).

Factors influencing development of withdrawal effects

Although there has been limited research on the topic, there are several factors that are thought to have an effect on incidence, severity and duration of withdrawal symptoms. In general, a greater degree of adaptation to a drug is likely to lead to greater withdrawal effects, brought about, for example, by higher dose or longer use, as well as some variation among drugs and individual sensitivity to withdrawal effects.[6]

Physical dependence to psychiatric drugs resulting in a clinically significant withdrawal syndrome can occur within weeks of daily administration of some psychiatric medications.[6] Indeed, the FDA has warned that for some drugs, like benzodiazepines, physical dependence can occur within days of regular use.[11] Aspects of the pharmacology of a particular medication also plays a role – with short half-life medications more implicated in withdrawal than longer acting drugs, and specific receptor targets, such as noradrenergic effects (for example, with SNRIs) also particularly implicated.[6,12] There are a number of individual characteristics hypothesised to play a role, including variations in liver enzymes involved in the metabolism of psychiatric medications, sensitivity to adaption to the presence of a drug, but this has received little research attention.[6,13]

In general women have been observed to experience greater severity of withdrawal symptoms for a variety of psychotropic medications.[6] Age plays some role in withdrawal effects, with children more likely to demonstrate visual hallucinations, agitation, facial grimacing, myoclonus and other movement disorders in benzodiazepine withdrawal than adults.[6] Older adults are more likely to demonstrate confusion, disorientation and, sometimes, hallucinations than younger people.[6]

References

1. Reidenberg MM. Drug discontinuation effects are part of the pharmacology of a drug. *J Pharmacol Exp Ther* 2011; 339: 324–8.
2. Turton S, Lingford-Hughes A. Neurobiology and principles of addiction and tolerance. *Medicine* 2016; 44: 693–6.
3. Hyman SE, Nestler EJ. Initiation and adaptation: a paradigm for understanding psychotropic drug action. *Am J Psychiatry* 1996; 153: 151–62.
4. Silvestri S, Seeman MV, Negrete JC, et al. Increased dopamine D2receptor binding after long-term treatment with antipsychotics in humans: a clinical PET study. *Psychopharmacology* 2000; 152: 174–80.
5. Gray NA, Milak MS, DeLorenzo C, et al. Antidepressant treatment reduces serotonin-1A autoreceptor binding in major depressive disorder. *Biol Psychiatry* 2013; 74: 26–31.
6. Lerner A, Klein M. Dependence, withdrawal and rebound of CNS drugs: an update and regulatory considerations for new drugs development. *Brain Commun* 2019; 1: fcz025.
7. Bhagwagar Z, Rabiner EA, Sargent PA, Grasby PM, Cowen PJ. Persistent reduction in brain serotonin1A receptor binding in recovered depressed men measured by positron emission tomography with [11C]WAY-100635. *Mol Psychiatry* 2004; 9: 386–92.
8. Caroff SN, Ungvari GS, Cunningham Owens DG. Historical perspectives on tardive dyskinesia. *J Neurol Sci* 2018; 389: 4–9.
9. Joyce J. D2 but not D3 receptors are elevated after 9 or 11 months chronic haloperidol treatment: influence of withdrawal period. *Synapse* 2001; 40: 137–44.
10. Horowitz MA, Taylor D. How to reduce and stop psychiatric medication. *Eur Neuropsychopharmacol* 2021; 55: 4–7.
11. FDA Drug Safety Communication. FDA requiring boxed warning updated to improve safe use of benzodiazepine drug class. 2020. www.fda.gov/drugs/drug-safety-and-availability/fda-requiring-boxed-warning-updated-improve-safe-use-benzodiazepine-drug-class#:~:text=FDA is requiring the boxed, and life-threatening side effects (accessed 15 June 2023).
12. Framer A. What I have learnt from helping thousands of people taper off psychotropic medications. *Ther Adv Psychopharmacol* 2021; 11: 204512532199127.
13. Horowitz MA, Taylor D. Tapering of SSRI treatment to mitigate withdrawal symptoms. *Lancet Psychiatry* 2019; 6: 538–46.

Clinical aspects of psychiatric drug withdrawal

Distinguishing withdrawal symptoms from relapse

As mentioned, withdrawal symptoms, which include poor mood, anxiety, insomnia, agitation and a range of other psychological symptoms may be often mistaken for relapse of the underlying disorder for which the patient was prescribed psychiatric medication.[1,2] A thorough history can allow identification of several characteristics that help to distinguish withdrawal effects from relapse:

■ time of onset
■ presence of distinctive – often physical, though sometimes psychological - symptoms
■ response to re-instatement

The presence of severe symptoms that are long-lasting is not as helpful for distinction as once thought as it is now recognised that these symptoms can be characteristic of withdrawal and not just of relapse.[3]

Time of onset

Withdrawal symptoms usually occur hours or days after skipping, reducing or stopping a psychiatric drug.[4] There is some variability in this depending on the half-life of elimination such that longer half-life medications can have delays in onset of symptoms by weeks.[5] It has also been reported that some symptoms of psychiatric drug withdrawal may not manifest for weeks or longer after discontinuation, even for drugs with short half-lives, although the mechanism for this is not well understood.[6] A delayed decrease in central receptor occupancy, lagging behind plasma concentration decline, is one suggested explanation.[7]

Since withdrawal syndromes are recognised to last for months, or even years in some patients symptom duration past a few weeks is not an indication of relapse rather than withdrawal.[6,8,9] Relapse would be expected to have onset weeks, or months after drug cessation, depending on the usual frequency of episodes in the individual's original condition and be similar in nature to the original mental health episode.[10]

Characteristic symptomology of withdrawal

Symptoms that differentiate withdrawal from relapse may be revealed by taking a careful history inquiring after the more common symptoms of withdrawal. If physical symptoms co-occur with psychological symptoms, this indicates a high likelihood of a withdrawal syndrome.[3] For example, if a patient were to experience a surge of anxiety and lowered mood on stopping a psychiatric medication, and this was also accompanied by nausea, dizziness or electric-shock sensations or 'zaps', it is more likely that this represents a withdrawal syndrome rather than relapse of a depressive condition.[3] Some commentators have suggested that withdrawal symptoms and relapse may co-occur and while this is a possibility, Occam's razor suggests that it is more likely that a single condition will cause several symptoms, rather than several conditions co-occurring.[11] Some symptoms are so distinctive – such as the electric 'zaps' (head sensations some experience, especially on lateral eye movements)[12] that they could be considered pathognomonic of psychiatric drug withdrawal.[3]

Even when symptoms on stopping psychiatric drugs are solely psychological in nature, these can be quite distinct from the symptoms of the original condition, or more severe in nature.[13] For example, if a patient experiences agitation and panic on stopping a psychiatric medication when the patient's original condition involved depressed mood and poor appetite after a loss, the diagnosis of a withdrawal syndrome should be strongly considered,[3,14] rather than onset of a new mental health condition co-incidentally occurring at just the moment that the mediction was stopped. Withdrawal symptoms can be new and qualitatively different from the patient's original condition, while relapse is reminiscent of it.[13] Sometimes, the patient will provide the clue themselves when they say 'This is nothing like my original condition.'[4]

However, sometimes the symptoms experienced in withdrawal are very difficult to differentiate from the patient's underlying condition. This may be because some people are prone to characteristic symptoms – for example obsessive thinking or low mood – in periods of stress, whether that stress is psychological, or physiological, such as in medication withdrawal. This presentation of worsening of underlying symptoms in withdrawal is often referred to as 'rebound symptoms' (see below).[15]

Response to re-instatement

Another means of distinction is the time taken for symptoms to resolve on re-instatement of a psychiatric medication: for withdrawal symptoms this will be more rapid than for relapse, as demonstrated by resolution within a few days of re-instatement of an antidepressant (after several days of placebo treatment) in a large study[16] – withdrawal symptoms may even improve within a few hours of re-instatement. However, re-instatement might be less successful when it is delayed for months after the onset of withdrawal symptoms.[6]

The major distinguishing features between withdrawal and relapse are summarised in Table 1.2. Of course, a clinician should continue to be vigilant for genuine

Table 1.2 Distinguishing features between psychiatric drug withdrawal symptoms and relapse of an underlying condition.

	Withdrawal symptoms	Relapse
Time of onset	Often within hours or days of reducing or stopping a psychiatric medication (but can be delayed for long-acting drugs – and sometimes even for short-acting medications as well)	Usually weeks or months after stopping a psychiatric drug (depending on the characteristic periodicity of the condition)
Duration	Can range from days to months (or, sometimes, years)	Variable
Response to re-instatement	Improvement can be within hours or days (especially if re-instatement occurs soon after symptoms onset)	Usually delayed
Distinctive symptoms	Characteristic accompanying symptoms e.g. dizziness, headache, sweating, muscle ache; brain 'zaps' may be pathognomonic. Any symptoms not present in the underlying condition (including psychological symptoms)	Episodes of individual patients have typical characteristics

relapse of the patient's underlying condition, which may come on weeks or months after treatment is stopped and may have characteristics that are quite typical for the patient.

Distinguishing withdrawal symptoms from new onset of a psychiatric or medical condition

In addition to withdrawal effects being diagnosed as a relapse of an underlying mental health condition, many patients report that they have had withdrawal symptoms mis-diagnosed as the onset of a new psychiatric condition.[4,17,18] As symptoms of psychiatric drug withdrawal can include agitation, anxiety, depressed mood, panic, obsessive thoughts and in some cases manic and psychotic symptoms (in people who have not experienced these symptoms previously) as well as a range of behavioural disturbances, these can be mis-diagnosed as a variety of mental health conditions including agitated depression, bipolar disorder, psychotic disorders, psychosomatic disorders, panic and other anxiety disorders.[4,15,17] It should be considered that the onset of a de novo psychiatric disorder that happens to coincide with the process of stopping medication is less likely than experiencing quite typical withdrawal symptoms on stopping.[17]

Withdrawal symptoms can also be mis-diagnosed as a new-onset medical condition, or placed in the category of 'medically unexplained symptoms' or functional neurological disorder, or even attributed to malingering (Table 1.3).[17] This interpretation likely arises because of the wide array of symptoms that psychiatric drug withdrawal can produce and a lack of familiarity with withdrawal symptoms.[17] There are numerous overlapping symptoms of psychiatric drug withdrawal with these conditions: tremor, weakness (functional neurological disorder); fatigue, tiredness (chronic fatigue syndrome) and numerous symptoms that could be grouped under the category of 'medically unexplained symptoms' when the symptoms are not attributed to psychiatric drug withdrawal.[17] These misdiagnoses can lead to a failure to recommend appropriate treatment, extensive medical investigation and a feeling on behalf of patients that they were not listened to.[17]

Table 1.3 Potential mis-diagnoses of drug withdrawal syndromes.

Mis-diagnosis of psychiatric drug withdrawal	Psychiatric drug withdrawal symptoms which overlap with diagnostic criteria
Onset of new psychiatric diagnosis (e.g. agitated depression, mania, anxiety disorder, depression, psychotic episode)	New onset of anxiety, depression, panic attacks, agitation, obsessive thinking, insomnia, worry, suicidality, and more rarely, de novo manic or psychotic symptoms
Chronic fatigue syndrome	Fatigue, insomnia, muscle aches
Medically unexplained symptoms/ Functional neurological disorder	Tremor, muscle weakness, muscle spasm, pain, fatigue
Stroke, neurological disorder	Muscle weakness, 'electric zaps', tremor, headache, visual changes, vertigo, unsteadiness on feet, sensory changes

References

1. Groot PC, van Os J. Antidepressant tapering strips to help people come off medication more safely. *Psychosis* 2018; 10: 142–5.
2. Young A, Haddad P. Discontinuation symptoms and psychotropic drugs. *Lancet* 2000; 355: 1184–5.
3. Horowitz MA, Taylor D. Distinguishing relapse from antidepressant withdrawal: clinical practice and antidepressant discontinuation studies. *BJPsych Advances* 2022; 28: 297–311.
4. Framer A. What I have learnt from helping thousands of people taper off psychotropic medications. *Ther Adv Psychopharmacol* 2021; 11: 204512532199127.
5. Zajecka J, Fawcett J, Amsterdam J, et al. Safety of abrupt discontinuation of fluoxetine: a randomized, placebo-controlled study. *J Clin Psychopharmacol* 1998; 18: 193–7.
6. Hengartner MP, Schulthess L, Sorensen A, Framer A. Protracted withdrawal syndrome after stopping antidepressants: a descriptive quantitative analysis of consumer narratives from a large internet forum. *Ther Adv Psychopharmacol* 2020; 10: 2045125320980573.
7. Sørensen A, Ruhé HG, Munkholm K. The relationship between dose and serotonin transporter occupancy of antidepressants—a systematic review. *Mol Psychiatry* 2021; 27(1): 1–10.
8. Stockmann T, Odegbaro D, Timimi S, Moncrieff J. SSRI and SNRI withdrawal symptoms reported on an internet forum. *Int J Risk Saf Med* 2018; 29: 175–80.
9. Davies J, Regina P, Montagu L. All-Party Parliamentary Group for Prescribed Drug Dependence Antidepressant Withdrawal: a survey of patients' experience by the All-Party Parliamentary Group for Prescribed Drug Dependence. All-Party Parliamentary Group for Prescribed Drug Dependence, 2018 http://prescribeddrug.org/wp-content/uploads/2018/10/APPG-PDD-Survey-of-antidepressant-withdrawal-experiences.pdf (accessed 24 April 2022).
10. Haddad PM, Anderson IM. Recognising and managing antidepressant discontinuation symptoms. *Adv Psychiatr Treat* 2007; 13: 447–57.
11. Wildner M. In memory of William of Occam. *Lancet* 1999; 354: 2172.
12. Papp A, Onton JA. Brain zaps: An underappreciated symptom of antidepressant discontinuation. *The Primary Care Companion for CNS Disorders* 2018; 20. doi:10.4088/PCC.18m02311.
13. Chouinard G, Chouinard VA. New classification of selective serotonin reuptake inhibitor withdrawal. *Psychother Psychosom* 2015; 84: 63–71.
14. Warner CH, Bobo W, Warner C, Reid S, Rachal J. Antidepressant discontinuation syndrome. *Am Fam Physician* 2006; 74: 449–56.
15. Cosci F, Chouinard G. Acute and persistent withdrawal syndromes following discontinuation of psychotropic medications. *Psychother Psychosom* 2020; 89: 283–306.
16. Rosenbaum JF, Fava M, Hoog SL, Ascroft RC, Krebs WB. Selective serotonin reuptake inhibitor discontinuation syndrome: A randomized clinical trial. *Biol Psychiatry* 1998; 44: 77–87.
17. Guy A, Brown M, Lewis S, Horowitz MA. The 'patient voice' – patients who experience antidepressant withdrawal symptoms are often dismissed, or mis-diagnosed with relapse, or onset of a new medical condition. *Ther Adv Psychopharmacol* 2020; 10: 204512532096718.
18. White E, Read J, Julo S. The role of Facebook groups in the management and raising of awareness of antidepressant withdrawal: is social media filling the void left by health services? *Ther Adv Psychopharmacol* 2021; 11: 2045125320981174.

Specific issues in psychiatric drug withdrawal

Rebound symptoms

A specific sub-set of withdrawal symptoms identified by many commentators are rebound withdrawal symptoms, which are defined as a rapid return of the patient's original symptoms at greater intensity than before treatment.[1,2] This phenomenon may occur because people have characteristic patterns of thoughts or feelings that are triggered by the process of withdrawal. For example, on exposure to an anxiogenic substance (such as high doses of caffeine), many people are likely to experience anxiety, but the nature of that anxiety is likely to be expressed idiosyncratically for each individual and influenced by their usual expression of anxiety (e.g. health-related, obsessive), despite being clearly chemically induced. This seems to apply in the process of withdrawal as well where typical patterns of thoughts and feelings are stimulated by the withdrawal process.[3,4] This may present a particularly confusing presentation for both the clinician and patient to distinguish from relapse. Quick resolution on dose increase, resolution over time with no change to medication dose and the accompaniment of these familiar symptoms with other symptoms (physical or psychological) of withdrawal can help to characterise these symptoms as rebound withdrawal symptoms rather than relapse[4,5] – but sometimes this distinction may be challenging.

Delayed onset withdrawal effects

Delayed onset withdrawal effects are widely recognised for drugs with long half-lives such as fluoxetine,[6] because the onset of symptoms is delayed by the long elimination half-life of its active metabolite norfluoxetine (7–15 days). However, it has also been observed that withdrawal effects from other psychiatric drugs, even those with short half-lives can also emerge for the first time after weeks and sometimes months.[6,7] For example, in one analysis, the mean time to onset of withdrawal symptoms following discontinuation or reduction of dose of SSRIs was 4.5 weeks, with a standard deviation of 13 weeks, indicating that some patients experienced onset of withdrawal symptoms up to 4 months after stopping their antidepressant.[7] Vigilance for withdrawal effects should be maintained even weeks after psychiatric drugs are ceased, especially when typical physical symptoms are reported. A lack of recognition of delayed onset withdrawal effects is likely responsible for mis-diagnosis in some patients.[4]

Withdrawal akathisia

Although there are myriad psychological and physical withdrawal symptoms from psychiatric drugs, perhaps the most distressing potential consequence is akathisia, a neuropsychiatric condition, characterised by severe agitation, restlessness and a sense of terror.[8-11] This condition is most often recognised as a side effect of antipsychotic use, but it has also been observed to occur in withdrawal from various psychiatric medications, including antidepressants and benzodiazepines.[8-12] Patients report a very distressing subjective feeling of restlessness and dysphoria, and they often fidget, pace, rock and are unable to sit or stand still. However, akathisia can also manifest more subtly without obvious motor symptoms, typified by terror and a subjective feeling of restlessness.[13]

The pathophysiology is poorly understood, with leading theories implicating a reduction in dopaminergic activity in the mesocortical pathway projecting from the ventral tegmental area to the limbic system and prefrontal cortex, leading to suppression of the usual inhibitory effects on motor function, producing unwanted involuntary movements.[12] Other theories implicate changes to serotonin and noradrenaline levels that can have indirect effects on dopaminergic activity.[14]

This pronounced state of agitation can be mis-diagnosed as a manic state,[10] an anxiety disorder, a panic disorder, a personality disorder, ADHD, health anxiety, restless leg disorder and functional neurological disorder, or a factitious disorder by clinicians unfamiliar with the syndrome in psychiatric drug withdrawal.[12,15,16] It has been associated with increased suicidality because of the distress and agitation it engenders.[12,15,17]

Protracted withdrawal syndrome

Severe and persistent withdrawal syndromes (months or years) are recognised for a range of psychotropic medications, including benzodiazepines, antipsychotics and antidepressants.[2,3,9,17] Protracted withdrawal syndrome, sometimes called post-acute withdrawal syndrome (PAWS) or persistent post-withdrawal syndrome (PPWS) or prolonged withdrawal syndrome, occurs in an unknown proportion of patients after stopping psychiatric medications.[9,17,18] This syndrome has long been neglected or minimised,[17] with poor education about its existence leading to mis-attribution of these symptoms to relapse or the emergence of new mental health conditions.[4,5,17,19] Protracted withdrawal symptoms are thought to be caused by changes to the brain secondary to exposure (generally long-term) to psychiatric drugs, which persist for months and years after stopping;[2,17,20] with speculation that for some patients these effects may be permanent, or very slowly reversible.[2] The long-lasting brain changes that persist after long-term psychiatric drug use has ceased is consistent with these clinical observations.[21,22] These long-lasting symptoms may cause considerable disruption and disability in people's lives and the lack of recognition by clinicians often compounds the difficulties experienced by such patients.[9,17]

Withdrawal symptoms during maintenance treatment

Missed doses causing withdrawal symptoms

Although psychiatric drug withdrawal symptoms are most often discussed when the dose is being deliberately reduced or medication stopped, it is a common occurrence even during maintenance treatment. After a patient has been taking a psychiatric medication daily for only a few weeks, doses that are accidentally missed, skipped, taken in the wrong dosage or even taken a few hours late (depending on the half-life of the medication) may result in withdrawal symptoms.[23-26] These odd withdrawal symptoms might be reported to the clinician as sudden onset psychological or physical symptoms (e.g. dizziness, headache or mood changes).

Insomnia or other psychological withdrawal effects might be mis-identified as emerging treatment resistance or worsening of the original condition.[27,28] If not recognised, intermittent dosing may bring about the additional risk and expense of inappropriate medical care and prescriptions.[29] Departures from a regular dosing schedule are common among patients, with estimates for irregular dosing being 50% or more.[30,31]

Withdrawal symptoms after switching psychiatric medications

Withdrawal symptoms may also emerge after a switch from one psychiatric drug to another, although there has been almost no research on the incidence of withdrawal symptoms in the process of switching.[4] Various techniques for switching have been suggested,[32] though evidence is lacking for the best way to switch psychiatric medications to minimise the risk of withdrawal and other adverse effects.[6] The more dis-similar the pharmacodynamic actions (receptor targets) of two psychiatric drugs the more likely they are to give rise to withdrawal symptoms on switching. Care should be taken not to mistake withdrawal symptoms from the psychiatric drug being stopped for adverse reactions to the new drug or manifestation of new psychiatric symptoms.[33] Slower cross-titration of psychiatric drugs may minimise the risk of withdrawal effects.

References

1. Chouinard G, Chouinard VA. New classification of selective serotonin reuptake inhibitor withdrawal. *Psychother Psychosom* 2015; 84: 63–71.

2. Lerner A, Klein M. Dependence, withdrawal and rebound of CNS drugs: an update and regulatory considerations for new drugs development. *Brain Commun* 2019; 1: fcz025.

3. Cosci F, Chouinard G. Acute and persistent withdrawal syndromes following discontinuation of psychotropic medications. *Psychother Psychosom* 2020; 89: 283–306.

4. Framer A. What I have learnt from helping thousands of people taper off psychotropic medications. *Ther Adv Psychopharmacol* 2021; 11: 204512532199127.

5. Horowitz MA, Taylor D. Distinguishing relapse from antidepressant withdrawal: clinical practice and antidepressant discontinuation studies. *BJPsych Advances* 2022; 28: 297–311.

6. Fava GA, Gatti A, Belaise C, Guidi J, Offidani E. Withdrawal symptoms after selective serotonin reuptake inhibitor discontinuation: A systematic review. *Psychother Psychosom* 2015; 84: 72–81.

7. Stockmann T, Odegbaro D, Timimi S, Moncrieff J. SSRI and SNRI withdrawal symptoms reported on an internet forum. *Int J Risk Saf Med* 2018; 29: 175–80.

8. Hirose S. Restlessness related to SSRI withdrawal. *Psychiatry Clin Neurosci* 2001; 55: 79–80.

9. Guy A, Brown M, Lewis S, Horowitz MA. The 'patient voice' – patients who experience antidepressant withdrawal symptoms are often dismissed, or mis-diagnosed with relapse, or onset of a new medical condition. *Ther Adv Psychopharmacol* 2020; 10: 204512532096718.

10. Narayan V, Haddad PM. Antidepressant discontinuation manic states: a critical review of the literature and suggested diagnostic criteria. *J Psychopharmacol* 2010; 25: 306–13.

11. Sathananthan GL, Gershon S. Imipramine withdrawal: an akathisia-like syndrome. *Am J Psychiatry* 1973; 130: 1286–7.

12. Tachere RO, Modirrousta M. Beyond anxiety and agitation: A clinical approach to akathisia. *Aust Fam Physician* 2017; 46: 296–8.

13. Sachdev P. Acute and tardive drug-induced akathisia. In: Sethi KD, ed. *Drug Induced Movement Disorders*. Neurological Disease and Therapy Series. New York, USA: Macel Dekker, 2004: 129–64.

14. Lane RM. SSRI-induced extrapyramidal side-effects and akathisia: implications for treatment. *J Psychopharmacol* 1998; 12: 192–214.

15. Akathisia Alliance for Education and Research. https://akathisiaalliance.org/about-akathisia/ (accessed September 17, 2022).

16. Lohr, J., Eidt, C., Abdulrazzaq Alfaraj, A., & Soliman, M. (2015). The clinical challenges of akathisia. CNS Spectrums, 20(S1), 1–16. doi:10.1017/S1092852915000838

17. Hengartner MP, Schulthess L, Sorensen A, Framer A. Protracted withdrawal syndrome after stopping antidepressants: a descriptive quantitative analysis of consumer narratives from a large internet forum. *Ther Adv Psychopharmacol* 2020; 10: 2045125320980573.

18. Davies J, Read J. A systematic review into the incidence, severity and duration of antidepressant withdrawal effects: are guidelines evidence-based? *Addict Behav* 2019; 97: 111–21.

19. White E, Read J, Julo S. The role of Facebook groups in the management and raising of awareness of antidepressant withdrawal: is social media filling the void left by health services? *Ther Adv Psychopharmacol* 2021; 11: 2045125320981174.

20. Reidenberg MM. Drug discontinuation effects are part of the pharmacology of a drug. *J Pharmacol Exp Ther* 2011; 339: 324–8.

21. Bhagwagar Z, Rabiner EA, Sargent PA, Grasby PM, Cowen PJ. Persistent reduction in brain serotonin1A receptor binding in recovered depressed men measured by positron emission tomography with [11C]WAY-100635. *Mol Psychiatry* 2004; 9: 386–92.

22. Joyce J. D2 but not D3 receptors are elevated after 9 or 11 months chronic haloperidol treatment: influence of withdrawal period. *Synapse* 2001; 40: 137–44.

23. Baldwin DS, Cooper JA, Huusom AKT, Hindmarch I. A double-blind, randomized, parallel-group, flexible-dose study to evaluate the tolerability, efficacy and effects of treatment discontinuation with escitalopram and paroxetine in patients with major depressive disorder. *Int Clin Psychopharmacol* 2006; 21: 159–69.

24. Bauer R, Glenn T, Alda M, et al. Antidepressant dosage taken by patients with bipolar disorder: factors associated with irregularity. *Int J Bipolar Disord* 2013; 1: 26.

25. Demyttenaere K, Haddad P. Compliance with antidepressant therapy and antidepressant discontinuation symptoms. *Acta Psychiatr Scand Suppl* 2000; 403: 50–6.

26. Jha MK, Rush AJ, Trivedi MH. When discontinuing SSRI antidepressants is a challenge: management tips. *Am J Psychiatry* 2018; 175: 1176–84.

27. Fava GA, Cosci F, Guidi J, Rafanelli C. The deceptive manifestations of treatment resistance in depression: a new look at the problem. *Psychother Psychosom* 2020; 89: 265–73.

28. Howes OD, Thase ME, Pillinger T. Treatment resistance in psychiatry: state of the art and new directions. *Mol Psychiatry* 2022; 27: 58–72.

29. Steinman MA. Reaching out to patients to identify adverse drug reactions and nonadherence: necessary but not sufficient. *JAMA Intern Med* 2013; 173: 384–5.

30. Ho SC, Chong HY, Chaiyakunapruk N, Tangiisuran B, Jacob SA. Clinical and economic impact of non-adherence to antidepressants in major depressive disorder: A systematic review. *J Affect Disord* 2016; 193: 1–10.

31. Meijer WE, Bouvy ML, Heerdink ER, Urquhart J, Leufkens HG. Spontaneous lapses in dosing during chronic treatment with selective serotonin reuptake inhibitors. *Br J Psychiatry* 2001; 179: 519–22.

32. Keks N, Hope J, Keogh S. Switching and stopping antidepressants. *Aust Prescr* 2016; 39: 76–83.

33. Haddad PM, Anderson IM. Recognising and managing antidepressant discontinuation symptoms. *Adv Psychiatr Treat* 2007; 13: 447–57.

How to Deprescribe Psychiatric Medications Safely

Although there is somewhat limited research evidence on how to stop psychiatric drugs, some advice can be offered by using data from existing studies, an understanding of the pharmacology of psychiatric drugs as well as lessons from practical clinical experience (including patient-reported experience).[1–5] In light of a lack of definitive empirical evidence, shared decision making between the patient and clinician may be the best approach to managing the uncertainty.[6,7]

Stopping psychiatric medications can be a difficult process for a significant proportion of patients.[1,8–11] However, by applying pharmacological principles and taking care to modify the rate of reduction to manage withdrawal effects for a given patient, the tapering process can often be made more tolerable. The broad principles for tapering off psychiatric drugs are:

- taper gradually (over months more often than weeks, and sometimes longer) unless there are urgent risks to manage;
- taper at a rate that the individual finds tolerable;
- taper in a hyperbolic pattern of dose decrements (so that dose reductions become smaller and smaller as total dosage gets lower); and
- taper to low doses before stopping, so that the final reduction to zero in not greater (in terms of effect on target receptors) than the reductions previously tolerated[3] (example for a generic drug shown in Figure 1.2).

In this section, we examine the practical aspects of tapering in clinical practice using receptor occupancy as a guide to enable tapering in a pharmacologically rational manner with the following steps:

- Step 1: estimate the size of the initial reduction and implement this;
- Step 2: monitor subsequent withdrawal symptoms;
- Step 3: make decisions about further dose reductions based on this experience; and
- Step 4: continue this iterative process through to discontinuation or partial reduction.

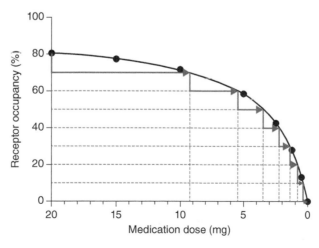

Figure 1.2 Example of hyperbolic tapering of a psychiatric medication. Dose reductions are shown on the x-axis, with increasingly small reductions producing equal-sized reductions in receptor occupancy (on the y-axis).

We also review the practical issues of making up small doses or doses that are intermediate between existing tablet dosages of psychiatric medications from liquid preparations, or alternatives, as well as some of the psychological issues encountered during tapering.

The neurobiology of tapering

As described previously, during long-term use of a psychiatric drug, the brain and body make adaptations to the drug to maintain homeostasis.[12,13] These adaptations are the key component of physical dependence.[13,14] The particular adaptations made in response to different psychiatric drugs depend on the receptor targets of the drug, and whether they are antagonists or agonists. There is evidence that these changes can persist for months or years after stopping in some patients,[15,16] a suggestion supported by findings in animal studies.[15,17]

Gradual tapering – theoretical aspects

These adaptations explain why when a psychiatric drug is stopped abruptly (as in Figure 1.3a), withdrawal symptoms are likely to occur. This action produces a large discrepancy between the level of drug the system 'expects' and the reduced level of actual drug action.[13,18] The duration of withdrawal symptoms is largely determined by the time required for adaptations to the presence of the drug to resolve (i.e. to re-adjust to the absence of the drug),[18] and not the time taken for the drug to be eliminated from the system.[15,19,20]

Alternatively, if the drug is reduced by small amounts and adequate time permitted before the next reduction in order for the brain to adjust to this lesser amount of drug (i.e. a new homeostatic equilibrium to be established), the risk of withdrawal effects (and their severity) is likely to be minimised (Figure 1.3b).[2] This can be thought of the difference between jumping from the top of a building to the ground (stopping a drug abruptly) versus going down storey by storey from the top of a building (tapering a drug).

Theoretically, lesser amounts of homeostatic disruption brought about by more gradual dose reductions result in reduced risk of severe (and, perhaps, long-lasting) withdrawal symptoms;[1,20] a principle which is now supported by some empirical studies.[21,22] Psychiatric drugs or formulations with longer half-lives may lessen withdrawal symptom risk further by minimising the degree of homeostatic disruption (e.g. drugs delivered in depot formulations).[23,24] Even smaller reductions of dose may further reduce withdrawal symptoms (Figure 1.3c) – analogous to taking even smaller steps down from the top of a building, allowing the brain to make small re-adjustments in its homeostatic equilibrium over a period of time.

Another useful analogy may be 'the bends' that is experienced by scuba divers when rising too quickly to the surface after a deep dive. Their bodies adapt to the greater depth and on rising to the surface of the water they experience uncomfortable symptoms called 'the bends'. The condition is prevented by slowly rising to the surface, allowing time for the body to adapt to the lower pressure conditions. The faster one rises the more likely 'the bends' are to occur. Successful prevention involves a stepped titration to sea-level pressure based on the person's response. If symptoms of 'the bends'

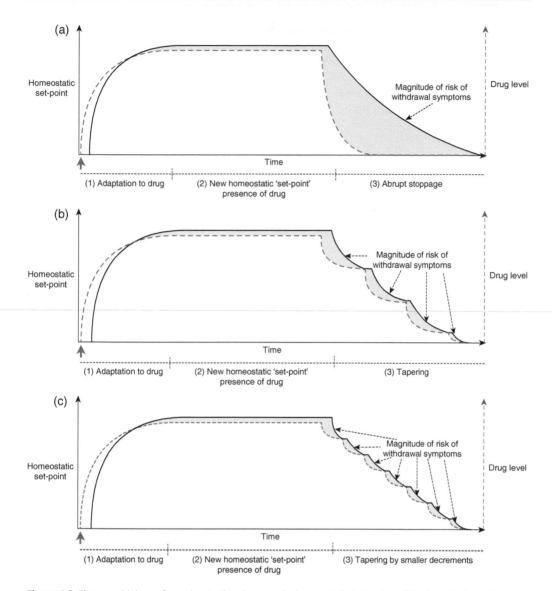

Figure 1.3 The neurobiology of tapering. In this diagram, the homeostatic 'set-point' of the brain is shown in black and psychiatric drug levels are shown in purple dashed lines. Adapted from Horowitz and Taylor (2021).[2] The shaded grey regions represent the degree of risk of withdrawal symptoms: the larger the area the greater the risk of withdrawal. (a) (1) and (2) The brain adapts to levels of a drug used over time. (3) The medication is abruptly ceased and plasma drug levels drop to zero (exponentially, according to the elimination half-life of the drug). This difference between the homeostatic set-point (the 'expectations' of the system) and the level of drug in the system (dashed purple line) is experienced as withdrawal symptoms. (b) (3) Tapering: when a drug is reduced step-wise, drug levels reduce exponentially to lower levels. At each step, there is a lag as the system adapts to a new level of drug, causing withdrawal symptoms (dashed arrows), but of lesser intensity (shaded area under the small, cupped curves) than the abrupt discontinuation shown in (a). A new (lower) homeostatic 'set-point' is established before further dose reductions are made. Drugs with longer half-lives may lessen withdrawal symptoms further by minimising the difference between the shifting homeostatic 'set-point' and plasma levels. (c) (3) An even more gradual step-wise reduction, with even smaller risk of withdrawal symptoms (shaded area under the smaller, cupped curves). With permission of Elsevier.

do occur the treatment is increasing pressure again and making even more gradual reductions subsequently. Similarly, for psychiatric drug withdrawal the more abrupt the change in level of drug the more pronounced the symptoms. An ounce of prevention is also worth a pound of cure because once significant disruption to the system is produced it is more difficult to reverse. If unpleasant symptoms arise, returning to a higher dose followed by more gradual dose reductions is generally the best approach.

Empirical support for gradual tapering

The evidence for gradual tapering for specific drug classes will be explored more closely in the relevant chapters, but, generally, in studies in which psychiatric drugs are stopped more slowly, there is a smaller risk of relapse. Many of these analyses were performed by Baldessarini and colleagues: they demonstrated that relapse rates are higher for patients who stop their antidepressants, mood stabilisers or antipsychotics abruptly or rapidly compared to those who stopped them more slowly.[25,26] For example, patients tapered off antidepressants rapidly had higher relapse rates than those tapered more gradually.[26] These findings are supported by more modern studies that find that relapse rates are lower in people who taper off a variety of psychiatric drugs more slowly.[3,4,27,28] For example, in one meta-analysis, a small number of studies found that the relapse rate in people who taper off antidepressants over several months is no different to the relapse rate in people who maintain antidepressants, while it is increased in those who taper off over weeks.[28]

These studies tell us two things: the first is that tapering more slowly seems to produce better outcomes. The second is that withdrawal effects must contribute to the reason that relapse rates are different when the rate of drug tapering is different. If relapse was simply the consequence of unmasking the untreated natural history of a patient's underlying condition, the rate at which a drug was stopped would be immaterial.[2] The rate at which, say, insulin is stopped has no bearing on relapse rates. For psychiatric drugs the nature of the process of discontinuation itself must be causally related to relapse.[29] If it is agreed that it is not plausible that rate of tapering can worsen an underlying condition, it is therefore more likely that rapidly stopping induces withdrawal effects (including effects on sleep, appetite, mood, anxiety and other psychiatric symptoms) which register on symptom rating scales as deterioration and are detected as relapse.[2,29–31] In addition to this, and perhaps at the same time, abrupt withdrawal can de-stabilise an individual, leading to genuine relapse.[25]

Overall, tapering more gradually is likely to reduce the relapse rate, if only because withdrawal symptoms are minimised. This notion is strengthened by findings that more gradual tapering can reduce the risk of withdrawal effects with a number of psychiatric drug classes.[3,13,32] The probability that withdrawal effects are contributing to an increase in apparent relapse rate is also supported by the pattern of relapses that occur in discontinuation studies where a disproportionate number of relapses occur in the first few weeks after stopping drugs.[30,33–35] As there should be no intrinsic reason why patients should relapse at the same time (they would each presumably have their own idiosyncratic periodicity of relapse), the early disproportionate preponderance of relapses suggests a withdrawal effect (withdrawal being most likely to occur at an early time point).[30,33–35] Gradual tapering may therefore minimise withdrawal effects and risk of relapse.

Hyperbolic tapering – theoretical aspects

In addition to the speed of tapering, the pattern of dose reduction is also likely to be important when trying to minimise withdrawal effects, and perhaps relapse, because of the pharmacology of psychiatric drugs.[2-4] The law of mass action dictates that when few molecules of a drug are present, every additional milligram of the drug will have large additional effects, because of the large number of unoccupied receptors to act upon, whilst when larger amounts of the drug are present, receptors are increasingly saturated and so each additional milligram of the drug will have smaller and smaller incremental effects.[36] This leads to a typical hyperbolic relationship between the dose of a psychiatric drug and its effect on target receptors, as revealed by PET imaging of various psychiatric drugs: GABA-A occupancy in benzodiazepines, D_2 dopaminergic blockade in antipsychotics and SERT occupancy for antidepressants. A generic relationship between a psychiatric drug and its target receptor is shown in Figure 1.4. The relationship between the dose of a psychiatric drug and its effect on its target receptors is very steep at small doses, with the curve flattening out at higher doses (often corresponding to the doses commonly employed clinically).

This hyperbolic relationship between the dose of a psychiatric drug and the effect on its major target receptors is not restricted to a single receptor target but applies to all targets of psychiatric drugs, including noradrenergic, dopaminergic, cholinergic, histaminergic and serotonergic receptors (which may each be responsible for the pathogenesis of some withdrawal effects),[37] as the law of mass action dictates the nature of the effect on all these receptors.[36,38] This relationship is sometimes obscured in textbooks and academic papers by plotting dose–response relationships with drug dose on a logarithmic axis, giving the impression of a linear relationship between drug dose and effect, especially at intermediate doses.[36,39] For some classes of drugs, including antipsychotics, antidepressants and benzodiazepines, clinical effects – such as on symptom scores and adverse effects – have also been demonstrated to follow this hyperbolic relationship with dose.[40-42] This is mirrored in cellular processes – for example, extracellular

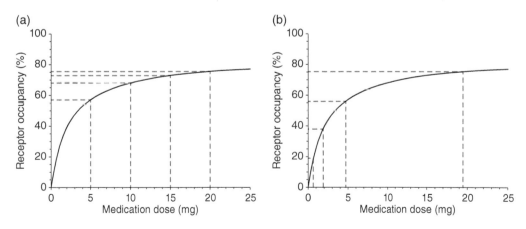

Figure 1.4 Linear versus hyperbolic tapering (a) Linear reductions of dose cause increasingly large reductions in effect on receptor targets, possibly associated with more withdrawal effects. (b) 'Even' reductions of effect at target receptors requires hyperbolic dose reductions. The final dose before stopping will need to be very small so that this step down is not larger (in terms of effect on the brain) than previous reductions.

serotonin levels show a hyperbolic relationship with dosage of antidepressants[43] as do GABA-gated currents in response to diazepam in cellular models[44] – suggesting that the effects of psychiatric drugs from the molecular level to the clinical level are all similarly hyperbolic in pattern.

Therefore, although tapering psychiatric drugs by linear amounts (for example, 20mg, 15mg, 10mg, 5mg, 0mg) seems intuitively appealing (and practical, through splitting tablets), however, because of the hyperbolic relationship between dose of psychiatric drug and effect on its receptor targets, this linear pattern of tapering will produce increasingly large reductions in effect on the target receptors (Figure 1.4a).

Whilst it is true that the relationship between dose of psychiatric drugs and effect on target receptor occupancy has not yet been shown to have a direct relationship to withdrawal effects, such a relationship remains highly plausible because all studied biochemical and clinical effects follow a hyperbolic relationship with psychiatric drug dosage. This is also consistent with patient accounts, who report that withdrawal effects worsen as the total dose becomes lower.[1,45] Given the pharmacology of psychiatric drugs, it is difficult to put forward a rationale for linear tapering.

It makes more sense to reduce the drug in such a way that produces an 'even' amount of reduction in effect on target receptors – which entails hyperbolic dose reductions (Figure 1.4b). In this figure reductions of 20 percentage points of receptor occupancy are shown. It can be seen that reducing in a manner that produces the same-sized reductions in receptor occupancy requires making dose reductions by smaller and smaller amounts. Note how small the final doses are required to be so that the final 'step down' from the lowest dose to zero is not larger (in terms of effect at target receptors) than the prior reductions in dose that have been tolerable for the patient (in Figure 1.4, this is 0.6mg). This is comparable to the manner in which planes land: they follow a hyperbolic pattern of descent, flattening out the angle of descent as they approach the ground to enable a soft landing.

> Note: A percentage point means one point on a scale. For example, 80% receptor occupancy when reduced by 20 percentage points will produce 60% receptor occupancy. This is distinct from reducing 80% by 20% which will give 64% receptor occupancy.

The reduction regimens shown in the chapters dedicated to individual drugs follow this pattern of hyperbolic reductions, with more or less widely spaced steps in between doses. For each suggested regimen, the difference in receptor occupancy is preserved between the given steps, producing a pharmacologically rational regimen. This can be thought of as similar to the bellows on an accordion – where the steps are equally spaced apart but can be compressed (analogous to tapering more quickly) or dilated (analogous to tapering more slowly) according to the degree to which the patient tolerates the withdrawal process.

> To taper at an 'even' rate, dose decreases are made such that the degree of receptor occupancy is reduced by the same number of percentage points of receptor occupancy at each step of the reduction regimen.

Empirical support for hyperbolic tapering

Although there has been limited research into tapering practice, there is some empirical support for tapering according to this hyperbolic pattern of dose reduction for some psychiatric drugs using 'tapering strips'.[32,46] 'Tapering strips' are composed of compounded tablet formulations of small doses of psychiatric medication – for example 5mg, 2mg, 1mg, 0.5mg, 0.2mg and 0.1mg of a drug – packaged into plastic pouches (similar to the way in which different change is made up by small denominations of coins) in such a way as to produce very gradual dose reductions (with the reductions slowing down at lower doses): for example 20mg, 19mg, 18mg, 17mg ... 1mg, 0.7mg, 0.5mg, 0.2mg, 0mg. These tapering strips are arranged in a hyperbolic pattern so that reductions are made by smaller and smaller amounts as total dosage gets lower. Several studies have now demonstrated that many patients on long-term antidepressants who have been unable to taper using conventional approaches are able to stop their antidepressants when following this pattern of hyperbolic dose reduction[32,46,47] and are able to remain off their medication at long periods of follow up (1–5 years).[47]

Other studies have shown that the risk of relapse when reducing dose of antipsychotic follows a hyperbolic pattern – when dose reductions are made from high doses there is only a minor increase in risk of relapse, but as doses become lower the risk of relapse increases hyperbolically, mirroring the receptor occupancy of antipsychotics.[48,49] This suggests that tapering of antipsychotics that adjusts for this effect (i.e. tapering hyperbolically) might minimise the risk of relapse. Some evidence for this suggestion exists in an antipsychotic reduction study performed with exponential reductions (i.e. reducing by one-quarter of the most recent dose every 6 months), which showed many patients were able to reduce their dose of antipsychotic by half or three-quarters without an increased risk of relapse.[50]

In the UK, NICE recommends tapering according to a proportionate pattern – that is, by a proportion of the most recent dose, so that the size of dose reductions becomes increasingly smaller as the total dose gets lower, a simple approximation of hyperbolic tapering – for several psychiatric medications, including antidepressants, benzodiazepines, and z-drugs, as well as opioids.[51]

CHAPTER 1

References

1. Framer A. What I have learnt from helping thousands of people taper off psychotropic medications. *Ther Adv Psychopharmacol* 2021; 11: 204512532199127.

2. Horowitz MA, Taylor D. How to reduce and stop psychiatric medication. *Eur Neuropsychopharmacol* 2021; 55: 4–7.

3. Horowitz MA, Taylor D. Tapering of SSRI treatment to mitigate withdrawal symptoms. *Lancet Psychiatry* 2019; 6: 538–46.

4. Horowitz MA, Jauhar S, Natesan S, Murray RM, Taylor DM. A method for tapering antipsychotic treatment that may minimize the risk of relapse. *Schizophr Bull* 2021; 47: 1116–29.

5. Gupta S, Cahill JD, Miller R. Deprescribing antipsychotics: a guide for clinicians. *BJPsych Advances* 2018; 24: 295–302.

6. Groot PC, van Os J. How user knowledge of psychotropic drug withdrawal resulted in the development of person-specific tapering medication. *Ther Adv Psychopharmacol* 2020; 10: 204512532093245.

7. Ruhe H, Horikx A, van Avendonk M, Groeneweg B, Woutersen-Koch H. Multidisciplinary recommendations for discontinuation of SSRIs and SNRIs. *Lancet Psychiatry* 2019.

8. Guy A, Brown M, Lewis S, Horowitz M. The 'patient voice': patients who experience antidepressant withdrawal symptoms are often dismissed, or misdiagnosed with relapse, or a new medical condition. *Ther Adv Psychopharmacol* 2020; 10: 2045125320967183.

9. Davies J, Read J. A systematic review into the incidence, severity and duration of antidepressant withdrawal effects: are guidelines evidence-based? *Addict Behav* 2019; 97: 111–21.

10. Brandt L, Bschor T, Henssler J, et al. Antipsychotic withdrawal symptoms: a systematic review and meta-analysis. *Front Psychiatry* 2020; 11: 569912.

11. Read J. The experiences of 585 people when they tried to withdraw from antipsychotic drugs. *Addict Behav Rep* 2022; 15: 100421.

12. Walewski JW, Filipa JA, Hagen CL, Sanders ST. Standard single-mode fibers as convenient means for the generation of ultrafast high-pulse-energy super-continua. *Appl Phys B* 2006; 83: 75–9.

13. Lerner A, Klein M. Dependence, withdrawal and rebound of CNS drugs: an update and regulatory considerations for new drugs development. *Brain Commun* 2019; 1: fcz025.

14. Brunton LL, Chabner BA, Knollmann BC. *Goodman & Gilman's The Pharmacological Basis of Therapeutics*, 12e. McGraw-Hill Education, 2011.

15. Bhagwagar Z, Rabiner EA, Sargent PA, Grasby PM, Cowen PJ. Persistent reduction in brain serotonin1A receptor binding in recovered depressed men measured by positron emission tomography with [11C]WAY-100635. *Mol Psychiatry* 2004; 9: 386–92.

16. Silvestri S, Seeman MV, Negrete JC, et al. Increased dopamine D2receptor binding after long-term treatment with antipsychotics in humans: a clinical PET study. *Psychopharmacology* 2000; 152: 174–80.

17. Joyce J. D2 but not D3 receptors are elevated after 9 or 11 months chronic haloperidol treatment: Influence of withdrawal period. *Synapse* 2001; 40: 137–44.

18. Reidenberg MM. Drug discontinuation effects are part of the pharmacology of a drug. *J Pharmacol Exp Ther* 2011; 339: 324–8.

19. Cosci F, Chouinard G. Acute and persistent withdrawal syndromes following discontinuation of psychotropic medications. *Psychother Psychosom* 2020; 89: 283–306.

20. Hengartner MP, Schulthess L, Sorensen A, Framer A. Protracted withdrawal syndrome after stopping antidepressants: a descriptive quantitative analysis of consumer narratives from a large internet forum. *Ther Adv Psychopharmacol* 2020; 10: 2045125320980573.

21. Moncrieff J, Read J, Horowitz M. Severity of antidepressant withdrawal effects versus symptoms of underlying conditions. (in preparation).

22. Horowitz M, Flanigan R, Cooper R, Moncrieff J. The determinants of outcome from antidepressant withdrawal in a large survey of patients. (in preparation).

23. Schoretsanitis G, Kane JM, Correll CU, Rubio JM. Predictors of lack of relapse after random discontinuation of oral and long-acting injectable antipsychotics in clinically stabilized patients with schizophrenia: a re-analysis of individual participant data. *Schizophr Bull* 2021;: 1–11.

24. Horowitz MA, Murray RM, Taylor D. Confounding of antipsychotic discontinuation studies by withdrawal-related relapse. *Schizophr Bull* 2022; 48: 294–5.

25. Baldessarini RJ, Tondo L. Effects of treatment discontinuation in clinical psychopharmacology. *Psychother Psychosom* 2019; 88: 65–70.

26. Baldessarini RJ, Tondo L, Ghiani C, Lepri B. Illness risk following rapid versus gradual discontinuation of antidepressants. *Am J Psychiatry* 2010; 167: 934–41.

27. Bogers JPAM, Hambarian G, Michiels M, Vermeulen J, de Haan L. Risk factors for psychotic relapse after dose reduction or discontinuation of antipsychotics in patients with chronic schizophrenia: a systematic review and meta-analysis. *Schizophr Bull Open* 2020; 1. DOI:10.1093/schizbullopen/sgaa002.

28. Gøtzsche, P. C., & Demasi, M. (2023). Interventions to help patients withdraw from depression drugs: A systematic review. *The International Journal of Risk & Safety in Medicine*. https://doi.org/10.3233/JRS-230011

29. Récalt AM, Cohen D. Withdrawal confounding in randomized controlled trials of antipsychotic, antidepressant, and stimulant drugs, 2000–2017. *Psychother Psychosom* 2019; 88: 105–13.

30. Hengartner MP, Plöderl M. Prophylactic effects or withdrawal reactions? An analysis of time-to-event data from antidepressant relapse prevention trials submitted to the FDA. *Ther Adv Psychopharmacol* 2021; 11: 20451253211032052.

31. Horowitz MA, Taylor D. Distinguishing relapse from antidepressant withdrawal: clinical practice and antidepressant discontinuation studies. *BJPsych Advances* 2022; 28: 297–311.

32. Groot PC, van Os J. Successful use of tapering strips for hyperbolic reduction of antidepressant dose: a cohort study. *Ther Adv Psychopharmacol* 2021; 11: 20451253211039330.

33. Moncrieff J, Jakobsen JC, Bachmann M. Later is not necessarily better: limitations of survival analysis in studies of long-term drug treatment of psychiatric conditions. *BMJ Evid Based Med* 2022; 27: 246–50.

34. Viguera AC, Baldessarini RJ, Hegarty JD, Van Kammen DP, Tohen M. Clinical risk following abrupt and gradual withdrawal of maintenance neuroleptic treatment. *Arch Gen Psychiatry* 1997; 54: 49–55.

35. Suppes T, Baldessarini R, Faedda G, Tohen M. Risk of recurrence following discontinuation of lithium treatment in bipolar disorder. *Arch Gen Psychiatry* 1991; 48: 1082–8.

36. Holford N. Pharmacodynamic principles and the time course of delayed and cumulative drug effects. *Translational and Clinical Pharmacology* 2018; 26: 56.

37. Horowitz MA, Framer A, Hengartner MP, Sørensen A, Taylor D. Estimating risk of antidepressant withdrawal from a review of published data. CNS Drugs. 2023;37: 143–157.

38. Meyer JH, Wilson AA, Sagrati S, et al. Serotonin transporter occupancy of five selective serotonin reuptake inhibitors at different doses: an [11C]DASB positron emission tomography study. *Am J Psychiatry* 2004; 161: 826–35.

39. Horowitz MA, Taylor D. Tapering of SSRI treatment to mitigate withdrawal symptoms – Authors' reply. *Lancet Psychiatry* 2019; 6: 562–3.

40. Furukawa TA, Cipriani A, Cowen PJ, Leucht S, Egger M, Salanti G. Optimal dose of selective serotonin reuptake inhibitors, venlafaxine, and mirtazapine in major depression: a systematic review and dose-response meta-analysis. *Lancet Psychiatry* 2019; 6: 601–9.

41. Leucht S, Crippa A, Siafis S, Patel MX, Orsini N, Davis JM. Dose-response meta-analysis of antipsychotic drugs for acute schizophrenia. *Am J Psychiatry* 2020; 177: 342–53.

42. Bottlaender M, Brouillet E, Varastet M, et al. In vivo high intrinsic efficacy of triazolam: a positron emission tomography study in nonhuman primates. *J Neurochem* 1994; 62: 1102–11.

43. Beyer CE, Boikess S, Luo B, Dawson LA. Comparison of the effects of antidepressants on norepinephrine and serotonin concentrations in the rat frontal cortex: an in-vivo microdialysis study. *J Psychopharmacol* 2002; 16: 297–304.

44. Atack JR. Subtype-selective GABA(A) receptor modulation yields a novel pharmacological profile: the design and development of TPA023. *Adv Pharmacol*. 2009; 57: 137–85.

45. Stockmann T. What it was like to stop an antidepressant. *Ther Adv Psychopharmacol* 2019; 9: 2045125319884834.

46. Groot PC, van Os J. Antidepressant tapering strips to help people come off medication more safely. *Psychosis* 2018; 10: 142–5.

47. Groot PC, van Os J. Outcome of antidepressant drug discontinuation with taperingstrips after 1–5 years. *Ther Adv Psychopharmacol* 2020; 10: 204512532095460.

48. Horowitz MA, Macaulay A, Taylor D. Limitations in research on maintenance treatment for individuals with schizophrenia. *JAMA Psychiatry* 2021; published online 24 November. doi:10.1001/jamapsychiatry.2021.3400.

49. Leucht S, Bauer S, Siafis S, et al. Examination of dosing of antipsychotic drugs for relapse prevention in patients with stable schizophrenia: a meta-analysis. *JAMA Psychiatry* 2021; 78: 1238–48.

50. Liu CC, Takeuchi H. Achieving the lowest effective antipsychotic dose for patients with remitted psychosis: a proposed guided dose-reduction algorithm. *CNS Drugs* 2020; 34: 117–26.

51. National Institute for Health and Care Excellence (NICE). Medicines associated with dependence or withdrawal symptoms: safe prescribing and withdrawal management for adults | Guidance | NICE. https://www.nice.org.uk/guidance/ng215/chapter/Recommendations (accessed 27 June 2022).

Practical options for prescribing gradually tapering doses

The dose forms available for psychiatric drugs are those marketed for therapeutic use, not for hyperbolic tapering. For many drugs, it is therefore difficult to find dose forms that are anywhere near small enough for such tapers. The smallest available tablets produce high receptor occupancy such that going from this tablet (or even a quarter of the smallest available tablet) to zero would cause a very large reduction in effect, producing substantial withdrawal symptoms for some patients.[1,2] NICE guidance on stopping antidepressants recommends, for example, 'if once very small doses have been reached, slow tapering cannot be achieved using tablets or capsules, consider using liquid preparations if available'.[3] The Royal College of Psychiatrists' guidance on 'Stopping antidepressants' provides examples throughout involving splitting tablets or using liquid versions of antidepressants to make up doses that cannot be made up by splitting existing tablet formulations.[4] This approach can be usefully applied to other psychiatric drugs as well.

To prepare dosages that allow steps in between or lower than doses widely available in tablet formulations, one or more of the following licensed methods can be used to facilitate gradual tapering:

- splitting tablets using a tablet cutter
- using manufacturers' liquid preparations

There are also off-licence methods that many patients use to make up these small doses including:[5-8]

- custom compounding of medications into tablets, capsules or liquids
- opening capsules to count or weigh beads
- dispersing (or sometimes dissolving) medication available in tablet or powdered (in capsules) form in water or other diluents

Every-other-day dosing

As current tablet formulations of many psychiatric medications do not permit pharmacologically informed tapering regimens as outlined above it is tempting to make dose reductions by having patients take their dose every other day or every third day so that their average dose each day is reduced. However, this method is not recommended for most psychiatric drugs, other than those with long elimination half-lives.[5,9] The half-lives of many psychiatric drugs are 24 hours or less, so dosing every second day will cause plasma levels of the drug to fall to one-quarter, or less, of peak levels before the next dose. It is widely recognised that skipping doses can induce withdrawal effects from psychiatric drugs,[10,11] something which patients routinely report,[5] and every-other-day dosing to taper has similar consequences. Some exceptions to this rule, such as drugs with longer half-lives (or metabolites with longer half-lives), for example, fluoxetine or diazepam, are discussed in the relevant chapters.

Splitting tablets using a tablet cutter

Many tablets can be easily divided into halves (or quarters if they are round) using cheaply available tablet cutters.[12] Using tablet cutters is more accurate for dividing tablets than either splitting by hand (for scored tablets), cutting with scissors or using a kitchen knife (for unscored tablets).[13] Although in older methods of manufacturing, active medication was not evenly distributed throughout a tablet, this is no longer the case.[14] Tablet splitting is widely employed with almost one quarter of all drugs administered in primary care being split.[15] Although there are concerns that the splitting process may not be completely accurate,[16] this can be mitigated by storing the remainder of the tablet fragment to be used over subsequent days, meaning that the correct dose will be received over 2 or 4 days. Tablet cutters have the advantage of closing as they are used and so retain both halves of the tablet being cut.

This technique may be helpful for the first few steps of a reduction regimen but may not be suitable after this stage as the doses required will be smaller than one-quarter of the smallest available tablet for some medications. Small variation in dose from day to day whilst at higher doses of medication is unlikely to cause withdrawal issues for most people (although these differences can become more critical at lower doses). Sustained-release, and extended-release tablets can also be split, with the understanding that splitting these types of tablets to some extent compromises their sustained-release properties, and may in some cases convert them to immediate-release formulations, which may need to be taken in divided doses two (or three) times a day, depending on their elimination half-lives.[8]

Solutions and suspensions

The difference between solutions and suspensions should be noted. When a substance is soluble enough in a solvent it will dissolve and form a solution. The substance will be evenly distributed in the solution once it is completely dissolved. An example is sugar in hot tea. When a substance is not very soluble in a solvent it will form a suspension, which is a heterogenous mixture of a fluid (usually called a 'vehicle') with solid particles spread throughout. An example is fine particles of sand suspended in a bucket of water. The particles will eventually settle if it is left to sit long enough. The speed of settling depends upon the size of the particles and the viscosity of the vehicle. Often suspensions are made with a viscous vehicle, like syrup (e.g. Ora Plus), as this slows down the process of settling.[6] Psychiatric drug tablets will often form suspensions in water as they are often only partially soluble.[7] In this case there may be visible material in the suspension, composed of both tablet filler and active medication. Vigorous shaking of such a suspension will cause the suspended drug particles to be more evenly distributed throughout the suspension so that each given volume contains equal amounts of drug. This is why it is so important to vigorously shake suspensions before any manipulation – such as removing a volume, or diluting it further – and before consuming a portion. Drug molecules will not be damaged by vigorous shaking.

Manufacturers' liquids

The most widely available option for making up doses that are smaller than those available in tablets is liquid versions of a drug. For some psychiatric drugs, liquid versions are available. These bottles of liquid usually contain a fixed amount of drug in 5mLs of liquid but sometimes come with a droplet mechanism which generally provide small drops (often 0.1mL) when the bottle is held upside down. This droplet mechanism allows only specific doses to be given – for example, 2mg per drop, so multiples of 2mg can be administered, but

CHAPTER 1

half drops cannot. Alternatively, the droplet mechanism from these bottles is removable, and this allows the use of a small oral syringe to draw up small amounts of liquid, giving greater precision (for example, using a 1mL syringe, with 0.01mL gradations).

Some – but not all – liquid formulations are more expensive than tablets. For those liquid formulations that are more expensive, short-term use of this formulation might lead to a reduction in aversive effects from the discontinuation process and longer-term savings if the medication is successfully ceased[17] as well as a reduction in the burden of adverse effects to the patient and healthcare system.[18]

Off-licence options for making small doses of medications

Regulatory authorities approve formulations of drugs on the basis that these formulations provide a precise and accurate dosage and are stable, both chemically and biologically, over the period indicated by the stated expiry or expiration date. Any alteration to these approved formulations renders use 'off-label'. This includes the crushing of tablets and dilution of liquid formulations. It is important to note that dose precision and stability often cannot be formally guaranteed by the manufacturer in these situations. However, some manufacturers do assure stability for some situations and in other cases research has confirmed chemical stability.

Whilst it may represent an unlicensed ('off-label') use to open capsules, crush tablets or make extemporaneous suspensions, the General Medical Council (GMC) guidance on this matter states that doctors are permitted to prescribe medications off-licence when 'the dosage specified for a licensed medicine would not meet the patient's need'.[19] In the UK, for example, a medical practitioner can authorise the use of unlicensed medication (according to the Medicines Act 1968).[7] This is echoed by the NHS Pharmaceutical Quality Assurance Committee in their *Handbook of Extemporaneous Solutions*: 'some patients have special clinical needs that cannot be met by licensed medicinal products or by a viable alternative option. In these circumstances it would be inappropriate to curtail the patient's treatment, as this would have a detrimental effect on their condition'.[6] In the USA, such usage is also considered 'off-label' or 'unapproved' use by the FDA, which, however, explains that 'healthcare providers generally may prescribe the drug for an unapproved use when they judge that it is medically appropriate for their patient'.[20]

Dilutions of manufacturers' liquids

The manufacturers' liquid versions of some psychiatric drugs are often quite concentrated – for example citalopram comes as a 40mg/mL solution.[21] As greater errors are found when measuring less than 20% of the labelled capacity of a syringe[22] and the smallest syringe widely available is a 1mL syringe, the smallest dose that could be measured accurately with a syringe is 8mg (0.2mL). This means that dilution of these liquids is often necessary to make the small doses needed by some patients. Citalopram, for example, can be diluted in water or juice according to their Summary of Product Characteristics (SmPC) approved by the Medicines and Healthcare products Regulatory Agency (MHRA) in the UK.[21] The FDA also recommends that sertraline liquid is diluted in water or juices before administration.[23] This allows formulation of

> **Box 1.1** Steps required to measure out a small dose of a psychiatric medications, by diluting a manufacturer's oral solution. Other doses can be made following similar rules. Pharmacists will be a useful source of advice on these issues.
>
> To deliver a psychiatric drug at a dose of 2mg from a liquid concentration of 40mg/mL made by the manufacturer:
>
> - First verify the biological equivalence between the liquid version and the tablet version of the drug as sometimes different salts are used.
> - In the case of equal bio-availability 2mg of liquid drug is equivalent to 2mg of drug in tablet form (otherwise a bio-equivalence calculation should be made).
> - Volume of liquid drug required = mass/concentration = 2mg/ (40mg/mL) = 0.05mL.
> - The smallest volume that can be accurately measured with a 1mL syringe is 0.2mL; therefore a dilution is required.
> - Most liquid drugs (which are dissolved in water) can be mixed with water, or juice.[21]
> - 0.5mL of this solution can be mixed with 4.5mLs of water to produce a solution with a concentration of 4mg/mL (a 1 in 10 dilution).
> - Concentration = mass/volume. Therefore, volume = mass/concentration.
> - Volume of this diluted solution required = 2mg/ (4mg/mL) = 0.5mL (which can be measured accurately with a 1mL syringe).
> - Many drug labels for liquid versions of drugs recommends that this solution is consumed 'immediately',[21] which might be interpreted as meaning within an hour of preparation.

the very small doses suggested to facilitate tolerable tapering of different psychiatric medications (Box 1.1). The SmPC and FDA guidance both advise that such dilutions be consumed 'immediately', which may be interpreted as within an hour of preparation.[21,23]

It is likely that this recommendation is based on the remote possibility that chemical stability is compromised by dilution. Studies have found that there was less than 5% degradation over 8 weeks for fluoxetine solution in fruit juice, or other common diluents, as assessed by high-performance liquid chromatography.[24] Similarly, citalopram solution in water showed no significant degradation over 30 days when stored in the dark.[25]

The biological stability (referring to a drug's susceptibility to microbial contamination) of psychiatric drug dilutions has not been formally evaluated but this is likely to be unproblematic if solutions are stored in a refrigerator for several days. Some of the manufacturers' labels do not specifically state that a solution of a psychiatric drug can be diluted in water but if these drugs are dissolved in water, further dilution in water should be acceptable in terms of drug solubility.

Custom compounding of individualized dosages

Compounded liquids (e.g. 'Specials' in the UK)

For some psychiatric medications that are not made by their manufacturer into liquid formulations, liquid versions can be compounded at specialist pharmacies (for example, some psychiatric medications are available as prescription 'Specials' in the UK).

Compounded capsules or tablets

Some pharmacies are able to make up custom-made doses of medication in tablet or capsule form. Sometimes this will remove slow-release characteristics of the medication, which will have to be taken in immediate release form, sometimes necessitating dosing more than once a day. This should be verified with the pharmacy.

One such option is pre-packaged customised formulations of tablets that allow gradual reductions, made by a Dutch compounding pharmacy that produces 'tapering strips', as an unlicensed medication.[26,27] As mentioned above, these 'tapering strips' involve making up smaller formulations of many psychiatric medications than are currently available in tablet form, for example, 0.1mg or 0.5mg of a medication and preparing pouches of medication that contain a number of small tablets in order to make up hyperbolically decreasing dose regimens that are able to go down to very small final doses before stopping (e.g. 0.1mg of citalopram). Additionally, this compounding pharmacy also allows doctors to order customised reduction regimens, which facilitate any desired reduction trajectory.

Dispersing tablets

When liquid formulations are not available, many tablets that are not enterically coated or sustained- or extended-release can be crushed to a powdered form and/or dispersed in water, as indicated by guidance for patients with swallowing difficulties.[7,28] The contents may sometimes taste bitter and some drugs may have a local anaesthetic effect on the tongue.[7] Crushing and dispersing will not greatly alter these medications' pharmacokinetic properties (their rate of gastrointestinal absorption will be increased as they are more easily absorbed), according to the FDA medication guide[8] and the Royal Pharmaceutical Society (RPS) guidance on crushing, opening or splitting oral dosage forms.[12]

Many immediate-release tablets will simply disperse in water after a few minutes, aided by stirring or shaking.[29] Some formulations of psychiatric medications come as orodispersible tablets, such as mirtazapine or olanzapine. These tablets are designed to rapidly disintegrate on the tongue without the need for water. However, guidelines for people who have swallowing difficulties, like the NEWT guidelines in the UK,[7] and similar guidance in the USA[30] indicate that they will also disperse in water (generally quickly) and the suspension formed can be used to administer the drug to the patient.[7]

The Specialist Pharmacy Service in the NHS provides instructions on how to administer antidepressants to people with swallowing difficulties, recommending that citalopram, escitalopram, paroxetine and sertraline can all be crushed and/or dispersed in water and that fluoxetine capsules can be opened and dispersed in water.[28] Crushing can be performed with a spoon or a mortar and pestle and will help the drug to dissolve more quickly. For example, application of the above principles for gradual tapering could involve dispersing a 10mg tablet in 100mL of water (by shaking or stirring) and then discarding 5mL of the suspension with a syringe to administer a dose of 9.5mg when the remaining 95mL is consumed.

As some psychiatric medications are poorly soluble in water, it should be noted that mixtures made by dispersing a tablet in water are often suspensions (not solutions). Flakes or particles visible in a suspension are a combination of excipients (or 'fillers') and active drug. Care should be taken to vigorously shake a suspension to ensure even dispersion of drug.[29] Some sustained-release and extended-release drug forms contain a binder that will thicken when added to liquid and so cannot be crushed and dissolved in an aqueous solution. If an enteric coating, which protects a drug from the acidic environment in the stomach, is removed by crushing the tablet, the in vivo drug degradation will increase, with less drug available to produce the desired clinical effect.[12] Issues regarding specific drugs are discussed in subsequent chapters.

Opening capsules to count beads

The extended-release forms of various psychiatric drugs, when delivered as gelatine capsules filled with tiny beads, may be opened and the beads emptied out, as suggested by guidelines for patients with difficulty swallowing tablets or capsules.[7] The pharmacokinetic properties of beads are retained if the capsules are opened and the beads are exposed to air for medications like duloxetine and venlafaxine.[31,32] These drugs can then be tapered by progressively removing more beads at designated intervals to gradually reduce the dose. This method requires some amount of manual dexterity and so will not be appropriate for all patients. The beads can be weighed or counted. This should be done with clean and dry hands (or using an instrument like a ruler or pair of tweezers). The number of beads to be taken will need to be placed back into the original capsule or another gelatine capsule bought from a pharmacy or online. The beads should not be swallowed without a capsule as there are some reports of throat irritation occurring.[33]

Each capsule contains the same weight of drug but, because the beads vary in size, they may have different numbers of beads. The average number of beads in three capsules might be used to estimate the number in each capsule. Doses in milligrams can then be converted into the number of beads required. For example, if a 30mg capsule contains, on average, 250 beads, then to achieve a dose of 6mg 50 beads are needed. Beads can be kept in a suitable container for a couple of days as their enteric coating is stable in air.[34] This is an off-label use of the drug.

References

1. Horowitz MA, Taylor D. Tapering of SSRI treatment to mitigate withdrawal symptoms. *Lancet Psychiatry* 2019; 6: 538–46.
2. Horowitz MA, Taylor D. How to reduce and stop psychiatric medication. *Eur Neuropsychopharmacol* 2021; 55: 4–7.
3. National Institute for Health and Care Excellence (NICE). Depression in adults (Draft for consultation, November 2021). https://www.nice.org.uk/guidance/indevelopment/gid-cgwave0725/consultation/html-content-3 (accessed 28 November 2021).
4. Burn W, Horowitz M, Roycroft G, Taylor D. Stopping antidepressants. 2020. https://www.rcpsych.ac.uk/mental-health/treatments-and-wellbeing/stopping-antidepressants (accessed 22 April 2022).
5. Framer A. What I have learnt from helping thousands of people taper off psychotropic medications. *Ther Adv Psychopharmacol* 2021; 11: 204512532199127.
6. Jackson M, Lowey A. *Handbook of Extemporaneous Preparation*. Pharmaceutical Press, 2010.
7. Smyth J. The NEWT guidelines for administration of medication to patients with enteral feeding tubes or swallowing difficulties. 2011. https://www.newtguidelines.com/index.html (accessed 7 September 2022).
8. Bostwick JR, Demehri A. Pills to powder: a clinician's reference for crushable psychotropic medications. *Curr Psychiatr* 2014; 13.
9. Ruhe H, Horikx A, van Avendonk M, Groeneweg B, Woutersen-Koch H. Multidisciplinary recommendations for discontinuation of SSRIs and SNRIs. *Lancet Psychiatry* 2019.
10. National Institute for Health and Care Excellence (NICE). Depression in adults: treatment and management | Guidance | NICE. 2022; published online June. https://www.nice.org.uk/guidance/ng222 (accessed 16 July 2022).
11. Kaplan EM. Antidepressant noncompliance as a factor in the discontinuation syndrome. *J Clin Psychiatry* 1997; 58 Suppl 7: 31–5; discussion 36.
12. Root T, Tomlin S, Erskine D, Lowey A. Pharmaceutical issues when crushing, opening or splitting oral dosage forms. *Royal Pharmaceutical Society* 2011; 1: 1–7.
13. Verrue C, Mehuys E, Boussery K, Remon J-P, Petrovic M. Tablet-splitting: a common yet not so innocent practice. *J Adv Nurs* 2011; 67: 26–32.
14. Hisada H, Okayama A, Hoshino T, et al. Determining the distribution of active pharmaceutical ingredients in combination tablets using near IR and low-frequency Raman spectroscopy imaging. *Chem Pharm Bull* 2020; 68: 155–60.
15. Chaudhri K, Kearney M, Di Tanna GL, Day RO, Rodgers A, Atkins ER. Does splitting a tablet obtain the accurate dose?: A systematic review protocol. *Medicine* 2019; 98: e17189.
16. Center for Drug Evaluation, Research. Best practices for tablet splitting. U.S. Food and Drug Administration. https://www.fda.gov/drugs/ensuring-safe-use-medicine/best-practices-tablet-splitting (accessed 22 September 2022).
17. Davies J, Cooper RE, Moncrieff J, Montagu L, Rae T, Parhi M. The costs incurred by the NHS in England due to the unnecessary prescribing of dependency-forming medications. *Addict Behav* 2021; 125: 107143.
18. Moriarty F, Cahir C, Bennett K, Fahey T. Economic impact of potentially inappropriate prescribing and related adverse events in older people: a cost-utility analysis using Markov models. *BMJ Open* 2019; 9: e021832.
19. General Medical Council. Prescribing unlicensed medicines. 2021.
20. Office of the Commissioner. Understanding unapproved use of approved drugs 'off label'. U.S. Food and Drug Administration. https://www.fda.gov/patients/learn-about-expanded-access-and-other-treatment-options/understanding-unapproved-use-approved-drugs-label (accessed 22 September 2022).
21. Electronic Medicines Compendium. Citalopram 40mg/ml Oral Drops, solution. 2021. https://www.medicines.org.uk/emc/product/3349/smpc#gref.
22. Jordan MA, Choksi D, Lombard K, Patton LR. Development of guidelines for accurate measurement of small volume parenteral products using syringes. *Hosp Pharm* 2021; 56: 165–71.
23. Pfizer. ZOLOFT (sertraline hydrochloride) Label. Accessdata.fda.gov. 2016; published online December. www.accessdata.fda.gov/drugsatfda_docs/label/2016/019839S74S86S87_20990S35S44S45lbl.pdf (accessed 9 September 2022).
24. Peterson JA, Risley DS, Anderson PN, Hostettler KF. Stability of fluoxetine hydrochloride in fluoxetine solution diluted with common pharmaceutical diluents. *Am J Hosp Pharm* 1994; 51: 1342–5.
25. Kwon JW, Armbrust KL. Degradation of citalopram by simulated sunlight. *Environ Toxicol Chem* 2005; 24: 1618–23.
26. Groot PC, van Os J. How user knowledge of psychotropic drug withdrawal resulted in the development of person-specific tapering medication. *Ther Adv Psychopharmacol* 2020; 10: 204512532093245.
27. Groot PC, van Os J. Outcome of antidepressant drug discontinuation with taperingstrips after 1–5 years. *Ther Adv Psychopharmacol* 2020; 10: 204512532095460.
28. Brennan K. Selective serotonin reuptake inhibitor (SSRI) formulations suggested for adults with swallowing difficulties. SPS – Specialist Pharmacy Service. 2021; published online 1 July. https://www.sps.nhs.uk/articles/selective-serotonin-reuptake-inhibitor-ssri-formulations-suggested-for-adults-with-swallowing-difficulties/ (accessed 14 July 2022).
29. White R, Bradnam V. *Handbook of Drug Administration via Enteral Feeding Tubes*, 3rd ed. Padstow: Pharmaceutical Press, 2015.
30. Bostwick JR, Pharm D, Demehri A. Pills to powder: an updated clinician's reference for crushable psychotropics. *Curr Psychiat* 2017; 16: 46–9.
31. Wells KA, Losin WG. In vitro stability, potency, and dissolution of duloxetine enteric-coated pellets after exposure to applesauce, apple juice, and chocolate pudding. *Clin Ther* 2008; 30: 1300–8.
32. Jain RT, Panda J, Srivastava A. Two formulations of venlafaxine are bioequivalent when administered as open capsule mixed with applesauce to healthy subjects. *Indian J Pharm Sci* 2011; 73: 510–16.
33. FDA. Memorandum: DMETS Medication Error Postmarketing Safety Review: Cymbalta. Fda.gov. 2007; published online 8 March. www.fda.gov/media/74134/download (accessed 9 September 2022).
34. Kuang C, Sun Y, Li B, et al. Preparation and evaluation of duloxetine hydrochloride enteric-coated pellets with different enteric polymers. *Asian J Pharm Sci* 2017; 12: 216–26.

Psychological aspects of tapering

Tapering off psychiatric drugs can be a difficult process, leading to numerous withdrawal symptoms described in subsequent chapters, as well as risking relapse. Although there are ways of coping with specific distressing withdrawal symptoms, which will be discussed, it is generally best to avoid overly distressing symptoms because they can impair social and professional functioning, precipitate relapse and cause a patient to become fearful of the process of reducing their medication or of ever stopping it.[1] Although there may be exceptions, most people do not do well by 'white-knuckling' through the process of very severe withdrawal effects. Furthermore, while there has been limited research in the area, it seems to be the case that more severe withdrawal symptoms arising from rapid reductions may increase the risk of a protracted withdrawal syndrome in the long run.[1–3]

Many people cannot tolerate severe withdrawal effects and will return to a full dose of medication, or seek other medications to manage their symptoms, and occasionally severe withdrawal effects can lead to hospital admissions or suicidality because they are so aversive.[4–6] So the main approach to manage withdrawal symptoms during the process of discontinuing psychiatric medications should be to reduce the dose gradually enough to avoid severe withdrawal symptoms in the first place. Generally, if symptoms are too severe, the reduction schedule should be halted until these symptoms resolve. In the case of intolerable withdrawal symptoms then the dose should be increased and held there until the symptoms resolve, before progressing at a more gradual rate (with smaller dose reductions, and/or longer periods between dose reductions).

There are several techniques that may be helpful to cope with withdrawal symptoms – derived from both the academic literature and extensive patient experience.[1,7–9] There are a few interventions which have some evidence in supporting patients during tapering – for example mindfulness based cognitive therapies in antidepressant withdrawal.[9,10] While these forms of therapy, especially mindfulness, seem to be helpful with the process of discontinuation, it is unlikely that any psychological therapy can substitute for gradual tapering titrated to the ability of the individual patient to tolerate the process,[1] as evidenced by some negative findings for these interventions.[11,12]

Many patients report that it is useful to be clear, and to be reminded, that the symptoms that are experienced during the withdrawal process are of a physiological origin due to decreasing the drug rather than conferring on these symptoms an existential weight they do not merit.[7] In peer-led withdrawal communities these symptoms are referred to as 'neuro-emotions', denoting emotions that arise because of withdrawal-associated neurological processes, as distinct from 'endogenous' emotions that relate to events in the person's life.[1] This may be thought of as similar to the negative emotions that are well recognised to occur in withdrawal states from recreational substances.[1,13] A guide book for therapists on how to support patients undergoing psychiatric drug withdrawal suggests to therapists that they 'suspend customary assumptions about the source of distress and associated interventions (i.e. emotional processing or analysis) for the duration of withdrawal'(p.95).[7] Other coping techniques are outlined in Box 1.2.

This advice relates to patients without significant risk of harm to themselves or others and in cases where these risks are unmanageable in the process of withdrawal then sensible clinical management should be followed. Clinicians need to stay vigilant for genuine relapse as well, using guides outlined in subsequent chapters for how to distinguish withdrawal effects from relapse. A previously agreed-upon plan for how to approach relapse with the patient is useful in such circumstances.

> **Box 1.2** Coping techniques during tapering.
>
> ■ Often patients will require some preparation for psychiatric drug tapering. This might include devising a list of existing coping skills for dealing with difficult emotions and sensations.
> ■ Patients may also consider developing new coping skills before or during tapering. For example, mindfulness based cognitive therapy (MB-CT) appears helpful in the process of stopping antidepressants.[9]
> ■ Sometimes practical arrangements for reducing work or family duties can be worth exploring.
> ■ Patients may require more psychological support during the process; professional or otherwise.[7] This could be via more frequent contact with a physician, nurse, counsellor or peer group.
> ■ Some patients will find monitoring their symptoms to be helpful in giving them some perspective that symptoms come and go, often with a predictable pattern after dose reductions. This can help to counter fears about relapse and help people to plan their lives around withdrawal symptoms.
> ■ Patients may benefit from being directed to useful written or online resources.[8]
> ■ For difficulties with sleep, which are common during withdrawal, maintaining a fixed sleep–wake cycle, avoiding light for an hour or two before bed (especially electronic equipment) or using different means to restrict blue light from devices, exposure to bright light in the morning, avoiding caffeine in the afternoon and exercise (more than 3 hours before bed ideally) can be helpful.[14]
> ■ There are a number of other coping techniques that people report are useful summarised in a guidebook for therapists[7] as well as other sites.[8] They include:
>   ● Acceptance/non-resistance – maintaining a non-resisting attitude involving staying with painful experiences rather than struggling with them or attempting to stop or fix them
>   ● Breathing exercises – one form of intentional relaxation
>   ● Exercise – if tolerable and appropriate to the person's capacity
>   ● Healthy distraction
>   ● Keeping a diary – can help patients to get a sense of how reductions in dose affect their symptoms
>   ● De-catastrophising – trying to avoid worst case scenario thinking

References

1. Framer A. What I have learnt from helping thousands of people taper off psychotropic medications. *Ther Adv Psychopharmacol* 2021; 11: 204512532199127.
2. Moncrieff J, Read J, Horowitz M. Severity of antidepressant withdrawal effects versus symptoms of underlying conditions. (in preparation).
3. Horowitz M, Flanigan R, Cooper R, Moncrieff J. The determinants of outcome from antidepressant withdrawal in a large survey of patients. (in preparation).
4. Valuck RJ, Orton HD, Libby AM. Antidepressant discontinuation and risk of suicide attempt. *J Clin Psychiatry* 2009; 70: 1069–77.
5. Guy A, Brown M, Lewis S, Horowitz M. The 'patient voice': patients who experience antidepressant withdrawal symptoms are often dismissed, or misdiagnosed with relapse, or a new medical condition. *Ther Adv Psychopharmacol* 2020; 10: 2045125320967183.
6. Hengartner MP, Schulthess L, Sorensen A, Framer A. Protracted withdrawal syndrome after stopping antidepressants: a descriptive quantitative analysis of consumer narratives from a large internet forum. *Ther Adv Psychopharmacol* 2020; 10: 2045125320980573.
7. Guy A, Davies J, Rizq R. *Guidance for Psychological Therapists: Enabling Conversations with Clients Taking or Withdrawing from Prescribed Psychiatric Drugs*. London: APPG for Prescribed Drug Dependence, 2019.
8. Outro Library. https://learn.outro.com/home (accessed July 5, 2023).
9. Maund E, Stuart B, Moore M, et al. Managing antidepressant discontinuation: a systematic review. *Ann Fam Med* 2019; 17: 52–60.
10. Breedvelt JJF, Warren FC, Segal Z, Kuyken W, Bockting CL. Continuation of antidepressants vs sequential psychological interventions to prevent relapse in depression: an individual participant data meta-analysis. *JAMA Psychiatry* 2021; 78: 868–75.
11. Fava GA, Belaise C. Discontinuing antidepressant drugs: lesson from a failed trial and extensive clinical experience. *Psychother Psychosom* 2018; 87: 257–67.
12. Scholten WD, Batelaan NM, Van Oppen P, et al. The efficacy of a group CBT relapse prevention program for remitted anxiety disorder patients who discontinue antidepressant medication: a randomized controlled trial. *Psychother Psychosom* 2018; 87: 240–2.
13. Lerner A, Klein M. Dependence, withdrawal and rebound of CNS drugs: an update and regulatory considerations for new drugs development. *Brain Commun* 2019; 1: fcz025.
14. Lack LC, Wright HR. Treating chronobiological components of chronic insomnia. *Sleep Med* 2007; 8: 637–44.

Tapering psychiatric drugs in practice

The practical steps for deprescribing are similar across different classes of psychiatric drugs, although there will be wide variation on the details depending on the medication type and the patient's pre-existing condition.

These steps are explored in more detail for each relevant drug class in subsequent chapters, but some general principles are outlined below.

Considerations before tapering

Education about benefits and harms of continuing or stopping medication

- Discuss the patient's circumstances and motivation for reducing or stopping. More stable life circumstances are generally more conducive towards reducing medication. Patients who are ambivalent about the process may benefit from more information.
- Patients should be informed about the risks and benefits of reducing or stopping their psychiatric drug. The major risks are withdrawal and relapse. The risk of relapse might be mitigated by slowly tapering the medication, and by alternative means for managing an underlying mental health condition. For some patients a past stressor will have resolved such that relapse is less of a concern. For other patients with a greater number of risk factors or severe conditions relapse will be a much greater concern. The risks and benefits of medication continuation are outlined in subsequent chapters.
- Some patients may have queries about prescribing decisions made previously. Explain that our understanding of the balance of risks and benefits of a medicine can change over time.
- The adverse effects of being on a psychiatric drug need to be weighed against the potentially aversive consequences of stopping a psychiatric drug too quickly. If the adverse effects of a psychiatric medication are life-threatening or severe, then this will need to take precedence over slow tapering. In other circumstances the risks will need to be balanced for each individual case.[1] Most of the advice below relates to patients who do not have life-threatening or urgent adverse effects.

Addressing potential barriers and facilitators

- Recognise that patients may have fears and concerns about stopping their psychiatric drugs (both relapse and withdrawal effects) and will need support to withdraw successfully, particularly if previous attempts have been difficult. Details for online or written resources may be useful[2] as will increased support from a clinician or therapist (for example, check-in phone calls, more frequent appointments and specific advice about major hurdles that might arise, such as insomnia).[3]
- If possible it is useful to engage support networks in the process – including family and friends, and other professionals involved in care.[4,5] These people can have strong opinions regarding continuing or stopping medication that can be barriers or facilitators of the process. Much of the information given to patients about withdrawal effects, the distinction from relapse, and the harms and benefits of continuing versus stopping medication can be useful for these stakeholders as well.

- Existing beliefs about medication should be explored including the patient's understanding of the role of medication, and alternative options.[4,6] For example, in an intervention designed to help patients to stop unnecessary antidepressants, one element was educating patients that there is no evidence that antidepressants correct an underlying chemical imbalance in depression, identified as an important barrier to stopping medications.[6]

Education about withdrawal symptoms and their management

- All patients should be informed of the risk of withdrawal symptoms on reducing the dose or stopping any psychiatric drug.[1] These symptoms arise because the brain has become accustomed to the medication and when the drug dose is lowered, the difference between what the brain expects and what input the drugs provide is experienced as withdrawal symptoms, as for many other substances like caffeine, or nicotine.

- In order that patients do not mistake withdrawal symptoms for a return of their underlying condition, it is useful to inform patients which withdrawal symptoms they might experience. Specific symptoms for each class of medication are provided in subsequent chapters. For all classes of psychiatric drugs withdrawal symptoms can manifest as both psychological and physical symptoms because of the myriad effects of the medications on different bodily systems. It is the psychological symptoms of withdrawal that cause the most confusion regarding relapse, as there is much overlap in these sets of symptoms.

- Reassure the patient that although there seems to be an intimidating list of symptoms these symptoms are most likely to occur or to be severe when people stop their psychiatric drugs abruptly or too quickly. The entire process outlined below is aimed to minimise the chance of experiencing these unpleasant withdrawal symptoms.

- Explain that it is not fully understood what factors determine risk of withdrawal symptoms for an individual. However, there is evidence that the risks are increased for longer term use, higher doses, specific drugs (for example, short-acting drugs or those with specific receptor targets, such as paroxetine and venlafaxine). People who have experienced withdrawal symptoms previously when tapering or on forgetting their dose are more likely to experience withdrawal symptoms in the future.

- The patient's past experience of stopping should be explored as this can be informative for predicting which symptoms may arise again on tapering. Careful exploration of past attempts to stop may detect withdrawal symptoms being mis-diagnosed as relapse (e.g. by the presence of dizziness, electric 'zaps' or symptoms quite distinct from the original condition for which the drug was prescribed).

- Explain that withdrawal symptoms often occur within a few days of reducing or stopping psychiatric drugs, although they can be delayed in onset, especially with medications with a long half-life like fluoxetine, which can take several weeks to arise.[7] For reasons that are not completely understood (but may relate to the time taken for drug levels in the brain to calibrate to peripheral plasma levels), medications with shorter half-lives can also have delayed onset of withdrawal symptoms, sometimes by several weeks, or longer.[8-10]

- Withdrawal symptoms vary greatly in duration and severity. Some people experience minimal withdrawal effects that last for a few days, but severe withdrawal effects are also possible, although there has been little research into what proportion of patients may experience this.[10]
- Withdrawal symptoms are thought to be more severe and long-lasting when psychiatric drugs are stopped quickly and lessened when they are stopped more gradually.[9,11,12] Withdrawal symptoms can last for months or years in some cases.[10] Long-lasting withdrawal symptoms are often termed post-acute withdrawal symptoms (PAWS). Patients should therefore be warned not to stop psychiatric drugs abruptly. This is ample reason to approach the rate of taper cautiously; if there are no withdrawal symptoms the rate of taper can always be increased.
- Patients should also be made aware that if they experience unpleasant psychological and physical symptoms during withdrawal, this does not necessarily indicate that they need the drug, but rather it may be withdrawal symptoms that instead indicate the need to taper the drug more slowly (after a period of stabilisation).[10] Patients often report that withdrawal symptoms they have experienced in the past have been perceived as relapse.[13,14] Familiarity of the patient and the prescriber with the wide variety of withdrawal symptoms may help to mitigate unnecessary anxiety when symptoms arise.

Outline the process of reducing and/or stopping the medication

- Reassure patients that the some of the negative consequences of tapering can be managed by regular and frequent monitoring. If withdrawal symptoms become too severe then the taper can be halted, or the dose increased. Withdrawal symptoms will then normally resolve over time and the rate of taper can be slowed down to prevent further symptoms arising.[9,15,16]
- Tapering according to a pattern that matches the action of the drugs on the brain might also minimise withdrawal effects. A clinician may explain to the patient that the relationship between the dose of a psychiatric drug and its effect on the brain is hyperbolic, meaning that at small doses, every extra milligram of drug has a large additive effect, whereas at commonly used doses every extra milligram has less and less additive effect. It is thought that this can inform the process of tapering, where patients can reduce their dose by greater amounts when at higher doses but need to reduce by smaller and smaller decrements as they get down to lower doses. Tapering according to a hyperbolic pattern down to low final doses before completely stopping can reduce the risk of withdrawal symptoms.[15,17]
- Patients often find it helpful to see a picture of the relationship between their drug and its effect on the brain so that they understand the rationale for tapering in a hyperbolic manner. On seeing the relationship between the dose of their medication and its effect on target receptors some patients may understand why past attempts were not successful as they stopped at doses that produce high receptor occupancy, leading to significant withdrawal symptoms. These graphs are presented for many commonly used psychiatric drugs in the drug-specific chapters.

- Although it is difficult to predict the exact period required for an individual to taper off their medication most patients take months or even years after long-term use,[1,17,18] depending on the characteristics of their medication use and the individual. This may help to set expectations. Suggested reduction regimens that span these time-lines are given for commonly used medications in later chapters. Some patients might find the prospect of long periods to taper off their medication unappealing, but will sometimes understand as the process unfolds that more gradual tapering gives them a better chance of reducing and stopping their medication in a sustainable manner. Generally, patients should proceed as fast as they can tolerate, but as slow as they need to balance the harm of staying on unnecessary medication against the harm of tapering too quickly.
- Often patients will require some preparation for tapering. This might include devising a list of existing coping skills that the patient possesses for dealing with difficult emotions and sensations, for example acceptance, breathing exercises, mindfulness, exercise, time with friends and family, hobbies, diary keeping and de-catastrophising (see previous section).
- Patients may require more psychological support during the process, which might be professional or otherwise. This could be in the form of a group or via more frequent contact with a physician, nurse, counsellor or peer group.[4,19]
- A plan should also be agreed upon for how to approach a deterioration in mental state, or early signs of relapse – ranging from pausing or slowing down the taper, to more targeted management including increased contact, non-pharmacological management, admission to hospital, or re-instatement of medication, depending on the preference of the patient, and the degree of past and present risk.

Choosing a medication in the case of polypharmacy

- In the case of polypharmacy, although there is limited research, it is generally best to start with a single drug first so that the process of tapering can be optimised before a second drug is also considered for tapering. In terms of selecting a specific drug, there is limited research[20] but there are several pertinent factors to consider. Perhaps the most important is which drug the patient feels is causing them the most pronounced adverse effects and the least benefit. In case the patient is unsure, more objective criteria such as those medications with the least favourable balance of recognised adverse effects and benefit for the patient's condition should be prioritised. Suggestions can be adapted from the STOPP (Screening Tool of Older Persons' Prescriptions) criteria, which although aimed at older people, espouses general principles applicable to other patient groups such as prioritising deprescribing of any drug without an evidence-based clinical indication, or a drug prescribed beyond its recommended duration, or where there is a duplication of prescription from the same drug class.[21] The patient's wishes and aims should be prioritised in any decision.
- Other considerations might be to choose the drug most recently started on the premise that this might be the most easily stopped as adaptation to the drug will be most limited for this medication. Related to this, the drug that the patient thinks might be the easiest to come off might be worth choosing, to build confidence in the process of stopping. Other commentators recommend postponing cessation of medications that can help with sleep in order that these drugs may help to minimise insomnia, which is a very common and sometimes troubling withdrawal symptom.[9]

CHAPTER 1

The process of dose reduction

Once there has been agreement to reduce the dose of a medication, the key elements of a programme of tapering are:

■ that it is flexible and can be adjusted so that the process is tolerable for the patient;
■ that it involves close monitoring of withdrawal symptoms to facilitate timely adjustments to the rate of taper;
■ that patients are provided with preparations of their medication to make the process of creating doses that are not easily able to be made with currently available tablet doses (e.g. access to liquid formulations of their medication or smaller formulations of tablets).

The actual process of tapering involves the following four steps (Figure 1.5):

■ Step 1: estimation of risk of withdrawal for the patient and from this estimate the size of the initial dose reduction.
■ Step 2: monitoring of the withdrawal symptoms resulting from this initial reduction.
■ Step 3: determination of the size of the next reduction based on how tolerable this reduction was for the patient.
■ Step 4: repetition of Steps 2 and 3 until a dose is reached that is small enough so that the reduction to zero is not a larger step down (in terms of effect on the brain) than the reductions that have been previously tolerated.

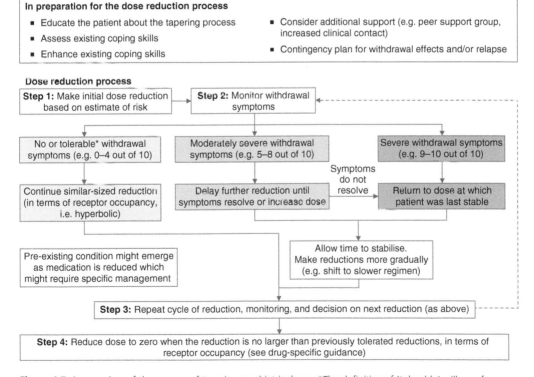

Figure 1.5 An overview of the process of tapering psychiatric drugs. *The definition of 'tolerable' will vary from patient to patient.

These steps are explored in greater depth in subsequent chapters (see Chapter 2), but, in general, a rate of reduction is selected based on the suspected risk of withdrawal effects, erring on the side of caution, but taking into account the patient's preferences (Step 1). There are several options provided for each medication in the drug-specific chapters.

After the first dose reduction patients should be monitored for symptoms of withdrawal. Common withdrawal symptoms can be found in each relevant chapter. Some patients will be aware of their distinctive withdrawal symptoms from previous reduction attempts. Monitoring should normally occur for a period of two to four weeks but may be longer in patients for which there is greater uncertainty about the response (Step 2). Based on the response to this first reduction the next reduction can be made according to a similar reduction in receptor occupancy (along the same reduction schedule), slowed down (or sometimes sped up) (Step 3). The next reduction should occur when withdrawal effects from the previous reduction have resolved or largely resolved.

This process should be repeated – involving repeated cycles of dose reduction, symptom monitoring and adjustment of the next reduction based on these symptoms (Step 4). As circumstances change and symptoms can vary, the trajectories suggested in subsequent chapters should not be seen as 'set-and-forget' regimens but require active monitoring and feedback with adjustment of the rate of taper in order to make the process tolerable. Many patients will find a rate of taper that they can tolerate around their lives. The drug can be stopped when a reduction to zero will not cause a greater decrease in effect (in terms of receptor occupancy) than previous reductions. Patients should be monitored after they have stopped medication for several weeks or longer in case of delayed-onset withdrawal effects or relapse, and these conditions managed appropriately.

References

1. National Institute for Health and Care Excellence (NICE). Medicines associated with dependence or withdrawal symptoms: safe prescribing and withdrawal management for adults I Guidance I NICE. www.nice.org.uk/guidance/ng215/chapter/Recommendations (accessed 27 June 2022).

2. Inner Compass Initiative. The Withdrawal Project. 2021. https://withdrawal.theinnercompass.org/ (accessed 22 November 2022).

3. National Institute for Health and Care Excellence (NICE). Depression in adults: treatment and management I Guidance I NICE. 2022; published online June. www.nice.org.uk/guidance/ng222 (accessed 16 July 2022).

4. Gupta S, Cahill JD, Miller R. Deprescribing antipsychotics: a guide for clinicians. *BJPsych Advances* 2018; 24: 295–302.

5. Moncrieff J, Gupta S, Horowitz MA. Barriers to stopping neuroleptic (antipsychotic) treatment in people with schizophrenia, psychosis or bipolar disorder. *Ther Adv Psychopharmacol* 2020; 10: 2045125320937910.

6. Bowers HM, Kendrick T, Glowacka M, et al. Supporting antidepressant discontinuation: the development and optimisation of a digital intervention for patients in UK primary care using a theory, evidence and person-based approach. *BMJ Open* 2020; 10: e032312.

7. Horowitz MA, Taylor D. Distinguishing relapse from antidepressant withdrawal: clinical practice and antidepressant discontinuation studies. *BJPsych Advances* 2022; 28: 297–311.

8. Stockmann T. What it was like to stop an antidepressant. *Ther Adv Psychopharmacol* 2019; 9: 2045125319884834.

9. Framer A. What I have learnt from helping thousands of people taper off psychotropic medications. *Ther Adv Psychopharmacol* 2021; 11: 204512532199127.

10. Cosci F, Chouinard G. Acute and persistent withdrawal syndromes following discontinuation of psychotropic medications. *Psychother Psychosom* 2020; 89: 283–306.

11. Moncrieff J, Read J, Horowitz M. Severity of antidepressant withdrawal effects versus symptoms of underlying conditions. (in preparation).

12. Horowitz M, Flanigan R, Cooper R, Moncrieff J. The determinants of outcome from antidepressant withdrawal in a large survey of patients. (in preparation).

13. Morant N, Long M, Jayacodi S, et al. The role of Facebook groups in the management and raising of awareness of antidepressant withdrawal: is social media filling the void left by health services? *Ther Adv Psychopharmacol* 2021; 11. 2045125320981174.

14. Morant N, Long M, Jayacodi S, et al. Experiences of reduction and discontinuation of antipsychotics: a qualitative investigation within the 'RADAR' trial (in press).

15. Horowitz MA, Taylor D. Tapering of SSRI treatment to mitigate withdrawal symptoms. *Lancet Psychiatry* 2019; 6: 538–46.

16. Horowitz MA, Taylor D. How to reduce and stop psychiatric medication. *Eur Neuropsychopharmacol* 2021; 55: 4–7.

17. Horowitz MA, Jauhar S, Natesan S, Murray RM, Taylor DM. A method for tapering antipsychotic treatment that may minimize the risk of relapse. *Schizophr Bull* 2021; 47: 1116–29.

18. Burn W, Horowitz M, Roycroft G, Taylor D. Stopping antidepressants. 2020. www.rcpsych.ac.uk/mental-health/treatments-and-wellbeing/stopping-antidepressants (accessed 22 April 2022).

19. Gupta S, Cahill JD. A prescription for 'deprescribing' in psychiatry. *Psychiatric Services* 2016; 67: 904–7.

20. Halli-Tierney AD, Scarbrough C, Carroll D. Polypharmacy: evaluating risks and deprescribing. *Am Fam Physician* 2019; 100: 32–8.

21. O'Mahony D, O'Sullivan D, Byrne S, O'Connor MN, Ryan C, Gallagher P. STOPP/START criteria for potentially inappropriate prescribing in older people: version 2. *Age Ageing* 2015; 44: 213–18.

Further topics

Troubleshooting

If withdrawal symptoms become intolerable at any point – and risk is manageable – it is worth repeating that the best approach is to either hold the current dose for longer to allow symptoms to resolve, or increase to the last dose at which the symptoms were tolerable, remaining there until they resolve (which can sometimes take much longer than expected – weeks or months in some cases).[1] Sometimes patients will need to increase their dose further in order to stabilise after severe withdrawal effects. After this stabilisation, further tapering will need to be performed more gradually with smaller reductions and/or longer periods between them. Patients, and clinicians, are often surprised at how long a tolerable taper can take – sometimes more than a year and in some cases over several years.[1] Some patients find they cannot reduce at a rate quicker than that equivalent to a reduction of 1 percentage point of receptor occupancy every 4 weeks (equivalent to approximately 5–10% dose reductions every 4 weeks), or sometimes by even smaller amounts. Most people through some trial and error can find a rate that is tolerable for them. If a patient experiences distressing withdrawal symptoms, this does not necessarily indicate that they cannot stop a psychiatric medication, but might mean that they need to taper more slowly. If complete cessation is too difficult, being on a smaller dose may be a worthwhile goal as patients will be exposed to less adverse effects.

It is not generally advisable to use other medications that can themselves cause physical dependence and withdrawal in order to manage withdrawal symptoms from psychiatric medications.[2] These medications include benzodiazepines, antidepressants, gabapentinoids, opioids and antipsychotics.[3,4] Use of these medications to manage withdrawal can lead to switching from one medication to another, rather than stopping the first medication. It is generally better to slow down a taper to produce tolerable withdrawal effects than substitute a different medication.

Psychological effects of psychiatric drug withdrawal

As mentioned, the withdrawal process per se can involve intense emotions, ranging from despair, to anger, anxiety, emotional lability, hypomania and suicidal thoughts, often unrelated or out of proportion to events or circumstances.[1,3,5] These can sometimes be familiar to the patient, and other times be quite novel, and can be distressing and confusing.[1] Like the physical symptoms of withdrawal, these can often come in intense waves.[1,6]

Sometimes withdrawal symptoms from psychiatric drugs can be difficult to distinguish from an underlying condition not just for the clinician but also for the patient.[1] The Royal College of Psychiatrists' guidance on 'Stopping Antidepressants' specifically cautions patients on this point, highlighting that 'Some withdrawal symptoms can feel like the symptoms you had before you started the antidepressant. The low mood and difficulty in sleeping of withdrawal can feel like the symptoms of depression.'[7] Although timing and associated physical symptoms can be helpful to discern this distinction the subjective similarity of symptoms to the original condition can be confusing for some.[1] Such symptoms have been designated rebound withdrawal symptoms, because they involve the effects of withdrawal causing previously present symptoms to be exaggerated.[8]

Many patients go through a phase of shock when they contemplate the effects of withdrawal on their lives, including worries about the impact on their financial, work and personal affairs, involving feelings of regret, self-blame and anger.[1,9] They may feel unhappy that they were not properly informed about the difficulties in stopping medication. Another common emotional symptom in withdrawal is the opposite of intense emotion: rather it is the complete absence of emotions, sometimes referred to as 'emotional anaesthesia', or as anhedonia, numbness, apathy or 'dysthymia' following drug withdrawal.[1,3,10,11] This effect, like other withdrawal effects, seems to fade over time but can take months or years in some patients.[3]

There are patient support groups, in person or online,[6,12] that might provide helpful support for patients going through this process. Techniques such as distraction, acceptance and re-orientation to recognising these symptoms as temporary products of the withdrawal process that resolve in time like other symptoms can all be helpful.[1] Some patients find that learning to manage and cope with withdrawal symptoms, also translates to being able to manage better the mental health conditions that first prompted medication prescriptions.[1]

Approach to withdrawal akathisia

As mentioned, one of the worst outcomes of psychiatric drug withdrawal, generally when it is too rapid, is akathisia.[13–16] Although this has been more often associated with an adverse effect of antipsychotic exposure it can be induced by withdrawal from antidepressants and benzodiazepines.[13–16] Gradual tapering is thought to minimise the risk of this event, but there have been no trials looking specifically at this topic. As people can be agitated and quite disordered in their behaviour (pacing, restless, grimacing, etc.) it is often mis-diagnosed as mania, psychosis or agitated depression,[15,17,18] and can sometimes lead to suicide.[19,20] Once a patient is in such a state it is very difficult to treat. This state can be prolonged in some patients.[17]

Although there has been little in the way of research on this topic, the most successful approach to this condition is, as for other withdrawal symptoms, a return to the dose of the medication being tapered at which the patient was last stable. If this approach is unsuccessful, then other agents may be required. The drugs most commonly reported to be useful are beta-blockers like propranolol, $5HT_{2A}$ receptor antagonists (e.g. mirtazapine, cyproheptadine), anti-histamines and benzodiazepines (e.g. clonazepam and diazepam).[17] However, patient groups who advocate for greater awareness of akathisia report that even these medications, including benzodiazepines, antidepressants and antipsychotics can all exacerbate akathisia in some people.[19] Consequently, a cautious approach to treatment is recommended. This should involve exposure to one medication at a time, followed by close observation to assess response, with cessation if unhelpful, before trialling additional medication.[17,19] Some patient advocacy groups suggest that the best management may be conservative – that is, not introducing further pharmacological agents – allowing symptoms to resolve over time with minimal intervention, although this can sometimes be difficult for patients to tolerate.[19] Movement is widely found to be helpful by patients, who often find that pacing somewhat lessens unpleasant sensations, with a (stationary) cycling intervention supported by a case study.[21]

Management of protracted withdrawal syndrome

Protracted withdrawal (sometimes called PAWS) occurs in an unknown proportion of patients after stopping psychiatric medications.[3,14,20,22] Its risk is thought to be minimised by gradual tapering.[23,24] Some patients may present for assistance in protracted withdrawal from previous rapid reductions. There is a dearth of research on the best management approach but two methods are suggested: conservative management or re-instatement of the original medication.

Limited research and clinical experience suggest people do recover spontaneously from protracted withdrawal without specific intervention, albeit over sometimes long periods. So, a conservative approach to management may be reasonable.[1,20] Patients often require reassurance that they will improve in time. They also need support, often including financial assistance, if such states are prolonged, as they can sometimes be debilitating.[1,14,20]

The second option is re-instatement of the original medication.[20] When re-instatement is performed shortly after cessation of a psychiatric drug, this almost universally leads to symptom resolution. However, when there is a longer delay in re-instatement after the onset of withdrawal effects (e.g. months or longer) the response is less certain. Re-instatement can still be successful. For example, in an analysis of patients with protracted withdrawal syndromes from antidepressants, it was found that re-instatement of the original drug was the most common approach trialled and was successful in about half of people who attempted it, even when it was initiated months or years after the drug had been stopped.[20]

However, there is great variation in response to re-instatement in people with protracted withdrawal syndromes. Some of these patients report improvement in their symptoms soon after re-instatement. Some report initial worsening of their symptoms, followed by improvement. Some report no discernible change and some patients report paradoxical worsening.[1] These responses have not been systematically studied and there is a poor understanding of the relevant factors. Paradoxical worsening is most well-recognised in re-instatement of benzodiazepines long after cessation.[1] These paradoxical responses have been linked to a process called kindling, involving sensitisation to the ceased medication, which is analogous to the kindling effect recognised in repeated cycles of exposure to and cessation of several psychoactive substances, especially alcohol.[1,25,26]

Given this uncertainty one suggested approach to mitigate the possibility of negative outcomes whilst trialling re-instatement is to re-instate a very small dose of the original medication (as small as 5% of usual doses).[1] This provides a test dose to monitor response, and can be successful in some cases of long-standing protracted withdrawal.[1,20] If this test dose has positive effects, a further increase in dose may be cautiously trialled;[1] if a negative response is produced the drug may be stopped.

Initiation of other medications is of mixed utility for most patients with this condition, perhaps because of increased sensitivity to psychoactive substances in this state (see subsequent section).[1,20] Response to the initiation of novel psychiatric medications is somewhat unpredictable with some reported cases of improvement, as well as deterioration, but in the absence of clear factors allowing prediction of response.[1,20] Caution is recommended in the trial of any novel psychotropic medication in this population.

Sensitivity to other substances during withdrawal

Patients can become highly sensitive to neurologically active substances in the process of withdrawal, thought to be related to an increased sensitivity to stimuli secondary to the de-stabilisation produced by the drug withdrawal process,[1,27,28] though the mechanism is not fully understood. People can respond to a wide variety of substances with activation or other paradoxical effects, including alcohol, neurologically active antibiotics,[29] caffeine, St John's Wort, and sometimes even to specific foods, supplements and herbs,[1,30] in addition to sensitivities to light and sound, more generally recognised.[3] Exposure to these substances can exacerbate withdrawal symptoms, and in this case it can be useful to restrict exposure during the discontinuation process depending on the clinical circumstances.[1] These sensitivities can resolve or improve when the patient recovers from the withdrawal process.[1]

References

1. Framer A. What I have learnt from helping thousands of people taper off psychotropic medications. *Ther Adv Psychopharmacol* 2021; 11: 204512532199127.
2. National Institute for Health and Care Excellence (NICE). Depression in adults: treatment and management I Guidance I NICE. 2022; published online June. www.nice.org.uk/guidance/ng222 (accessed 16 July 2022).
3. Cosci F, Chouinard G. Acute and persistent withdrawal syndromes following discontinuation of psychotropic medications. *Psychother Psychosom* 2020; 89: 283–306.
4. Lerner A, Klein M. Dependence, withdrawal and rebound of CNS drugs: an update and regulatory considerations for new drugs development. *Brain Commun* 2019; 1: fcz025.
5. Fava GA, Gatti A, Belaise C, Guidi J, Offidani E. Withdrawal symptoms after selective serotonin reuptake inhibitor discontinuation: A systematic review. *Psychother Psychosom* 2015; 84: 72–81.
6. White E, Read J, Julo S. The role of Facebook groups in the management and raising of awareness of antidepressant withdrawal: is social media filling the void left by health services? *Ther Adv Psychopharmacol* 2021; 11: 2045125320981174.
7. Burn W, Horowitz M, Roycroft G, Taylor D. Stopping antidepressants. 2020. www.rcpsych.ac.uk/mental-health/treatments-and-wellbeing/stopping-antidepressants (accessed 22 April 2022).
8. Chouinard G, Chouinard VA. New classification of selective serotonin reuptake inhibitor withdrawal. *Psychother Psychosom* 2015; 84: 63–71.
9. National Institute for Health and Care Excellence (NICE). Medicines associated with dependence or withdrawal symptoms: safe prescribing and withdrawal management for adults I Guidance I NICE. www.nice.org.uk/guidance/ng215/chapter/Recommendations (accessed 27 June 2022).
10. El-Mallakh RS, Briscoe B. Studies of long-term use of antidepressants: how should the data from them be interpreted? *CNS Drugs* 2012; 26: 97–109.
11. Renoir T, Pang TY, Lanfumey L. Drug withdrawal-induced depression: serotonergic and plasticity changes in animal models. *Neurosci Biobehav Rev* 2012; 36: 696–726.
12. Outro Library. https://learn.outro.com/home (accessed July 5, 2023).
13. Hirose S. Restlessness related to SSRI withdrawal. *Psychiatry Clin Neurosci* 2001; 55: 79–80.
14. Guy A, Brown M, Lewis S, Horowitz MA. The 'patient voice' – patients who experience antidepressant withdrawal symptoms are often dismissed, or mis-diagnosed with relapse, or onset of a new medical condition. *Ther Adv Psychopharmacol* 2020; 10: 2045125320967183.
15. Narayan V, Haddad PM. Antidepressant discontinuation manic states: a critical review of the literature and suggested diagnostic criteria. *J Psychopharmacol* 2010; 25: 306–13.
16. Sathananthan GL, Gershon S. Imipramine withdrawal: an akathisia-like syndrome. *Am J Psychiatry* 1973; 130: 1286–7.
17. Tachere RO, Modirrousta M. Beyond anxiety and agitation: a clinical approach to akathisia. *Aust Fam Physician* 2017; 46: 296–8.
18. Lohr JB, Eidt CA, Abdulrazzaq Alfaraj A, Soliman MA. The clinical challenges of akathisia. *CNS Spectr* 2015; 20 Suppl 1: 1–14; quiz 15–6.
19. Akathisia Alliance for education and research. Akathisia Alliance for education and research. https://akathisiaalliance.org/about-akathisia/ (accessed 17 September 2022).

20. Hengartner MP, Schulthess L, Sorensen A, Framer A. Protracted withdrawal syndrome after stopping antidepressants: a descriptive quantitative analysis of consumer narratives from a large internet forum. *Ther Adv Psychopharmacol* 2020; 10: 2045125320980573.

21. Taubert M, Back I. The akathisic cyclist – An unusual symptomatic treatment. 2007. https://orca.cardiff.ac.uk/id/eprint/117286/ (accessed 24 September 2022).

22. Davies J, Read J. A systematic review into the incidence, severity and duration of antidepressant withdrawal effects: are guidelines evidence-based? *Addict Behav* 2019; 97: 111–21.

23. Moncrieff J, Read J, Horowitz M. Severity of antidepressant withdrawal effects versus symptoms of underlying conditions. (in preparation).

24. Horowitz M, Flanigan R, Cooper R, Moncrieff J. The determinants of outcome from antidepressant withdrawal in a large survey of patients. (in preparation).

25. Becker HC. Kindling in alcohol withdrawal. *Alcohol Health Res World* 1998; 22: 25–33.

26. Flemenbaum A. Postsynaptic supersensitivity and kindling: further evidence of similarities. *Am J Drug Alcohol Abuse* 1978; 5: 247–54.

27. Otis HG, King JH. Unanticipated psychotropic medication reactions. *J Ment Health Couns* 2006; 28: 218–40.

28. Smith SW, Hauben M, Aronson JK. Paradoxical and bidirectional drug effects. *Drug Saf* 2012; 35: 173–89.

29. Bangert MK, Hasbun R. Neurological and psychiatric adverse effects of antimicrobials. *CNS Drugs* 2019; 33: 727–53.

30. Parker G. Psychotropic drug intolerance. *J Nerv Ment Dis* 2018; 206: 223–5.

Safe Deprescribing of Antidepressants

When and Why to Stop Antidepressants

Antidepressants are used by approximately 1 in every 6 people in western countries, and prescription rates continues to rise year on year,[1-3] while rates of depression and anxiety have remained fairly constant.[4] For example, in England 1 in 10 of the adult population takes an antidepressant in any given month,[5] with approximately 40% of use exceeding 2 years and 24% exceeding 3 years.[5] In the USA, the mean duration of use of antidepressants is more than 5 years.[2,3] There is also relatively greater prescribing for various groups in the UK: women, people in socioeconomically disadvantaged areas of the country and older people.[5]

Surveys of long-term antidepressant users in the UK, Holland and Australia have found that 30–50% of users have no evidence-based indication to continue them and so might consider stopping treatment.[6-8] A portion of antidepressant use thus extends beyond that which is thought to be helpful,[6,8,9] potentially exposing patients to needless harms and causing significant avoidable costs for the healthcare system. In the UK, it is estimated that around £40 million is wasted on unnecessary treatment each year.[10]

The increase in use of antidepressants has been thought to occur largely because people are using these medications for longer.[11] There is concern that one reason for this continued use is because of the difficulties people have in stopping them,[12] and that these difficulties, which may relate to withdrawal symptoms, are being mis-diagnosed as relapse of an underlying condition or, in some cases, onset of a new physical or mental health condition.[13,14] The debate around the short-term efficacy of antidepressants has continued, with general consensus that the benefits of medication are small compared with placebo (which itself shows a substantial effect) for most patients,[15-17] with larger short-term benefits for a small minority.[18] There is also debate over the extent of their ability to prevent relapse.[19,20]

Many but not all patients who are on antidepressants for longer than guidelines suggest may be able to stop their medications without increasing their chance of relapse.[21-23] Even those patients who are on antidepressants for a duration consistent with guidelines may wish to attempt stopping their antidepressant because their situation has changed,

The Maudsley® Deprescribing Guidelines: Antidepressants, Benzodiazepines, Gabapentinoids and Z-drugs, First Edition. Mark Horowitz and David Taylor.
© 2024 John Wiley & Sons Ltd. Published 2024 by John Wiley & Sons Ltd.

the adverse effects outweigh the benefits, their condition has improved or they have changed their preference about treatment.[24] Another valid reason for considering stopping is that the antidepressant was not effective in the first place. Commentators have been concerned that an important proportion of people remain on antidepressants in the absence of any benefit.[4,6,7,25,26]

At the time of writing, there is more attention being paid to discontinuing long-term antidepressants in the UK, with new NICE guidelines[24,27] and guidance from the Royal College of Psychiatrists (RCPsych)[28] on this topic, although many other countries have not updated their guidance in 2023.[29] NICE recommends regular review of ongoing antidepressant prescriptions at least every 6 months,[27] especially if there are adverse effects, the patient becomes pregnant or is planning pregnancy.[24] These reviews should involve mood monitoring, side effect review, reviewing perpetuating factors (and efforts made to help rectify these issues) and exploring the patient's preferences.[27]

Deprescribing antidepressants which are no longer needed safely should be a component of high-quality prescribing practice. Some of the considerations regarding reasons to stop antidepressants, who should contemplate stopping antidepressants, and when to do so are outlined. There are several reasons why stopping antidepressants may be a reasonable clinical decision, explored below:

- no ongoing benefit derived from medication,
- completion of treatment course,
- uncertainty about the extent of the relapse prevention properties of antidepressants,
- patient preference,
- preference for alternative treatments, and
- adverse effects, tolerability and quality of life.

No ongoing benefit derived from medication

Some patients do not derive benefit from antidepressants. Based on response rates after several weeks of treatment, a Cochrane review derived a number needed to treat (NNT) for SSRIs of seven (i.e. if seven people receive antidepressants one extra person will respond over those given placebo).[30] An analysis of individual patient data has found that 15% of patients will experience a substantial improvement in their depression score from antidepressants at 8 weeks.[18] These analyses suggest a large proportion of patients will not derive significant benefit from the acute use of antidepressants. Despite these rather poor acute response rates many patients continue treatment for months or years. Part of the reason for this is that prescribers are willing to wait for 4 weeks or more to see the emergence of response. Another part is that partial improvement is sometimes considered a success worth persisting with. Notably, in one large-scale RCT, almost half (44%) of patients with multiple episodes of depression on long-term treatment (>2 years) who stopped antidepressants (quite rapidly – over 4–8 weeks) were able to do so without experiencing a relapse.[22]

Additionally, some patients who did derive initial benefit from antidepressants will have had their circumstances change or their condition improved and will therefore no longer need medication. Lastly, some patients who benefited from antidepressants will experience a return of depression owing to tolerance effects[31] (called 'poop out' in America), a phenomenon linked to medications that cause withdrawal effects[32] although this idea has been considered somewhat controversial with regards antidepressants.

Completion of treatment course

Antidepressants are recommended in the treatment of a number of different mental health conditions, with many guidelines recommending minimum periods of treatment, as well as periods when treatment could be ceased (Table 2.1). The basis for these recommendations is that trials generally show higher relapse rates when antidepressants are stopped than when they are continued at these time points.

Table 2.1 Longer-term use or relapse prevention advice in official guidelines.

Condition	USA	UK
Major depressive disorder	'Patients who have been treated successfully with antidepressant medications should continue the medication for 4–9 months' (APA)[33] 'Consider maintenance treatment for higher risk patients' (APA)[33]	'Usually taken for at least 6 months (and for some time after symptoms remit)' (NICE)[27] 'Discuss with people that continuation of treatment (antidepressants or psychological therapies) after full or partial remission may reduce their risk of relapse and may help them stay well. (NICE)[27]
Generalised anxiety disorder	'The recommended duration of treatment can vary but may be as short as 3–6 months, or up to 1–2 years or even longer.'[34]	'If the drug is effective, advise the person to continue taking it for at least a year as the likelihood of relapse is high' (NICE)[35] 'Review the effectiveness and side effects of the drugs every 2 to 4 weeks during the first 3 months of treatment and every 3 months thereafter' (NICE)[35] 'Continue drug treatment for up to 18 months in patients who have responded' (BAP)[36]
Panic disorder	'Pharmacotherapy should generally be continued for 1 year or more after acute response to promote further symptom reduction and decrease risk of recurrence. (APA)[37]	'If the person is showing improvement on treatment with an antidepressant, the medication should be continued for at least 6 months after the optimal dose is reached, after which the dose can be tapered' (NICE)[35] 'Continue drug treatment for at least 6 months in patients who have responded' (BAP)[36]
Social anxiety disorder	'The recommended duration of treatment can vary but may be as short as 3–6 months, or up to 1–2 years or even longer.'[34]	'If the person's symptoms of social anxiety disorder have responded well to a pharmacological intervention in the first 3 months, continue it for at least a further 6 months' (NICE)[38] 'Continue drug treatment for at least 6 months in patients who have responded' (BAP)[36]

(Continued)

Table 2.1 (*Continued*)

Condition	USA	UK
Post-traumatic stress disorder	'Patients who respond favorably will generally need to continue taking medication in order to maintain clinical gains' (APA)[39]	'Consider venlafaxine or a selective serotonin reuptake inhibitor (SSRI), such as sertraline, for adults with a diagnosis of PTSD if the person has a preference for drug treatment. Review this treatment regularly' (NICE, 2018)[40]
		'Continue drug treatment for at least 12 months in patients who have responded to treatment' (BAP)[36]
Obsessive compulsive disorder	'Successful medication treatment should be continued for 1–2 years before considering a gradual taper by decrements of 10–25% every 1–2 months while observing for symptom return or exacerbation' (APA)[41]	'When an adult with OCD... has taken an SSRI for 12 months after remission (symptoms are not clinically significant and the person is fully functioning for at least 12 weeks), healthcare professionals should review with the patient the need for continued treatment' (NICE)[42]
		'Continue drug treatment for at least 12 months in patients who have responded to treatment (BAP)'[36]

APA = American Psychiatric Association, BAP = British Association of Psychopharmacology, NICE = National Institute for Health and Care Excellence

As previously described, surveys of long-term antidepressant users have found that 30–50% of users have no evidence-based indication to continue treatment.[6–8] Guidelines for antidepressant use in depression in the UK and US generally recommend that patients with an episode of depression should use antidepressants for several months (Table 2.1). The Canadian Network for Mood and Anxiety Treatments (CANMAT) guidelines recommend treatment for 6 to 9 months after remission.[43] For anxiety disorders, there is more variation in guidelines with suggestions of several months of treatment, or up to 1–2 years (Table 2.1).'[25]

Guidelines generally reserve longer term use of antidepressants for relapse prevention for people with severe or recurrent depressive disorders, who are at higher risk of relapse.[27,33] These guidelines also identify people with partial response, ongoing stressors and unhelpful coping styles as candidates for ongoing treatment.[27] Similarly, the APA suggests that maintenance treatment is reserved for this higher risk group, recommending maintenance treatment for people with 3 or more prior major depressive episodes or for those with chronic disorders.[33] The CANMAT guidelines identify that there is limited research for the recommendations to extend treatment to 2 years or beyond.[43]

The NICE guidelines on depression also highlight the risks of ongoing treatment – particularly, increased bleeding risks, long-term effects on sexual function, and difficulty stopping antidepressants – recognising that even in people at high risk for relapse there might be 'good reason to reduce it (such as side effects)'.[27] The importance of taking patient preference into account in these decisions is emphasised.[27] NICE suggests that group CBT or mindfulness-based CBT may be a substitute for those 'who do not wish to continue on antidepressants'.[27] The APA also highlights that maintenance cognitive therapy delivered over 2 years was as effective as maintenance medication for recurrent major depressive disorder.[33]

Uncertainty about the extent of the relapse prevention properties of antidepressants

There are limitations to the evidence underlying these recommendations for long-term continuation of antidepressants for relapse prevention.[20,44] The advice on duration of maintenance treatment with antidepressants is based upon antidepressant discontinuation studies. In discontinuation studies patients who have responded to antidepressants are randomised to either continue or to stop antidepressant treatment and relapse measured using depression symptom scales over the following period.[21,27,44]

An influential study by Geddes and colleagues in 2003 forms the core of evidence relating to duration of treatment. In this meta-analysis of 37 discontinuation studies, the most common method for stopping antidepressants was to do so abruptly, and the mean period for tapering was 5 days.[44] We now know that this method of stopping medication is likely to produce withdrawal symptoms for some patients, including some with severe symptoms (see further sections). These withdrawal symptoms will register on the symptom scales employed to detect relapse (e.g. the MADRS or HAM-D) as many withdrawal symptoms overlap with the domains measured.[19,20,44] As a result, the rate of relapse in the discontinuation group will be artificially elevated, indirectly exaggerating the relapse prevention properties of continued antidepressants.[44]

A 2021 study (the ANTLER study) attempted to mitigate these issues by tapering patients off antidepressants over 8 weeks but neglected to distinguish withdrawal symptoms from relapse symptoms and so suffers from some of the same limitations as previous studies.[22,45,46] Given this confounding, the true extent of the relapse prevention properties of antidepressants is difficult to establish. Even so, in this study almost half (44%) of patients with recurrent depression on long-term antidepressants were able to stop antidepressants without relapsing.[22] Some authors have argued that the vast majority of relapses in discontinuation trials are probably due to withdrawal effects because these relapses are seen soon after stopping.[20,47]

Gradual tapering may lower the chance of relapse on stopping. Recently it has been found that discontinuing antidepressants (when compared to continuation of antidepressants) only increases the chance of relapse when it is conducted rapidly (over less than 8 weeks).[48] In studies where tapering is conducted over a longer period of time (up to 6 months) there was no increased risk of relapse compared to continuation of antidepressants (risk difference = –6%, 95% CI: –13% to 1%, $I^2 = 0$, p = 0.08, three trials) – that is, a non-significant lower risk of relapse with discontinuation.[48] Further, a recent individual patient meta-analysis found that there was no significant difference in time to relapse in people who were either given preventative cognitive therapy or mindfulness-based cognitive therapy during or after antidepressant tapering compared with continuing on their antidepressant treatment (four RCTs, hazard ratio 0.86, 95% CI: 0.60 – 1.23).[23]

This suggests that if antidepressants are tapered more gradually than the methods used in most discontinuation trials that there might be little or no excess relapse compared with continuation of antidepressants. The risk may also be minimised by providing mindfulness-based cognitive therapy or preventative cognitive therapy. Almost certainly, the advice in guidelines based on discontinuation studies might over-estimate the relapse prevention properties of antidepressants.[44]

Patient preference

Patients may express a number of reasons for preferring to stop antidepressants. In the UK the NICE guidelines highlight this as an important factor to consider when evaluating continuing versus discontinuing antidepressants, especially in the context of alternative options.[27] Guidelines from the APA also emphasise the importance of patient choice: 'the psychiatrist should identify the patient's wishes for treatment and collaborate with the patient in choosing among effective treatments'(p.23).[33]

In a survey in England, patients reported the following reasons for wanting to stop antidepressants (more than one answer was permissible):[49]

- a desire to see whether they can live without the medication (52%);
- concerns about the long-term effect on their health (37%);
- feeling better (17%);
- a perceived lack of efficacy (10%);
- side effects (14%);
- concern over being reliant/dependent or feeling 'addicted' to their antidepressant (48%); and
- wanting to stop antidepressants before becoming pregnant (10%).

Preference for alternative treatments

Arguably, there has been widespread acceptance of the idea amongst the general population that antidepressants are necessary to reverse a 'chemical imbalance' (the colloquial term for the hypothesis that depression is caused by low serotonin levels or serotonin activity) in depressed people.[50,51] Despite ongoing interest in the area, there is now general consensus that a simple relationship between low serotonin and depression is unsupported by evidence.[52-55] Consequently, patients should not be told that antidepressants 'correct a chemical imbalance' especially as it is known that patients who believe this are reluctant to stop medication even when it is no longer indicated.[55,56]

There are a number of other treatments that are effective in depression as outlined in the recent NICE update to the depression guidelines,[27] reflecting other guidance around the world, which patients may wish to explore. For 'less severe depression' (the name now given to mild depression and subthreshold symptoms) the following were found to be as effective (and cost-effective) as antidepressants in the short term (with likely lesser adverse effects):

- guided self-help;
- individual and group cognitive behavioural therapy;

- individual and group behavioural activation;
- group exercise;
- group mindfulness and meditation;
- interpersonal or short-term psychodynamic psychotherapy; and
- counselling.

These guidelines specifically recommend that patients are not offered antidepressants as a first-line treatment for less severe depression, unless they have a stated preference.

For 'more severe depression' (the name now used for moderate and severe depression) the following are as effective (and cost-effective) as antidepressants (with likely fewer adverse effects) according to NICE:

- individual cognitive behavioural therapy,
- individual behavioural activation,
- individual problem solving,
- counselling,
- interpersonal or short-term psychodynamic psychotherapy,
- guided self-help, and
- group exercise.

In particular, group CBT and mindfulness-based cognitive therapy are supported for relapse prevention as alternatives to antidepressants.[27] The APA guidelines for depression also recommend that a number of non-pharmacological treatments are effective including cognitive behavioural therapy, interpersonal psychotherapy, psychodynamic therapy and problem-solving therapy for individuals and in groups.[33] The CANMAT guidelines point out that 'the magnitude of benefit for psychological treatment appears to increase with increasing severity, although there is evidence that psychological treatments are beneficial even for subthreshold depressive symptoms.'[57]

References

1. NHS Digital. Prescriptions dispensed in the community – statistics for England, 2007–2017. 2018. https://digital.nhs.uk/data-and-information/publications/statistical/prescriptions-dispensed-in-the-community/prescriptions-dispensed-in-the-community-england---2007---2017 (accessed 15 January 2023).

2. Pratt LA, Brody DJ, Gu Q. Antidepressant use among persons aged 12 and over: United States, 2011–2014. *NCHS Data Brief* 2017; 283: 1–8.

3. Mojtabai R, Olfson M. National trends in long-term use of antidepressant medications: results from the US National Health and Nutrition Examination Survey. *J Clin Psychiatry* 2014; 75: 169–77.

4. Kendrick T. Strategies to reduce use of antidepressants. *Br J Clin Pharmacol* 2021; 87: 23–33.

5. Public Health England. Dependence and withdrawal associated with some prescribed medicines. An evidence review. 2019. https://www.gov.uk/government/publications/prescribed-medicines-review-report (accessed 25 May 2021).

6. Ambresin G, Palmer V, Densley K, Dowrick C, Gilchrist G, Gunn JM. What factors influence long-term antidepressant use in primary care? Findings from the Australian diamond cohort study. *J Affect Disord* 2015; 176: 125–32.

7. Eveleigh R, Grutters J, Muskens E, et al. Cost-utility analysis of a treatment advice to discontinue inappropriate long-term antidepressant use in primary care. *Fam Pract* 2014; 31: 578–84.

8. Cruickshank G, MacGillivray S, Bruce D, Mather A, Matthews K, Williams B. Cross-sectional survey of patients in receipt of long-term repeat prescriptions for antidepressant drugs in primary care. *Ment Health Fam Med* 2008; 5: 105–9.

9. Piek E, van der Meer K, Hoogendijk WJG, Penninx BWJH, Nolen WA. Most antidepressant use in primary care is justified; results of the Netherlands study of depression and anxiety. *PLoS One* 2011; 6: 1–8.

10. Davies J, Cooper RE, Moncrieff J, Montagu L, Rae T, Parhi M. The costs incurred by the NHS in England due to the unnecessary prescribing of dependency-forming medications. *Addict Behav* 2021; 107143.

11. Moore M, Yuen H, Dunn N, Mullee MA, Maskell J, Kendrick T. Explaining the rise in antidepressant prescribing: A descriptive study using the general practice research database. *BMJ* 2009; 339: 956.

12. Healy D, Aldred G. Antidepressant drug use and the risk of suicide. *Int Rev Psychiatry* 2005; 17: 163–72.

13. Guy A, Brown M, Lewis S, Horowitz MA. The 'patient voice' – patients who experience antidepressant withdrawal symptoms are often dismissed, or mis-diagnosed with relapse, or onset of a new medical condition. *Ther Adv Psychopharmacol* 2020; 10: 204512532096718.

14. Davies J, Read J. A systematic review into the incidence, severity and duration of antidepressant withdrawal effects: Are guidelines evidence-based? *Addict Behav* 2019; 97: 111–21.

15. Munkholm K, Paludan-Müller AS, Boesen K. Considering the methodological limitations in the evidence base of antidepressants for depression: a reanalysis of a network meta-analysis. *BMJ Open* 2019; 9: e024886.

16. Cipriani A, Furukawa TA, Salanti G, et al. Comparative efficacy and acceptability of 21 antidepressant drugs for the acute treatment of adults with major depressive disorder: a systematic review and network meta-analysis. *Lancet* 2018; 391: 1357–66.

17. Horowitz M, Taylor D. How do we determine whether antidepressants are useful or not? *The Lancet Psychiatry* 2019; 6: 888.

18. Stone MB, Yaseen ZS, Miller BJ, Richardville K, Kalaria SN, Kirsch I. Response to acute monotherapy for major depressive disorder in randomized, placebo controlled trials submitted to the US Food and Drug Administration: individual participant data analysis. *BMJ* 2022; 378: e067606.

19. Hengartner MP. How effective are antidepressants for depression over the long term? A critical review of relapse prevention trials and the issue of withdrawal confounding. *Ther Adv Psychopharmacol* 2020; 10: 2045125320921694.

20. Hengartner MP, Plöderl M. Prophylactic effects or withdrawal reactions? An analysis of time-to-event data from antidepressant relapse prevention trials submitted to the FDA. *Ther Adv Psychopharmacol* 2021; 11: 20451253211032052.

21. Geddes JR, Carney SM, Davies C, et al. Relapse prevention with antidepressant drug treatment in depressive disorders: A systematic review. *Lancet* 2003; 361: 653–61.

22. Lewis G, Marston L, Duffy L, et al. Maintenance or discontinuation of antidepressants in primary care. *N Engl J Med* 2021; 385: 1257–67.

23. Breedvelt JJF, Warren FC, Segal Z, Kuyken W, Bockting CL. Continuation of antidepressants vs sequential psychological Interventions to prevent relapse in depression: An individual participant data meta-analysis. *JAMA Psychiatry* 2021; 78: 868–75.

24. National Institute for Clinical Excellence. Medicines associated with dependence or withdrawal symptoms: Safe prescribing and withdrawal management for adults | Guidance | NICE. 2022. https://www.nice.org.uk/guidance/ng215/chapter/Recommendations (accessed 27 June 2022).

25. Wallis KA, Donald M, Moncrieff J. Antidepressant prescribing in general practice: A call to action. *Aust J Gen Pract* 2021; 50: 954–6.

26. Byng R. Should we, can we, halt the rise in prescribing for pain and distress? *Br J Gen Pract* 2020; 70: 432–3.

27. National Institute of Health and Social Care (NICE). Depression in adults: Treatment and management | Guidance | NICE. 2022; published online June. https://www.nice.org.uk/guidance/ng222 (accessed 16 July 2022).

28. Burn W, Horowitz M, Roycroft G, Taylor D. Stopping antidepressants. Stopping Antidepressants 2020. https://www.rcpsych.ac.uk/mental-health/treatments-and-wellbeing/stopping-antidepressants (accessed 15 January 2023).

29. Sørensen A, Juhl Jørgensen K, Munkholm K. Clinical practice guideline recommendations on tapering and discontinuing antidepressants for depression: a systematic review. *Ther Adv Psychopharmacol* 2022; 12: 2045125321067656.

30. Arroll B, Elley CR, Fishman T, et al. Antidepressants versus placebo for depression in primary care. *Cochrane Database Syst Rev* 2009; CD007954.

31. Kinrys G, Gold AK, Pisano VD, et al. Tachyphylaxis in major depressive disorder: A review of the current state of research. *J Affect Disord* 2019; 245: 488–97.

32. Fava GA, Offidani E. The mechanisms of tolerance in antidepressant action. *Prog Neuropsychopharmacol Biol Psychiatry* 2011; 35: 1593–602.

33. American Psychiatric Association. Practice guideline for the treatment of patients with major depressive disorder. 2010.

34. Garakani A, Murrough JW, Freire RC, et al. Pharmacotherapy of anxiety disorders: Current and emerging treatment pptions. *Focus* 2021; 19: 222–42.

35. NICE. Generalised anxiety disorder and panic disorder in adults: Management. *NICE Clinical Guideline CG113* 2011. https://www.nice.org.uk/guidance/cg113/chapter/2-Research-recommendations#the-effectiveness-of-physical-activity-compared-with-waiting-list-control-for-the-treatment-of-gad (accessed 15 January 2023).

36. Baldwin DS, Anderson IM, Nutt DJ, et al. Evidence-based pharmacological treatment of anxiety disorders, post-traumatic stress disorder and obsessive compulsive disorder: A revision of the 2005 guidelines from the British Association for Psychopharmacology. *J Psychopharmacol* 2014; 28: 403–39.

37. American Psychiatric Association. Practice Guideline for the Treatment of Patients With Panic Disorder. 2009. https://psychiatryonline.org/pb/assets/raw/sitewide/practice_guidelines/guidelines/panicdisorder.pdf (accessed 23 January 2023).

38. Recommendations | Social anxiety disorder: Recognition, assessment and treatment | Guidance | NICE. 2013. https://www.nice.org.uk/guidance/cg159/chapter/Recommendations (accessed 21 January 2023).

39. American Psychiatric Association. Practice guideline for the treatment of patients with Acute Stress Disorder and Post-traumatic Stress Disorder. 2004. https://psychiatryonline.org/pb/assets/raw/sitewide/practice_guidelines/guidelines/acutestressdisorderptsd.pdf (accessed 15 January 2023).

40. National Institute for Health and Social Care. Post-traumatic stress disorder guideline. 2018. https://www.nice.org.uk/guidance/ng116/chapter/Recommendations (accessed January 21, 2023).

41. American Psychiatric Association. Practice guideline for the treatment of patients with obsessive-compulsive disorder. 2007. https://psychiatryonline.org/pb/assets/raw/sitewide/practice_guidelines/guidelines/ocd.pdf (accessed 15 January 2023).

42. Recommendations | Obsessive compulsive disorder and body dysmorphic disorder: treatment | Guidance | NICE. 2005. https://www.nice.org.uk/guidance/cg31/chapter/Recommendations (accessed 21 January 2023).

43. Kennedy SH, Lam RW, McIntyre RS, et al. Canadian Network for Mood and Anxiety Treatments (CANMAT) 2016 clinical guidelines for the management of adults with major depressive disorder: Section 3. Pharmacological treatments. *Can J Psychiatry* 2016; 61: 540–60.

44. Horowitz MA, Taylor D. Distinguishing relapse from antidepressant withdrawal: Clinical practice and antidepressant discontinuation studies. *BJPsych Advances* 2022; 28: 297–311.

45. Horowitz, MA Moncrieff, J. Antidepressant discontinuation trial misleading as it likely mis-interprets withdrawal effects as relapse. *British Medical Journal* 2021; published online 14 December. https://www.bmj.com/content/374/bmj.n2403/rr-4 (accessed 19 December 2021).

46. Liang C-S, Tseng P-T, Chen M-H. Maintenance or discontinuation of antidepressants in primary care. *N Engl J Med* 2021. https://www.nejm.org/doi/full/10.1056/NEJMoa2106356#article_citing_articles (accessed 15 January 2023).

47. Moncrieff J, Jakobsen JC, Bachmann M. Later is not necessarily better: Limitations of survival analysis in studies of long-term drug treatment of psychiatric conditions. *BMJ Evid Based Med* 2022; 27: 246–50.

48. Gøtzsche PC, Demasi M. Interventions to help patients withdraw from depression drugs: A systematic review. *Int J Risk Saf Med*. 2023 September 13. doi: 10.3233/JRS-230011. Epub ahead of print.

49. Horowitz M, Moncrieff J. Experience of using and stopping antidepressants in patients enrolled in a public therapy program. (In preparation).

50. Pilkington PD, Reavley NJ, Jorm AF. The Australian public's beliefs about the causes of depression: Associated factors and changes over 16 years. *J Affect Disord* 2013; 150: 356–62.

51. France CM, Lysaker PH, Robinson RP. The 'chemical imbalance' explanation for depression: Origins, lay endorsement and clinical implications. *Prof Psychol Res Pr* 2007; 38: 411–20.

52. Healy D. Serotonin and depression. *BMJ: British Medical Journal* 2015; 350: h1771.

53. Lacasse JR, Leo J. Serotonin and depression: A disconnect between the advertisements and the scientific literature. *PLoS Med* 2005; 2: 1211–6.

54. Moncrieff J, Cooper RE, Stockmann T, Amendola S, Hengartner MP, Horowitz MA. The serotonin theory of depression: A systematic umbrella review of the evidence. *Mol Psychiatry* 2022; published online 20 July. doi:10.1038/s41380-022-01661 0.

55. Kendrick T, Collinson S. Antidepressants and the serotonin hypothesis of depression. *BMJ* 2022; 378: o1993.

56. Eveleigh R, Speckens A, van Weel C, Oude Voshaar R, Lucassen P. Patients' attitudes to discontinuing not-indicated long-term antidepressant use: barriers and facilitators. *Ther Adv Psychopharmacol* 2019; 9: 204512531987234.

57. Parikh SV, Quilty LC, Ravitz P, et al. Canadian Network for Mood and Anxiety Treatments (CANMAT) 2016 Clinical guidelines for the management of adults with major depressive disorder: Section 2. Psychological treatments. *Can J Psychiatry* 2016; 61: 524–39.

Adverse effects of antidepressants

The adverse (or side) effects of antidepressants include numerous physical and psychological symptoms and for some patients the burden of these effects may exceed the benefit of medication. One naturalistic study looking at adverse effects in 1,000 patients with a median duration of antidepressant use of one year found that two-thirds reported at least one side effect, with a third having three or more, and with risk of side effects increasing with each year of use (Table 2.2).[1]

Table 2.2 Adverse effects of antidepressants reported by 1,000 patients in primary- or secondary-care settings. These self-attributed adverse effects need to be viewed with some caution, especially in the absence of a placebo group to allow 'placebo-adjusted' figures to be derived.

Type of antidepressant	SSRIs (%)	TCA (%)	Venlafaxine (%)	Mirtazapine (%)
Type of adverse effect ascribed to medication				
Sleeplessness	7	5	10	5
Sleepiness during the day	21	14	20	30
Restlessness	9	6	10	12
Muscle spasms, twitching	9	12	15	7
Dry mouth	22	49	23	22
Profuse sweating	20	20	32	14
Sexual dysfunction	23	20	31	10
Nausea	10	4	9	5
Constipation	8	20	10	2
Diarrhoea	7	4	5	5
Weight gain	19	22	17	29
Dizziness	12	11	19	12

Emotional numbing and related effects

In surveys of a convenience sample of people who were on antidepressants for a longer period (most for more than three years), and who may not be representative of all antidepressant users, rates of adverse effects were even higher:

- emotional numbness (71%),
- feeling foggy or detached (70%),
- feeling not like myself (66%),
- drowsiness (63%), and
- reduction in positive feelings (60%).[2]

Emotional blunting seems to be a common, and dose-dependent, consequence of antidepressant use.[3,4] Although this effect has sometimes been attributed to the underlying condition a double-blind placebo-controlled study in healthy volunteers found clear evidence of emotional blunting in the patients administered an SSRI for three weeks.[5] One survey found about 46% of patients on antidepressants reported emotional blunting.[6,7] Some patients report that emotional blunting (which indicates that both positive and negative emotions are blunted) can have detrimental effects on their well-being and relationships.[3] Some observers have suggested that use of antidepressants might undermine a person's autonomy and resilience, increasing their dependence on medical help.[8]

Weight gain

Long-term use of antidepressants may cause a greater degree of weight gain than that suggested in short-term trials. In one case-control observational study with almost 2 million patient years of follow-up, with patients taking SSRIs, SNRIs and other commonly used antidepressants such as mirtazapine and tricyclics there was a 30% increased risk of people of normal weight becoming overweight or obese in 10 years of follow-up, compared to people not taking antidepressants.[9] There was also a 30% increased chance of overweight people taking antidepressants becoming obese in 10 years compared with overweight people not taking antidepressants.[9] It is possible that residual confounding might contribute to these associations. The effects were most marked for mirtazapine (50% increased risk of greater than 5% weight gain).[9]

Cognitive effects

Meta-analysis has also found that some antidepressants produce cognitive impairment in healthy controls, on tests of information processing, memory, hand–eye co-ordination, concentration, as well as higher order functions.[10] There was variation between different antidepressants with SSRIs producing between 1% and 16% impairments (where proportions referred to the number of test points where impairment was found), while venlafaxine produced 9% impairment, mirtazapine produced 35% impairment, and older tricyclics producing between 19% and 47% impairment (highest for amitriptyline).[10] These studies are useful in that they exclude confounding by an underlying disorder by studying the effects of antidepressants in healthy controls. Small studies find that MMSE scores (a crude measure of cognition that detects coarse changes in cognitive ability) decreased over consecutive weeks of follow-up in people with OCD given antidepressants.[11] The long-term consequences of these cognitive impairments have not been investigated or quantified.

Risks in older people

For older people adverse effects can be more overt. A retrospective cohort study of over 61,000 patients found the following absolute increased risks over 1 year of exposure to SSRIs compared with not being on an antidepressant (adjusted for comorbidities and a range of potential confounding variables):

- 2.2% for falls,
- 0.38% for stroke/TIA,

- 0.1% for upper gastrointestinal bleeding,
- 0.98% for fractures, and
- 0.15% for hyponatraemia.[12]

Absolute risk over 1 year for all-cause mortality was 7.04% for patients not taking antidepressants, 8.12% for those taking TCAs, 10.61% for SSRIs and 11.43% for other antidepressants.[12] This observational research is susceptible to confounding by indication, and residual confounding, so differences in characteristics between patients prescribed different antidepressants could account for some of the associations between them and the adverse outcomes.[12]

Most antidepressants have been associated with hyponatraemia, likely due to the syndrome of inappropriate secretion of antidiuretic hormone (SIADH), generally with onset within 30 days of starting treatment.[13] Risk of hospitalisation with hyponatraemia is elevated from 1 in 1,600 in the general population to 1 in 300 for those starting an antidepressant,[14] and is associated with increased mortality (at any severity).[15]

Cardiovascular risks

There exist no long-term placebo-controlled trials of antidepressants in order to assess their long-term health effects, so observational studies comparing people on and not on antidepressants are the only source of evidence we have for determining long-term health risks, with the issues of confounding such studies entail. One study found that people on SSRIs had an increased hazard ratio of 1.34 at 10 years for risk of cardiovascular diseases, a hazard ratio of 1.73 for mortality due to cardiovascular disease and a hazard ratio of 1.73 for all-cause mortality, and that the effects were dose-dependent.[16] Other antidepressants increased the risk of coronary heart disease by a hazard ratio of 1.99, cardiovascular disease in general of 1.99 and all-cause mortality of 2.20, with some evidence of a dose–response relationship.[16] Although a wide range of confounders were adjusted for, residual confounding cannot be ruled out, especially as baseline depression scores were not available.

Potential increase in risk of dementia

There is also evidence that antidepressants may increase risk of dementia. A large nested case-control study of 225,000 people found a dose–response relationship between total exposure to antidepressants and risk of diagnosis with dementia.[17] Those patients with the highest exposure to antidepressants – more than 3 years of daily use of standard doses – had a 34% increased chance of dementia over those patients not exposed at all to antidepressants. Another nested case-control study of 40,000 people found similar results, with antidepressants with the strongest anticholinergic properties (amitriptyline, dosulepin and paroxetine) producing a 10% increased risk of dementia.[18] Other antidepressants (largely SSRIs), with lesser or no anticholinergic effects were also associated with dementia but associations were greater for prescriptions closer to dementia incidence suggesting reverse causation as a possible explanation.[18] Although efforts were taken in these studies to control for confounding variables, there is the possibility that residual confounding may explain some of these associations.

Bleeding risks

SSRIs and SNRIs inhibit the uptake of serotonin into platelets. Serotonin plays a role in the response to vascular injury, promoting vasoconstriction and morphological changes in platelets leading to aggregation.[19] Depletion of platelet serotonin leads to a reduced ability to form clots and therefore an increase in the risk of bleeding. The relative risk of any bleeding event on an SSRI/SNRI compared with no use is 1.4, with the absolute risk being between 0.5% and 6% (depending on a variety of factors, including length of treatment).[20] SSRIs also increase gastric acid secretion and may therefore increase the risk of peptic ulcer.[21]

A population-based study found that SSRIs increase the rate of upper gastrointestinal bleeds (UGIB) with a hazard ratio of 1.97, and low gastrointestinal bleeds (LGIB) with a hazard ratio of 2.96, after adjusting for all relevant risk factors.[22] A meta-analysis of 22 studies concluded that current users of SSRIs are 55% more at risk of UGIB compared with those who do not take SSRIs.[23] The absolute risk of an UGIB while on long-term SSRIs is 2% and of an LGIB it is 1%.[22,24]

Risk of intracranial haemorrhage is increased in people on SSRIs – with an absolute annual risk of 0.42% in older patients.[25] The prevalence of menstrual disorder (unusual or excessive bleeding, irregular menstruation, menorrhagia, etc.) is doubled in women on antidepressants compared with women not taking antidepressants (24.6% vs 12.2%).[26] In addition, the absolute risk of post-partum haemorrhage was 18% for women using SSRIs, compared to 8.7% for women not using antidepressants.[27] The MHRA in the UK issued a warning regarding the use of SSRIs and post-partum blood loss in 2021.[28] Use of SSRIs in the pre-operative period is associated with a 20% increase in inpatient mortality (absolute risk 1 in 1,000).[29] In coronary artery bypass graft (CABG) procedures, there is a 50% increase risk of mortality in users of serotonergic antidepressants compared with non-users.[30]

Withdrawal effects

Withdrawal effects from antidepressants occur commonly and can be severe in some people.[31] The likelihood and severity seem to increase with longer term use.[32] This may be a sufficient reason on its own to limit the duration of antidepressant use. Withdrawal symptoms are discussed in detail in subsequent sections.

Withdrawal effects increase in both likelihood and severity with longer term use, probably because the brain and body adapt to a greater degree after longer exposure.[32] For example, in survey data, after 3 months of use, about 25% of patients reported withdrawal effects on stopping, with about 20% of patients reporting moderately severe or severe withdrawal effects. After 3 years of use, more than 60% of patients reported withdrawal effects on stopping, with about 50% of patients reporting moderately severe or severe withdrawal effects.[32] This may factor in to the decision to stop antidepressants sooner rather than later, in order to avoid more severe withdrawal effects.

Sexual effects

Sexual adverse effects can include a lack of desire as well as reduced sexual sensation, and failure to orgasm in both genders,[33] and occur in 25% to 80% of patients.[34] It is now recognised that these sexual effects can persist even after cessation of antidepressants in a minority of patients. This is called post-SSRI sexual dysfunction (PSSD), and was recently recognised by the European Medicines Agency.[35,36] Sexual side effects can negatively affect a person's self-esteem, quality of life and relationships.

Tardive dysphoria

Concerns have been raised that long-term use of antidepressants can itself induce dysphoria.[37,38] This has been thought related to the process of tolerance to these medications, involving serotonin receptor desensitisation, which can 'overshoot' leading to opposite effects to those originally produced by the medications.[37] This has been seen as analogous to opioid-induced hyperalgesia[39] and the increase in anxiety seen in long-term use of benzodiazepines.[40] For example, one observational study found that depressed people who used antidepressants long-term had poorer long-term outcomes compared with non-users or those who used them short-term, even after controlling for baseline depressive severity.[41]

References

1. Bet PM, Hugtenburg JG, Penninx BWJH, Hoogendijk WJG. Side effects of antidepressants during long-term use in a naturalistic setting. *Eur Neuropsychopharmacol* 2013; 23: 1443–51.
2. Read J, Williams J. Adverse effects of antidepressants reported by a large international cohort: Emotional blunting, suicidality, and withdrawal effects. *Curr Drug Saf* 2018; 13: 176–86.
3. Sansone RA, Sansone LA. SSRI-induced indifference. *Psychiatry* 2010; 7: 14–8.
4. Ma H, Cai M, Wang H. Emotional blunting in patients with major depressive disorder: a brief non-systematic review of current research. *Front Psychiatry* 2021; 12: 792960.
5. Langley C, Armand S, Luo Q, et al. Chronic escitalopram in healthy volunteers has specific effects on reinforcement sensitivity: a double-blind, placebo-controlled semi-randomised study. *Neuropsychopharmacology* 2023; published online 23 January. doi:10.1038/s41386-022-01523-x.
6. Goodwin GM, Price J, De Bodinat C, Laredo J. Emotional blunting with antidepressant treatments: a survey among depressed patients. *J Affect Disord* 2017; 221: 31–5.
7. Goldsmith L, Moncrieff J. The psychoactive effects of antidepressants and their association with suicidality. *Curr Drug Saf* 2011; 6: 115–21.
8. Kendrick T. Strategies to reduce use of antidepressants. *Br J Clin Pharmacol* 2021; 87: 23–33.
9. Gafoor R, Booth HP, Gulliford MC. Antidepressant utilisation and incidence of weight gain during 10 years' follow-up: population based cohort study. *BMJ* 2018; 361: k1951.
10. Hindmarch I. Cognitive toxicity of pharmacotherapeutic agents used in social anxiety disorder. *Int J Clin Pract* 2009; 63: 1085–94.
11. Sayyah M, Eslami K, AlaiShehni S, Kouti L. Cognitive function before and during treatment with selective serotonin reuptake inhibitors in patients with depression or obsessive-compulsive disorder. *Psychiatry J* 2016; 2016: 5480391.
12. Coupland C, Dhiman P, Morriss R, Arthur A, Barton G, Hippisley-Cox J. Antidepressant use and risk of adverse outcomes in older people: population-based cohort study. *BMJ* 2011; 343: d4551.
13. Egger C, Muehlbacher M, Nickel M, Geretsegger C, Stuppaeck C. A review on hyponatremia associated with SSRIs, reboxetine and venlafaxine. *Int J Psychiatry Clin Pract* 2006; 10: 17–26.
14. Gandhi S, Shariff SZ, Al-Jaishi A, et al. Second-generation antidepressants and hyponatremia risk: a population-based cohort study of older adults. *Am J Kidney Dis* 2017; 69: 87–96.
15. Selmer C, Madsen JC, Torp-Pedersen C, Gislason GH, Faber J. Hyponatremia, all-cause mortality, and risk of cancer diagnoses in the primary care setting: a large population study. *Eur J Intern Med* 2016; 36: 36–43.
16. Bansal N, Hudda M, Payne RA, Smith DJ, Kessler D, Wiles N. Antidepressant use and risk of adverse outcomes: population-based cohort study. *BJPsych Open* 2022; 8: e164.
17. Coupland CAC, Hill T, Dening T, Morriss R, Moore M, Hippisley-Cox J. Anticholinergic drug exposure and the risk of dementia: a nested case-control study. *JAMA Intern Med* 2019; 179: 1084–93.
18. Richardson K, Fox C, Maidment I, et al. Anticholinergic drugs and risk of dementia: case-control study. *BMJ* 2018; 361: k1315.
19. Skop BP, Brown TM. Potential vascular and bleeding complications of treatment with selective serotonin reuptake inhibitors. *Psychosomatics* 1996; 37: 12–6.
20. Laporte S, Chapelle C, Caillet P, et al. Bleeding risk under selective serotonin reuptake inhibitor (SSRI) antidepressants: a meta-analysis of observational studies. *Pharmacol Res* 2017; 118: 19–32.
21. Dall M, Schaffalitzky de Muckadell OB, Lassen AT, Hallas J. There is an association between selective serotonin reuptake inhibitor use and uncomplicated peptic ulcers: a population-based case-control study. *Aliment Pharmacol Ther* 2010; 32: 1383–91.

22. Cheng Y-L, Hu H-Y, Lin X-H, et al. Use of SSRI, but not SNRI, increased upper and lower gastrointestinal bleeding: a nationwide population-based cohort study in Taiwan. *Medicine* 2015; 94: e2022.

23. Jiang H-Y, Chen H-Z, Hu X-J, et al. Use of selective serotonin reuptake inhibitors and risk of upper gastrointestinal bleeding: a systematic review and meta-analysis. *Clin Gastroenterol Hepatol* 2015; 13: 42-50.e3.

24. Taylor D. *The Maudsley Prescribing Guidelines in Psychiatry*, 14th edn. Hoboken, NJ: Wiley-Blackwell, 2021, doi:10.1002/9781119870203.

25. Smoller JW, Allison M, Cochrane BB, et al. Antidepressant use and risk of incident cardiovascular morbidity and mortality among postmeno-pausal women in the Women's Health Initiative study. *Arch Intern Med* 2009; 169: 2128–39.

26. Uguz F, Sahingoz M, Kose SA, et al. Antidepressants and menstruation disorders in women: a cross-sectional study in three centers. *Gen Hosp Psychiatry* 2012; 34: 529–33.

27. Lindqvist PG, Nasiell J, Gustafsson LL, Nordstrom L. Selective serotonin reuptake inhibitor use during pregnancy increases the risk of post-partum hemorrhage and anemia: a hospital-based cohort study. *J Thromb Haemost* 2014; 12: 1986–92.

28. SSRI/SNRI antidepressant medicines: small increased risk of postpartum haemorrhage when used in the month before delivery. Gov.uk. 2021; published online 7 January https://www.gov.uk/drug-safety-update/ssri-slash-snri-antidepressant-medicines-small-increased-risk-of-postpartum-haemorrhage-when-used-in-the-month-before-delivery (accessed 21 January 2023).

29. Auerbach AD, Vittinghoff E, Maselli J, Pekow PS, Young JQ, Lindenauer PK. Perioperative use of selective serotonin reuptake inhibitors and risks for adverse outcomes of surgery. *JAMA Intern Med* 2013; 173: 1075–81.

30. Singh I, Achuthan S, Chakrabarti A, Rajagopalan S, Srinivasan A, Hota D. Influence of pre-operative use of serotonergic antidepressants (SADs) on the risk of bleeding in patients undergoing different surgical interventions: A meta-analysis. *Pharmacoepidemiol Drug Saf* 2015; 24: 237–45.

31. Davies J, Read J. A systematic review into the incidence, severity and duration of antidepressant withdrawal effects: are guidelines evidence-based? *Addict Behav* 2019; 97: 111–21.

32. Horowitz MA, Framer A, Hengartner MP, Sørensen A, Taylor D. Estimating risk of antidepressant withdrawal from a review of published data. *CNS Drugs* 2022; published online 14 December. doi:10.1007/s40263-022-00960-y.

33. Rothmore J. Antidepressant-induced sexual dysfunction. *Med J Aust* 2020; 212: 329–34.

34. Serretti A, Chiesa A. Treatment-emergent sexual dysfunction related to antidepressants: A meta-analysis. *J Clin Psychopharmacol* 2009; 29: 259–66.

35. Reisman Y. Post-SSRI sexual dysfunction. *BMJ* 2020; 368. doi:10.1136/bmj.m754.

36. Bala A, Nguyen HMT, Hellstrom WJG. Post-SSRI sexual dysfunction: A literature review. *Sexual Medicine Reviews* 2018; 6: 29–34.

37. Fava GA. May antidepressant drugs worsen the conditions they are supposed to treat? The clinical foundations of the oppositional model of tolerance. *Ther Adv Psychopharmacol* 2020; 10: 2045125320970325.

38. El-Mallakh RS, Gao Y, Jeannie Roberts R. Tardive dysphoria: the role of long-term antidepressant use in-inducing chronic depression. *Med Hypotheses* 2011; 76: 769–73.

39. Lee M, Silverman SM, Hansen H, Patel VB, Manchikanti L. A comprehensive review of opioid-induced hyperalgesia. *Pain Physician* 2011; 14: 145–61.

40. Ashton H. Benzodiazepine withdrawal: Outcome in 50 patients. *Br J Addict* 1987; 82: 665–71.

41. Hengartner MP, Angst J, Rössler W. Antidepressant use prospectively relates to a poorer long-term outcome of depression: Results from a prospective community cohort study over 30 years. *Psychother Psychosom* 2018; 87: 181–3.

CHAPTER 2

Discussing deprescribing antidepressants with patients

The role of the clinician

Given uncertainties regarding the decision to attempt stopping antidepressants, a frank and open discussion regarding what is known about the potential benefits and harms of ongoing use of antidepressants is warranted. Sometimes patients may have considered stopping an antidepressant but often the expectation is that the issue will be raised by the doctor when it is appropriate.[1,2]

The 2022 NICE guidance on deprescribing recommends that people taking antidepressants should be offered regular reviews that address the ongoing need to take the medication including reviewing adverse effects, ongoing benefits and the patient's preference.[3] Clinicians should be prepared to have these discussions because in the absence of action by a clinician the outcome is likely to be continuation of possibly unnecessary antidepressant treatment for many patients.[4] It has been found that simply prompting patients to consider stopping no longer necessary antidepressants is insufficient by itself (with only 7% of patients doing so),[5] and therefore a more comprehensive discussion regarding stopping and greater support for the patient during the process is probably required.[4]

NICE guidance encourages shared decision making about withdrawing antidepressants, in the following circumstances:

- it is no longer benefiting the person,
- the condition for which the medicine was prescribed has resolved,
- the harms of the medicine outweigh the benefits,
- the person wants to stop taking the medication.

NICE guidance recommends outlining the benefits a patient can expect from reducing the antidepressant including the mitigation of adverse effects outlined previously, as well as potential future adverse effects.[3] Each person's circumstances and preferences should be explored. Some patients may not be aware of the full array of adverse effects that antidepressants can cause and may not attribute these to the antidepressant. Outlining the range of potential adverse effects and their incidence may help patients to identify long-term issues that may be connected to the antidepressant. Sometimes the patient information leaflet (PIL) included with medication can be a helpful prompt to explore adverse effects the patient might be experiencing.

Pre-existing conceptions about antidepressant action

When discussing deprescribing there may be pre-existing ideas that the patient holds that may need to be addressed.[6,7] The following are some beliefs that patients might hold which may mean that they are disinclined to stop antidepressants, despite not meeting guideline indications for further treatment:[8]

- Belief that they have a chemical imbalance (or a serotonin deficiency);
- Belief that they need an antidepressant for depression like a diabetic needs insulin;
- Belief that they have a life-long condition and therefore need life-long treatment.

These patients may need to be gently informed that although this messaging was once widely disseminated, that there is no current evidence of a serotonin deficiency, and no evidence that anyone requires a life-long antidepressant to address a biochemical deficiency.[4,7,9,10] Patients who perceive that the cause of their depression is a long-term brain condition or biochemical in origin are less likely to stop medication.[2] NICE guidelines anticipate that some patients will be upset by hearing information that differs from what they have been told by clinicians in the past – it recommends in this case that clinicians should explain that our understanding of the balance of risks and benefits of a medicine can change over time and that past prescribing was done in the person's best interests using the knowledge available at the time.[3]

Some patients may believe antidepressants are highly effective at preventing relapse – and may need to appreciate better the reasonably small protective effects (e.g. an NNT of six from the ANTLER trial[11] without considering withdrawal confounding of relapse), as well as the considerable uncertainty regarding even these effects.[12] Patients can be re-assured that many people can stop antidepressants and not relapse and there are means to mitigate the risk of relapse – for example, by tapering more slowly, by pausing or increasing the dose if required or introducing other support or psychological therapies. For some patients the only way to establish whether the antidepressant is genuinely helpful is to gradually remove the medication and then compare the period off antidepressants (not the withdrawal period) with the medicated state.

Previous experience of difficulty on stopping

Patients may have had unpleasant experiences in the past when stopping an antidepressant and believe that to be evidence that they need to stay on the medication.[8] As discussed later, a clinician should explore the possibility that these symptoms were not in fact their underlying condition returning but withdrawal symptoms from stopping their medication (often undertaken too quickly).[15] A careful history may be able to identify symptoms from their past experience that mark this as distinct from relapse – such as dizziness, electric shocks or other symptoms not present in their underlying condition, or perhaps rapid resolution of symptoms on re-instatement of their antidepressant (further information in later sections).[15]

Other benefits of stopping

Other reasons to stop medication may include the benefits of preventing further cascades of prescribing where tolerance or adverse effects leads to the need for other medications.[16] The possibility of 'tardive dysphoria' may be another reason to avoid long-term use.[16,17] Some patients may be better able to engage in therapy or other useful non-drug modalities in the absence of medication, as cognitive impairment and emotional blunting may make aspects of therapy more difficult to access.[18] Lastly, the fact that being on antidepressants for longer will make them harder to stop may be a reason to try stopping sooner rather than later so as to avoid a more severe withdrawal reaction.[19]

Ambivalence

Many people are ambivalent about continuing or discontinuing long-term antidepressants;[7,8] with the default position often being to continue taking the medication ('if it ain't broke why fix it?'). There is a variety of barriers to considering stopping antidepressants that may make people ambivalent about doing so (Table 2.3).[2] In one trial of cessation of antidepressants not indicated by guidelines, some participants only needed a little 'nudge' while others refused to discontinue their antidepressant.[8] Motivational interviewing skills might be helpful to draw out the advantages and disadvantages of a different course of action.[7]

Table 2.3 Barriers and facilitators for patients to stop antidepressants. Adapted from Maund et al. (2019).[2]

Domain	Barriers	Facilitators
Psychological capabilities and physiological effects	Difficult life circumstances	Confidence in ability to discontinue
	Aversive experience of discontinuation in past	Life circumstances stable
	Lack of effective coping strategies	Well-informed about approach to tapering
	Physical dependence on antidepressants	
Perceived cause of depression	Long-term (perhaps life-long) condition requiring long-term treatment	Life circumstances
	Biochemical cause (particularly serotonin deficiency)	
Fears	Fear of relapse	Fear of 'addiction', physical dependence
	Fear of withdrawal effects	Fear of adverse effects
Personal goals/ motivations	Self-identity as 'disabled'	Self-identity as 'healthy'
	Stopping as threat to stability	Desire to function without an antidepressant
	Benefit of continuing to others around them	Feeling better
	Cure is not possible, only management	Dislike having to take an antidepressant
Perception of antidepressants	Positive effect	Ineffectual
	Natural or benign	Unacceptable adverse/side effects
	Lack of concern over adverse/side effects	Unnatural
		Unhappy about long-term use
Information about the discontinuation process	Inadequate information about the discontinuation process, and risks and benefits of this	Information on how to safely discontinue and what to expect
Support network (friends, family, professionals)	Pressure to stay on medication	Support to come off medication

References

1. Leydon GM, Rodgers L, Kendrick T. A qualitative study of patient views on discontinuing long-term selective serotonin reuptake inhibitors. *Fam Pract* 2007; 24: 570–5.

2. Maund E, Dewar-Haggart R, Williams S, et al. Barriers and facilitators to discontinuing antidepressant use: a systematic review and thematic synthesis. *J Affect Disord* 2019; 245: 38–62.

3. National Institute for Health and Care Excellence (NICE). Medicines associated with dependence or withdrawal symptoms: safe prescribing and withdrawal management for adults | Guidance | NICE. 2022. https://www.nice.org.uk/guidance/ng215/chapter/Recommendations (accessed 27 June 2022).

4. Kendrick T. Strategies to reduce use of antidepressants. *Br J Clin Pharmacol* 2021; 87: 23–33.

5. Eveleigh R, Muskens E, Lucassen P, et al. Withdrawal of unnecessary antidepressant medication: a randomised controlled trial in primary care. *BJGP Open* 2018; 1: bjgpopen17X101265.

6. National Institute for Health and Care Excellence (NICE). Medicines associated with dependence or withdrawal symptoms: safe prescribing and withdrawal management for adults (Draft for consultation, October 2021). 2021.

7. Karter JM. Conversations with clients about antidepressant withdrawal and discontinuation. *Ther Adv Psychopharmacol* 2020; 10: 2045125320922738.

8. Eveleigh R, Speckens A, van Weel C, Oude Voshaar R, Lucassen P. Patients' attitudes to discontinuing not-indicated long-term antidepressant use: barriers and facilitators. *Ther Adv Psychopharmacol* 2019; 9: 204512531987234.

9. Lacasse JR, Leo J. Serotonin and depression: a disconnect between the advertisements and the scientific literature. *PLoS Med* 2005; 2: 1211–6.

10. Moncrieff J, Cooper RE, Stockmann T, Amendola S, Hengartner MP, Horowitz MA. The serotonin theory of depression: a systematic umbrella review of the evidence. *Mol Psychiatry* 2022; published online 20 July. doi:10.1038/s41380-022-01661-0.

11. Lewis G, Marston L, Duffy L, et al. Maintenance or discontinuation of antidepressants in primary care. *N Engl J Med* 2021; 385: 1257–67.

12. Hengartner MP. How effective are antidepressants for depression over the long term? A critical review of relapse prevention trials and the issue of withdrawal confounding. *Ther Adv Psychopharmacol* 2020; 10: 2045125320921694.

13. Gøtzsche PC, Demasi M. Interventions to help patients withdraw from depression drugs: A systematic review. *Int J Risk Saf Med.* 2023 September 13. doi: 10.3233/JRS-230011. Epub ahead of print.

14. Breedvelt JJF, Warren FC, Segal Z, Kuyken W, Bockting CL. Continuation of antidepressants vs sequential psychological interventions to prevent relapse in depression: an individual participant data meta-analysis. *JAMA Psychiatry* 2021; 78: 868–75.

15. Horowitz MA, Taylor D. Distinguishing relapse from antidepressant withdrawal: Clinical practice and antidepressant discontinuation studies. *BJPsych Advances* 2022; 28: 297–311.

16. Fava GA. May antidepressant drugs worsen the conditions they are supposed to treat? The clinical foundations of the oppositional model of tolerance. *Ther Adv Psychopharmacol* 2020; 10: 2045125320970325.

17. El-Mallakh RS, Gao Y, Briscoe BT, Roberts RJ. Antidepressant-induced tardive dysphoria. *Psychother Psychosom* 2011; 80: 57–9.

18. Sotsky M, Glass DR, Ph D, et al. Patient predictors of response to psychotherapy and pharmacotherapy: findings in the NIMH treatment of depression collaborative research program. *Am J Psychiatry* 1991; 148: 997–1008.

19. Horowitz MA, Framer A, Hengartner MP, Sørensen A, Taylor D. Estimating risk of antidepressant withdrawal from a review of published data. *CNS Drugs* 2022; published online 14 December. doi:10.1007/s40263-022-00960-y.

CHAPTER 2

CHAPTER 2

Withdrawal Effects from Antidepressants

Recent developments in the understanding of antidepressant withdrawal

There have been significant developments in the understanding of antidepressant withdrawal in recent years. Before this period, for many years guidelines reported that antidepressant discontinuation symptoms are 'mild and self-limiting', for example, by NICE[1] in the UK. In the USA, the depression guidelines from the APA, published in 2010, still suggest 'discontinuation-emergent symptoms … typically resolve without specific treatments over 1–2 weeks'.[2] The APA guidelines do identify that 'some patients do experience more protracted discontinuation syndromes, particularly those treated with paroxetine'.[2]

In a systematic analysis of worldwide clinical practice guidelines for depression withdrawal symptoms were mostly described as mild, brief and self-limiting, and severe in a minority of cases.[3] Estimates of the duration and incidence were included in only a quarter of guidelines and the values given were in all cases lower than those reported in systematic review.[3] This systematic analysis concluded that clinical practice guidelines from most countries provide scarce and inadequate information on antidepressant withdrawal symptoms and only limited guidance for distinguishing withdrawal symptoms from symptoms of relapse.[3]

In recent years there has been more widespread recognition in some countries that withdrawal symptoms from antidepressants are common, can be severe and may be long-lasting, over months or years.[1,4,5] RCPsych in the UK issued a position statement emphasising that 'There should be greater recognition of the potential in some people for severe and long-lasting withdrawal symptoms',[6] and a corresponding update to the NICE guidelines highlighted '[antidepressant withdrawal] symptoms lasting much longer (sometimes months or more) and being more severe for some patients'.[1]

There has been perhaps less obvious acknowledgement of this change in characterisation of withdrawal in other countries, including the USA.[7] There are some exceptions. The Therapeutics Initiative (TI) in Canada, which produces guidance on medications independent from drug company sponsorship, based at the University of British Columbia, points out that for antidepressants 'severe and prolonged withdrawal symptoms have been reported lasting weeks to months'.[8] The TI guidance also recognises that 'antidepressants should be added to the list of drugs associated with tolerance, dependence and a withdrawal syndrome' and that withdrawal symptoms occur in at least one-third of patients who stop.[4] TI also points out that patients must be informed of the possibility of withdrawal symptoms before starting an antidepressant, drawing a comparison to opioid treatment: 'the requirements for informed consent are analogous to recommendations before initiating long-term opioid therapy'.[8] RCPsych and NICE in the UK both recommend that providing information on withdrawal symptoms from stopping antidepressants should be a part of informed consent when an antidepressant is being considered.[6]

Patients often report that withdrawal symptoms from antidepressants are under-recognised, or minimised by clinicians,[9–11] probably as a result of official guidance minimising the frequency and severity of antidepressant withdrawal symptoms.[3] One consequence of this has been that many patients are forced to seek help outside the medical system from peer support websites[11] or social media sites, including private Facebook groups.[10]

Withdrawal symptoms can be somewhat different from those of depression and anxiety but there are important similarities.[12] Withdrawal should now be carefully considered by clinicians as an important differential diagnosis whenever antidepressant doses are reduced or missed – especially given that patients commonly report that their withdrawal symptoms from antidepressants are mis-diagnosed as relapse.[10,12] A quarter of clinical practice guidelines around the world highlight the risk of mis-diagnosing antidepressant withdrawal symptoms as a relapse of the underlying condition.[3] The TI underlines the risk of mis-diagnosing withdrawal symptoms as a return of a mental health condition by pointing out that on stopping antidepressants 'depressive symptoms or increased suicidality may represent withdrawal or re-emergence of the original condition'.[8] Patients report that the lack of understanding or recognition of withdrawal symptoms by clinicians compounds the problems that arise on stopping antidepressants and adds unnecessary distress.[9]

Physical dependence vs addiction

The term 'dependence' has recently come to be used interchangeably with 'addiction' (to mean uncontrolled drug-seeking behaviour). Inevitably this has led to some unfortunate confusion.[13] This choice of language was made in DSM-III-R because the term 'addiction' was thought to be pejorative while the word 'dependence' was thought more neutral.[13] However, the original usage of the word 'dependence' referred to 'physiological adaptation that occurs when medications acting on the central nervous system are ingested with rebound when the medication is abruptly discontinued'.[13] The National Institute on Drug Abuse (NIDA) in the USA states

'Dependence means that when a person stops using a drug, their body goes through "withdrawal": a group of physical and mental symptoms that can range from mild (if the drug is caffeine) to life-threatening ... Many people who take a prescription medicine every day over a long period of time can become dependent; when they go off the drug, they need to do it gradually, to avoid withdrawal discomfort. But people who are dependent on a drug or medicine are not necessarily addicted.'[14]

In addition, Goodman and Gilman's textbook of pharmacology points out 'The appearance of a withdrawal syndrome when administration of the drug is terminated is the only actual evidence of physical dependence.'[15]

All major classes of antidepressants SSRIs, SNRIs, monoamine oxidase inhibitors (MAOIs), tricyclic antidepressants (TCAs), noradrenaline and specific serotonergic antidepressants (NaSSAs)) can be associated with withdrawal symptoms on cessation or dose reduction. These symptoms occur in a substantial proportion of patients, most likely as a result of physical dependence (a normal neurobiological response to drugs that act on the central nervous system) in these patients.[13,16–20] Physical dependence on antidepressants arises because the body and brain undergo adaptations to the presence of a drug, countering its effect in order to maintain homeostasis.[13,21,22] The only evidence necessary for a state of physical dependence to be diagnosed is the appearance of withdrawal symptoms on reducing or stopping the drug.[15] It is also clear that the vast majority of antidepressants – with the possible exceptions of tranylcypromine and aminéptine – do not cause addiction, as they do not induce compulsion, craving and other symptoms of addiction.[23,24]

Some patients may be uninterested in academic distinctions between dependence and addiction and more interested in the reality that they cannot stop their antidepressants because of unpleasant withdrawal effects. They may therefore describe them colloquially as 'addictive',[25,26] though antidepressants do not fit the strict definition of this. Some patients may also not be happy being described as 'dependent' on antidepressants (which they may still associate with the concept of addiction), and in this case, it may be better to talk in terms of 'neuroadaptation' or 'adaptation'.

Withdrawal symptoms vs discontinuation symptoms

The term 'discontinuation symptom' was promoted by drug manufacturers to minimise patient concerns regarding their product and to prevent association with the idea of addiction.[27,28] There is now widespread recognition that this euphemism is misleading and that its use minimises the potential adverse consequences of stopping antidepressants.[28–30] The more pharmacologically accurate term is 'withdrawal symptoms', now adopted by RCPsych,[6,28] the British Medical Association[28] and NICE in the UK.[1,31] In Canada, the TI has updated its language as well: 'The effects of stopping any antidepressant should be more precisely termed "withdrawal syndrome" instead of "antidepressant discontinuation syndrome".'[8] There has been limited official acknowledgement of this in the USA.

References

1. Iacobucci G. NICE updates antidepressant guidelines to reflect severity and length of withdrawal symptoms. *BMJ* 2019; 367: l6103.

2. Gelenberg AJ, Freeman MP, Markowitz JC, et al. American Psychiatric Association Practice Guideline for the Treatment of Patients With Major Depressive Disorder, Third Edition. Am J Psychiatry. 2010;167(suppl):1–152.

3. Sørensen A, Jørgensen KJ, Munkholm K. Description of antidepressant withdrawal symptoms in clinical practice guidelines on depression: a systematic review. *J Affect Disord* 2022; published online 11 August. doi:10.1016/j.jad.2022.08.011.

4. Davies J, Read J. A systematic review into the incidence, severity and duration of antidepressant withdrawal effects: are guidelines evidence-based? *Addict Behav* 2019; 97: 111–21.

5. National Institute of Health and Social Care (NICE). Depression in adults: Treatment and management | Guidance | NICE. 2022; published online June. https://www.nice.org.uk/guidance/ng222 (accessed 16 July 2022).

6. Royal College of Psychiatrists. Position statement on antidepressants and depression. 2019. https://www.rcpsych.ac.uk/docs/default-source/improving-care/better-mh-policy/position-statements/ps04_19---antidepressants-and-depression.pdf?sfvrsn=ddea9473_5 (accessed 18 January 2023).

7. Mangin D. Breaking up can be hard to do: practical approaches to how and when to stop antidepressants in primary care. Therapeutics Initiative. 2022; published online 9 March. https://www.ti.ubc.ca/2022/03/09/mar-9-best-evidence-webinar-breaking-up-can-be-hard-to-do-practical-approaches-to-how-and-when-to-stop-antidepressants-in-primary-care/ (accessed 16 July 2022).

8. Therapeutics Initiative. Antidepressant withdrawal syndrome. 2018; published online June. https://www.ti.ubc.ca/2018/07/23/112-antidepressant-withdrawal-syndrome/#:~:text=Symptoms%20include%20anxiety%2C%20crying%2C%20dizziness,%2C%20imbalance%2C%20and%20sensory%20disturbances (accessed 4 July 2022).

9. Guy A, Brown M, Lewis S, Horowitz MA. The 'patient voice' – patients who experience antidepressant withdrawal symptoms are often dismissed, or mis-diagnosed with relapse, or onset of a new medical condition. *Ther Adv Psychopharmacol* 2020; 10: 204512532096718.

10. White E, Read J, Julo S. The role of Facebook groups in the management and raising of awareness of antidepressant withdrawal: is social media filling the void left by health services? *Ther Adv Psychopharmacol* 2021; 11: 2045125320981174.

11. Framer A. What I have learnt from helping thousands of people taper off psychotropic medications. *Ther Adv Psychopharmacol* 2021; 11: 204512532199127.

12. Horowitz MA, Taylor D. Distinguishing relapse from antidepressant withdrawal: clinical practice and antidepressant discontinuation studies. *BJPsych Advances* 2022; 28: 297–311.

13. O'Brien C. Addiction and dependence in DSM-V. *Addiction* 2011; 106: 866–7.

14. National Institute on Drug Abuse. Is there a difference between physical dependence and addiction? National Institute on Drug Abuse. https://nida.nih.gov/publications/principles-drug-addiction-treatment-research-based-guide-third-edition/frequently-asked-questions/there-difference-between-physical-dependence-addiction (accessed 31 May 2022).

15. Brunton LL, Chabner BA, Knollmann BC. *Goodman & Gilman's The Pharmacological Basis of Therapeutics*, 12edn. McGraw Hill Education, 2011.

16. Howland RH. Potential adverse effects of discontinuing psychotropic drugs: part 2: antidepressant drugs. *J Psychosoc Nurs Ment Health Serv* 2010; 48: 9–12.

17. Haddad PM, Anderson IM. Recognising and managing antidepressant discontinuation symptoms. *Advances in Psychiatric Treatment* 2007; 13: 447–57.

18. Public Health England. Dependence and withdrawal associated with some prescribed medicines. An evidence review. 2019. https://www.gov.uk/government/publications/prescribed-medicines-review-report (accessed 25 May 2021).

19. Taylor D, Stewart S, Connolly A. Antidepressant withdrawal symptoms–telephone calls to a national medication helpline. *J Affect Disord* 2006; 95: 129–33.

20. Lerner A, Klein M. Dependence, withdrawal and rebound of CNS drugs: an update and regulatory considerations for new drugs development. *Brain Commun* 2019; 1: fcz025.

21. Turton S, Lingford-Hughes A. Neurobiology and principles of addiction and tolerance. *Medicine* 2016; 44: 693–6.

22. Hyman SE, Nestler EJ. Initiation and adaptation: a paradigm for understanding psychotropic drug action. *Am J Psychiatry* 1996; 153: 151–62.

23. Haddad P. Do antidepressants have any potential to cause addiction? *J Psychopharmacol* 1999; 13: 300–7.

24. Jauhar S, Hayes J, Goodwin GM, Baldwin DS, Cowen PJ, Nutt DJ. Antidepressants, withdrawal, and addiction; where are we now? *J Psychopharmacol* 2019; 33: 655–9.

25. Read J, Williams J. Adverse effects of antidepressants reported by a large international cohort: emotional blunting, suicidality, and withdrawal effects. *Curr Drug Saf* 2018; 13: 176–86.

26. Burn W, Horowitz M, Roycroft G, Taylor D. Stopping antidepressants. 2020. https://www.rcpsych.ac.uk/mental-health/treatments-and-wellbeing/stopping-antidepressants (accessed 18 January 2023).

27. Nielsen M, Hansen EH, Gotzsche PC. What is the difference between dependence and withdrawal reactions? A comparison of benzodiazepines and selective serotonin re-uptake inhibitors. *Addiction* 2012; 107: 900–8.

28. Massabki I, Abi-Jaoude E. Selective serotonin reuptake inhibitor 'discontinuation syndrome' or withdrawal. *Br J Psychiatry* 2020; 1–4.

29. Lugg W. The case for discontinuation of the 'discontinuation syndrome'. *Aust N Z J Psychiatry* 2021 January; 56(1): 93–5. doi:10.1177/00048674211043443.

30. Fava GA, Gatti A, Belaise C, Guidi J, Offidani E. Withdrawal symptoms after selective serotonin reuptake inhibitor discontinuation: a systematic review. *Psychother Psychosom* 2015; 84: 72–81.

31. National Institute for Health and Care Excellence (NICE). Depression in adults: recognition and management (NICE Guideline 90). London: NICE., 2009 https://www.nice.org.uk/guidance/cg90.

Pathophysiology of antidepressant withdrawal symptoms

Drug discontinuation effects are effectively part of the pharmacology of any drug when the body eliminates that drug faster than adaptations to the presence of the drug can subside.[1] Following this idea, any evidence of persisting adaptation to a drug strongly suggests that withdrawal symptoms will occur when the drug is stopped.[1]

Homeostatic adaptation to antidepressants

The brain adapts to the presence of all classes of antidepressants, countering the effect of the drug in order to maintain homeostasis (Figure 2.1).[2-4] This process will lead to physical (or physiological) dependence.[5] Adaptation to the antidepressant may be associated with tolerance or loss of effect. In one longitudinal study it was observed that 25% of patients required increased dosages of antidepressant over time,[6] consistent with the development of tolerance. A systematic review found that rates of tachyphylaxis occurred in about 10% to 30% of patients with depression treated with antidepressants.[7]

During ongoing administration of antidepressants, as for other drugs acting on the central nervous system, neuroadaptation establishes a new homeostatic equilibrium, in which the system accommodates to alterations produced by the drug. When the medication is reduced or stopped, the homeostasis is perturbed, resulting in withdrawal symptoms.[1,3] Adaptations to the presence of the drug predict withdrawal effects because these adaptations often do not resolve instantaneously upon stopping the drugs but will persist for some period. The 'mis-match' between the level of drug action to which the body has been adapted to and the lesser amount of drug action it receives (upon dose reduction or cessation) gives rise to withdrawal effects.[1]

It is thought that antidepressants that increase synaptic serotonin, like SSRIs, and SNRIs lead to down-regulation of serotonergic receptors.[8] This is a homeostatic response to higher levels of synaptic serotonin arising as a consequence of serotonin transporter (SERT) antagonism, the primary target of many antidepressants.[8] The drugs may also affect pathways downstream of these receptors.[9]

PET binding studies demonstrate that short-term SSRI use reduces the sensitivity of cortical $5\text{-}HT_{2A}$ receptors[10] and down-regulates $5\text{-}HT_{1A}$ receptors[11] in depressed patients, and $5\text{-}HT_4$ receptors in healthy controls.[12] There is also evidence that $5\text{-}HT_{1A}$ down-regulation can persist for months and years after antidepressants are ceased.[11] In one neuroimaging study, patients who had been previously treated with antidepressants showed $5\text{-}HT_{1A}$ down-regulation in 38 out of 40 brain regions analysed, on average, 29 months after antidepressants were ceased (range 8–60 months).[13]

Animal studies have found a number of alterations to the serotonergic system that persist after SSRI cessation following weeks of treatment with antidepressants.[14] These brain changes are found in conjunction with behavioural withdrawal effects (e.g. increased acoustic startle reflex).[14] The following neurobiological changes have been detected in animals after stopping antidepressants: lowered serotonin and serotonin metabolites in the hippocampus and frontal cortex, reduced SERT binding, a reduction in the expression of SERT and $5\text{-}HT_{1B}$ receptors in the raphe nucleus, and reduced $5\text{-}HT_{2C}$ expression in the frontal cortex.[14] Animals also show reduced oxytocin

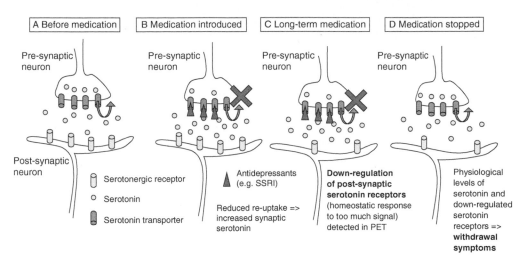

Figure 2.1 Neuro-adaptation to the presence of antidepressants and the effects on reduction or stopping antidepressants. A – serotonin is released from the pre-synaptic neuron into the synapse where it then activates serotonergic receptors on the post-synaptic neuron. The serotonin transporter undertakes reuptake of synaptic serotonin, producing an equilibrium level. B – introduction of an antidepressant blocks about 60–80% of serotonin transporter activity, causing less reuptake of serotonin into the pre-synaptic neuron. This leads to an increase in synaptic levels of serotonin, which increases the activation of the post-synaptic serotonergic receptors. C – due to homeostasis, the excess activation of post-synaptic serotonergic receptors leads to down-regulation of receptors, changes evident after short-term use of antidepressants on nuclear imaging,[10,12] which can persist for long periods.[13] D – when the antidepressant is removed (or reduced) after long-term use the serotonin transporter is unblocked and serotonin is now removed from the synapse and returns to physiological levels. The down-regulation of the post-synaptic receptors persists for some time after antidepressant cessation. The system registers the effect of physiological levels of serotonin on the down-regulated receptors as a diminished effect, likely related to antidepressant withdrawal symptoms. These symptoms will persist for as long as it take the serotonergic receptors to be up-regulated back to their 'pre-drug' configuration. Note: the serotonergic system is focused on primarily in this diagram but similar effects will apply to other neurotransmitter systems that are affected by antidepressants, or exist downstream of serotonergic effects.

response (to a 5-HT_{1A} receptor agonist), and reduced 5-HT_{1A} sensitivity after antidepressant cessation.[14] Notably, many of these changes persisted for up to 2 weeks in rodent models after antidepressants were stopped[14] (17 rat days being equivalent to a human year).[15]

In one study that measured changes for longer, 14 days of fluoxetine treatment in rats produced a reduced oxytocin response that was still present 60 days after drug cessation – four times longer than the period of treatment.[14,16] Using a widely cited means of drawing equivalencies between rat time and human time, 60 days is equivalent to approximately 3 human years, although this equivalence has not been specifically verified in regards to the duration of adaptations to antidepressant treatment.[15,16] This is consistent with the time period demonstrated in neuroimaging of patients who had previously used antidepressants. These observations suggest several ways in which the brain adapts to long-term use of antidepressants that persist after cessation and may give rise to withdrawal symptoms.

Homeostatic disruption on antidepressant discontinuation

When an antidepressant taken long-term is reduced in dose or stopped, the homeostatic equilibrium that had been established is perturbed. The difference between the 'expected' level of activity by the system and the actual 'input' by the drug is responsible for withdrawal symptoms as shown in Figure 2.2.[1-3] The duration of withdrawal symptoms is largely determined by the time required for adaptations to the drug to resolve.[1]

It is sometimes erroneously believed that withdrawal symptoms last for the time taken for the drug to be eliminated from the system. This misunderstanding sometimes leads clinicians to tell patients that they could not be experiencing long-lasting withdrawal symptoms because 'the drug is out of their system'. However, Figure 2.2 illustrates that while the onset of withdrawal symptoms is strongly determined by the elimination half-life of a drug (shorter half-life, quicker onset), the duration of withdrawal is determined by the plasticity of the system in returning to a 'pre-drug' homeostatic equilibrium (that is to become accustomed to the presence of less drug in the system).

An analogy might be made to the experience of walking out of a loud concert (more signal as with the increased synaptic serotonin during antidepressant treatment) into a quiet street (physiological levels of serotonin after drug removal), where sounds appear muted because of adaptation of tympanic sensitivity (as with serotonergic sensitivity) for a few minutes while your tympanic membrane re-accommodates to a different average amount of sound (an analogous delay for the serotonergic system to re-adapt to less signal, although it seems to take much longer than a few minutes). The time for the sound to dissipate (or for synaptic serotonin levels to normalise on removal of the drug) is trivial; it is the time taken for tympanic re-accommodation that determines the

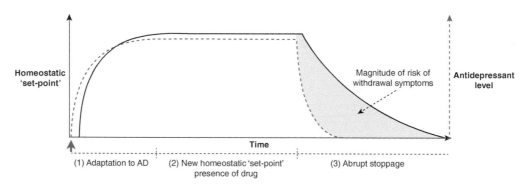

Figure 2.2 The neurobiology of antidepressant withdrawal. In this diagram, the homeostatic 'set-point' is shown in black and antidepressant drug levels are shown in purple dashed lines. (1) The system is at baseline. At the Solid purple arrow, an antidepressant is administered; drug plasma levels increase. Physiological adaptations of the system to the presence of the drug begin. (2) At the plateau, drug plasma levels (and target receptor activation) have reached a steady state with a new homeostatic set-point of the system established. (3) The antidepressant is abruptly ceased and plasma drug levels drop to zero (exponentially, according to the elimination half-life of the drug). This difference between the homeostatic set-point (the 'expectations' of the system) and the level of drug in the system (dashed purple line) is experienced as withdrawal symptoms. Hence, withdrawal symptoms may worsen or peak even long after the drug has been eliminated from the system. The shaded area under the curve, representing the difference between the homeostatic set-point and the level of the drug, indicates the degree of risk of withdrawal symptoms: the larger the area the greater the risk.

duration of the withdrawal effects (as for re-adaptation of the processes affected by long-term antidepressant use). Due to wide-ranging adaptations in the brain and body to antidepressants, withdrawal symptoms can manifest in both physical and psychological symptoms.[17,18]

It is also unlikely that withdrawal symptoms are mediated simply through serotonergic receptors, as there are many other downstream effects including adrenergic, dopaminergic, cholinergic, glutamatergic and other pathways, which may also adapt to long-term administration of antidepressants.[2,14,17,19,20] For example, rapid reversal of the inhibition of noradrenergic function in the locus coeruleus (caused by the inhibitory influence of increased serotonin levels during antidepressant treatment when antidepressants are stopped) may explain some symptoms of antidepressant withdrawal.[21] Paroxetine's anti-cholinergic effects may lead to cholinergic rebound on cessation, partly accounting for the severity of its withdrawal syndrome.[21] Withdrawal symptoms have also been attributed to increased glutamatergic neurotransmission on cessation,[22] as well as dopaminergic neurotransmission and effects on the hypothalamic-pituitary adrenal axis.[14,22]

Minor role for psychosomatic (or nocebo) effects

Some commentators have suggested that withdrawal symptoms may be a psychosomatic response rather than genuine physiological symptoms.[23] These authors have hypothesised that patients have negative expectations of the consequence of stopping their antidepressants, leading to nocebo withdrawal effects (the opposite of the placebo effect).[23] However, the presence of antidepressant withdrawal symptoms in both animals[14] and neonates of antidepressant-using mothers[24] suggests that the process is primarily physiological rather than psychosomatic. Randomised controlled trials conducted to detect withdrawal symptoms used double-blind placebo-controlled designs so that participants and researchers were unaware whether the participant was receiving a continuation of their antidepressant or identical placebo pills for several days.[25,26] This design minimises the role of psychological expectation or nocebo effects and therefore suggests that withdrawal effects are physiological consequences of stopping the medication.[25] It is also worth stating that patients would need to be aware of the range of effects possible in order for psychosomatic symptoms to arise in the same form as 'real' symptoms – who would guess that brain zaps are a symptom of withdrawal?

The rate of nocebo withdrawal effects has been explored in six double-blind randomised controlled trials in two ways: either by cessation of placebo or continuation of antidepressants unbeknownst to the patient. Excluding an outlier value, these studies yield a weighted average of nocebo withdrawal effects of 11.8%,[8,27] much less than the incidence of withdrawal when stopping antidepressants of 40–50% (see later sections).[28,29] A limitation to the analysis of nocebo effects is that the severity of withdrawal symptoms is not measured in these studies, and it is not clear that 'dizziness' or 'nausea' reported in the nocebo group is the same as such symptoms in the withdrawal group (there are case reports of such symptoms being severe enough to prompt investigation of stroke).[30] Furthermore, withdrawal effects from placebo do not show a relationship with duration of treatment, in the same way that withdrawal effects from

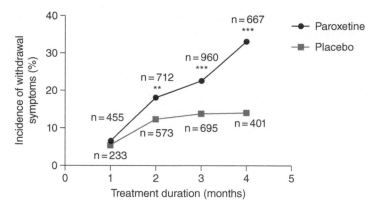

Figure 2.3 The relationship between duration of treatment and proportion of patients who experienced withdrawal effects on stopping either paroxetine or placebo (overall trend p-value <0.001).[33] Adapted from Horowitz et al. (2023)[10]

antidepressants do (Figure 2.3).[31] As with all health symptoms, there may be a psychological component to withdrawal effects but this is likely to be a minor contribution.[8,27]

Pathogenesis of specific withdrawal effects

As discussed, mechanisms of antidepressant withdrawal symptoms are thought to arise from a mis-match in expected inputs to the system and actual inputs from the drug, involving serotonergic, noradrenergic, glutamatergic and dopaminergic effects, as well as other systems such as the HPA axis.[8,9,14,22]

The hypothesised role of serotonin in coordinating sensory and autonomic function with motor activity has been proposed as a possible mechanism for the withdrawal syndrome.[32] In particular, a link has been hypothesised between dizziness, vertigo, nausea and lethargy, which resemble motion sickness, and dysmodulation of the raphe $5HT_{1A}$ receptors, known to be involved in this phenomenon.[33] Withdrawal-induced dysregulation of somatosensory functions may cause paraesthesia, while altered dopaminergic function may be responsible for the movement disorders (for example, dystonia) occasionally experienced in SSRI withdrawal.[34] The electric shock or 'zap' sensations of withdrawal have been attributed to serotonergic or noradrenergic effects, as they are also present in withdrawal from MDMA.[35,36] Analogies have been made to Lhermitte's sign, also an electric-shock like phenomenon, seen in multiple sclerosis and vitamin B12 deficiency and from iatrogenic causes, conceptualised as arising from demyelination of cervical spinal cord axons.[37,38]

That many antidepressant withdrawal symptoms appear to be autonomic suggests the homeostatic disturbance of withdrawal may extend to dysregulation of the autonomic nervous system.[39,40] Many antidepressants can affect heart rhythm, blood pressure, sleep and other autonomic functions (accounting for some of the adverse effects of antidepressants),[41,42] and removal of these effects may lead to disruption of this system. Further research is required to understand the pathogenesis of the wide variety of withdrawal symptoms experienced.

References

1. Reidenberg MM. Drug discontinuation effects are part of the pharmacology of a drug. *J Pharmacol Exp Ther* 2011; 339: 324–8.
2. Hyman SE, Nestler EJ. Initiation and adaptation: A paradigm for understanding psychotropic drug action. *Am J Psychiatry* 1996; 153: 151–62.
3. Turton S, Lingford-Hughes A. Neurobiology and principles of addiction and tolerance. *Medicine* 2016; 44: 693–6.
4. O'Brien C. Addiction and dependence in DSM-V. *Addiction* 2011; 106: 866–7.
5. Lerner A, Klein M. Dependence, withdrawal and rebound of CNS drugs: an update and regulatory considerations for new drugs development. *Brain Commun* 2019; 1: fcz025.
6. Solomon DA, Leon AC, Mueller TI, et al. Tachyphylaxis in unipolar major depressive disorder. *J Clin Psychiatry* 2005; 66: 283–90.
7. Kinrys G, Gold AK, Pisano VD, et al. Tachyphylaxis in major depressive disorder: A review of the current state of research. *J Affect Disord* 2019; 245: 488–97.
8. Horowitz MA, Framer A, Hengartner MP, Sørensen A, Taylor D. Estimating risk of antidepressant withdrawal from a review of published data. *CNS Drugs*. 2023;37: 143–157.
9. Jha MK, Rush AJ, Trivedi MH. When discontinuing SSRI antidepressants is a challenge: Management tips. *Am J Psychiatry* 2018; 175: 1176–84.
10. Meyer JH, Kapur S, Eisfeld B, et al. The effect of paroxetine on 5-HT$_{2A}$receptors in depression: An [^{18}F]setoperone PET imaging study. *Am J Psychiatry* 2001; 158: 78–85.
11. Gray NA, Milak MS, DeLorenzo C, et al. Antidepressant treatment reduces serotonin-1A autoreceptor binding in major depressive disorder. *Biol Psychiatry* 2013; 74: 26–31.
12. Haahr ME, Fisher PM, Jensen CG, et al. Central 5-HT4receptor binding as biomarker of serotonergic tonus in humans: A [11C]SB207145 PET study. *Mol Psychiatry* 2014; 19: 427–32.
13. Bhagwagar Z, Rabiner EA, Sargent PA, Grasby PM, Cowen PJ. Persistent reduction in brain serotonin1A receptor binding in recovered depressed men measured by positron emission tomography with [11C]WAY-100635. *Mol Psychiatry* 2004; 9: 386–92.
14. Renoir T. Selective serotonin reuptake inhibitor antidepressant treatment discontinuation syndrome: A review of the clinical evidence and the possible mechanisms involved. *Front Pharmacol* 2013; 4 April: 1–10.
15. Quinn R. Comparing rat's to human's age: How old is my rat in people years? *Nutrition* 2005; 21: 775–7.
16. Raap DK, Garcia F, Muma NA, Wolf WA, Battaglia G, van de Kar LD. Sustained desensitization of hypothalamic 5-Hydroxytryptamine1A receptors after discontinuation of fluoxetine: Inhibited neuroendocrine responses to 8-hydroxy-2-(Dipropylamino)Tetralin in the absence of changes in Gi/o/z proteins. *J Pharmacol Exp Ther* 1999; 288: 561–7.
17. Schatzberg AF, Haddad P, Kaplan EM, et al. Serotonin reuptake inhibitor discontinuation syndrome: A hypothetical definition. Discontinuation consensus panel. *J Clin Psychiatry* 1997; 58 Suppl 7: 5–10.
18. Haddad PM, Anderson IM. Recognising and managing antidepressant discontinuation symptoms. *Advances in Psychiatric Treatment* 2007; 13: 447–57.
19. Harvey BH, Slabbert FN. New insights on the antidepressant discontinuation syndrome. *Hum Psychopharmacol* 2014; 29: 503–16.
20. Warner CH, Bobo W, Warner C, Reid S, Rachal J. Antidepressant discontinuation syndrome. *Am Fam Physician* 2006; 74: 449–56.
21. Blier P, Tremblay P. Physiologic mechanisms underlying the antidepressant discontinuation syndrome. *J Clin Psychiatry* 2006; 67 Suppl 4: 8–13.
22. Harvey BH, McEwen BS, Stein DJ. Neurobiology of antidepressant withdrawal: implications for the longitudinal outcome of depression. *Biol Psychiatry* 2003; 54: 1105–17.
23. Jauhar S, Hayes J, Goodwin GM, Baldwin DS, Cowen PJ, Nutt DJ. Antidepressants, withdrawal, and addiction; where are we now? *J Psychopharmacol* 2019; 33: 655–9.
24. Levinson-Castiel R, Merlob P, Linder N, Sirota L, Klinger G. Neonatal abstinence syndrome after in utero exposure to selective serotonin reuptake inhibitors in term infants. *Arch Pediatr Adolesc Med* 2006; 160: 173–6.
25. Rosenbaum JF, Fava M, Hoog SL, Ascroft RC, Krebs WB. Selective serotonin reuptake inhibitor discontinuation syndrome: a randomized clinical trial. *Biol Psychiatry* 1998; 44: 77–87.
26. Hindmarch I, Kimber S, Cockle SM. Abrupt and brief discontinuation of antidepressant treatment: effects on cognitive function and psychomotor performance. *Int Clin Psychopharmacol* 2000; 15: 305–18.
27. Horowitz MA, Taylor D. Distinguishing relapse from antidepressant withdrawal: clinical practice and antidepressant discontinuation studies. *BJPsych Advances* 2022; 28: 297–311.
28. Davies J, Read J. A systematic review into the incidence, severity and duration of antidepressant withdrawal effects: are guidelines evidence-based? *Addict Behav* 2019; 97: 111–21.
29. Fava GA, Gatti A, Belaise C, Guidi J, Offidani E. Withdrawal symptoms after selective serotonin reuptake inhibitor discontinuation: a systematic review. *Psychother Psychosom* 2015; 84: 72–81.
30. Haddad P, Devarajan S, Dursun S. Antidepressant discontinuation (withdrawal) symptoms presenting as 'stroke'. *J Psychopharmacol* 2001; 15: 139–41.
31. Weller I, Ashby D, Chambers M, et al. Report of the CSM Expert Working Group on the Safety of Selective Serotonin Reuptake Inhibitors Antidepressants. MHRA, 2005.
32. Maixner SM, Greden JF. Extended antidepressant maintenance and discontinuation syndromes. *Depress Anxiety* 1998; 8 Suppl 1: 43–53.
33. Coupland NJ, Bell CJ, Potokar JP. Serotonin reuptake inhibitor withdrawal. *J Clin Psychopharmacol* 1996; 16: 356–62.
34. Olver JS, Burrows GD, Norman TR. Discontinuation syndromes with selective serotonin reuptake inhibitors are there clinically relevant differences? *CNS Drugs* 1999; 12: 171–7.

35. Boland B, Mitcheson L, Wolff K. Lhermittes sign, electric shock sensations and high dose ecstasy consumption: Preliminary findings. *J Psychopharmacol* 2010; 24: 213–20.

36. Cortes JA, Radhakrishnan R. A case of amelioration of venlafaxine-discontinuation brain shivers with atomoxetine. *The Primary Care Companion for CNS Disorders* 2013; 15: PCC.12l01427.

37. Haddad P. The SSRI discontinuation syndrome. *J Psychopharmacol* 1998; 12: 305–13.

38. Khare S, Seth D. Lhermitte's Sign: The current status. *Ann Indian Acad Neurol* 2015; 18: 154–6.

39. Coulson J, Routledge PA. Adverse reactions to drug withdrawal. *Adverse Drug React Bull* 2008; NA: 967–70.

40. Chouinard G, Chouinard VA. New classification of selective serotonin reuptake inhibitor withdrawal. *Psychother Psychosom* 2015; 84: 63–71.

41. Licht CMM, Penninx BWJH, de Geus EJC. Effects of antidepressants, but not psychopathology, on cardiac sympathetic control: a longitudinal study. *Neuropsychopharmacology* 2012; 37: 2487–95.

42. Wichniak A, Wierzbicka A, Jernajczyk W. Sleep and antidepressant treatment. *Curr Pharm Des* 2012; 18: 5802–17.

Clinical aspects of antidepressant withdrawal

The major risks in stopping antidepressants are of course relapse or recurrence of the underlying condition and the emergence of withdrawal symptoms. Withdrawal symptoms can make stopping antidepressants difficult and can sometimes be debilitating.[1,2] All classes of antidepressants (including TCAs, MAO-Is, SSRIs, SNRIs, NaSSAs, SARIs) are associated with physical dependence and withdrawal symptoms on stopping or reducing the dose.[3–5]

Recognising antidepressant withdrawal symptoms

Some excerpts from qualitative papers examining withdrawal effects from antidepressants are perhaps illustrative:

I am currently trying to wean myself off of Venlafaxine, which honestly is the most awful thing I have ever done. I have horrible dizzy spells and nausea whenever I lower my dose.[6]

I forgot to take my Citalopram for two days and woke up one morning with severe dizziness. It was so extreme that I fell over when I tried to get out of bed and I threw up.[7]

The withdrawal effects if I forget to take my pill are severe shakes, suicidal thoughts, a feeling of too much caffeine in my brain, electric shocks, hallucinations, insane mood swings ... kinda stuck on them now coz I'm too scared to come off it.[8]

The adverse effects have been devastating – when I have tried to withdraw – with 'head zaps', agitation, insomnia and mood changes. This means that I do not have the option of managing the depression any other way because I have a problem coming off this medication.[9]

It took me almost two years to get off Paroxetine and the side effects were horrendous. I even had to quit my job because I felt sick all the time. Even now that I am off of it, I still feel electric shocks in my brain.[6]

Whilst on and trying to get off these meds (mainly SSRIs) I've experienced incredible denial and confusion amongst GPs and psychiatrists. At the point where four different psychiatrists gave me four different diagnoses and prescriptions in the same month this became very clear. You're essentially on your own on this journey, and no, your friends and family probably won't understand.[10]

The first time that I felt some sort of control over my condition was when we went for the second opinion – and everything that I said was believed. That ... is vital to coping with dependence and, again, in withdrawal.[10]

Nature of withdrawal symptoms

There are at least 80 antidepressant withdrawal symptoms described, involving many bodily systems.[11–13] This variety of symptoms probably arises because of the wide-ranging effects of antidepressants on multiple targets. This array of physical and psychological symptoms can be confusing to both patients and clinicians unfamiliar with the syndrome, leading commonly to mis-diagnosis of relapse of an underlying psychiatric condition, or onset of a new physical or mental health problem[10] (Table 2.4).

Table 2.4 Withdrawal symptoms from SSRIs and SNRIs.*

PHYSICAL

General	Neuromuscular	Sensory	Gastrointestinal
Dizziness (65%)	Myoclonus	Electric shock sensations ('zaps')	*Nausea (44%)*
Headache (53%)	Tremor	Tinnitus	Anorexia
Fatigue (45%)	Coordination problems	Blurred vision	Vomiting
Malaise	Numbness	Visual changes (e.g. palinopsia)	Diarrhoea
Tiredness	Myalgia	Hyperesthesia	Abdominal pain/cramp
Lethargy	Ataxia	Altered taste	
Sweating	Muscular spams	Pruritis	
Flu-like symptoms	Neuralgia	Buzzing noise within the head	
Flushing chills	Arthralgias	Prickling sensations	
Pain	Cramp	Paraesthesiae	
Akathisia	Seizures		

Cognitive	Cardiovascular	Sexual
Confusion (53%)	Tachycardia	Premature ejaculation
Amnesia/memory difficulty (34%)	Light-headedness	Genital hypersensitivity
Impaired concentration	Chest pain	
Impaired attention	Hypertension	
Disorientation	Postural hypotension	
Lethargy/drowsiness	Vertigo	
	Syncope	
	Dyspnoea	

(Continued)

Table 2.4 (*Continued*)

PSYCHOLOGICAL

Affective	Behavioural	Sleep	Psychotic
Depression/worsened mood (60%)	Restlessness	*Vivid dreams (51%)*	Visual/auditory hallucinations
Irritability (60%)	Aggressive behaviour	*Insomnia (50%)*	Delirium
Agitation (56%)	Impulsivity	Nightmares	Catatonia
Weeping (54%)	Bouts of crying/ outbursts of anger	Hypersomnia	
Nervousness (53%)			
Mood swings/emotional lability (47%)			
Tension/Anger (47%)			
Anxiety			
Panic			
Dysphoria			
Suicidal ideations/attempts			
Depersonalisation			
Derealisation			
Fear			
Hypomania/euphoria			

* Derived from Cosci and Chouinard (2020),[15] Fava et al. (2015),[16] Guy et al. (2020)[10] and Rosenbaum et al. (1998).[12] The 15 most common withdrawal symptoms from SSRIs are shown in italics with incidence rates. Data is the average incidence of symptoms in patients who abruptly stopped sertraline and paroxetine for 5–8 days in Rosenbaum et al. (1998), rounded to the nearest per cent.

One guide that may be helpful for clinicians is a list of the most discriminatory withdrawal symptoms (the Discriminatory Antidepressant Withdrawal Symptom Scale (DAWSS)) (Table 2.5).[14] This set of symptoms was derived from a large-scale survey of patients with antidepressant withdrawal syndrome who were asked about the incidence and severity of symptoms before starting antidepressants (i.e. the symptoms that prompted prescription of an antidepressant) and symptoms experienced during or after stopping antidepressants (i.e. withdrawal effects).[14] This set of 15 symptoms represents the symptoms that showed the greatest increase in severity and incidence during withdrawal compared with before starting to yield the symptoms that most discriminate between these two conditions.

In severe cases antidepressant withdrawal can be so unpleasant that it provokes suicidality.[10,17] Indeed, in the first 14 days of the discontinuation period is associated with a 60% increase in suicide attempts compared with previous users of antidepressants[18] – as it is improbable that these suicide attempts arose as a consequence of relapse (as relapse is generally thought to be delayed in onset for more than 2 weeks after stopping antidepressants),[19] this increase has been attributed to withdrawal effects.[20]

Table 2.5 Most discriminatory withdrawal symptoms, in order.[14]

Order	Most discriminatory withdrawal symptoms
1	Electric shocks ('brain zaps')
2	Akathisia/ internal sensation of buzzing or tension causing need to move
3	Dizziness/light-headedness
4	Vomiting
5	Vertigo
6	Nausea
7	Gait and coordination problems
8	Increased sensitivity (to light, noise etc)
9	Tinnitus
10	Psychotic symptoms
11	Diarrhoea
12	Muscular problems (cramps, twitches, spasm, pain)
13	Palpitations
14	Vivid dreams
15	Memory problems

Akathisia

Perhaps the other most distressing consequence of antidepressant withdrawal is akathisia, a neuropsychiatric condition (ICD-10-CM Code G25.71), characterised by severe agitation, restlessness and a sense of terror.[10,21–23] Patients report a very distressing subjective feeling of restlessness and dysphoria; they are often fidgeting, pacing, rocking and often have an inability to sit or stand still, although sometimes the manifestations are only subjective, sometimes referrred to as 'inner akathisia'.[24,25] Although this condition is most often recognised as a side effect of antipsychotic use, it has also been observed to occur in SSRI and TCA withdrawal.[10,21–23,25] The pathophysiology is poorly understood, with leading theories implicating a reduction in dopaminergic activity in the mesocortical pathway projecting from the ventral tegmental area to the limbic system and prefrontal cortex, resulting in suppression of the usual inhibitory effects on motor function, leading to unwanted involuntary movements.[25] Other theories implicate changes to serotonin and noradrenaline levels, which can have indirect effects on dopaminergic activity.[26]

This pronounced state of agitation can be mis-diagnosed as a manic state,[22] an anxiety disorder, a panic disorder, a personality disorder, ADHD, health anxiety, restless leg disorder and functional neurological disorder, or a factitious disorder by clinicians unfamiliar with the syndrome in antidepressant withdrawal.[24,25,27] It has been associated with suicidality because of the distress and agitation it engenders.[24,25,28]

References

1. Davies J, Read J. A systematic review into the incidence, severity and duration of antidepressant withdrawal effects: are guidelines evidence-based? *Addict Behav* 2019; 97: 111–21.

2. Groot PC, van Os J. Antidepressant tapering strips to help people come off medication more safely. *Psychosis* 2018; 10: 142–5.

3. Howland RH. Potential adverse effects of discontinuing psychotropic drugs: part 2: antidepressant drugs. *J Psychosoc Nurs Ment Health Serv* 2010; 48: 9–12.

4. Taylor D, Stewart S, Connolly A. Antidepressant withdrawal symptoms–telephone calls to a national medication helpline. *J Affect Disord* 2006; 95: 129–33.

5. Public Health England. Dependence and withdrawal associated with some prescribed medicines. An evidence review. 2019. https://www.gov.uk/government/publications/prescribed-medicines-review-report (accessed 25 May 2021).

6. Pestello FG, Davis-Berman J. Taking anti-depressant medication: a qualitative examination of internet postings. *J Ment Health* 2008; 17: 349–60.

7. Read J, Cartwright C, Gibson K. How many of 1829 antidepressant users report withdrawal effects or addiction? *Int J Ment Health Nurs* 2018; 27: 1805–15.

8. Gibson K, Cartwright C, Read J. 'In my life antidepressants have been ...': A qualitative analysis of users' diverse experiences with antidepressants. *BMC Psychiatry* 2016; 16: 1–7.

9. Cartwright C, Gibson K, Read J, Cowan O, Dehar T. Long-term antidepressant use: Patient perspectives of benefits and adverse effects. *Patient Prefer Adherence* 2016; 10: 1401–7.

10. Guy A, Brown M, Lewis S, Horowitz MA. The 'Patient voice' – Patients who experience antidepressant withdrawal symptoms are often dismissed, or mis-diagnosed with relapse, or onset of a new medical condition. *Ther Adv Psychopharmacol* 2020; 10: 204512532096718.

11. Black K, Shea C, Dursun S, Kutcher S. Selective serotonin reuptake inhibitor discontinuation syndrome: Proposed diagnostic criteria. *J Psychiatry Neurosci* 2000; 25: 255–61.

12. Rosenbaum JF, Fava M, Hoog SL, Ascroft RC, Krebs WB. Selective serotonin reuptake inhibitor discontinuation syndrome: A randomized clinical trial. *Biol Psychiatry* 1998; 44: 77–87.

13. Haddad PM, Anderson IM. Recognising and managing antidepressant discontinuation symptoms. *Advances in Psychiatric Treatment* 2007; 13: 447–57.

14. Moncrieff J, Read J, Horowitz M. The nature and impact of antidepressant withdrawal symptoms and development of the Discriminatory Antidepressant Withdrawal Symptoms Scale (DAWSS) (in preparation).

15. Cosci F, Chouinard G. Acute and persistent withdrawal syndromes following discontinuation of psychotropic medications. *Psychother Psychosom* 2020; 89: 283–306.

16. Fava GA, Gatti A, Belaise C, Guidi J, Offidani E. Withdrawal symptoms after selective serotonin reuptake inhibitor discontinuation: a systematic review. *Psychother Psychosom* 2015; 84: 72–81.

17. Read J. How common and severe are six withdrawal effects from, and addiction to, antidepressants? The experiences of a large international sample of patients. *Addict Behav* 2020; 102: 106157.

18. Valuck RJ, Orton HD, Libby AM. Antidepressant discontinuation and risk of suicide attempt. *J Clin Psychiatry* 2009; 70: 1069–77.

19. Rosenbaum JF, Zajecka J. Clinical management of antidepressant discontinuation. *J Clin Psychiatry* 1997; 58 Suppl 7: 37–40.

20. Horowitz MA, Framer A, Hengartner MP, Sørensen A, Taylor D. Estimating risk of antidepressant withdrawal from a review of published data. *CNS Drugs* 2023; 37: 143–57.

21. Hirose S. Restlessness related to SSRI withdrawal. *Psychiatry Clin Neurosci* 2001; 55: 79–80.

22. Narayan V, Haddad PM. Antidepressant discontinuation manic states: A critical review of the literature and suggested diagnostic criteria. *J Psychopharmacol* 2010; 25: 306–13.

23. Sathananthan GL, Gershon S. Imipramine withdrawal: an akathisia-like syndrome. *Am J Psychiatry* 1973; 130: 1286–7.

24. Akathisia Alliance for Education and Research. Akathisia Alliance for Education and Research. https://akathisiaalliance.org/about-akathisia/ (accessed 17 September 2022).

25. Tachere RO, Modirrousta M. Beyond anxiety and agitation: a clinical approach to akathisia. *Aust Fam Physician* 2017; 46: 296–8.

26. Lane RM. SSRI-induced extrapyramidal side-effects and akathisia: implications for treatment. *J Psychopharmacol* 1998; 12: 192–214.

27. Lohr JB, Eidt CA, Abdulrazzaq Alfaraj A, Soliman MA. The clinical challenges of akathisia. *CNS Spectr* 2015; 20 Suppl 1: 1–14; quiz 15–6.

28. Hengartner MP, Schulthess L, Sørensen A, Framer A. Protracted withdrawal syndrome after stopping antidepressants: a descriptive quantitative analysis of consumer narratives from a large internet forum. *Ther Adv Psychopharmacol* 2020; 10: 2045125320980573.

CHAPTER 2

How common, severe and long-lasting are withdrawal symptoms from antidepressants?

Incidence of antidepressant withdrawal after discontinuation

There is ongoing debate about the incidence of withdrawal effects from antidepressants. A 2019 systematic review identified 14 relevant studies from which to calculate the incidence of antidepressant withdrawal symptoms.[1] The incidence rates ranged from 27% to 86%, with a median of 55% and a weighted average of 56.4%.[1] Restricting the analysis only to double-blind RCTs captured in this review the incidence of withdrawal syndrome was 53.9% (six RCTs, 731 participants), where the majority of studies used an increase in discontinuation-emergent signs and symptoms (DESS)[2] of ≥ 4 to define a withdrawal syndrome (Table 2.6). Restricting analysis to studies of SSRIs, withdrawal syndromes occurred with a median rate of 53.6%, and a weighted average of 50.5%.[1]

Table 2.6 Incidence of withdrawal in double-blind randomised controlled trials captured in Davies and Read (2019).[1] Table is adapted from Horowitz et al. (2023)[3]

Double-blind RCTs	Period of treatment before cessation	Period of observation	Definition of withdrawal syndrome	People with withdrawal syndromes	Total stopped from medication	Proportion with withdrawal (%)
Oehrberg 1995[4]	12 weeks	2 weeks	'any adverse effect on discontinuation'	19	55	34.6
Rosenbaum 1998[2]	11.4 months	5–8 days	DESS ≥ 4	86	185	46.5
Zajecka 1998[5]	12 weeks	6 weeks	'new or worsened events'	64	95	67.4
Hindmarch 2000[6]	'At least 3 months'	4–7 days	DESS ≥ 4	66	86	76.7
Montgomery 2005[7]	12 weeks	2 weeks	DESS ≥ 4	49	181	27.1
Sir 2005[8]	8 weeks	2 weeks	Any discontinuation-emergent symptom	110	129	85.3
Total				394	731	53.9

DESS = Discontinuation-Emergent Signs and Symptoms Checklist.

As these studies provided single-arm frequencies for antidepressant withdrawal, these estimates may need to be adjusted for the nocebo effects (symptoms that arise from negative expectations on stopping medication) that may occur when stopping placebo or continuing antidepressants. Subtracting the weighted average of nocebo effects derived previously[3,9] of 11.8% from the overall detected rate in double-blind RCTs (53.9%–11.8%) might therefore give a more reasonable estimate of 42.1%, and 38.7% for SSRIs specifically (50.5%–11.8%).[3]

Severity of withdrawal symptoms

The severity of antidepressant withdrawal symptoms varies widely, ranging from mild, short-lasting cases that can be managed with education and reassurance, to severe cases that cause significant disruption to normal functioning, job loss, relationship breakdown and even suicide.[1,10–12] This variability presumably relates to differing degrees of neurobiological adaptation to antidepressants among individuals.[3] In its severe form, the antidepressant withdrawal syndrome has been reported to be associated with ataxia leading to falls, electric shock sensations and disorientation that impair walking and driving,[10,13] and urgent consultations at emergency departments.[14,15] Some patients experience such severe withdrawal effects that they become bed-bound, debilitated, suicidal[11,16] and others can experience akathisia, which can be highly distressing.[11,17,18]

A systematic review identified five studies that evaluated the severity of post-discontinuation withdrawal effects, with nearly half of participants who had experienced them choosing the most extreme option in a scale to describe the severity of those effects.[1] For example, in response to the question 'How severely do you feel withdrawal has affected your life?' on a scale of 0–10 given to 580 people who had attempted withdrawal from antidepressants, mostly SSRIs, the mean response was 8.35 (SD 2.05), indicating that the majority experienced severe reactions, with 43% (249) of participants choosing 10, the highest level of the scale.[19] The online survey method employed by four of these studies may be biased by a self-selected subject group with more negative experiences than average. However, somewhat more than half of the participants surveyed in these studies had used antidepressants for more than 3 years,[20] mirroring the wider UK population, where about half of antidepressant users have been on them for more than two years.[21] In the USA about half of antidepressant users take the medication for at least five years.[22]

The remaining study, conducted by Pfizer, found that 34.3% of patients treated with sertraline for only 8 weeks experienced moderately severe symptoms (as rated by an investigator on global assessment) upon discontinuation, 23.9% of them experienced a mild withdrawal reaction, while 23.9% reported a minimal one.[8] For venlafaxine, after 8 weeks of use, 38.7% of patients were rated by study researchers as experiencing moderately severe withdrawal symptoms, with 3.2% as 'severe' and 1.6% as 'very severe'.[8] As longer duration of treatment appears to be associated with a greater incidence and severity of withdrawal symptoms (see below), patients who are on antidepressants for longer than the 8 weeks of this study are more likely to suffer more severe withdrawal symptoms.[20,23]

Duration of post-discontinuation withdrawal symptoms

Some studies report that withdrawal symptoms can be self-limiting over a couple of weeks, especially when the medications are only used for several weeks.[24] However there is also significant evidence that withdrawal symptoms can persist for months or even years,[1] sometimes referred to as protracted withdrawal syndrome or post-acute withdrawal symptoms (PAWS).[12,25,26] As mentioned earlier, although protracted withdrawal symptoms have been regarded as pharmacologically implausible in the past ('the drug is out of your system'), this understanding has been updated to recognise that drug-induced neuro-adaptations may require an extended period to return to their pre-drug state, rather than resolve when the drug is eliminated from the body.[12,27] Consistent with this, RCPsych has updated its position,[28] and a corresponding update was made to the NICE guidelines,[29] to indicate that withdrawal symptoms can last for 'months, or longer'.

This has been confirmed by a large (n = 478) double-blind randomised controlled discontinuation trial in which participants who had been on antidepressants for 2 years or longer and felt well enough to consider stopping were randomised to be maintained on their antidepressant or have it stopped over a period of 4 to 8 weeks.[30] In this trial those patients in the discontinuation group reported an increase in withdrawal symptoms that were present for at least 7 months after medications were stopped.[30] Withdrawal symptoms were most numerous at 4 weeks after antidepressants were ceased with more than a doubling in the number of symptoms compared with maintenance patients, but remained elevated at 7 months. Severity of withdrawal symptoms was not measured in this trial.

This is consistent with findings in surveys. A RCPsych online survey found that for the 512 users who experienced withdrawal, a quarter of the group reported withdrawal symptoms that lasted more than 12 weeks.[1] In another survey of 580 people who had withdrawn from antidepressant medication, 86.7% responded that the syndrome had lasted at least two months, 58.6% at least one year and 16.2% for more than three years,[19] although this study may have surveyed a self-selected population with a more severe experience of withdrawal than average. Other studies also report longer durations of withdrawal symptoms – in at least some cases symptoms (outlined in Table 2.6) can persist for years, which can be debilitating.[11,12,25,31,32]

It is difficult to establish to what extent these very long-lasting syndromes represent outliers, as it is not possible to establish that these are representative populations of antidepressant users, but it is clear now from double-blind RCTs that withdrawal symptoms persist for months for many people, significantly longer than the one- or two-week periods that have been previously ascribed to them.[33] It remains to be established exactly what proportion of patients experience debilitating, multi-year withdrawal.

There is also debate about whether very prolonged withdrawal syndromes represent a syndrome distinct from the acute antidepressant withdrawal syndrome or merely a continuation of these symptoms.[12,26,34] Another perspective is that these long-lasting effects should be seen more similarly to tardive dyskinesia – that is, possibly years-long or even permanent neurological alterations produced by exposure to the drug (that might improve over time).[35]

References

1. Davies J, Read J. A systematic review into the incidence, severity and duration of antidepressant withdrawal effects: are guidelines evidence-based? *Addict Behav* 2019; 97: 111–21.
2. Rosenbaum JF, Fava M, Hoog SL, Ascroft RC, Krebs WB. Selective serotonin reuptake inhibitor discontinuation syndrome: a randomized clinical trial. *Biol Psychiatry* 1998; 44: 77–87.
3. Horowitz MA, Framer A, Hengartner MP, Sørensen A, Taylor D. Estimating risk of antidepressant withdrawal from a review of published data. *CNS Drugs* 2023; 37: 143–57.
4. Oehrberg S, Christiansen PE, Behnke K, et al. Paroxetine in the treatment of panic disorder. A randomised, double-blind, placebo-controlled study. *Br J Psychiatry* 1995; 167: 36–42.
5. Zajecka J, Fawcett J, Amsterdam J, et al. Safety of abrupt discontinuation of fluoxetine: a randomized, placebo-controlled study. *J Clin Psychopharmacol* 1998; 18: 193–7.
6. Hindmarch I, Kimber S, Cockle SM. Abrupt and brief discontinuation of antidepressant treatment: effects on cognitive function and psycho-motor performance. *Int Clin Psychopharmacol* 2000; 15: 305–18.
7. Montgomery SA, Nil R, Durr-Pal N, Loft H, Boulenger J-P. A 24-week randomized, double-blind, placebo-controlled study of escitalopram for the prevention of generalized social anxiety disorder. *J Clin Psychiatry* 2005; 66: 1270–8.
8. Sir A, D'Souza RF, Uguz S, et al. Randomized trial of sertraline versus venlafaxine XR in major depression: efficacy and discontinuation symptoms. *J Clin Psychiatry* 2005; 66: 1312–20.
9. Horowitz MA, Taylor D. Distinguishing relapse from antidepressant withdrawal: clinical practice and antidepressant discontinuation studies. *BJPsych Advances* 2022; 28: 297–311.
10. Haddad PM, Anderson IM. Recognising and managing antidepressant discontinuation symptoms. *Adv Psychiatr Treat* 2007; 13: 447–57.
11. Guy A, Brown M, Lewis S, Horowitz MA. The 'patient voice' – patients who experience antidepressant withdrawal symptoms are often dismissed, or mis-diagnosed with relapse, or onset of a new medical condition. *Ther Adv Psychopharmacol* 2020; 10: 204512532096718.
12. Hengartner MP, Schulthess L, Sørensen A, Framer A. Protracted withdrawal syndrome after stopping antidepressants: a descriptive quantitative analysis of consumer narratives from a large internet forum. *Ther Adv Psychopharmacol* 2020; 10: 2045125320980573.
13. Campagne DM. Venlafaxine and serious withdrawal symptoms: Warning to drivers. *MedGenMed* 2005; 7: 22.
14. Pacheco L, Malo P, Aragues E, Etxebeste M. More cases of paroxetine withdrawal syndrome. *BJPsych* 1996; 169: 384.
15. Haddad P, Devarajan S, Dursun S. Antidepressant discontinuation (withdrawal) symptoms presenting as 'stroke'. *J Psychopharmacol* 2001; 15: 139–41.
16. Valuck RJ, Orton HD, Libby AM. Antidepressant discontinuation and risk of suicide attempt. *J Clin Psychiatry* 2009; 70: 1069–77.
17. Narayan V, Haddad PM. Antidepressant discontinuation manic states: a critical review of the literature and suggested diagnostic criteria. *J Psychopharmacol* 2010; 25: 306–13.
18. Akathisia Alliance for Education and Research. https://akathisiaalliance.org/about-akathisia/ (accessed 17 September 2022).
19. Davies J, Regina P, Montagu L. All-Party Parliamentary Group for Prescribed Drug Dependence Antidepressant Withdrawal: A Survey of Patients' Experience by the All-Party Parliamentary Group for Prescribed Drug Dependence. 2018. http://prescribeddrug.org/wp-content/uploads/2018/10/APPG-PDD-Survey-of-antidepressant-withdrawal-experiences.pdf (accessed 18 January 2023).
20. Read J, Williams J. Adverse effects of antidepressants reported by a large international cohort: emotional blunting, suicidality, and withdrawal effects. *Curr Drug Saf* 2018; 13: 176–86.
21. Johnson CF, Macdonald HJ, Atkinson P, Buchanan AI, Downes N, Dougall N. Reviewing long-term antidepressants can reduce drug burden: a prospective observational cohort study. *Br J Gen Pract* 2012; 62: e773–9.
22. Mojtabai R, Olfson M. National trends in long-term use of antidepressant medications: results from the U.S. National Health and Nutrition Examination Survey. *J Clin Psychiatry* 2014; 75: 169–77.
23. Weller I, Ashby D, Chambers M, et al. Report of the CSM Expert Working Group on the Safety of Selective Serotonin Reuptake Inhibitors Antidepressants. 2005.
24. Baldwin DS, Montgomery SA, Nil R, Lader M. Discontinuation symptoms in depression and anxiety disorders. *Int J Neuropsychopharmacol* 2007; 10: 73–84.
25. Framer A. What I have learnt from helping thousands of people taper off psychotropic medications. *Ther Adv Psychopharmacol* 2021; 11: 204512532199127.
26. Cosci F, Chouinard G. Acute and persistent withdrawal syndromes following discontinuation of psychotropic medications. *Psychother Psychosom* 2020; 89: 283–306.
27. Reidenberg MM. Drug discontinuation effects are part of the pharmacology of a drug. *J Pharmacol Exp Ther* 2011; 339: 324–8.
28. Royal College of Psychiatrists. Position statement on antidepressants and depression. 2019; published online May. https://www.rcpsych.ac.uk/docs/default-source/improving-care/better-mh-policy/position-statements/ps04_19---antidepressants-and-depression.pdf?sfvrsn=ddea9473_5 (accessed 18 January 2023).
29. Iacobucci G. NICE updates antidepressant guidelines to reflect severity and length of withdrawal symptoms. *BMJ* 2019; 367: l6103.
30. Lewis G, Marston L, Duffy L, et al. Maintenance or discontinuation of antidepressants in primary care. *N Engl J Med* 2021; 385: 1257–67.
31. Fava GA, Bernardi M, Tomba E, Rafanelli C. Effects of gradual discontinuation of selective serotonin reuptake inhibitors in panic disorder with agoraphobia. *Int J Neuropsychopharmacol* 2007; 10: 835–8.
32. Bhanji NH, Chouinard G, Kolivakis T, Margolese HC. Persistent tardive rebound panic disorder, rebound anxiety and insomnia following paroxetine withdrawal: a review of rebound-withdrawal phenomena. *Can J Clin Pharmacol* 2006; 13: e69–74.
33. Davies J, Read J, Hengartner MP, et al. Clinical guidelines on antidepressant withdrawal urgently need updating. *BMJ* 2019; 365: l2238.
34. Lerner A, Klein M. Dependence, withdrawal and rebound of CNS drugs: An update and regulatory considerations for new drugs development. *Brain Commun* 2019; 1: fcz025.
35. Fava GA, Cosci F. Understanding and managing withdrawal syndromes after discontinuation of antidepressant drugs. *J Clin Psychiatry*. 2019; 80. doi:10.4088/jcp.19com12794.

Protracted antidepressant withdrawal syndrome

Severe and persistent (for months or years) withdrawal syndromes are recognised for a range of psychotropic medications, including antidepressants.[1-4] Post-acute withdrawal syndrome (PAWS) occurs in an unknown proportion of patients after stopping antidepressants.[3-5] This syndrome has long been neglected or minimised,[3] with poor education about its existence leading to mis-attribution of these symptoms to relapse or the emergence of new mental health conditions.[3,6-8] Protracted withdrawal symptoms are thought to be caused by changes to the brain during exposure (generally long term) to antidepressants, which persist for months and years after stopping the drugs.[2,3,9] Indeed, there is PET imaging which demonstrates changes to serotonergic receptor sensitivity for months and years after the medication is stopped;[10] some have postulated that these changes may be irreversible, though recovery seems possible for people in the long term.[1-3,7] Its risk is thought to be minimised by gradual tapering.[7,11,12] There is great similarity between symptoms in acute withdrawal from antidepressants and in protracted withdrawal but some authors have considered them separate (but related) syndromes.[3,13] Some patients experience onset of severe, long-lasting withdrawal symptoms (many of quite typical characteristics, for example, electric shock sensations, altered sensorium and psychological symptoms quite distinct from their underlying condition)[3] after several weeks of mild withdrawal symptoms following stopping an antidepressant, possibly suggesting different pathophysiological mechanisms.[3]

In an analysis of patient narratives, protracted withdrawal is characterised by similar symptoms to those recognised in acute withdrawal, with the most common symptoms reported being general (headache, fatigue), balance (dizziness), sensory symptoms (electric shock sensations ('brain zaps')), neuromotor symptoms (muscle aches, muscle tremor), gastrointestinal symptoms (nausea, diarrhoea), affective symptoms (anxiety, depressed mood, emergent suicidality), insomnia and decreased concentration ('brain fog').[3] Less commonly, new-onset psychotic symptoms and persistent sexual problems were also reported in this cohort.[3]

In a survey of a convenience sample of 1,150 patients regarding their protracted withdrawal symptoms the following consequences were reported: 68.9% reported reduced social activities, 55.7% reported impaired work function, 40.9% reported family discord, 33.1% reduced work time or responsibilities, 26.8% took sick leave, 25.3% reported relationship breakdown, 21.6% left or lost their job during withdrawal and 12.8% had physical accidents.[11] In analyses of patient reports there has been increased suicidality[3,4] and completed suicides, attributed to withdrawal effects.[3] Protracted withdrawal can have devastating consequences for patients and their families, especially when accurate diagnosis is rare. Increased awareness of this condition could lead to improved outcomes for sufferers.[7]

References

1. Cosci F, Chouinard G. Acute and persistent withdrawal syndromes following discontinuation of psychotropic medications. *Psychother Psychosom* 2020; 89: 283–306.
2. Lerner A, Klein M. Dependence, withdrawal and rebound of CNS drugs: an update and regulatory considerations for new drugs development. *Brain Commun* 2019; 1: fcz025.
3. Hengartner MP, Schulthess L, Sørensen A, Framer A. Protracted withdrawal syndrome after stopping antidepressants: A descriptive quantitative analysis of consumer narratives from a large internet forum. *Ther Adv Psychopharmacol* 2020; 10: 2045125320980573.
4. Guy A, Brown M, Lewis S, Horowitz MA. The 'patient voice' – patients who experience antidepressant withdrawal symptoms are often dismissed, or mis-diagnosed with relapse, or onset of a new medical condition. *Ther Adv Psychopharmacol* 2020; 10: 204512532096718.
5. Davies J, Read J. A systematic review into the incidence, severity and duration of antidepressant withdrawal effects: are guidelines evidence-based? *Addict Behav* 2019; 97: 111–21.
6. White E, Read J, Julo S. The role of Facebook groups in the management and raising of awareness of antidepressant withdrawal: is social media filling the void left by health services? *Ther Adv Psychopharmacol* 2021; 11: 2045125320981174.
7. Framer A. What I have learnt from helping thousands of people taper off psychotropic medications. *Ther Adv Psychopharmacol* 2021; 11: 204512532199127.
8. Horowitz MA, Taylor D. Distinguishing relapse from antidepressant withdrawal: Clinical practice and antidepressant discontinuation studies. *BJPsych Advances* 2022; 28: 297–311.
9. Reidenberg MM. Drug discontinuation effects are part of the pharmacology of a drug. *J Pharmacol Exp Ther* 2011; 339: 324–8.
10. Bhagwagar Z, Rabiner EA, Sargent PA, Grasby PM, Cowen PJ. Persistent reduction in brain serotonin1A receptor binding in recovered depressed men measured by positron emission tomography with [11C]WAY-100635. *Mol Psychiatry* 2004; 9: 386–92.
11. Moncrieff J, Read J, Horowitz M. The nature and impact of antidepressant withdrawal symptoms and development of the Discriminatory Antidepressant Withdrawal Symptoms Scale (DAWSS) (in preparation).
12. Horowitz M, Flanigan R, Cooper R, Moncrieff J. The determinants of outcome from antidepressant withdrawal in a large survey of patients (in preparation).
13. Chouinard G, Chouinard VA. New classification of selective serotonin reuptake inhibitor withdrawal. *Psychother Psychosom* 2015; 84: 63–71.

CHAPTER 2

Post-SSRI sexual dysfunction

PSSD is a protracted state that persists in an unknown proportion of people after stopping antidepressants that may be related to other protracted withdrawal syndromes, and can cause significant distress to sufferers.[1] The condition was first characterised in 2006,[2] and in 2019 the European Medicines Agency recommended that the product information on SSRIs and SNRIs be updated after a review of pharmacovigilance data.[1,3] The symptoms include genital numbness, decreased libido, erectile dysfunction, failure to become aroused or orgasm, and pleasureless or weak orgasm. The sensory changes may extend beyond the genital area to a more general dampening or numbing of emotions.[1,4] The pathophysiology is poorly understood but genital numbing might be related to the action of SSRIs at sodium channels in the cell membrane.[1] Case reports show that it can occur after differing periods of exposure to antidepressants, and sometimes spontaneously resolves (sometimes taking months or years to do so).[1] Some people experience brief remissions, suggesting that the effects may not be permanent.[1]

References

1. Reisman Y. Post-SSRI sexual dysfunction. *BMJ* 2020; 368. doi:10.1136/bmj.m754.
2. Csoka AB, Shipko S. Persistent sexual side effects after SSRI discontinuation. *Psychother Psychosom* 2006; 75: 187–8.
3. European Medicines Agency. New product information wording – extracts from PRAC recommendations on signals. European Medicines Agency. 2019. https://www.ema.europa.eu/en/documents/other/new-product-information- (accessed 23 September 2022).
4. Healy D, Le Noury J, Mangin D. Enduring sexual dysfunction after treatment with antidepressants, 5α-reductase inhibitors and isotretinoin: 300 cases. *Int J Risk Saf Med* 2018; 29: 125–34.

Factors influencing development of withdrawal effects

Although there has been limited research on the topic, there are several factors that are thought to have an effect on incidence, severity and duration of withdrawal symptoms. In general, greater adaptation (or physical dependence) to the drug is likely to lead to greater withdrawal effects, brought about, for example, by higher dose or longer use, as well as some variation among drugs and individual neurobiology.[1]

Duration of use

Risk of withdrawal increases after 4–6 weeks of daily use.[2] Longer duration of use would be expected to produce greater adaptation to the presence of the drug and therefore present a greater risk of withdrawal.

Although no RCTs have examined the role of treatment duration in incidence or severity of withdrawal symptoms, surveys have done so.[3,4] Of course, these surveys may have captured a skewed sample (of patients with more severe withdrawal effects than the average patient), however, these studies suggest a clear gradient between duration of use of antidepressants (mostly SSRIs and SNRIs) and both incidence of withdrawal effects and their severity (Table 2.7).[4] This suggests that for patients who have been on antidepressants for more than 3 years, about half will experience severe withdrawal symptoms, while only a small proportion of patients will experience withdrawal effects after only a few weeks of use.[4] A recent analysis also found that longer use of antidepressants was associated with longer periods of withdrawal effects.[5]

Table 2.7 The relationship between duration of treatment with an antidepressant and incidence and severity of withdrawal symptoms from surveys of antidepressant users. Data is derived from Read et al. (2018).[4]

Duration of antidepressant use	Withdrawal effects – any severity (%)	Withdrawal effects – moderate or severe (%)
<3 months	28.0	17.0
3–6 months	28.3	19.2
6–12 months	40.4	24.2
1–2 years	48.2	31.1
2–3 years	62.9	48.3
>3 years	66.9	56.2

There were five studies for which duration of antidepressant use and duration of withdrawal symptoms were available (Table 2.8).[6–10] Although a relationship appears to exist between duration of use and duration of withdrawal symptoms, the data was heterogenous. Both studies with a longer duration of use involved samples of patients who self-identified as having trouble with withdrawal, likely to represent a more severe group than average.[7,9] Additionally, such data are susceptible to the ecological fallacy (that is, an effect on group averages might not apply to the individuals in the

Table 2.8 The relationship between duration of treatment and duration of withdrawal effects of studies included in the 2019 systematic review. Adapted from Davies and Read (2019).[11]

Duration of antidepressant use (months)	Duration of withdrawal symptoms (weeks)	Study
3	4	Zajecka et al., 1998[8]
3	6	Narayan and Haddad, 2010[10]
23	1	Bogetto et al., 2002[6]
24	50	Davies et al., 2018[9]
60	79	Stockmann et al., 2018[7]

group). However, it does appear that a portion of patients will experience withdrawal symptoms for several months or longer than a year, perhaps related to length of treatment.

Drug type

It has been suggested that differences among antidepressants explain differences in withdrawal effects from antidepressants. It is thought that drugs with short half-lives would produce more precipitous drops in 'input' expected by the system causing greater withdrawal effects (see Figure 2.2).[12] This is supported by the finding that percentage reductions in plasma concentration of fluoxetine, sertraline and paroxetine, following cessation, showed a significant correlation with the appearance of withdrawal symptoms.[13] Consistent with this, cessation of paroxetine for several days causes withdrawal symptoms in 66–100% of patients,[14,15] cessation of sertraline in 59–60% of patients,[14,15] and fluoxetine in 14–77% of patients (although the value of 77% is likely to be an outlier).[14,15] In surveys, which may include a self-selected population, these differences among common SSRIs are roughly preserved: 69%, 62% and 44% of patients stopping paroxetine, sertraline and fluoxetine, respectively, report withdrawal symptoms.[11]

Paroxetine and fluoxetine are both metabolised by cytochrome P450 2D6 (while fluoxetine's active metabolite, norfluoxetine, is metabolised by P450 3A4) and inhibit their own metabolism, resulting in non-linear kinetics.[16] This predicts disproportionate declines in plasma concentrations during dose reduction as metabolism accelerates as the drug leaves the body. While this effect may not be clinically significant for fluoxetine because of its long half-life, it may be a significant factor in withdrawal effects for paroxetine.[17]

In addition, paroxetine may produce a more severe withdrawal syndrome than other SSRIs because it exhibits the highest known binding affinity for the central site of SERT,[18] and demonstrates muscarinic antagonist effects and moderate norepinephrine transporter-inhibiting effects as well.[17,19] Antidepressants with pronounced noradrenergic effects in addition to serotonergic tend to be associated with more severe withdrawal – for example, venlafaxine, and duloxetine.[12,20]

Tiers of risk based on drug type

The relative risk of withdrawal symptoms from different antidepressants (Table 2.9)[1] was derived from several analyses including a recent structured analysis of the published literature,[12] an analysis of calls to an English medication helpline for issues related to withdrawal, normalised to prescription numbers,[20] as well as comparative studies of withdrawal effects from the WHO pharmacovigilance database.[21,22] However, for some of the antidepressants outlined here only case reports were available[12] so this summary can only be considered preliminary.

Table 2.9 Common antidepressants stratified by risk of withdrawal symptoms, derived from Henssler et al. (2019)[12], calls to a withdrawal helpline, normalised to prescription numbers,[20] and analyses of reports to the WHO pharmacovigilance service.[21,22]

Likelihood of withdrawal and severity of withdrawal	Antidepressant
Severe/frequent withdrawal	**SNRIs:** venlafaxine, desvenlafaxine, duloxetine
	paroxetine
	MAO-Is: tranylcypromine, phenelzine, isocarboxazid
	moclobemide
	Other: mirtazapine
Moderately severe/moderately frequent withdrawal	**SSRIs:** citalopram, escitalopram, sertraline, fluvoxamine, fluoxetine, vilazodone
	TCAs: nortriptyline, clomipramine, imipramine, amitriptyline, desipramine, doxepin
	SARIs: nefazodone, trazodone
	Other: milnacipran, reboxetine, bupropion
Less severe/less frequent withdrawal	vortioxetine, mianserin, dosulepin, trimipramine
Minimal/lowest withdrawal risk	agomelatine, lofepramine

Higher drug dosage

There is some evidence that higher doses of antidepressants are associated with greater risks of withdrawal effects, though not to a very large degree, nor in a linear manner. There was a higher incidence of withdrawal effects for higher dosages of paroxetine in an analysis by the Committee on the Safety of Medicines (CSM),[23] although the effect reached a threshold at 20mg (Table 2.10). There was a more pronounced dose-dependent relationship for venlafaxine withdrawal effects (Table 2.10),[23] with increased incidence at higher dosages possibly related to greater noradrenergic effects at these dosages.[24,25] Fluvoxamine and mirtazapine did not demonstrate clear dose-dependent effects, however the data was not well-suited to detect these effects.[23] Overall, dosage does appear to have some relationship to risk of withdrawal symptoms (where higher doses were associated with increased risk of withdrawal), but its influence may not be as strong as duration of use, perhaps because higher dosages have only small additional pharmacological effects over minimum clinically employed dosages because of the hyperbolic shape of their dose–response curves, leading to ceiling effects.[26–30]

Table 2.10 The relationship between dosage of antidepressants and incidence of withdrawal effects. Adapted from Horowitz et al. (2023).[1]

Study	Medication	Dose			
		Proportion of patients with withdrawal effects/(number of patients in group)			
CSM[23]	Paroxetine	10mg	20mg	30mg	40mg
		9% (46)	16% (55)	18% (61)	17% (60)
CSM[23]	Venlafaxine	37.5mg	75mg	150mg	
		13% (92)	11% (92)	24% (98)	
Lader et al. (2004)[31,32]	Escitalopram	5mg	10mg	20mg	
		15.1% (124)	17.1% (125)	21.7% (111)	
Baldwin et al (2006, 2007)[32,33]	Escitalopram	5mg	10mg		
		6.9% (116)	12.2% (115)		

Individual characteristics determining withdrawal risk

One question often asked is: why do some people get withdrawal symptoms and others do not? It is likely that myriad individual neurobiological, physiological (and perhaps psychological) differences, as yet poorly understood, determine vulnerability to withdrawal.[34,35] Although there has not been much empirical examination of these questions, there are a number of possible variations that might affect the degree to which an individual's brain might adapt in response to the drug – and thereby increase the risk of withdrawal effects on stopping. These include sensitivity of SERT to inhibition,[34,35] and it has been hypothesised that different rates of metabolism of drugs (determined by cytochrome P450 polymorphisms) may affect risk of withdrawal[36] but no studies have investigated this relationship. The likelihood of withdrawal symptoms has been associated with the C(-1019)G polymorphism of the $5HT_{1A}$ receptor gene, known to be affected by long-term antidepressant treatment.[37] The use of other medications that induce or inhibit the speed of metabolism of antidepressants may also affect risk of withdrawal.[38]

One clinical indication of likelihood of withdrawal is past experience of withdrawal – either when accidentally forgetting medication (for example, when going on holiday) or on previous attempts to stop.[39–42] Indeed some authors have thought that inconsistent dosing itself increases the chance of withdrawal effects on stopping (in addition to revealing the propensity of an individual to experience withdrawal effects).[42] It is possible that the difficulty of withdrawal tends to increase with each subsequent attempt at withdrawal through a process similar to the neurological kindling phenomenon observed in repeated cycles of use and cessation of illicit drugs and alcohol.[43–47] Similarly, intermittent dosing of antipsychotics is also thought to increase the risk of tardive dyskinesia.[48]

There is also evidence that patients who experience adverse reactions in the early phase of treatment are more likely to experience withdrawal effects on stopping, perhaps indicative of greater susceptibility to their effects, including adaptation to their presence, leading to greater difficulties with withdrawal.[38,49] Although there has been limited research into the topic, analyses conducted so far indicate that there is no difference in risk of withdrawal effects in respect to the diagnosis for which the medication was commenced.[32] This is consistent with the understanding that it is the effect of the drug on the brain that determines withdrawal effects.[50]

References

1. Horowitz MA, Framer A, Hengartner MP, Sørensen A, Taylor D. Estimating risk of antidepressant withdrawal from a review of published data. *CNS Drugs* 2023; 37: 143–57.

2. Jha MK, Rush AJ, Trivedi MH. When discontinuing SSRI antidepressants is a challenge: management tips. *Am J Psychiatry* 2018; 175: 1176–84.

3. Read J, Cartwright C, Gibson K. Adverse emotional and interpersonal effects reported by 1829 New Zealanders while taking antidepressants. *Psychiatry Res* 2014; 216: 67–73.

4. Read J, Cartwright C, Gibson K. How many of 1829 antidepressant users report withdrawal effects or addiction? *Int J Ment Health Nurs* 2018; 27: 1805–15.

5. Moncrieff J, Read J, Horowitz M. The nature and impact of antidepressant withdrawal symptoms and development of the Discriminatory Antidepressant Withdrawal Symptoms Scale (DAWSS) (in preparation).

6. Bogetto F, Bellino S, Revello RB, Patria L. Discontinuation syndrome in dysthymic patients treated with selective serotonin reuptake inhibitors: a clinical investigation. *CNS Drugs* 2002; 16: 273–83.

7. Stockmann T, Odegbaro D, Timimi S, Moncrieff J. SSRI and SNRI withdrawal symptoms reported on an internet forum. *Int J Risk Saf Med* 2018; 29: 175–80.

8. Zajecka J, Fawcett J, Amsterdam J, et al. Safety of abrupt discontinuation of fluoxetine: A randomized, placebo-controlled study. *J Clin Psychopharmacol* 1998; 18: 193–7.

9. Davies J, Regina P, Montagu L. All-Party Parliamentary Group for Prescribed Drug Dependence Antidepressant Withdrawal: a Survey of Patients' Experience by the All-Party Parliamentary Group for Prescribed Drug Dependence. All-Party Parliamentary Group for Prescribed Drug Dependence, 2018 http://prescribeddrug.org/wp-content/uploads/2018/10/APPG-PDD-Survey-of-antidepressant-withdrawal-experiences.pdf (accessed 18 January 2023).

10. Narayan V, Haddad PM. Antidepressant discontinuation manic states: a critical review of the literature and suggested diagnostic criteria. *J Psychopharmacol* 2010; 25: 306–13.

11. Davies J, Read J. A systematic review into the incidence, severity and duration of antidepressant withdrawal effects: are guidelines evidence-based? *Addict Behav* 2019; 97: 111–21.

12. Henssler J, Heinz A, Brandt L, Bschor T. Antidepressant withdrawal and rebound phenomena. *Dtsch Arztebl Int* 2019; 116: 355–61.

13. Michelson D, Fava M, Amsterdam J, et al. Interruption of selective serotonin reuptake inhibitor treatment. Double blind, placebo-controlled trial. *Br J Psychiatry* 2000; 176: 363–8.

14. Rosenbaum JF, Fava M, Hoog SL, Ascroft RC, Krebs WB. Selective serotonin reuptake inhibitor discontinuation syndrome: a randomized clinical trial. *Biol Psychiatry* 1998; 44: 77–87.

15. Hindmarch I, Kimber S, Cockle SM. Abrupt and brief discontinuation of antidepressant treatment: effects on cognitive function and psychomotor performance. *Int Clin Psychopharmacol* 2000; 15: 305–18.

16. Preskorn SH. Clinically relevant pharmacology of selective serotonin reuptake inhibitors. An overview with emphasis on pharmacokinetics and effects on oxidative drug metabolism. *Clin Pharmacokinet* 1997; 32 Suppl 1: 1–21.

17. Olver JS, Burrows GD, Norman TR. Discontinuation syndromes with selective serotonin reuptake inhibitors. Are there clinically relevant differences? *CNS Drugs* 1999; 12: 171–7.

18. Coleman JA, Navratna V, Antermite D, Yang D, Bull JA, Gouaux E. Chemical and structural investigation of the paroxetine-human serotonin transporter complex. *Elife* 2020; 9: e56427.

19. Renoir T. Selective serotonin reuptake inhibitor antidepressant treatment discontinuation syndrome: a review of the clinical evidence and the possible mechanisms involved. *Front Pharmacol* 2013; 4 April: 1–10.

20. Taylor D, Stewart S, Connolly A. Antidepressant withdrawal symptoms – telephone calls to a national medication helpline. *J Affect Disord* 2006; 95: 129–33.

21. Quilichini J-B, Revet A, Garcia P, et al. Comparative effects of 15 antidepressants on the risk of withdrawal syndrome: a real-world study using the WHO pharmacovigilance database. *J Affect Disord* 2021; 297: 189–93.

22. Gastaldon C, Schoretsanitis G, Arzenton E, et al. Withdrawal syndrome following discontinuation of 28 antidepressants: pharmacovigilance analysis of 31,688 reports from the WHO spontaneous reporting database. *Drug Saf* 2022; 45: 1539–49.

23. Weller I, Ashby D, Chambers M, et al. Report of the CSM Expert Working Group on the Safety of Selective Serotonin Reuptake Inhibitors Antidepressants. MHRA, 2005.

24. Debonnel G, Saint-André É, Hébert C, De Montigny C, Lavoie N, Blier P. Differential physiological effects of a low dose and high doses of venlafaxine in major depression. *Int J Neuropsychopharmacol* 2007; 10: 51–61.

CHAPTER 2

25. Owens MJ, Krulewicz S, Simon JS, et al. Estimates of serotonin and norepinephrine transporter inhibition in depressed patients treated with paroxetine or venlafaxine. *Neuropsychopharmacology* 2008; 33: 3201–12.
26. Holford N. Pharmacodynamic principles and the time course of delayed and cumulative drug effects. *Transl Clin* 2018; 26: 56.
27. Horowitz MA, Taylor D. Tapering of SSRI treatment to mitigate withdrawal symptoms – authors' reply. *The Lancet Psychiatry* 2019; 6: 562–3.
28. Furukawa TA, Cipriani A, Cowen PJ, Leucht S, Egger M, Salanti G. Optimal dose of selective serotonin reuptake inhibitors, venlafaxine, and mirtazapine in major depression: a systematic review and dose-response meta-analysis. *The Lancet Psychiatry* 2019; 6: 601–9.
29. Moncrieff J, Gupta S, Horowitz MA. Barriers to stopping neuroleptic (antipsychotic) treatment in people with schizophrenia, psychosis or bipolar disorder. *Ther Adv Psychopharmacol* 2020; 10: 2045125320937910.
30. Horowitz MA, Murray RM, Taylor D. Tapering antipsychotic treatment. *JAMA Psychiatry* 2021; 78: 125–6.
31. Lader M, Stender K, Bürger V, Nil R. Efficacy and tolerability of escitalopram in 12- and 24-week treatment of social anxiety disorder: randomised, double-blind, placebo-controlled, fixed-dose study. *Depress Anxiety* 2004; 19: 241–8.
32. Baldwin DS, Montgomery SA, Nil R, Lader M. Discontinuation symptoms in depression and anxiety disorders. *Int J Neuropsychopharmacol* 2007; 10: 73–84.
33. Baldwin DS, Huusom AKT, Maehlum E. Escitalopram and paroxetine compared to placebo in the treatment of generalised anxiety disorder (GAD). *BJPsych* 2006; 189: 264–72.
34. Haddad PM, Anderson IM. Recognising and managing antidepressant discontinuation symptoms. *Adv Psychiatr Treat* 2007; 13: 447–57.
35. Bitter I, Filipovits D, Czobor P. Adverse reactions to duloxetine in depression. *Expert Opin Drug Saf* 2011; 10: 839–50.
36. Horowitz MA, Taylor D. Tapering of SSRI treatment to mitigate withdrawal symptoms. *The Lancet Psychiatry* 2019; 6: 538–46.
37. Murata Y, Kobayashi D, Imuta N, et al. Effects of the serotonin 1A, 2A, 2C, 3A, and 3B and serotonin transporter gene polymorphisms on the occurrence of paroxetine discontinuation syndrome. *J Clin Psychopharmacol* 2010; 30: 11–7.
38. Ruhe H, Horikx A, van Avendonk M, Groeneweg B, Woutersen-Koch H. Multidisciplinary recommednations for discontinuation of SSRIs and SNRIs. *The Lancet Psychiatry* 2019.
39. Lejoyeux M, Ades J. Antidepressant discontinuation: a review of the literature. *J Clin Psychiatry* 1997; 58 Suppl 7: 11–5; discussion 16.
40. Harvey BH, Slabbert FN. New insights on the antidepressant discontinuation syndrome. *Hum Psychopharmacol* 2014; 29: 503–16.
41. Muzina. Discontinuing an antidepressant? Tapering tips to ease distressing symptoms. *Curr Psychiatr*; 9: 50–7.
42. Schatzberg AF, Haddad P, Kaplan EM, et al. Serotonin reuptake inhibitor discontinuation syndrome: a hypothetical definition. Discontinuation consensus panel. *J Clin Psychiatry* 1997; 58 Suppl 7: 5–10.
43. Framer A. What I have learnt from helping thousands of people taper off psychotropic medications. *Ther Adv Psychopharmacol* 2021; 11: 204512532199127.
44. Allison C, Pratt JA. Neuroadaptive processes in GABAergic and glutamatergic systems in benzodiazepine dependence. *Pharmacol Ther* 2003; 98: 171–95.
45. Becker HC. Kindling in alcohol withdrawal. *Alcohol Health Res World* 1998; 22: 25–33.
46. Flemenbaum A. Postsynaptic supersensitivity and kindling: further evidence of similarities. *Am J Drug Alcohol Abuse* 1978; 5: 247–54.
47. Kraus JE. Sensitization phenomena in psychiatric illness: lessons from the kindling model. *J Neuropsychiatry Clin Neurosci* 2000; 12: 328–43.
48. Duncan D, McConnell H, Taylor D. Tardive dyskinesia – how is it prevented and treated? *Psychiatr Bull R Coll Psychiatr* 1997; 21: 422–5.
49. Himei A, Okamura T. Discontinuation syndrome associated with paroxetine in depressed patients: A retrospective analysis of factors involved in the occurrence of the syndrome. *CNS Drugs* 2006; 20: 665–72.
50. Hyman SE, Nestler EJ. Initiation and adaptation: a paradigm for understanding psychotropic drug action. *Am J Psychiatry* 1996; 153: 151–62.

Stratfiying risk of antidepressant withdrawal

Based on the above characteristics, a preliminary means of stratifying patients with regards to their risk of withdrawal symptoms has been derived.[1] From clinical experience, one of the strongest predictors of withdrawal symptoms is past experience of withdrawal symptoms (in a previous attempt at discontinuation, a drug switch or after skipped doses),[2] as recognised in similar efforts to determine risk,[3] and so this was given strong weighting (3 points) (Table 2.11). Duration of use appears to have a strong effect on risk of withdrawal symptoms, including their severity and possibly their duration and therefore this was given strong emphasis (3 points). Antidepressant type (4 points) has been associated with varying risk, as have higher doses (1 point) though to a lesser extent. This approach can only be seen as preliminary and will need to be further clarified with empirical data. However, this approach might offer a useful starting point in clinical practice to begin to stratify patients (Table 2.12), building on earlier approaches to this issue.[3,4]

Table 2.11 Preliminary tool for evaluation of risk of withdrawal for an individual patient, adapted from Horowitz et al. 2022.[1]

Determinant of withdrawal risk	Weighting
Duration of use[a]	
■ Short term (1–6 months)	0 points
■ Intermediate term (6–12 months)	1 point
■ Long term (1–3 years)	2 points
■ Very long-term use (>3 years)	3 points
Antidepressant type	
■ Lowest risk (e.g. agomelatine)	0 points
■ Low risk (e.g. vortioxetine, trimipramine, dosulepin)	1 point
■ Moderate risk (e.g. SSRIs: citalopram, escitalopram, sertraline, fluvoxamine, fluoxetine; TCAs: amitriptyline, nortriptyline, clomipramine, imipramine; other: bupropion)	2 points
■ High risk (e.g. SNRIs: desvenlafaxine, duloxetine, venlafaxine; MAOIs: phenelzine, moclobemide; Other: paroxetine, mirtazapine)	4 points
Dosage	
■ Minimum therapeutic dosage or lower	0 points
■ Greater than the minimum therapeutic dosage	1 point
Past experience of withdrawal symptoms	
■ Stopped antidepressant in past with no withdrawal symptoms/unknown	0 points
■ Mild to moderate withdrawal symptoms	1 point
■ Severe withdrawal symptoms	2 points
■ Very severe withdrawal symptoms	3 points

[a] Note that very short-term use (<4 weeks) is not normally associated with significant risk of withdrawal.
MAOI monoamine oxidase inhibitor, SSRI selective serotonin reuptake inhibitor, SNRI serotonin and norepinephrine reuptake inhibitor, TCA tricyclic antidepressant

Table 2.12 Estimation of risk category for withdrawal for an individual patient, adapted from Horowitz et al. 2023.[1]

Risk category	Low	Medium	High	Very high
Point score	0	1–4	5–8	≥ 9

References

1. Horowitz MA, Framer A, Hengartner MP, Sørensen A, Taylor D. Estimating risk of antidepressant withdrawal from a review of published data. *CNS Drugs* 2023; 37: 143–57.
2. Schatzberg AF, Haddad P, Kaplan EM, et al. Serotonin reuptake inhibitor discontinuation syndrome: A hypothetical definition. Discontinuation consensus panel. *J Clin Psychiatry* 1997; 58 Suppl 7: 5–10.
3. Ruhe H, Horikx A, van Avendonk M, Groeneweg B, Woutersen-Koch H. Multidisciplinary recommendations for discontinuation of SSRIs and SNRIs. *The Lancet Psychiatry* 2019.
4. Fava G. Discontinuing antidepressant medications. In: *Discontinuing Antidepressant Medications*, 1st edn. Oxford University Press, 2021. doi:10.1093/med/9780192896643.001.0001.

Distinguishing antidepressant withdrawal symptoms from relapse

Withdrawal symptoms, which include poor mood, anxiety and insomnia, may be often mistaken for relapse of the underlying disorder for which the patient was prescribed antidepressants, although this has not been systematically studied.[1,2] In general, physicians have been poor at recognising withdrawal from psychotropic medications.[3] When antidepressant withdrawal symptoms were widely believed to be mild and brief (as promulgated by most guidance), the assumption was that any severe and/or long-lasting psychological symptoms reported after stopping or reducing the dose of an antidepressant were likely to represent relapse of an underlying condition.[4] However, as we now understand that withdrawal symptoms are common, can be severe and/or long-lasting, distinguishing these symptoms from relapse becomes clinically important.[4]

The tendency to confound relapse with withdrawal effects has been widely discussed: nearly 15 years ago it was observed that antidepressant '[withdrawal] symptoms may be diagnosed as a relapse or recurrence of the underlying affective illness for which the antidepressant was originally prescribed' (p.449).[5] Several clinical practice guidelines around the world identify the overlap between symptoms of depression and withdrawal symptoms,[6] including guidance by the APA[7] and NICE.[8]

Mis-diagnosis of withdrawal as relapse can have several negative consequences including unnecessary long-term re-instatement of the antidepressant, with ongoing exposure to the adverse effects of the medication, and a more negative prognosis.[5] This mis-diagnosis can result in patients internalising the notion that they require antidepressants, and that they have a severe condition and lead to 'significant social implications' (p.449).[5] Mis-diagnosis of withdrawal effects as relapse by their prescribers was the most common reason people cited for seeking advice on social media sites on how to stop antidepressants.[9,10]

A thorough history will allow identification of several characteristics that allow distinction of withdrawal effects from relapse:

- time of onset,
- presence of distinctive, often physical, symptoms, and
- response to re-instatement.

The presence of severe symptoms that are long-lasting – now recognised to be characteristic of some instances of withdrawal – may also help distinguish withdrawal from relapse in the case when the underlying condition was not characterised by severe symptomatology.[4]

Time of onset

Withdrawal symptoms usually occur hours or days after skipping, reducing or stopping an antidepressant. There is some variability in this – fluoxetine has an effective half-life of 7–15 days and so withdrawal symptoms might be delayed for weeks.[11] It has also been reported that some symptoms of antidepressant withdrawal may not manifest for weeks or longer after discontinuation, even for drugs with short half-lives, although the mechanism for this is not well understood.[12] A delayed decrease in SERT occupancy, lagging plasma concentration decline, is one hypothesised explanation.[13]

CHAPTER 2

Since the withdrawal syndrome is recognised to last for months, or even years, in some patients, symptom duration past a few weeks is not a clear indication of relapse rather than withdrawal.[12,14,15] Relapse would be expected to have onset weeks, months or years later and be much like the original mental health episode, depending on the usual frequency of episodes in the individual's original condition (for some patients, the index episode may relate to a temporary stressor in which case relapse might be unlikely).[5]

For example, NICE says that patients should be told that 'relapse does not usually happen as soon as you stop taking an antidepressant medication or lower the dose', whereas withdrawal symptoms are common soon after dose reductions.[8] As withdrawal symptoms can be reported as being similar to those of relapse, differentiation by symptomology can be diffcult.[16] Rather, the clinician must take into account the chronology: if the symptoms newly arise after missed or decreased doses, even if some time later, as one guidance for GPs puts it, maintain a 'high index of suspicion' (p.449)[17] for a withdrawal syndrome rather than relapse.[4,17,18]

Characteristic symptomology of withdrawal

The distinctive symptoms that differentiate withdrawal symptoms from relapse may be revealed by taking a careful history asking about some of the more common symptoms in Table 2.4 or those in Table 2.5. If physical symptoms co-occur with psychological symptoms, this likely indicates a withdrawal syndrome.[4] For example, if a patient were to experience a surge of anxiety and lowered mood on stopping an antidepressant, and this was also accompanied by nausea, dizziness or electric shock sensations/ 'zaps' (a neurological symptom of withdrawal), we should much more readily conclude that these are withdrawal symptoms rather than relapse of a depressive condition.[4] Occam's razor suggests that, although an episode of relapse and a withdrawal syndrome may co-occur, it is more likely that one condition will cause several symptoms, rather than several conditions co-occurring.[19] Some symptoms are so distinctive, such as the electric 'zaps' – head sensations often experienced on lateral eye movements[20] – which they could be considered pathognomonic of antidepressant withdrawal;[4] dizziness, the most common symptom of antidepressant withdrawal, may also fit into this category.

Even when symptoms on stopping antidepressants are solely psychological in nature, these can be quite distinct from the symptoms of the original condition.[18] For example, if a patient's original condition involved depressed mood and poor appetite, but after stopping antidepressants they now report agitation, anxiety and insomnia, the diagnosis of a withdrawal syndrome should be strongly considered,[4,17] rather than onset of a new mental health condition co-incidentally occurring just at the moment an antidepressant was stopped. Withdrawal symptoms can often be new and qualitatively different from the patient's original condition, while relapse is reminiscent of it.[18] Sometimes, the patient will provide the clue themselves when they say 'this is nothing like my original condition'.[16]

Response to re-instatement

Another means of distinction is the time taken for symptoms to resolve on re-instatement of the antidepressant: for withdrawal symptoms this will be more rapid than for relapse, as demonstrated by resolution within a few days of re-instatement (after several days of

Table 2.13 Distinguishing features between antidepressant withdrawal symptoms and relapse of an underlying condition.

	Withdrawal symptoms	Relapse
Time of onset	Often within hours or days of reducing or stopping antidepressant (but can be delayed for drugs such as fluoxetine – and sometimes for antidepressants with shorter half-lives as well, for reasons that are poorly understood)	Usually weeks or months after stopping an antidepressant (may not be a characteristic if original condition was due to a temporary, resolved stressor)
Duration	Can range from days to months or years	Variable
Response to re-instatement	Improvement can be within hours or days (especially if re-instatement occurs soon after symptoms onset)	Usually delayed by weeks
Distinctive symptoms	Characteristic accompanying symptoms e.g. dizziness, 'brain fog', increased sensitivity to sensory stimuli, depersonalisation/derealisation, muscle cramps. The presence of brain 'zaps' may be pathognomonic. Any symptoms not present in the underlying condition (e.g. patient treated for depression/lethargy developed anxiety, agitation, insomnia on stopping medication). The patient may say 'this is nothing like my original condition'	Not commonly associated – core symptoms are psychological and cognitive; neuro-vegetative symptoms can be a feature. Episodes of individual patients may have typical characteristics

CHAPTER 2

placebo treatment) in a large study.[21] Unlike relapse, withdrawal symptoms commonly will resolve quickly when dosage is restored while tapering[5] and even when antidepressants are recommenced weeks after cessation.[16] However, re-instatement might be less successful when it is delayed for months after the onset of withdrawal symptoms.[12]

The major distinguishing features between withdrawal and relapse are summarised in Table 2.13. Of course, one should continue to be vigilant for genuine relapse of the patient's underlying condition, which may come on weeks or months after treatment is stopped and may have characteristics that are quite typical for the patient.

References

1. Groot PC, van Os J. Antidepressant tapering strips to help people come off medication more safely. *Psychosis* 2018; 10: 142–5.

2. Young A, Haddad P. Discontinuation symptoms and psychotropic drugs. *The Lancet* 2000; 355: 1184–5.

3. Frank D. 'I'm pretty sure it's either food poisoning or Covid-19': lived experience versus medical knowledge in diagnosing substance use problems. *Int J Drug Policy* 2021; 98: 103348.

4. Horowitz MA, Taylor D. Distinguishing relapse from antidepressant withdrawal: clinical practice and antidepressant discontinuation studies. *BJPsych Advances* 2022; 28: 297–311.

5. Haddad PM, Anderson IM. Recognising and managing antidepressant discontinuation symptoms. *Adv Psychiatr Treat* 2007; 13: 447–57.

6. Sørensen A, Jørgensen KJ, Munkholm K. Description of antidepressant withdrawal symptoms in clinical practice guidelines on depression: A systematic review. *J Affect Disord* 2022; published online 11 August. doi:10.1016/j.jad.2022.08.011.

7. Gelenberg AJ, Freeman MP, Markowitz JC, et al. American Psychiatric Association practice guideline for the treatment of patients with major depressive disorder, third edition. *Am J Psychiatry* 2010; 167(suppl): 1–152.

8. National Institute of Health and Social Care (NICE). Depression in adults: Treatment and management I Guidance I NICE. 2022; published online June. https://www.nice.org.uk/guidance/ng222 (accessed 16 July 2022).

9. Guy A, Brown M, Lewis S, Horowitz MA. The 'patient voice' – patients who experience antidepressant withdrawal symptoms are often dismissed, or mis-diagnosed with relapse, or onset of a new medical condition. *Ther Adv Psychopharmacol* 2020; 10: 204512532096718.

10. White E, Read J, Julo S. The role of Facebook groups in the management and raising of awareness of antidepressant withdrawal: is social media filling the void left by health services? *Ther Adv Psychopharmacol* 2021; 11: 2045125320981174.

11. Zajecka J, Fawcett J, Amsterdam J, et al. Safety of abrupt discontinuation of fluoxetine: a randomized, placebo-controlled study. *J Clin Psychopharmacol* 1998; 18: 193–7.

12. Hengartner MP, Schulthess L, Sørensen A, Framer A. Protracted withdrawal syndrome after stopping antidepressants: a descriptive quantitative analysis of consumer narratives from a large internet forum. *Ther Adv Psychopharmacol* 2020; 10: 2045125320980573.

13. Sørensen A, Ruhé HG, Munkholm K. The relationship between dose and serotonin transporter occupancy of antidepressants – a systematic review. *Mol Psychiatry* 2022; 27: 192–201.

14. Stockmann T, Odegbaro D, Timimi S, Moncrieff J. SSRI and SNRI withdrawal symptoms reported on an internet forum. *Int J Risk Saf Med* 2018; 29: 175–80.

15. Davies J, Regina P, Montagu L. All-Party Parliamentary Group for Prescribed Drug Dependence Antidepressant Withdrawal: A Survey of Patients' Experience by the All-Party Parliamentary Group for Prescribed Drug Dependence. 2018. http://prescribeddrug.org/wp-content/uploads/2018/10/APPG-PDD-Survey-of-antidepressant-withdrawal-experiences.pdf (accessed 18 January 2023).

16. Framer A. What I have learnt from helping thousands of people taper off psychotropic medications. *Ther Adv Psychopharmacol* 2021; 11: 204512532199127.

17. Warner CH, Bobo W, Warner C, Reid S, Rachal J. Antidepressant discontinuation syndrome. *Am Fam Physician* 2006; 74: 449–56.

18. Chouinard G, Chouinard VA. New classification of selective serotonin reuptake inhibitor withdrawal. *Psychother Psychosom* 2015; 84: 63–71.

19. Wildner M. In memory of William of Occam. *The Lancet* 1999; 354: 2172.

20. Papp A, Onton JA. Brain zaps: an underappreciated symptom of antidepressant discontinuation. *The Primary Care Companion for CNS Disorders* 2018; 20. doi:10.4088/PCC.18m02311.

21. Rosenbaum JF, Fava M, Hoog SL, Ascroft RC, Krebs WB. Selective serotonin reuptake inhibitor discontinuation syndrome: a randomized clinical trial. *Biol Psychiatry* 1998; 44: 77–87.

Distinguishing antidepressant withdrawal symptoms from new onset of a physical or mental health condition

Distinguishing withdrawal symptoms from new onset of a physical health condition

In addition to withdrawal effects being diagnosed as a relapse of an underlying mental health condition, many patients report that they have had their symptoms mistaken for a new physical health condition, or placed in the category of 'medically unexplained symptoms'.[1] This response is likely because of the wide array of symptoms that antidepressant withdrawal can produce (Table 2.4) and a lack of familiarity with antidepressant withdrawal amongst most physicians.[1] In one survey of (self-selected) patients with antidepressant withdrawal symptoms, about 25% were diagnosed with 'medically unexplained symptoms' or functional neurological disorder (FND), with chronic fatigue syndrome (CFS) also often diagnosed.[1] Antidepressant withdrawal symptoms can also be mis-diagnosed as conditions such as stroke, other neurological disorders, gastrointestinal diseases and adverse effects of other medication that the patient is taking.[2,3]

This is likely to be due to numerous overlapping symptoms of antidepressant withdrawal with these conditions (Table 2.14): tremor, weakness (functional neurological disorder); fatigue, tiredness (CFS) and numerous symptoms that could be grouped under the category of 'medically unexplained symptoms' when the symptoms are not attributed to antidepressant withdrawal.[1] In these cases, these misdiagnoses led to a failure to recommend appropriate treatment (i.e. re-instatement of the antidepressant, followed by a more gradual taper), extensive medical investigation and a feeling on behalf of the patients that they were not listened to.[1] Greater familiarity with the wide variety of symptoms possible in antidepressant withdrawal could prevent this unfortunate mis-diagnosis and consequent mis-management.

Table 2.14 Conditions for which antidepressant withdrawal symptoms are mis-diagnosed.

Condition mis-diagnosed	Antidepressant withdrawal symptoms that overlap with symptoms of conditon
Chronic fatigue syndrome	Fatigue, insomnia, muscle aches
Medically unexplained symptoms/ functional neurological disorder	Tremor, muscle weakness, muscle spasm, pain, fatigue
Gastrointestinal condition	Diarrhoea, constipation, nausea
Stroke/neurological disorder	Muscle weakness, 'electric zaps', tremor, headache, visual changes, sensory changes
Onset of new psychiatric disorder	Anxiety, depression, panic attacks, insomnia, worry, crying attacks, agitation, suicidality

Patients have commented:

I got no help from my doctors. Due to the extreme involuntary movements, my neurologists diagnosed me with a "functional movement disorder", migraines, and chronic fatigue syndrome. I had none of these issues before taking and stopping the venlafaxine.[1]

My psychiatrist wouldn't entertain the idea of protracted withdrawal. My psychiatrist kept saying my symptoms were somatic or medically unexplained.[1]

Distinguishing withdrawal symptoms from new onset of a mental health condition

Another related issue is the possibility of antidepressant withdrawal symptoms being mis-diagnosed as onset of a new mental health condition (Table 2.14).[4] As mentioned above, new onset of symptoms like anxiety or panic that the patient has not previously experienced before antidepressant cessation are more likely to be withdrawal symptoms than onset of a new anxiety or panic disorder that just happen to coincide with drug cessation.[5] The same reasoning can be applied to novel depressed mood. Antidepressant withdrawal symptoms can include manic symptoms,[6] irritability, sleeplessness and anxiety or agitation, leading to inappropriate diagnosis of bipolar disorder.[2] Antidepressant withdrawal-induced akathisia can also be mis-diagnosed as a manic state.[6] Rarely, antidepressant withdrawal symptoms can include psychotic symptoms,[7] which might leading to mis-diagnosis of a new-onset psychotic disorder. Sometimes antidepressant withdrawal symptoms can be attributed to a somatising disorder or other psychosomatic condition, or even a delusional disorder.

References

1. Guy A, Brown M, Lewis S, Horowitz MA. The 'patient voice' – patients who experience antidepressant withdrawal symptoms are often dismissed, or mis-diagnosed with relapse, or onset of a new medical condition. *Ther Adv Psychopharmacol* 2020; 10: 204512532096718.
2. Warner CH, Bobo W, Warner C, Reid S, Rachal J. Antidepressant discontinuation syndrome. *Am Fam Physician* 2006; 74: 449–56.
3. Haddad P, Devarajan S, Dursun S. Antidepressant discontinuation (withdrawal) symptoms presenting as 'stroke'. *J Psychopharmacol* 2001; 15: 139–41.
4. Gabriel M, Sharma V. Antidepressant discontinuation syndrome. *CMAJ* 2017; 189: E747.
5. Horowitz MA, Taylor D. Distinguishing relapse from antidepressant withdrawal: clinical practice and antidepressant discontinuation studies. *BJPsych Advances* 2022; 28: 297–311.
6. Narayan V, Haddad PM. Antidepressant discontinuation manic states: a critical review of the literature and suggested diagnostic criteria. *J Psychopharmacol* 2010; 25: 306–13.
7. Cosci F, Chouinard G. Acute and persistent withdrawal syndromes following discontinuation of psychotropic medications. *Psychother Psychosom* 2020; 89: 283–306.

Withdrawal symptoms during antidepressant maintenance treatment or switching medication

Missed doses causing withdrawal symptoms

Although antidepressant withdrawal symptoms are most often discussed when the dose is being deliberately reduced or medication stopped, it is a common occurrence even during maintenance treatment. After a patient has been taking an antidepressant daily for only a few weeks, doses that are accidentally missed, skipped, taken in the wrong dosage or even taken a few hours late (depending on the half-life of the medication) may result in withdrawal symptoms.[1-4] These odd withdrawal symptoms might be reported as sudden onset psychological or physical symptoms (e.g. dizziness, headache, mood changes).

A potential outcome of inconsistent dosing is the appearance of anxiety, depressed mood and insomnia as withdrawal effects, which might be mis-identified as treatment resistance (i.e. the medication is no longer effective).[5,6] If not recognised, intermittent dosing may bring about the additional risk and expense of inappropriate medical care and prescriptions.[7] Departures from a regular dosing schedule are common among patients, with estimates for irregular dosing being 50% or more.[8,9]

Withdrawal symptoms after switching antidepressants

Withdrawal symptoms may also emerge after a switch from one antidepressant to another, although there has been almost no research on the incidence of withdrawal symptoms in the process of switching.[10] Switching antidepressants is generally employed to remedy non-response or drug adverse reaction.[11] Various techniques for switching have been suggested,[12] though evidence is lacking for the best way to change antidepressants while minimising risk of withdrawal and other adverse effects.[13] The more dissimilar the pharmacodynamic actions (receptor targets) of the two antidepressants, the more likely they are to give rise to withdrawal symptoms on switching. Care should be made not to mistake withdrawal symptoms from the antidepressant being stopped for adverse reactions to the new drug or manifestation of new psychiatric symptoms.[14] Slower cross-titration of antidepressants may minimise the risk of withdrawal effects, but this has not been closely studied.

CHAPTER 2

References

1. Baldwin DS, Cooper JA, Huusom AKT, Hindmarch I. A double-blind, randomized, parallel-group, flexible-dose study to evaluate the toler-ability, efficacy and effects of treatment discontinuation with escitalopram and paroxetine in patients with major depressive disorder. *Int Clin Psychopharmacol* 2006; 21: 159–69.
2. Bauer R, Glenn T, Alda M, et al. Antidepressant dosage taken by patients with bipolar disorder: factors associated with irregularity. *Int J Bipolar Disord* 2013; 1: 26.
3. Demyttenaere K, Haddad P. Compliance with antidepressant therapy and antidepressant discontinuation symptoms. *Acta Psychiatr Scand Suppl* 2000; 403: 50–6.
4. Jha MK, Rush AJ, Trivedi MH. When discontinuing SSRI antidepressants is a challenge: management tips. *Am J Psychiatry* 2018; 175: 1176–84.
5. Fava GA, Cosci F, Guidi J, Rafanelli C. The deceptive manifestations of treatment resistance in depression: a new look at the problem. *Psychother Psychosom* 2020; 89: 265–73.
6. Howes OD, Thase ME, Pillinger T. Treatment resistance in psychiatry: state of the art and new directions. *Mol Psychiatry* 2022; 27: 58–72.
7. Steinman MA. Reaching out to patients to identify adverse drug reactions and nonadherence: necessary but not sufficient. *JAMA Intern Med* 2013; 173: 384–5.
8. Ho SC, Chong HY, Chaiyakunapruk N, Tangiisuran B, Jacob SA. Clinical and economic impact of non-adherence to antidepressants in major depressive disorder: A systematic review. *J Affect Disord* 2016; 193: 1–10.
9. Meijer WE, Bouvy ML, Heerdink ER, Urquhart J, Leufkens HG. Spontaneous lapses in dosing during chronic treatment with selective sero-tonin reuptake inhibitors. *Br J Psychiatry* 2001; 179: 519–22.
10. Framer A. What I have learnt from helping thousands of people taper off psychotropic medications. *Ther Adv Psychopharmacol* 2021; 11: 204512532199127.
11. Carvalho AF, Berk M, Hyphantis TN, McIntyre RS. The integrative management of treatment-resistant depression: a comprehensive review and perspectives. *Psychother Psychosom* 2014; 83: 70–88.
12. Keks N, Hope J, Keogh S. Switching and stopping antidepressants. *Aust Prescr* 2016; 39: 76–83.
13. Fava GA, Gatti A, Belaise C, Guidi J, Offidani E. Withdrawal symptoms after selective serotonin reuptake inhibitor discontinuation: a systematic review. *Psychother Psychosom* 2015; 84: 72–81.
14. Haddad PM, Anderson IM. Recognising and managing antidepressant discontinuation symptoms. *Adv Psychiatr Treat* 2007; 13: 447–57.

How to Deprescribe Antidepressants Safely

The major risks when stopping antidepressants are withdrawal symptoms and relapse. Although there is somewhat limited research evidence on how to safely stop antidepressants,[1] some advice can be offered by using data from existing studies, an understanding of the pharmacology of antidepressants, and lessons learned from practical clinical experience (including patient-reported experience).[2,3] In light of a lack of definitive empirical evidence, shared decision making between the patient and clinician may be the best way to manage the uncertainty.[4,5] Although the principles outlined below apply to all classes of antidepressants, we have focused on the widely used newer generation of antidepressants. Many aspects of this advice will need to be clarified and updated through further research.

Stopping antidepressants can be a difficult process for a significant proportion of patients.[3,6,7] However, by applying pharmacological principles and taking care to modify rate of reduction to manage withdrawal effects for a given patient, the tapering process can be made much more tolerable – ideally just mildly unpleasant. As outlined in the introductory chapter the broad principles for tapering patients off long-term antidepressants are:

- taper gradually (months more often than weeks, and sometimes longer, for longer-term users);
- taper at a rate that the individual patient finds tolerable;
- taper in a hyperbolic pattern of dose decrements (so that dose reductions become smaller and smaller as total dosage gets lower); and
- taper to low doses before stopping, so that the final reduction to zero is not greater (in terms of effect on target receptors) than the reductions previously tolerated[2] (example for citalopram shown in Figure 2.4).

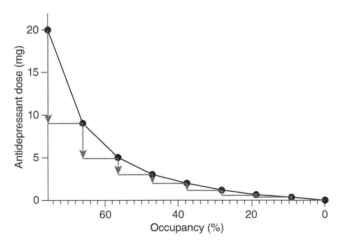

Figure 2.4 Example of hyperbolic tapering of citalopram. Dose reductions are shown on the y-axis, with increasingly small reductions producing equal-sized reductions in occupancy.

CHAPTER 2

In this section, we examine the practical aspects of tapering antidepressants in clinical practice using receptor occupancy as a guide to enable tapering in a pharmacologically rational manner with the following steps:

- estimate the size of the initial reduction and implement this;
- monitor subsequent withdrawal symptoms;
- make decisions about further dose reductions based on this experience; and
- continue this iterative process through to discontinuation.

We also review the practical issues of making up small or intermediary dosages of antidepressants from liquid preparations, or alternatives, as well as some of the psychological issues encountered during tapering.

Theoretical aspects of tapering antidepressants

During long-term use of an antidepressant, the brain and body make adaptations to the drug to maintain homeostasis,[8,9] as they do in response to many psychotropic medications (see introductory chapter). These adaptations are normally referred to as a state of physical dependence.[9,10] In long-term antidepressant use, several adaptations of the serotonergic system have been detected on PET imaging, including changes to serotonin receptor sensitivity, particularly reduced 5-HT_{1A} receptor sensitivity, which have been found to persist for months and years after antidepressants are stopped,[11] though other systems, which have received less attention may also be involved. These adaptations explain why when an antidepressant is stopped abruptly (as in Figure 2.5a), withdrawal symptoms are likely to occur,[7] due to a large discrepancy between the level of drug the system 'expects' and the reduced level of actual drug action.[9] The duration of withdrawal symptoms is largely determined by the time required for adaptations to the presence of the drug to resolve (i.e. to re-adjust to the absence of the drug),[12] and not the time taken for the drug to be eliminated from the system (Figure 2.5a). As there is evidence, from PET studies, that some of the adaptations to antidepressants can take months or years to resolve, this may explain the long duration of withdrawal effects reported by some patients.[11,13,14]

However, if the drug is reduced by small amounts and adequate time permitted before the next reduction so that the brain adjusts to this lesser amount of drug (i.e. a new homeostatic equilibrium is established), the risk of withdrawal effects (and their severity) is likely to be minimised (Figure 2.5b). This can be thought of the difference between jumping from the top of a building to the ground (stopping a drug abruptly) versus going down storey by storey, from the top of a building (tapering a drug with smaller reductions).

Theoretically, lesser amounts of homeostatic disruption brought about by more gradual dose reductions result in reduced risk of severe (and, perhaps, long-lasting) withdrawal symptoms,[3,14] which is supported by some empirical evidence.[15,16] Antidepressants with longer half-lives may also lessen withdrawal symptoms by minimising the degree of homeostatic disruption. Even smaller reductions of dose may further reduce withdrawal symptoms (Figure 2.5c) – analogous to taking even smaller steps down from the top of the building, allowing the brain to make small re-adjustments in its homeostatic equilibrium over a period of time. Another analogy might be made to landing a plane by taking the most direct route towards the ground (abrupt stoppage), versus slowly gliding in to land, flattening out its descent as it approaches the ground to make a soft landing (tapering).

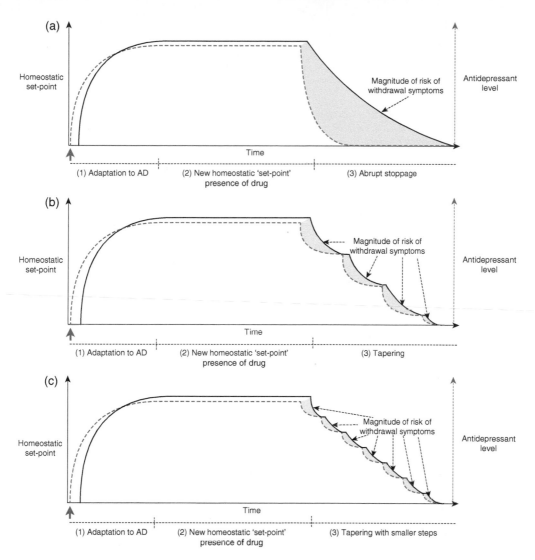

Figure 2.5 The neurobiology of tapering. In this diagram, the homeostatic 'set-point' of the brain is shown in black and antidepressant drug levels are shown in purple dashed lines. The shaded grey regions represent the degree of risk of withdrawal symptoms, the larger the area the greater the risk of withdrawal. (a) (1) and (2) As in the previous section, the brain adapts to levels of a drug used over time. (3) The antidepressant is abruptly ceased and plasma drug levels drop to zero (exponentially, according to the elimination half-life of the drug). This difference between the homeostatic set-point (the 'expectations' of the system) and the level of drug in the system (dashed purple line) is experienced as withdrawal symptoms. (b) (3) Tapering: when a drug is reduced stepwise, drug levels reduce exponentially (dependent on half-life) to lower levels. At each step, there is a lag as the system adapts to a new level of drug, causing withdrawal symptoms (dashed arrows), but of lesser intensity (shaded area under the small cupped curves) than the abrupt discontinuation shown in (a). A new (lower) homeostatic 'set-point' is established before further dose reductions are made. Drugs with longer half-lives may lessen withdrawal symptoms further by minimising the difference between the shifting homeostatic 'set-point' and plasma levels. (c) (3) An even more gradual stepwise reduction, with even smaller risk of withdrawal symptoms (shaded area under the smaller, cupped curves). AD: antidepressant. Adapted from Horowitz and Taylor (2021)[17].

References

1. Van Leeuwen E, Driel ML, Horowitz MA, et al. Approaches for discontinuation versus continuation of long-term antidepressant use for depressive and anxiety disorders in adults. *Cochrane Database Syst Rev* 2021. doi:10.1002/14651858.CD013495.pub2.

2. Horowitz MA, Taylor D. Tapering of SSRI treatment to mitigate withdrawal symptoms. *The Lancet Psychiatry* 2019; 6: 538–46.

3. Framer A. What I have learnt from helping thousands of people taper off psychotropic medications. *Ther Adv Psychopharmacol* 2021; 11: 204512532199127.

4. Groot PC, van Os J. How user knowledge of psychotropic drug withdrawal resulted in the development of person-specific tapering medication. *Ther Adv Psychopharmacol* 2020; 10: 204512532093245.

5. Ruhe H, Horikx A, van Avendonk M, Groeneweg B, Woutersen-Koch H. Multidisciplinary recommendations for discontinuation of SSRIs and SNRIs. *The Lancet Psychiatry* 2019.

6. Guy A, Brown M, Lewis S, Horowitz M. The 'patient voice': patients who experience antidepressant withdrawal symptoms are often dismissed, or misdiagnosed with relapse, or a new medical condition. *Ther Adv Psychopharmacol* 2020; 10: 2045125320967183.

7. Davies J, Read J. A systematic review into the incidence, severity and duration of antidepressant withdrawal effects: are guidelines evidence-based? *Addict Behav* 2019; 97: 111–21.

8. Walewski JW, Filipa JA, Hagen CL, Sanders ST. Standard single-mode fibers as convenient means for the generation of ultrafast high-pulse-energy super-continua. *Appl Phys B* 2006; 83: 75–9.

9. Lerner A, Klein M. Dependence, withdrawal and rebound of CNS drugs: an update and regulatory considerations for new drugs development. *Brain Commun* 2019; 1: fcz025.

10. Brunton LL, Chabner BA, Knollmann BC. *Goodman & Gilman's The Pharmacological Basis of Therapeutics*, 12edn. McGraw-Hill Education, 2011.

11. Bhagwagar Z, Rabiner EA, Sargent PA, Grasby PM, Cowen PJ. Persistent reduction in brain serotonin1A receptor binding in recovered depressed men measured by positron emission tomography with [11C]WAY-100635. *Mol Psychiatry* 2004; 9: 386–92.

12. Reidenberg MM. Drug discontinuation effects are part of the pharmacology of a drug. *J Pharmacol Exp Ther* 2011; 339: 324–8.

13. Cosci F, Chouinard G. Acute and persistent withdrawal syndromes following discontinuation of psychotropic medications. *Psychother Psychosom* 2020; 89: 283–306.

14. Hengartner MP, Schulthess L, Sørensen A, Framer A. Protracted withdrawal syndrome after stopping antidepressants: A descriptive quantitative analysis of consumer narratives from a large internet forum. *Ther Adv Psychopharmacol* 2020; 10: 2045125320980573.

15. Moncrieff J, Read J, Horowitz M. The nature and impact of antidepressant withdrawal symptoms and development of the Discriminatory Antidepressant Withdrawal Symptoms Scale (DAWSS) (in preparation).

16. Horowitz MA, Taylor D. How to reduce and stop psychiatric medication. *Eur Neuropsychopharmacol* 2021; 55: 4–7.

Tapering antidepressants gradually

Existing guidance

A 2021 systematic review of worldwide clinical practice guidelines on treating depression found that 70% recommended that antidepressants should be tapered gradually, but none provided guidance on dose reductions or specific advice on how to implement a tapering regimen.[1] No guideline provided guidance on how to distinguish withdrawal effects from relapse or how to deal with psychological challenges that occur in the tapering process.[1]

For many years guidelines in different countries have recommended that antidepressants be tapered over a few weeks. For example, in the UK, the NICE guidelines until 2022 recommended to 'gradually reduce the dose, normally over a 4-week period', pointing out that 'some people may require longer periods, particularly with drugs with a shorter half-life'. This recommendation was based on expert consensus in response to a study demonstrating that abruptly stopping antidepressants produced too great an incidence of withdrawal effects,[2] with the committee deciding that 4 weeks was a suitable time period.[3] There has been a recent update to this guidance where NICE now advises that the process of discontinuation 'may take weeks or months to complete successfully'.[4] Guidance from RCPsych advises that stopping antidepressants can take 'months or longer', providing examples of tapering regimens that can take 2 or 3 years, or longer.[5] It is known that for some people the process can take years to complete in a tolerable manner.[6] The APA guidelines, last updated in 2010, still recommend to 'taper over the course of at least several weeks', without details of how this should be implemented.[7]

Evidence for gradual tapering

Although there has been little attention paid to rate of tapering in the literature there is some existing evidence that gradual tapering can produce better outcomes than rapid tapering in terms of risk of relapse. A recent survey of specialised deprescribing services around the world, which help people to stop antidepressants, reported that most of their patients took between 3 months and 3 years to come off their antidepressants in a tolerable manner.[8] Note however that people seeking help from these organisations might be the more severe cases of withdrawal.

Speed of tapering and risk of relapse

A meta-analysis has found that discontinuing antidepressants (when compared to continuation of antidepressants) increases the chance of relapse only when it is conducted rapidly (in less than 8 weeks).[9] In studies where tapering is conducted over a longer period of time (up to 6 months) there was no increased chance of relapse compared with continuation of antidepressants (absolute risk difference = –6%, 95% CI –13% to 1%, three trials, n = 732).[9] This extends an earlier finding by Baldessarini and colleagues in which gradual tapering (over >14 days) reduced the overall relapse rate compared with quicker tapering (<14 days).[10] No studies have compared tapering over longer periods (months or years) with maintenance treatment but it may be expected that longer tapering periods might reduce the risk of relapse further.[11–13]

Speed of tapering and risk of withdrawal effects

There is also evidence that tapering more slowly can reduce the chance of intolerable withdrawal symptoms, perhaps by 'spreading out' symptoms over a longer period (Table 2.15).[14–16] Randomised studies show that tapering for up to 14 days either demonstrated no[17] or minimal[18] improvement in withdrawal symptom severity over abrupt discontinuation.[19] It has generally been concluded from these studies that longer tapering regimens are required.[20,21]

Table 2.15 Trials comparing the effects of different rates of antidepressant discontinuation on withdrawal symptoms. Adapted from Horowitz and Taylor (2019)[11].

Study (type)	Medication	Fast arm		Slow arm		Comment
		Taper period	Outcome (%withdrawal syndrome or DESS score)	Taper period	Outcome (% withdrawal syndrome or DESS score)	
Tint and colleagues (2008)[17] (RCT)	SSRIs, venlafaxine	3 days	46%	14 days	46%	No difference in tapering over 3 or 14 days
Baldwin and colleagues (2006)[18] (RCT)	Paroxetine, escitalopram	7 days	Paroxetine – DESS 5.4 Escitalopram – DESS 3.2	14 days	Paroxetine – DESS 5.4 Escitalopram – DESS 3.2	No difference in tapering over 7 or 14 days
Himei and Okamura (2006)[22] (Observ.)	Paroxetine	Abrupt discontinuation	33.8%	Tapering by 5–10mg every 2–4 weeks	4.6%	Large decrease in withdrawal symptoms when tapering over months rather than abruptly
Murata and colleagues (2010)[14] (Observ.)	Paroxetine	Abrupt discontinuation	78.2%	Average taper 39 weeks (range: 2–197 weeks)	6.1%	Tapering over months (and sometimes years) reduced incidence of withdrawal symptoms markedly
Van Geffen (2005)[16] (Observ.)	Fluvoxamine, fluoxetine, paroxetine, citalopram	Abrupt discontinuation	86%	2 weeks to 4 months	52%	Tapering over a few months reduced withdrawal symptoms compared to abrupt stopping

RCT = randomised controlled trials.
Observ. = observational trial

Tapering over months reduces the risk of withdrawal symptoms compared to stopping the drugs abruptly or quickly (over weeks).[14–16,22] In one observational study of patients stopping paroxetine in which the tapering rate was titrated according to the individual's experience of withdrawal symptoms, those patients gradually tapered had far lower rates of withdrawal effects.[14] In the gradual tapering group only 6% of patients experienced a withdrawal syndrome compared with almost 80% of those who stopped abruptly.[14] Notably, the average period for tapering patients was 9 months, with some patients able to taper in a number of weeks and others requiring up to 4 years to do so tolerably. Surveys of patients who have tapered over months using 'tapering strips' demonstrate much less severe withdrawal symptoms (mode 2 out of 7 for severity) compared to those experienced during faster tapering (mode 7 out of 7 for severity).[23]

Patients' anecdotal experience is consistent with this, with reports that some patients can take many months or years to taper off antidepressants in a tolerable manner – though it is not clear for what proportion of patients this will be relevant.[6] One study found that such peer-led community members coming off SSRIs and SNRIs with conventional short tapers (of weeks) experienced on average 79 weeks of withdrawal symptoms.[24] Another study of 600 people found that 87% of respondents experienced withdrawal symptoms for more than 2 months after coming off antidepressants, 59% for more than one year and 16% experienced withdrawal symptoms for more than 3 years.[25] While these patients may represent a more severe group than average (they are a self-selected population of people identifying as being in withdrawal) it does however suggest that the time period taken for some patients to taper off in a tolerable manner may be many months or years. These periods of time are also consistent with reports from professional deprescribing services.[8]

Success rates for different speeds of tapering

It is difficult to estimate the duration of tapering required for patients to stop the drugs without significant consequence. Existing evidence includes the ANTLER trial, which consisted of patients on sertraline, citalopram, fluoxetine and mirtazapine – 70% of whom had been on these medications for more than 3 years – either maintaining or discontinuing their antidepressants in a double-blind randomised controlled trial.[26] The reduction schedule in this trial consisted of halving the dose for those patients on fluoxetine for 4 weeks before stopping the drug, and, for the other antidepressants, halving the dose for 4 weeks, then giving half the dose every second day for another 4 weeks before completely stopping the drugs. Overall, 48% of those allocated to stop their medication dropped out of the trial, suggesting this tapering period of 4–8 weeks was too rapid for almost half of patients (or that they relapsed).[26] There were elevated levels of withdrawal symptoms for 7 months of follow up, further suggesting that this rate of reduction may have given rise to long-lasting withdrawal symptoms in the discontinuation group.[26,27] The severity of withdrawal symptoms was not measured in this study.[26] In this discontinuation group 44% of patients did not relapse – and it is possible that this proportion may have been improved by a slower taper. This study suggests that perhaps up to 44% of patients using antidepressants for more than 2 years may be able to taper off their antidepressant over 8 weeks without significant

CHAPTER 2

difficulty. However, it also possible that tapering over longer than the 8 weeks employed in this study may produce a more tolerable experience in terms of both relapse and withdrawal effects.

This idea is consistent with another randomised controlled trial in which patients with remitted anxiety were intended to reduce their antidepressant over 4 months ('according to a fixed schedule') but only 37% of patients were able to do so.[28] Patients were not surveyed to find out why they could not stop their antidepressants but the authors speculated it was because of withdrawal symptoms.[28,29] Another RCT had similar findings: patients on antidepressants were advised to taper off their antidepressants in 4 weeks (this being consistent with NICE guidance at the time) but this was not feasible for most patients – most (60% of patients) were only able to taper over a 6-month period, indicating that 4 weeks was too short for most patients.[30] As only 48% of participants were able to reduce their antidepressant dose by half or more at the end of this trial, this also suggests that 6 months was too short a period to completely stop medication for a large portion of patients.[30] Another study (also involving mindfulness-based cognitive therapy) found that only 53% of patients were able to completely discontinue antidepressants within 6 months, with a further 13% able to discontinue partially.[31]

Overall these studies suggest that about half of patients on long-term treatment are able to taper their antidepressants in 6 months (Table 2.16), with the remainder likely needing longer periods to taper, though this has not been studied empirically.[3] These findings are consistent with updated NICE guidance recommending that stopping antidepressants 'may take weeks or months to complete successfully',[4] and guidance from RCPsych suggesting it may take a year or longer.[5]

Table 2.16 Proportion of patients able to discontinue antidepressants in given timescale of different randomised controlled trials.

Study	Duration of antidepressant use	Tapering period	Proportion able to stop
Kuyken et al. 2008[32]	>6months	6 months	58–71% (completely)
			17% (reduced)
Kukyken et al. 2015[33]	>3 months	6 months	75%
Bockting et al. 2018[30]	>6 months	6 months	60%
Huijbers et al. 2020/2016[31]	>6 months	6 months	53% (completely)
			13% (reduced)
Scholten et al. 2018[28]	not available	4 months	37%
Lewis et al. 2021[26]	70% > 3 years	4 weeks (fluoxetine) 8 weeks (other ADs)	48% (but withdrawal symptoms elevated for 7 months)

References

1. Sørensen A, Juhl Jørgensen K, Munkholm K. Clinical practice guideline recommendations on tapering and discontinuing antidepressants for depression: a systematic review. *Ther Adv Psychopharmacol* 2022; 12: 20451253211067656.
2. Rosenbaum JF, Fava M, Hoog SL, Ascroft RC, Krebs WB. Selective serotonin reuptake inhibitor discontinuation syndrome: a randomized clinical trial. *Biol Psychiatry* 1998; 44: 77–87.
3. National Institute for Health and Care Excellence (NICE). Depression: The NICE guideline on the treatment and depression the treatment and management of depression. 2010.
4. National Institute for Health and Care Excellence (NICE). Depression in adults: Treatment and management | Guidance | NICE. 2022; published online June. https://www.nice.org.uk/guidance/ng222 (accessed 16 July 2022).
5. Burn W, Horowitz M, Roycroft G, Taylor D. Stopping antidepressants. Stopping antidepressants. 2020. https://www.rcpsych.ac.uk/mental-health/treatments-and-wellbeing/stopping-antidepressants (accessed 23 February 2023).
6. Framer A. What I have learnt from helping thousands of people taper off psychotropic medications. *Ther Adv Psychopharmacol* 2021; 11: 204512532199127.
7. Gelenberg AJ, Freeman MP, Markowitz JC, et al. American Psychiatric Association practice guideline for the treatment of patients with major depressive disorder, third edition. *Am J Psychiatry* 2010; 167(suppl): 1–152.
8. Cooper RE, Ashman M, Lomani J, et al. Stabilise-reduce, stabilise-reduce: a survey of the common practices of deprescribing services and recommendations for future services. *PLoS One* 2023; 18: e0282988.
9. Gøtzsche PC, Demasi M. Interventions to help patients withdraw from depression drugs: A systematic review. *Int J Risk Saf Med.* 2023 September 13. doi: 10.3233/JRS-230011. Epub ahead of print.
10. Baldessarini RJ, Tondo L, Ghiani C, Lepri B. Illness risk following rapid versus gradual discontinuation of antidepressants. *Am J Psychiatry* 2010; 167: 934–41.
11. Horowitz MA, Taylor D. Tapering of SSRI treatment to mitigate withdrawal symptoms. *The Lancet Psychiatry* 2019; 6: 538–46.
12. Horowitz MA, Taylor D. How to reduce and stop psychiatric medication. *Eur Neuropsychopharmacol* 2021; 55: 4–7.
13. Breedvelt JJF, Warren FC, Segal Z, Kuyken W, Bockting CL. Continuation of antidepressants vs sequential psychological interventions to prevent relapse in depression: an individual participant data meta-analysis. *JAMA Psychiatry* 2021; 78: 868–75.
14. Murata Y, Kobayashi D, Imuta N, et al. Effects of the serotonin 1A, 2A, 2C, 3A, and 3B and serotonin transporter gene polymorphisms on the occurrence of paroxetine discontinuation syndrome. *J Clin Psychopharmacol* 2010; 30: 11–7.
15. Groot PC, van Os J. Antidepressant tapering strips to help people come off medication more safely. *Psychosis* 2018; 10: 142–5.
16. Van Geffen ECGG, Hugtenburg JG, Heerdink ER, van Hulten RP, Egberts ACGG. Discontinuation symptoms in users of selective serotonin reuptake inhibitors in clinical practice: tapering versus abrupt discontinuation. *Eur J Clin Pharmacol* 2005; 61: 303–7.
17. Tint A, Haddad PM, Anderson IM. The effect of rate of antidepressant tapering on the incidence of discontinuation symptoms: A randomised study. *J Psychopharmacol* 2008; 22: 330–2.
18. Baldwin DS, Cooper JA, Huusom AKT, Hindmarch I. A double-blind, randomized, parallel-group, flexible-dose study to evaluate the tolerability, efficacy and effects of treatment discontinuation with escitalopram and paroxetine in patients with major depressive disorder. *Int Clin Psychopharmacol* 2006; 21: 159–69.
19. Montgomery SA, Kennedy SH, Burrows GD, Lejoyeux M, Hindmarch I. Absence of discontinuation symptoms with agomelatine and occurrence of discontinuation symptoms with paroxetine: a randomized, double-blind, placebo-controlled discontinuation study. *Int Clin Psychopharmacol* 2004; 19: 271–80.
20. Haddad PM, Anderson IM. Recognising and managing antidepressant discontinuation symptoms. *Adv Psychiatr Treat* 2007; 13: 447–57.
21. Phelps J. Tapering antidepressants: is 3 months slow enough? *Med Hypotheses* 2011; 77: 1006–8.
22. Himei A, Okamura T. Discontinuation syndrome associated with paroxetine in depressed patients: a retrospective analysis of factors involved in the occurrence of the syndrome. *CNS Drugs* 2006; 20: 665–72.
23. Groot PC, van Os J. Successful use of tapering strips for hyperbolic reduction of antidepressant dose: a cohort study. *Ther Adv Psychopharmacol* 2021; 11: 20451253211039330.
24. Stockmann T, Odegbaro D, Timimi S, Moncrieff J. SSRI and SNRI withdrawal symptoms reported on an internet forum. *Int J Risk Saf Med* 2018; 29: 175–80.
25. Davies J, Regina P, Montagu L. All-Party Parliamentary Group for Prescribed Drug Dependence Antidepressant Withdrawal: A Survey of Patients' Experience by the All Party Parliamentary Group for Prescribed Drug Dependence. All-Party Parliamentary Group for Prescribed Drug Dependence, 2018 http://prescribeddrug.org/wp-content/uploads/2018/10/APPG-PDD-Survey-of-antidepressant-withdrawal-experiences.pdf (accessed 23 February 2023).
26. Lewis G, Marston L, Duffy L, et al. Maintenance or discontinuation of antidepressants in primary care. *N Engl J Med* 2021; 385: 1257–67.
27. Lewis G, Lewis G. Half of people who stopped long term antidepressants relapsed within a year, study finds: rapid response. *BMJ* 2021; published online 20 October. https://www.bmj.com/content/374/bmj.n2403/rr-1 (Accessed 1st March, 2022).
28. Scholten WD, Batelaan NM, Van Oppen P, et al. The efficacy of a group CBT relapse prevention program for remitted anxiety disorder patients who discontinue antidepressant medication: a randomized controlled trial. *Psychother Psychosom* 2018; 87: 240–2.
29. Fava GA, Belaise C. Discontinuing antidepressant drugs: lesson from a failed trial and extensive clinical experience. *Psychother Psychosom* 2018; 87: 257–67.

CHAPTER 2

30. Bockting CLH, Klein NS, Elgersma HJ, et al. Effectiveness of preventive cognitive therapy while tapering antidepressants versus maintenance antidepressant treatment versus their combination in prevention of depressive relapse or recurrence (DRD study): A three-group, multicentre, randomised control. *The Lancet Psychiatry* 2018; 5: 401–10.

31. Huijbers MJ, Wentink C, Simons E, Spijker J, Speckens A. Discontinuing antidepressant medication after mindfulness-based cognitive therapy: a mixed-methods study exploring predictors and outcomes of different discontinuation trajectories, and its facilitators and barriers. *BMJ Open* 2020; 10: e039053.

32. Kuyken W, Byford S, Taylor RS, et al. Mindfulness-based cognitive therapy to prevent relapse in recurrent depression. *J Consult Clin Psychol* 2008; 76: 966–78.

33. Kuyken W, Hayes R, Barrett B, et al. Effectiveness and cost-effectiveness of mindfulness-based cognitive therapy compared with maintenance antidepressant treatment in the prevention of depressive relapse or recurrence (PREVENT): a randomised controlled trial. *The Lancet* 2015; 386: 63–73.

Hyperbolic tapering of antidepressants

Theoretical aspects

In addition to the speed of tapering, the pattern of dose reduction is also likely to be important when trying to minimise withdrawal effects for a patient, because of the pharmacology of antidepressants.[1] As outlined in the introductory chapter, the law of mass action dictates that when few molecules of a drug are present, every additional milligram of drug will have large additional effects, because of the large number of unoccupied receptors to act upon, while when larger amounts of the drug are present, receptors are increasingly saturated and so each additional milligram of drug will have smaller and smaller incremental effects.[2] This leads to a typical hyperbolic relationship between the dose of an antidepressant and the effect on target receptors, as revealed by PET imaging of SERT (and other targets such as the noradrenaline transporter (NET)) occupancy caused by SSRIs, SNRIs and other antidepressants using radiolabelled ligands (e.g. sertraline in Figure 2.6).[3,4] The relationship between the dose of drug and the effect on the brain (in this case inhibition of the serotonin transporter) is very steep at small doses, with the curve flattening out at doses commonly employed clinically.

This hyperbolic relationship between dose of antidepressant and occupancy of SERT is not particular to SERT occupancy but applies to the other targets of antidepressants, for example the NET,[5,6] or cholinergic, histaminergic and serotonergic receptors (which may also be responsible for the pathogenesis of withdrawal effects).[7] The law of mass action also describes the effect on these receptors.[2,3] This relationship is sometimes obscured in textbooks and academic papers by plotting dose–response relationships with drug dose on logarithmic axes, giving the impression of a linear relationship between drug dose and effect.[2,8] Both the clinical effects of antidepressants on symptom scores and adverse effects (as indicated by drop outs from studies) show a hyperbolic relationship with dose.[9] In animals, microdialysis studies show that extracellular serotonin levels show a hyperbolic relationship with dosage of antidepressants,[10] suggesting that the effects of antidepressants from the molecular level to the clinical level are all similarly hyperbolic in pattern, as they are for other drug classes.[11]

Although tapering antidepressants by linear amounts (for example, 50mg, 37.5mg, 25mg, 12.5mg, 0mg for sertraline) seems intuitively appealing (and practical, through splitting tablets), because of the hyperbolic relationship between dose of antidepressant and effect on its principal target, the SERT, this linear pattern of tapering will produce increasingly large reductions in effect on SERT occupancy (Figure 2.6a and Table 2.17).[1] This is likely to be associated with increasingly severe withdrawal symptoms, as patients often report when they reduce at lower doses of antidepressant.[12]

While the relationship between dose of antidepressant and effect on SERT occupancy has not yet been shown to have a direct relationship to withdrawal effects, such a relationship remains highly plausible because all studied biochemical and clinical effects follow a hyperbolic relationship with antidepressant dosage. A paper has reported that withdrawal effect shows a 'mirror-image' relationship with rate of tapering, suggesting that withdrawal effects may indeed correlate with receptor occupancy.[13] This is also consistent with patient accounts.[12,14] Given the pharmacology of antidepressants, it is difficult to put forward a rationale for linear tapering.

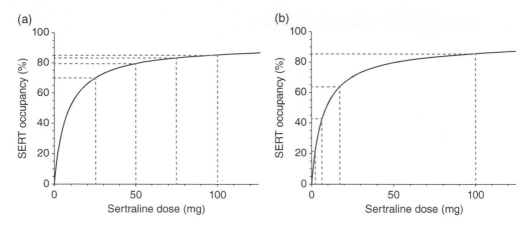

Figure 2.6 (a) Linear reductions of dose cause increasingly large reductions in effect on receptor targets, probably associated with more withdrawal effects. (b) Even reductions of effect at target receptors requires hyperbolic dose reductions. The final dose before stopping will need to be very small so that this step down is not larger (in terms of effect on the brain) than previous reductions.

Table 2.17 SERT occupancy produced by linear reductions of sertraline and the change in SERT produced by each step.

Dose (mg)	Serotonin transporter (SERT) occupancy (%)	Decrease in SERT occupancy from preceding step (%)
50	81.0	–
37.5	77.5	3.5
25	71.2	6.3
12.5	57.3	13.9
0	0	57.3

It seems more pharmacologically rational to reduce the drug in such a way that produces an 'even' amount of reduction in effect on target receptors with each step – which entails hyperbolic dose reductions (Figure 2.6b). In this figure reductions of 20 percentage points (Box 2.1) of SERT occupancy are shown, but smaller gradations can be made such as shown in Table 2.18. From Table 2.18 it can be seen that reducing in a manner that produces the same-sized reductions in SERT occupancy requires making dose reductions by smaller and smaller amounts. For example, the dose reduction from 50mg to 34mg of sertraline produces the same-sized reduction in SERT occupancy as the dose reduction from 2.1mg to 1.5mg. Note how small the final doses are required to be so that the final 'step down' from the lowest dose to zero is not larger (in terms of effect at target receptors) than the prior reductions in dose that have been tolerable for the patient – in this example it is 0.44mg. This, again, is comparable to the manner in which planes land: they follow a hyperbolic pattern of descent, flattening out the angle of descent as they approach the ground to make a soft landing. The NICE guidelines and RCPsych both recommend this pattern of tapering antidepressants (by making smaller and smaller sized reductions).

Box 2.1 Defintion of a percentage point.

Note: A percentage point means one point on a scale. For example, 80% receptor occupancy when reduced by 20 percentage points will produce 60% receptor occupancy. This is distinct from reducing 80% by 20% which will give 64% receptor occupancy.

Table 2.18 An example reduction schedule for sertraline consisting of 5 percentage point reductions.

SERT occupancy (%)	Amount of SERT occupancy decrease (percentage points)	Dose (mg)
80		50
75	5	34
70	5	25
65	5	19
60	5	14
55	5	11
50	5	9.2
45	5	7.4
40	5	5.9
35	5	4.7
30	5	3.7
25	5	2.9
20	5	2.1
15	5	1.5
10	5	0.94
5	5	0.44
0	5	0

Such reductions may be made every 2–4 weeks if tolerated by the patient. Such a schedule can be compressed (by taking every second, or third or fourth step) or dilated by placing further intermediate steps in between each reduction, while still retaining equal differences in terms of receptor occupancy between steps (as for the bellows on an accordion). Such a regimen preserves equal reductions in effect on SERT occupancy between each step. Doses are rounded to two significant figures.

The reduction regimens shown in the chapters dedicated to individual drugs follow this pattern of hyperbolic reductions, with more or less widely spaced steps in between doses. For each suggested regimen, the difference in SERT occupancy is preserved between the given steps, producing a pharmacologically rational regimen (Box 2.2). This can be thought of as something like the bellows on an accordion – where the steps are equally spaced apart but can be compressed (tapering quicker) or dilated (tapering more slowly) according to the degree to which the patient tolerates the withdrawal process.

CHAPTER 2

> **Box 2.2** Tapering according to receptor occupancy (e.g. SERT occupancy).
>
> To taper at an even rate, a dose decrease is made such that the degree of serotonin transporter occupancy is reduced by a certain number of percentage points of SERT occupancy. For example, reducing sertraline from 50mg by an amount equal to 5 percentage points of SERT occupancy will give a dose of 34mg (Table 2.17).

Empirical support for hyperbolic tapering

Although there has been limited research into tapering practice, there is some empirical support for tapering according to this hyperbolic pattern of dose reduction for antidepressants using 'tapering strips'.[15,16] 'Tapering strips' are composed of compounded formulations of small doses of antidepressants – for example 5mg, 2mg, 1mg, 0.5mg, 0.2mg and 0.1mg of citalopram – packaged into plastic pouches (similar to the way in which different change is made up by small denominations of coins) in such a way as to produce very gradual dose reductions (with the reductions slowing down at lower doses): e.g. 20mg, 19mg, 18mg, 17mg … 1mg, 0.7mg, 0.5mg, 0.2mg, 0mg. These tapering strips are arranged in a hyperbolic pattern so that reductions are made by smaller and smaller decrements as total dosage gets lower (Figure 2.7).

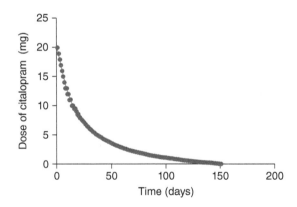

Figure 2.7 Hyperbolic pattern of dose reduction produced by tapering strips. These trajectories end at small fractions of commonly used doses – example for citalopram provided. Note the similarity with the suggested hypothetical tapering regime in Figure 2.4.

Several studies have now demonstrated that patients on long-term antidepressants who have been unable to taper using conventional approaches are able to taper off their antidepressants when following this pattern of hyperbolic dose reduction,[15-17] and are able to stay off their medication at long periods of follow up (1–5 years).[17] For example, one study involved surveying 824 individuals who used this hyperbolic method to taper off their antidepressants who had a median duration of use of 5–10 years. Most of these patients were using venlafaxine and paroxetine, and 71% had been unable to come off their antidepressants using conventional means.[15] With the help of tapering strips, 72%

of this group were able to discontinue their antidepressant when using a hyperbolic dose reduction schedule, which led to a final dose before stopping of about 0.5mg for paroxetine and 1mg for venlafaxine, in line with the small final doses predicted by the receptor occupancy curves.[1,18] In a similar population, 66% were able to stay off their antidepressant for 1–5 years (patients were sampled after differing periods of follow up).[17] Furthermore, most patients who used tapering strips reported that they mostly experienced mild withdrawal symptoms (most commonly rated at 2 out of 7 intensity) – this was in strong contrast to the largely severe withdrawal symptoms they experienced when tapering according to usual clinical practice (most commonly rated at 7 out of 7 intensity).[15]

Given a lack of RCTs in this area, another useful source of knowledge is from peer-led psychiatric drug tapering communities. From years of trial and error these groups have found that dose reductions made according to an exponential pattern (e.g. reductions of 10% of the most recent dose, so that the size of reductions gets progressively smaller as the total dosage becomes smaller),[12] derived originally from protocols for coming off benzodiazepines,[19] are the most helpful in getting people off their medication. Such regimens are strikingly close approximations to the hyperbolic dose reduction schedules derived from knowledge of receptor occupancy suggesting convergence between practical experience and theory (Figure 2.8).

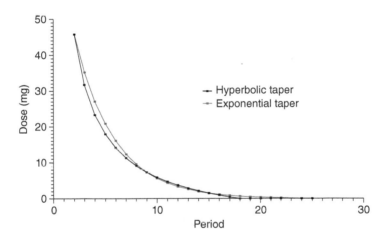

Figure 2.8 Exponential tapering (reducing dose according to a proportion of the most recent dose) and hyperbolic tapering (tapering according to the dose-effect relationship of the drugs) produce remarkably similar reduction regimens. It is striking that the pattern of dose reductions derived by trial and error by patients and clinicians like Professor Ashton[12,19,20] are so similar to the hyperbolic dose reductions predicted by the receptor occupancy of the drugs. There are discrepancies between these approaches at higher doses (exponential slower than hyperbolic) and at lower doses (exponential slower than hyperbolic and theoretically never meets zero but approaches it asymptotically).

CHAPTER 2

References

1. Horowitz MA, Taylor D. Tapering of SSRI treatment to mitigate withdrawal symptoms. *The Lancet Psychiatry* 2019; 6: 538–46.
2. Holford N. Pharmacodynamic principles and the time course of delayed and cumulative drug effects. *Translational and Clinical Pharmacology* 2018; 26: 56.
3. Meyer JH, Wilson AA, Sagrati S, et al. Serotonin transporter occupancy of five selective serotonin reuptake inhibitors at different doses: an [11C]DASB positron emission tomography study. *Am J Psychiatry* 2004; 161: 826–35.
4. Sørensen A, Ruhé HG, Munkholm K. The relationship between dose and serotonin transporter occupancy of antidepressants – a systematic review. *Mol Psychiatry* 2021; 1–10.
5. Moriguchi S, Takano H, Kimura Y, et al. Occupancy of norepinephrine transporter by duloxetine in human brains measured by positron emission tomography with (S,S)-[18F]FMeNER-D2. *Int J Neuropsychopharmacol* 2017; 20(12): 957–62.
6. Takano A, Halldin C, Farde L. SERT and NET occupancy by venlafaxine and milnacipran in nonhuman primates: a PET study. *Psychopharmacology* 2013; 226: 147–53.
7. Horowitz MA, Framer A, Hengartner MP, Sørensen A, Taylor D. Estimating risk of antidepressant withdrawal from a review of published data. *CNS Drugs* 2023; 37: 143–57.
8. Horowitz MA, Taylor D. Tapering of SSRI treatment to mitigate withdrawal symptoms – authors' reply. *The Lancet Psychiatry* 2019; 6: 562–3.
9. Furukawa TA, Cipriani A, Cowen PJ, Leucht S, Egger M, Salanti G. Optimal dose of selective serotonin reuptake inhibitors, venlafaxine, and mirtazapine in major depression: a systematic review and dose-response meta-analysis. *The Lancet Psychiatry* 2019; 6: 601–9.
10. Beyer CE, Boikess S, Luo B, Dawson LA. Comparison of the effects of antidepressants on norepinephrine and serotonin concentrations in the rat frontal cortex: An in-vivo microdialysis study. *J Psychopharmacol* 2002; 16: 297–304.
11. Leucht S, Crippa A, Siafis S, Patel MX, Orsini N, Davis JM. Dose-response meta-analysis of antipsychotic drugs for acute schizophrenia. *Am J Psychiatry* 2020; 177: 342–53.
12. Framer A. What I have learnt from helping thousands of people taper off psychotropic medications. *Ther Adv Psychopharmacol* 2021; 11: 204512532199127.
13. Van Os J, Groot P. Patterns and moderators of 'controlled' withdrawal in high-risk patients using taperingstrips for hyperbolic reduction of antidepressants. 2023; published online February
14. Stockmann T. What it was like to stop an antidepressant. *Ther Adv Psychopharmacol* 2019; 9: 2045125319884834.
15. Groot PC, van Os J. Successful use of tapering strips for hyperbolic reduction of antidepressant dose: A cohort study. *Ther Adv Psychopharmacol* 2021; 11: 20451253211039330.
16. Groot PC, van Os J. Antidepressant tapering strips to help people come off medication more safely. *Psychosis* 2018; 10: 142–5.
17. Groot PC, van Os J. Outcome of antidepressant drug discontinuation with taperingstrips after 1–5 years. *Ther Adv Psychopharmacol* 2020; 10: 204512532095460.
18. Ruhe H, Horikx A, van Avendonk M, Groeneweg B, Woutersen-Koch H. Multidisciplinary recommendations for discontinuation of SSRIs and SNRIs. *The Lancet Psychiatry* 2019.
19. Ashton H. Benzodiazepines: How they work and how to withdraw. *The Ashton Manual*. 2002. http://www.benzo.org.uk/manual/bzcha01.htm (accessed 18 January 2023).
20. Moncrieff J, Read J, Horowitz M. The nature and impact of antidepressant withdrawal symptoms and development of the Discriminatory Antidepressant Withdrawal Symptoms Scale (DAWSS) (in preparation).

Practical options in prescribing gradually tapering doses of antidepressants

The dose forms available for most antidepressants are those marketed for therapeutic use, not for hyperbolic tapering. For many drugs, it is difficult to find dose forms that are anywhere near small enough for such tapers. The smallest available tablets produce high receptor occupancy such that going from this tablet to zero would cause a very large reduction in effect, likely producing substantial withdrawal symptoms for some patients.[1] The NICE guidance on stopping antidepressants recommends, for example, 'if once very small doses have been reached, slow tapering cannot be achieved using tablets or capsules, consider using liquid preparations if available.'[2] The RCPsych guidance on 'Stopping antidepressants' provides examples throughout involving splitting tablets, or using liquid versions of antidepressants to make up doses that cannot be made up by splitting existing tablet formulations.[3]

To prepare dosages that allow steps in between or lower than doses widely available in tablet formulations, licensed and 'off-label' options are available, as outlined in the introductory chapter, in which the option of splitting tablets is discussed, as well as the difference between a solution and a suspension. Some specific remarks relevant to antidepressants are highlighted here.

Every-other-day dosing

In order to facilitate tapering it can be tempting to make dose reductions by having patients take a tablet every other day or every third day so that their overall dose per day is reduced. However, this method is not recommended for antidepressants other than fluoxetine.[4] The half-lives of most antidepressants are 24 hours or less, so dosing every second day will cause plasma levels of the drug to fall to one-quarter of peak levels before the next dose. It is widely recognised that skipping doses can induce withdrawal effects[5,6] from antidepressants, something which patients routinely report,[7] and every-other-day dosing to taper has similar consequences. This effect may be even more pronounced for antidepressants like paroxetine, which strongly inhibit its own metabolism (by inhibiting the P450 2D6 isoenzyme) and which therefore will demonstrate increasingly rapid elimination as doses get lower.[8]

The exception to this rule is fluoxetine, which has an active metabolite, norfluoxetine, which has a half-life of 7 to 15 days and so can be dosed as infrequently as once a week without a significant effect on steady state plasma levels or on trough levels. In general it is better to taper patients by prescribing the same small dose every day (using options outlined below) rather than increasing the time between doses.

Manufacturers' liquids

Apart from tablet splitting (covered in the introductory chapters), the most widely available option for making up doses that are smaller than those available in tablets is liquid versions of a drug. According to the British National Formulary (BNF),[9]

8 out of the 10 most commonly used antidepressants[10] in the UK are produced by their manufacturer in liquid (or dispersible tablet) form, which can facilitate the process of tapering (Table 2.19).[11] In the USA, 6 out of 10 of these antidepressants are available in liquid (or dispersible tablet) form (Table 2.20).[12]

These bottles of liquids usually contain a fixed amount of drug in 5mL of liquid but sometimes come with a droplet mechanism, which generally provides 0.1mL per drop when the bottle is held upside down. This allows only specific doses to be given – for example, citalopram drops give a dose of 2mg each, so multiples of 2mg can be given, but half drops cannot be administered. Alternatively, the droplet mechanism from these bottles is removable, and this allows the use of a small oral syringe to draw up small amounts of liquid, giving greater precision (for example, using a 1mL syringe, with 0.01mL gradations).

Some, but not all, liquid formulations are more expensive than tablets. For those liquid formulations that are more expensive, short-term use of this formulation might lead to a reduction in adverse effects from the process and longer-term savings when the medication is successfully ceased[13] (as well as a reduction in adverse effects to the patient and healthcare system).

Table 2.19 Manufacturer's liquid and dispersible tablet formulations available for the 10 most commonly used antidepressants in the UK for 2017–2018.[10]

Drug	Smallest oral tablet/capsule	Manufacturer's liquid preparation available (concentration, volume)	Dispersible tablet available (dose)
SSRIs			
Citalopram	10mg	Yes (40mg/mL, 15mL)	N/A
Escitalopram	5mg	Yes (20mg/mL, 15mL)	N/A
Fluoxetine	10mg	Yes (20mg/5mL, 70mL)	Yes (20mg)
Paroxetine	10mg	N/A*	N/A
Sertraline	25mg	Yes (100mg/5mL, 60mL)	N/A
SNRIs			
Duloxetine	20mg	N/A	N/A
Venlafaxine	37.5mg	Yes (37.5mg/5mL, 150mL)	N/A
TCAs			
Amitriptyline	10mg	Yes (25mg/5mL, 150mL)	N/A
Others			
Mirtazapine	15mg	Yes (15mg/mL, 66mL)	Yes (15mg)
Trazodone	50mg	Yes (50mg/5mL, 120mL)	N/A

These 10 drugs account for 96.5% of all antidepressant prescriptions. Only sertraline, duloxetine and paroxetine do not come in liquid or dispersible forms. All data from the British National Formulary.[9] Further information provided in drug-specific sections.

*Paroxetine is available as a liquid as a 'Special' in the UK.

Table 2.20 Options available for making up small dosage forms of antidepressants in the USA. Adapted from Bostwick and Demehri (2014),[12] the FDA Orange book[14] and the relevant FDA-approved labels (cited in the table).

Drug	Liquid preparation available	Dispersible tablet available	Crushable	Comment
SSRIs				
Citalopram	Yes	No	Yes	
Escitalopram	Yes	No	Yes	
Fluoxetine	Yes	No	Yes	
Fluvoxamine	No	No	Yes (Luvox)	Immediate-release form is crushable, controlled release form should not be crushed.
Paroxetine	Yes	No	Yes (Paxil)	Immediate-release form is crushable, if the controlled release form is crushed its controlled release properties are lost (and it should be treated as an immediate-release drug).
Sertraline	Yes	No	Yes	
SNRIs				
Duloxetine	No	No	No	Label states that the capsule should not be opened. Institute of Safe Medication Practices states contents of capsule can be added to apple sauce or apple juice.
Venlafaxine	No	No	Yes (Effexor)	The extended-release form should not be crushed. The FDA label allows carefully opening the capsule and sprinkling the spheroidal contents on a spoonful of apple sauce, advising this to be consumed immediately without chewing and followed by a glass of water.[15]
TCAs				
Amitriptyline	No	No	Yes	Crushing produced a local anaesthetic effect in the mouth.
Others				
Bupropion	No	No	Yes (Wellbutrin)	Label advises that the slow-release form of bupropion should not be crushed as this may lead to an increase risk of adverse effects, including seizures.[16]
Mirtazapine	No	Yes	Yes	
Trazodone	No	No	Yes	Crushing might result in poor taste and a local anaesthetic effect in the mouth.
Vortioxetine	No	No	Yes	

Dilutions of manufacturers' liquids

The manufacturers' liquid versions of antidepressants are often quite concentrated – for example citalopram comes as a 40mg/mL solution.[17] As greater errors are found when measuring less than 20% of the labelled capacity of a syringe[18] and the smallest syringe widely available is the 1mL syringe, the smallest dose that could be measured accurately with a syringe (after removing the dropper mechanism) is 8mg (0.2mL). This means that dilution of these liquids is often necessary to make the small doses needed by some patients. Citalopram, for example, can be mixed with water or juice according to the Summary of Product Characteristics (SmPC) approved by the MHRA.[17] In the USA, for example, the FDA advises that sertraline liquid must be diluted before use with water or acidic juices.[19] This allows formulation of the very small doses suggested to facilitate tolerable tapering of antidepressants (Box 2.3). The MHRA and FDA guidance both advise that such dilutions be consumed 'immediately', which may be interpreted as within an hour of preparation.[17]

It is likely that this recommendation is based on little more than guesswork. Studies have found that there was less than 5% degradation over 8 weeks of fluoxetine solution in fruit juice, or other common diluents, as assessed by high-performance liquid chromatography.[20] Similarly, citalopram solution in water showed no significant degradation over 30 days when stored in the dark.[21] The biological stability of other antidepressant dilutions has not been formally evaluated but this is likely to be unproblematic if solutions are stored in a refrigerator for several days. Some of the manufacturers' labels do not specifically state that a solution of an antidepressant can be diluted in water but as these drugs are frequently dissolved in water, further dilution in water should not be an issue. When the manufacturers' liquids are not aqueous solutions, then dilutions in water might have the effect of precipitating the drug and so a suspension might be formed. All dilutions need therefore to be shaken thoroughly before use.

Box 2.3 Steps required to make a dilution of citalopram oral drops equivalent to 2mg of citalopram in tablet form. Other doses can be made following similar rules. Pharmacists will be a useful source of advice on these issues.

To deliver citalopram solution equivalent to 2mg of citalopram in solid form from the manufacturer's drops:

- Citalopram drops (40mg/mL) have 25% more bio-availability than tablets so that 8mg of citalopram from oral drops is equivalent to 10mg of citalopram from a tablet (SmPC)[17]
- 2mg of citalopram (tablet) is equivalent to 1.6mg of citalopram (oral drops)
- Volume of citalopram = 1.6mg/ (40mg/mL) = 0.04mL
- The smallest volume that can be measured with a 1mL syringe is 0.2mL; therefore a dilution is required
- Citalopram oral drops can be mixed with water, orange or apple juice (according to its SmPC)[17]
- 0.5mL of citalopram oral drops in 4.5mL of water will produce a solution with a concentration of 4mg/mL
- Concentration = mass/volume
- Therefore, volume = mass/concentration
- Volume of this solution required = 1.6mg/ (4mg/mL) = 0.4mL (which can be measured accurately with a 1mL syringe)
- The SmPC for citalopram recommends that this solution is consumed 'immediately', which might be interpreted as meaning within an hour.
- Adding water to the original solution may have the effect of precipitating citalopram and so a suspension might be formed. All dilutions need therefore to be shaken thoroughly before use.

Custom compounding of individualised dosages

Compounded liquids (e.g. 'Specials' in the UK)

For some of those antidepressants that are not made by their manufacturer into liquid formulations, liquid versions can be compounded at specialist pharmacies (for example, paroxetine is available as a prescription 'Special' in the UK) (Table 2.21). In the UK, the only commonly used antidepressant not available as either a widely available liquid, dispersible tablet or as a 'Special' is duloxetine, which comes in a form that cannot be liquefied.

Table 2.21 Applicability of different options for sertraline, venlafaxine and duloxetine in the UK – including availability as a 'Special', solubility of the drug in water and stability of beads if emptied out of capsule.

Drugs	Available as Special liquid form (conc., volume)[9,*]	Solubility in water	Bead stability if emptied out of MR capsule	Comment
Duloxetine	No	'slightly soluble'[22] (suspension in 100mL of water)	Yes[23]	Eli Lilly study found that beads emptied from a capsule retained their slow-release properties when mixed with apple juice or apple sauce.[23] The drug label advises against sprinkling contents onto food or mixing with liquids because these actions might affect its enteric coating.[22]
Venlafaxine	Yes (75mg/5mL, 150mL)	572mg/mL[24] (solution in 100mL of water)	Yes[25]	Wyeth's product label allows opening capsules and sprinkling contents on a spoonful of apple sauce.[26] MR capsules can be opened and sprinkled onto soft food (North East Essex NHS guide).[27] Absorption profile is unaffected by this process.[25]
				Instant release tablets (as hydrochloride) disperse within 5 minutes when shaken in 10mL of water to form a dispersion with some larger granules (RPS enteral feeding guide).[28]
Sertraline	Yes (50mg/mL, 150mL)	'slightly soluble'[19]	N/A	Tablet will disintegrate if shaken in 10mL of water for a few minutes, giving a dispersion with some visible particles (RPS enteral feeding guide).[28] Pfizer does not have stability data and so advice is to administer immediately (RPS enteral feeding guide).[28]

*Paroxetine is also available as a liquid as a 'Special' in the UK.

Compounded capsules or tablets

As outlined in the introductory chapter some pharmacies are able to make up custom-made doses of antidepressants in tablet or capsule form. Sometimes this will remove slow-release characteristics of the medication, which will have to be taken in instant release form, sometimes necessitating dosing more than once a day. This should be verified with the pharmacy. One such option is pre-packaged customised formulations of tablets that allow gradual reductions, made by a Dutch compounding pharmacy that produces 'tapering strips', which are currently unlicensed medication so can only be prescribed 'off-label'.[29,30] These 'tapering strips' involve making up smaller formulations of an antidepressant than are currently available in tablet form, for example, 0.1mg or 0.5mg of citalopram and preparing pouches of medication that contain a number of small tablets in order to make up hyperbolically decreasing dose regimens that are able to go down to very small final doses before stopping (e.g. 0.1mg of citalopram). Additionally, this compounding pharmacy also allows doctors to order customised reduction regimens, which facilitate any desired reduction trajectory.

Other off-licence options for making small doses of medications

As outlined in the introductory chapter, while it may represent an unlicensed use to open capsules, crush tablets or make extemporaneous suspensions, the General Medical Council (GMC) guidance on this matter states that doctors are permitted to prescribe medications off-licence when 'the dosage specified for a licensed medicine would not meet the patient's need'.[31] In the USA, such usage is also considered 'off label' or 'unapproved' use by the FDA, which, however, explains that 'healthcare providers generally may prescribe the drug for an unapproved use when they judge that it is medically appropriate for their patient'.[32]

Dispersing tablets

As outlined in the introductory chapter, when liquid formulations are not available, many tablets that are not enterically coated or sustained- or extended-release can be crushed to a powdered form and/or dispersed in water, as indicated by guidance for patients with swallowing difficulties.[33,34] The contents may sometimes taste bitter. Crushed sertraline and paroxetine tablets may have a local anaesthetic effect on the tongue.[34] Crushing and dispersing will not greatly alter these medications' pharmacokinetic properties (their rate of gastrointestinal absorption will be increased), according to the FDA medication guide,[12] and the Royal Pharmaceutical Society (RPS) guidance on crushing, opening or splitting oral dosage forms.[35]

Many tablets, such as sertraline or escitalopram, simply disperse in water after a few minutes, aided by stirring or shaking.[28] Some formulations of antidepressants come as orodispersible tablets, such as mirtazapine. These tablets are designed to rapidly disintegrate on the tongue without the need for water. However, guidelines for people who have swallowing difficulties (like the NEWT guidelines in the UK)[33] indicate that they will also disperse in water (very quickly) and the suspension formed can be used to administer the drug to the patient. For example, application of the above principles for gradual taper could involve dispersing a 10mg citalopram tablet in 100mL water (by shaking or stirring) and then immediately removing and discarding 5mL of the suspension with a syringe to administer a dose of 9.5mg when the remaining solution is consumed. As some antidepressants, such as sertraline, are poorly soluble in water, it should be noted that mixtures made by dispersing a tablet in water are suspensions (not solutions) (Table 2.21). Flakes or particles visible in a suspension are a combination of excipients (or 'fillers') and active drug. Care should be taken to vigorously shake a suspension to ensure even dispersion of the drug.[28] In the absence of stability data, Pfizer, for instance, conservatively recommends suspensions of sertraline be consumed immediately,[28] which might be as interpreted as within an hour.

Sustained-release and extended-release drug forms often contain a binder that will thicken when added to liquid and so cannot be crushed and dissolved in an aqueous solution. For example, Venlafaxine XR in tablet form cannot be liquefied, as binders in the tablet will tend to gel.

Opening capsules to count beads

The extended-release forms of venlafaxine and duloxetine, often delivered as gelatine capsules filled with tiny beads, may be opened and the beads emptied out, as suggested by guidelines for patients with difficulty swallowing tablets or capsules.[33] The pharmacokinetic properties of beads are retained if the capsules are opened and the beads are exposed to air for both drugs.[23,25] These drugs can then be tapered by progressively removing more beads at designated intervals to gradually reduce the dose. This method requires some amount of manual dexterity and so will not be appropriate for all patients. The beads can be weighed or counted. This should be done with clean and dry hands (or using an instrument like a ruler or pair of tweezers). The number of beads to be taken will need to be placed back into the original capsule or another gelatine capsule bought from a pharmacy or online. The beads should not be swallowed without a capsule as there are some reports of throat irritation occurring.[36]

Each capsule contains the same weight of drug but, because the beads vary in size, they may have different numbers of beads. The average number of beads in three capsules might be used to estimate the number in each capsule. Doses in milligrams can then be converted into the number of beads required. For example, if a 30mg capsule contains, on average, 250 beads, then to achieve a dose of 6mg 50 beads are needed. Weighing the beads using a jeweller's scale may allow greater accuracy. Beads can be kept in a suitable container for a couple of days as their enteric coating is stable in air.[37]

This is an off-label use of the drug. The official drug label for duloxetine advises against sprinkling contents onto food or mixing with liquids because these actions might affect its enteric coating.[22] However, a formal analysis conducted by the manufacturer, Eli Lilly, concluded that duloxetine beads were stable and that their absorption profile was not altered by opening the capsule and mixing the beads with apple juice or apple sauce (but not chocolate pudding).[23] The NEWT guidelines in the UK recommend this approach as appropriate for people with difficulty swallowing,[33] and this may be extended to people tapering off medication. It has been demonstrated that beads emptied out of a capsule of venlafaxine, mixed with apple sauce, and swallowed with a glass of water, were bio-equivalent to normal administration in capsule form.[25]

It is possible to liquify this type of extended-release form of venlafaxine.[38] Utilising high-performance liquid chromatography, another study found that crushing extended-release microspheres of venlafaxine XR (removing their extended-release properties) into powder then dispersing it in either a specialist oral suspending vehicle (e.g. ORA-plus or Syrup BP) maintained stability for 28 days when stored in amber plastic bottles at either

CHAPTER 2

5 or 23 degrees Celsius.[39] However, one must take care with storing suspensions so that 'caking' does not occur – where a solid mass of aggregated particles form. Duloxetine beads cannot be crushed or liquefied; the enteric coating on the beads inside the capsules must be intact for proper drug delivery.[40]

References

1. Horowitz MA, Taylor D. Tapering of SSRI treatment to mitigate withdrawal symptoms. *The Lancet Psychiatry* 2019; 6: 538–46.

2. National Institute of Health and Social Care (NICE). Depression in adults (Draft for consultation, November 2021). https://www.nice.org.uk/guidance/-indevelopment/gid-cgwave0725/consultation/html-content-3 (accessed 28 November 2021).

3. Burn W, Horowitz M, Roycroft G, Taylor D. Stopping antidepressants. Stopping antidepressants. 2020. https://www.rcpsych.ac.uk/mental-health/treatments-and-wellbeing/stopping-antidepressants.

4. Ruhe H, Horikx A, van Avendonk M, Groeneweg B, Woutersen-Koch H. Multidisciplinary recommendations for discontinuation of SSRIs and SNRIs. *The Lancet Psychiatry* 2019.

5. National Institute of Health and Social Care (NICE). Depression in adults: treatment and management | Guidance | NICE. 2022; published online June. https://www.nice.org.uk/guidance/ng222 (accessed 16 July 2022).

6. Kaplan EM. Antidepressant noncompliance as a factor in the discontinuation syndrome. *J Clin Psychiatry* 1997; 58 Suppl 7: 31–5; discussion 36.

7. Framer A. What I have learnt from helping thousands of people taper off psychotropic medications. *Ther Adv Psychopharmacol* 2021; 11: 204512532199127.

8. Preskorn SH. Clinically relevant pharmacology of selective serotonin reuptake inhibitors. An overview with emphasis on pharmacokinetics and effects on oxidative drug metabolism. *Clin Pharmacokinet* 1997; 32 Suppl 1: 1–21.

9. Joint Formulary Committee. British National Formulary. 2021. https://bnf.nice.org.uk.

10. NHS Digital. Prescriptions dispensed in the community – Statistics for England, 2007–2017. 2018. https://digital.nhs.uk/data-and-information/publications/statistical/prescriptions-dispensed-in-the-community/prescriptions-dispensed-in-the-community-england---2007--2017 (accessed 5 January 2023).

11. Schuck RN, Pacanowski M, Kim S, Madabushi R, Zineh I. Use of titration as a therapeutic individualization strategy: an analysis of food and drug administration – approved drugs. *Clin Transl Sci* 2019; 12: 236–9.

12. Bostwick JR, Demehri A. Pills to powder: a clinician's reference for crushable psychotropic medications. *Curr Psychiatr* 2014; 13.

13. Davies J, Cooper RE, Moncrieff J, Montagu L, Rae T, Parhi M. The costs incurred by the NHS in England due to the unnecessary prescribing of dependency-forming medications. *Addict Behav* 2021; 107143.

14. U.S. Food and Drug Administration. Orange book: Approved drug products with therapeutic equivalence evaluations. 2021. https://www.accessdata.fda.gov/scripts/cder/ob/index.cfm?resetfields=1 (accessed 5 January 2023).

15. Pfizer Label for effexor XR (venlafaxine Extended-Release) capsules. 2017. https://www.accessdata.fda.gov/drugsatfda_docs/label/2017/020699s107lbl.pdf (accessed 5 January 2023).

16. GlaxoSmithKline. Wellbutrin (bupropion hydrochloride) tablets label. 2017. https://www.accessdata.fda.gov/drugsatfda_docs/label/2017/018644s052lbl.pdf (accessed 5 January 2023).

17. Advanz Pharma. Citalopram 40mg/ml Oral Drops, solution. 2021. https://www.medicines.org.uk/emc/product/3349/smpc#gref.

18. Jordan MA, Choksi D, Lombard K, Patton LR. Development of guidelines for accurate measurement of small volume parenteral products using syringes. *Hosp Pharm* 2021; 56: 165–71.

19. U.S. Food and drug administration. Zoloft (sertraline hydrochloride) tablets and oral concentrate. 2009.

20. Peterson JA, Risley DS, Anderson PN, Hostettler KF. Stability of fluoxetine hydrochloride in fluoxetine solution diluted with common pharmaceutical diluents. *Am J Hosp Pharm* 1994; 51: 1342–5.

21. Kwon JW, Armbrust KL. Degradation of citalopram by simulated sunlight. *Environ Toxicol Chem* 2005; 24: 1618–23.

22. Eli Lilly. Drug label: Cymbalta. 2020.

23. Wells KA, Losin WG. In vitro stability, potency, and dissolution of duloxetine enteric-coated pellets after exposure to applesauce, apple juice, and chocolate pudding. *Clin Ther* 2008; 30: 1300–8 (accessed 5 January 2023).

24. U.S. Food and Drug Administration. Effexor (venlafaxine hydrochloride) Tablets. 2017.

25. Jain RT, Panda J, Srivastava A. Two formulations of venlafaxine are bioequivalent when administered as open capsule mixed with applesauce to healthy subjects. *Indian J Pharm Sci* 2011; 73: 510–6.

26. Wyeth Pharmaceuticals. Drug label information: Effexor XR – venlafaxine hydrochloride capsule, extended release. 2019.

27. Information CM. NEEMMC Guidelines for tablet crushing and administration via enteral feeding tubes. 2013.

28. White R, Bradnam V. *Handbook of drug Administration via Enteral Feeding Tubes*, 3rd edn. Pharmaceutical Press, 2015.

29. Groot PC, van Os J. How user knowledge of psychotropic drug withdrawal resulted in the development of person-specific tapering medication. *Ther Adv Psychopharmacol* 2020; 10: 204512532093245.

30. Groot PC, van Os J. Outcome of antidepressant drug discontinuation with tapering strips after 1–5 years. *Ther Adv Psychopharmacol* 2020; 10: 204512532095460.

31. General Medical Council. Prescribing unlicensed medicines. 2021.

32. Office of the Commissioner. Understanding unapproved use of approved drugs 'off label'. U.S. Food and Drug Administration. https://www.fda.gov/patients/learn-about-expanded-access-and-other-treatment-options/understanding-unapproved-use-approved-drugs-label (accessed 22 September 2022).

33. Smyth J. The NEWT guidelines for administration of medication to patients with enteral feeding tubes or swallowing difficulties. 2011. https://www.newtguidelines.com/index.html (accesed 5 January 2023).

34. Brennan K. Selective serotonin reuptake inhibitor (SSRI) formulations suggested for adults with swallowing difficulties. SPS – Specialist Pharmacy Service. 2021; published online 1 July. https://www.sps.nhs.uk/articles/selective-serotonin-reuptake-inhibitor-ssri-formulations-suggested-for-adults-with-swallowing-difficulties/ (accessed 14 July 2022).

35. Root T, Tomlin S, Erskine D, Lowey A. Pharmaceutical issues when crushing, opening or splitting oral dosage forms. *Royal pharmaceutical society* 2011; 1: 1–7.

36. FDA. Memorandum: DMETS medication error postmarketing safety review: Cymbalta. Fda.gov. 2007; published online 8 March. www.fda.gov/media/74134/download (accessed 9 September 2022).

37. Kuang C, Sun Y, Li B, et al. Preparation and evaluation of duloxetine hydrochloride enteric-coated pellets with different enteric polymers. *Asian J Pharm Sci* 2017; 12: 216–26.

38. De Rosa NF, Sharley NA. Stability of venlafaxine hydrochloride liquid formulations suitable for administration via enteral feeding tubes. *J Pharm Pract* 2008; 38: 212–5.

39. Donnelly RF, Wong K, Goddard R, Johanson C. Stability of venlafaxine immediate-release suspensions. *Int J Pharm Compd* 2011; 15: 81–4.

40. Eli Lilly 30mg hard gastro-resistant capsules. https://www.medicines.org.uk/emc/product/3880/smpc (accessed 11 September 2022).

CHAPTER 2

Psychological aspects of antidepressant tapering

As outlined in the introductory chapter tapering off psychiatric medications like antidepressants can be a difficult process, leading to numerous withdrawal symptoms (or uncovering underlying mental health conditions). Although there are ways of coping with specific withdrawal symptoms, it is generally best to avoid overly distressing symptoms because they can impair social and professional functioning, precipitate relapse and cause the patient to become fearful of the process of reducing their medication or of ever being able to stop it. Although there may be exceptions, most people do not do well by 'white-knuckling' through the process of very severe withdrawal effects. Although there has been limited research in the area, it seems to be the case that more severe withdrawal symptoms from rapid reductions may also increase the risk of a protracted withdrawal syndrome in the long run.[1–3]

Most people cannot tolerate severe withdrawal effects and will return to a full dose of medication, or seek other medications to manage their symptoms; occasionally severe withdrawal effects will lead people to be admitted to hospital and in some cases to attempt suicide.[4–6] So although there are specific approaches to coping with withdrawal, the main tool to manage withdrawal symptoms during the process of discontinuing antidepressants should be to reduce the dose gradually enough to avoid severe withdrawal symptoms in the first place. Generally, if symptoms are too severe, the reduction schedule should be halted until these symptoms resolve or if intolerable then the dose should be increased and held there until symptoms resolve, before progressing at a more gradual rate (with smaller dose reductions, and/or longer periods between reductions).

There are some examples of methods of coping with withdrawal symptoms in the introductory chapters. For antidepressants, there are a few interventions that have some evidence in supporting patients during tapering. Using the rate of relapse after antidepressant discontinuation as the outcome measure, one systematic review found that mindfulness-based cognitive therapy reduced relapse during and after antidepressant tapering,[7] and an individual patient meta-analysis indicated preventative cognitive therapy or mindfulness-based cognitive therapy improved outcomes during and after antidepressant tapering.[8] While these forms of therapy, especially mindfulness, seem to be helpful with the process of antidepressant discontinuation, it is unlikely that any psychological therapy can substitute for gradual tapering titrated to the ability of the individual patient to tolerate the process.[1] A randomised controlled trial of antidepressant discontinuation over 4 months that found that cognitive behavioural therapy compared to treatment as usual did not affect any of the primary or secondary outcomes (including relapse and successful discontinuation) supports this advice.[9,10]

An analysis of several hundred people who came off antidepressants found that the following were used to cope with withdrawal symptoms while coming off antidepressants:

- seeking reassurance that symptoms were temporary (e.g. from friends, family or online communities) (92%),
- distraction (hobbies, other interests) (87%),
- exercise (86%),
- mindfulness (80%),
- breathing exercises (82%),
- monitoring symptoms (66.4%), and
- keeping a journal (44%), amongst a variety of others.[2]

Psychological effects of antidepressant withdrawal

The withdrawal process can involve intense emotions, some outlined previously, ranging from despair, to anger, anxiety, emotional lability, hypomania and suicidal thoughts, often unrelated to events or circumstances.[1,11,12] These can sometimes be familiar to the patient, and other times quite novel, and can be distressing and confusing.[1] Like the physical symptoms of withdrawal, these symptoms can often come in intense waves.[1] The emotional effects of antidepressant withdrawal are common in many drug withdrawal syndromes, perhaps most widely recognised from recreational drugs.[13] Some commentators have suggested that they may be best thought of as emotions of 'neurological origin', that is, emotions that arise from perturbations to the brain caused by withdrawal rather than 'endogenous' emotions, laden with existential meaning; they have been called 'neuro-emotions'.[1] In their more extreme forms they are very likely to attract mental health diagnoses from clinicians unfamiliar with this aspect of withdrawal.[1,14]

Sometimes withdrawal symptoms from antidepressants can be difficult to distinguish from an underlying condition not just for the clinician but also for the patient.[1] The RCPsych guidance on 'Stopping antidepressants' specifically cautions patients on this point, highlighting that 'the low mood and difficulty in sleeping of withdrawal can feel like the symptoms of depression'.[15] Although timing and associated physical symptoms can be helpful in achieving this distinction the subjective similarity of symptoms to the original condition can be confusing for some.[1] This may be because people have typical patterns of thoughts and emotions that are triggered by withdrawal symptoms. In the same way as anxiety triggered by an excess of caffeine in a given individual may have an idiosyncratic presentation depending on an individual's personality and habits of mind, withdrawal symptoms may interact with an individual's typical responses and therefore closely resemble an underlying condition (this is sometimes referred to as 'rebound' symptoms). In such cases, the pattern of symptoms over time (waxing and waning following reductions), co-incident symptoms that are not typical of the patient's mental health condition are most useful in helping to distinguish between these differentials.

Many patients go through a phase of shock when they contemplate the effects of withdrawal on their lives, including worries about the impact on their financial, work and personal affairs, involving feelings of regret, self-blame and anger.[1,16] They may feel anger that they were not properly informed about the difficulties in stopping medication. Another common emotional symptom in withdrawal is the opposite of intense emotion: rather it is the complete absence of emotions, sometimes referred to as 'emotional anaesthesia', or referred to as anhedonia, numbness, apathy or 'dysthymia' following drug withdrawal.[1,11,17,18] This effect, like other withdrawal effects, seems to fade over time but can take months or years in some patients.[11]

There are patient support groups that can provide helpful support for patients going through this process. Techniques such as distraction, acceptance and re-orientation to recognising these symptoms as temporary products of the withdrawal process that resolve in time like other symptoms can all be helpful.[1] Some patients find that learning to manage and cope with withdrawal symptoms, also translates to being better able to manage the mental health conditions that first prompted medication prescriptions.[1]

References

1. Framer A. What I have learnt from helping thousands of people taper off psychotropic medications. *Ther Adv Psychopharmacol* 2021; 11: 204512532199127.

2. Moncrieff J, Read J, Horowitz M. How patients taper off antidepressants in peer-led communities. (in preparation).

3. Horowitz M, Flanigan R, Cooper R, Moncrieff J. The determinants of outcome from antidepressant withdrawal in a large survey of patients (in preparation).

4. Valuck RJ, Orton HD, Libby AM. Antidepressant discontinuation and risk of suicide attempt. *J Clin Psychiatry* 2009; 70: 1069–77.

5. Guy A, Brown M, Lewis S, Horowitz M. The 'patient voice' – patients who experience antidepressant withdrawal symptoms are often dismissed, or misdiagnosed with relapse, or a new medical condition. *Ther Adv Psychopharmacol* 2020; 10: 2045125320967183.

6. Hengartner MP, Schulthess L, Sørensen A, Framer A. Protracted withdrawal syndrome after stopping antidepressants: a descriptive quantitative analysis of consumer narratives from a large internet forum. *Ther Adv Psychopharmacol* 2020; 10: 2045125320980573.

7. Maund E, Stuart B, Moore M, et al. Managing antidepressant discontinuation: A systematic review. *Ann Fam Med* 2019; 17: 52–60.

8. Breedvelt JJF, Warren FC, Segal Z, Kuyken W, Bockting CL. Continuation of antidepressants vs sequential psychological interventions to prevent relapse in depression: an individual participant data meta-analysis. *JAMA Psychiatry* 2021; 78: 868–75.

9. Fava GA, Belaise C. Discontinuing antidepressant drugs: lesson from a failed trial and extensive clinical experience. *Psychother Psychosom* 2018; 87: 257–67.

10. Scholten WD, Batelaan NM, Van Oppen P, et al. The efficacy of a group CBT relapse prevention program for remitted anxiety disorder patients who discontinue antidepressant medication: a randomized controlled trial. *Psychother Psychosom* 2018; 87: 240–2.

11. Cosci F, Chouinard G. Acute and persistent withdrawal syndromes following discontinuation of psychotropic medications. *Psychother Psychosom* 2020; 89: 283–306.

12. Fava GA, Gatti A, Belaise C, Guidi J, Offidani E. Withdrawal symptoms after selective serotonin reuptake inhibitor discontinuation: a systematic review. *Psychother Psychosom* 2015; 84: 72–81.

13. Lerner A, Klein M. Dependence, withdrawal and rebound of CNS drugs: An update and regulatory considerations for new drugs development. *Brain Commun* 2019; 1: fcz025.

14. White E, Read J, Julo S. The role of Facebook groups in the management and raising of awareness of antidepressant withdrawal: is social media filling the void left by health services? *Ther Adv Psychopharmacol* 2021; 11: 2045125320981174.

15. Burn W, Horowitz M, Roycroft G, Taylor D. Stopping antidepressants. Stopping antidepressants. 2020. https://www.rcpsych.ac.uk/mental-health/treatments-and-wellbeing/stopping-antidepressants (accessed 5 January 2023).

16. National Institute of Health and Social Care (NICE). Medicines associated with dependence or withdrawal symptoms: Safe prescribing and withdrawal management for adults | Guidance | NICE. 2022. https://www.nice.org.uk/guidance/ng215/chapter/Recommendations (accessed 27 June 2022).

17. El-Mallakh RS, Briscoe B. Studies of long-term use of antidepressants: how should the data from them be interpreted? *CNS Drugs* 2012; 26: 97–109.

18. Renoir T, Pang TY, Lanfumey L. Drug withdrawal-induced depression: serotonergic and plasticity changes in animal models. *Neurosci Biobehav Rev* 2012; 36: 696–726.

Tapering antidepressants in practice

This section provides a step-by-step guide to help clinicians guide patients through the process of reducing and stopping their antidepressants, starting with education before the process and then proceeding through cycles of dose reduction.

The considerations to be taken into account before making dose reductions are outlined in the introductory chapters, and they include:

- discussing with the patient the benefits and harms of continuing versus stopping one or more psychiatric medication;
- addressing potential barriers and facilitators, including existing beliefs, family and professional support (or otherwise), as well as existing coping skills;
- educating the patient about withdrawal symptoms from the medication and how this will be managed;
- outlining the process of reducing and/or stopping the medication, including the process of adjustment and monitoring.

Some particular considerations for antidepressants are outlined.

Before commencing dose reductions

- Patients should be informed about the risks and benefits of reducing or stopping antidepressants. The major risks are withdrawal and relapse. The risk of relapse might be mitigated by slowly tapering the medication, and by alternative means for managing an underlying mental health condition (for example mindfulness-based cognitive therapy and group CBT are both recommended for relapse prevention in depression by NICE).[1] For some patients a past stressor will have resolved such that relapse is less of a concern.
- The adverse effects of being on an antidepressant need to be weighed against the aversive consequences of stopping an antidepressant too quickly. If the adverse effects of an antidepressant are life-threatening or severe, then this will need to take precedence over slow tapering. In other circumstances, the risks will need to be balanced for each case.[2] Most of the advice below relates to patients who do not have life-threatening or urgent adverse effects.
- Recognise that patients may have fears and concerns about stopping their antidepressant (both relapse and withdrawal effects) and will need support to withdraw successfully, particularly if previous attempts have been difficult. Details for online or written resources may be useful,[3] as will increased support from a clinician or therapist (for example, check-in phone calls, more frequent appointments and specific advice about major hurdles that might arise such as insomnia).[1]
- Patients may have queries about prescribing decisions made previously. Explain that our understanding of the balance of risks and benefits of a medicine can change over time.[2]
- All patients should be informed of the risk of withdrawal symptoms on reducing the dose or stopping any antidepressant. These symptoms arise because the brain has become

accustomed to the medication and when the drug dose is lowered, the difference between what the brain 'expects' and what input the drugs provide is experienced as withdrawal symptoms, as for many other substances like caffeine, or nicotine.

- In order that patients do not mistake withdrawal symptoms for a return of their underlying condition, it is useful to inform patients what withdrawal symptoms they might experience. Patients should be told that antidepressant withdrawal symptoms can include:
  - Balance problems:
    – such as dizziness, which can be mild or can be so severe that people have difficulty standing up
    – loss of coordination, troubles with balance.
  - Sleep disorder:
    – difficulty in getting to and staying asleep
    – nightmares
  - Psychological symptoms:
    – anxiety which can come and go, sometimes in intense 'surges'
    – low mood, tearfulness, feeling unable to be interested in or enjoy things (anhedonia)
    – rapidly changing moods
    – anger, tension, irritability, agitation, restlessness
    – panic attacks, irrational fears, obsessive thoughts
    – suicidal thoughts and urges
    – hypomania and disinhibition
  - Sensory symptoms:
    – feeling of an electric shock-like sensations in the head (sometimes worse on turning the head to the side, often called 'zaps')
    – paraesthesia (pins and needles) and other altered sensations
    – palinopsia (prolonged after-images)
  - Neuro-cognitive symptoms:
    – the sensation that you are not real ('depersonalisation') or that the world is not real ('derealisation'), a dream-like sensation that can be disturbing for some people
    – memory difficulties
    – confusion, trouble concentrating, brain fog (people sometimes describe this as having 'cotton wool in their head')
  - Extrapyramidal/muscular symptoms:
    – muscle tremors, spasms, pain and tension, aches in joints
  - Gastrointestinal symptoms, like nausea, diarrhoea, constipation
  - General symptoms (flu-like):
    – a sense of being physically unwell
    – headache, lethargy, sweating
    – tiredness, loss of appetite, muscle pain
  - Other symptoms:
    – heart palpitations
    – pronounced fatigue
  - Some people may experience akathisia – a feeling that can vary from an inner restlessness and agitation, that can make them feel that they cannot sit still, to a feeling some people describe as their 'nervous system being on fire'.

A full list of withdrawal symptoms is given in Table 2.4. Patients should be reassured that these symptoms are most likely to occur to people who stop their antidepressants rapidly and that all care will be taken to minimise unpleasant withdrawal symptoms.

■ Explain that it is not fully understood what factors determine risk of withdrawal symptoms for an individual. However, there is evidence that the risks are increased for longer-term use, higher doses, specific antidepressants (such as SNRIs, and short-acting SSRIs). People who have experienced withdrawal symptoms previously when tapering or on forgetting their dose are more likely to experience withdrawal symptoms in the future. These risk factors have been combined to develop a preliminary tool to estimate risk of withdrawal for an individual wishing to stop an antidepressant (Table 2.11).

Distinguishing withdrawal symptoms from a return of an underlying condition

One of the most common issues that comes up in reducing or stopping an antidepressant is distinguishing between withdrawal symptoms and a relapse of an underlying condition (further details in 'Withdrawal effects from antidepressants'). This can be difficult for both clinicians and patients because of the pronounced overlap in symptoms. There are some useful clues that can help distinguish between the two:[4]

■ Withdrawal symptoms normally onset soon (e.g. days) after reducing the dose or stopping an antidepressant, whereas it can take weeks or months for an underlying condition to return. This is somewhat complicated by the fact that sometimes withdrawal effects from antidepressants can be delayed by weeks, for reasons that are not well understood.

■ Some withdrawal symptoms from antidepressants are distinct from the symptoms of anxiety or depression, especially physical symptoms, such as dizziness, headaches or unsteadiness. Some symptoms such as 'electric shock sensations' are so distinctive that they may be considered pathognomonic of withdrawal.[5]

■ Even new symptoms of anxiety and depression (not prior features of the underlying condition) should be regarded with a high index of suspicion as withdrawal effects (more likely than onset of a new mental health condition whose onset happened to coincide with the period of tapering). Patients might say 'I have never felt this way before' as the symptoms can be quite distinct from a usual mood state.[5] Sometimes the symptoms are difficult for patients to distinguish from relapse (see further below).[6]

■ More helpful in retrospect is that withdrawal symptoms normally resolve within days when the dose of the drug is increased (if done soon after withdrawal symptoms onset – resolution take longer if re-instatement is delayed). In contrast, it can take up to weeks for symptoms of depression or anxiety to respond to a medication.

■ If small reductions are made, a typical 'wave' pattern of symptoms are normally experienced, where symptoms onset, worsen, reach a peak and then improve and resolve: this is distinct from the pattern of a relapse (see further later).

Another, related problem is mis-diagnosis of withdrawal symptoms as onset of a new medical disorder, which many patients report (see further details in 'Withdrawal effects from antidepressants').

■ Muscle spasms, tremors or pain, and other neurological symptoms can attract a diagnosis of functional neurological disorder (FND) or medically unexplained symptoms (MUS) if clinicians are not familiar with these as symptoms of antidepressant withdrawal.

- Unsteadiness, and dizziness can sometimes be mis-diagnosed as stroke or other neuro-logical conditions.
- Fatigue, brain fog and difficulty concentrating can be mis-diagnosed as chronic fatigue syndrome (CFS).

Awareness of the myriad symptoms that antidepressant withdrawal can prevent mis-diagnosis (although, given it is possible for another disorder to be present at the same time, it can be prudent to rule out other pathology). Withdrawal symptoms can also be mis-diagnosed as new onset of a mental health condition, malingering or psychoso-matic conditions by clinicians unfamiliar with this syndrome.

Tapering in practice

The key elements of a programme of tapering are:

- that it is flexible and can be adjusted so that the process is tolerable for the patient;
- that it involves close clinician monitoring of withdrawal symptoms to facilitate timely adjustments to the rate of taper;
- that patients are provided with preparations of antidepressants to enable making doses that are not easily able to be made with currently available tablet doses (e.g. access to liquid formulations of antidepressants or smaller formulations of tablets).

The process of tapering in practice involves the following four steps (Figure 2.9):

- Step 1: Estimation of the risk of withdrawal for the patient and estimation of the size of the initial dose reduction

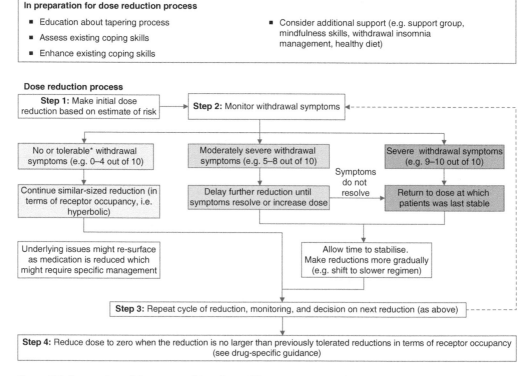

Figure 2.9 An overview of the process of tapering antidepressants.
*What constitutes tolerable symptoms will vary between patients but are generally symptoms that do not overly interfere with their lives.

- Step 2: Monitoring of withdrawal symptoms resulting from this initial reduction
- Step 3: Determination of the size of the next reduction based on how tolerable this reduction was for the patient
- Step 4: repetition of Steps 2 and 3 until a dose is reached that is small enough so that the reduction to zero is not a larger step down (in terms of receptor occupancy) than the reductions that have been previously tolerated

Step 1: Estimation of the risk of withdrawal and estimation of the size of the first reduction

- Patients may be risk stratified according to Table 2.11 and Table 2.12.
- This then allows broad categorisation of risk of withdrawal and an estimate of a reasonable initial dose reduction (Table 2.22).

Table 2.22 Estimation of tapering rate based on risk of withdrawal symptoms (see Tables 2.11 and 2.12).

Evaluation of risk	Initial tapering trajectory (see individual drug sections)	Initial dose reduction equivalent (approximately)*
Low risk = 0 points	Faster[a]	50% reduction
Medium risk = 1–4 points	Moderate[b]	25% reduction
High risk = 5–8 points	Slower[c]	10% reduction
Very high risk ≥ 9 points	Slowest[d]	5% reduction (or less)

*See further details in the drug-specific section but this value represents the approximate size of reduction from the lowest dose employed clinically
[a]Each step approximately equivalent to 10 percentage point reductions of SERT occupancy for SSRIs
[b]Each step approximately equivalent to 5 percentage point reductions of SERT occupancy for SSRIs
[c]Each step approximately equivalent to 2.5 percentage point reductions of SERT occupancy for SSRIs
[d]Each step approximately equivalent to 1 percentage point reductions of SERT occupancy for SSRIs. To make up this regimen will require adding intermediate steps to the 'slower' regimen outlined in the drug-specific chapters.

Specific guides for the dose reductions of commonly used antidepressants are given in the subsequent sections.

For example, a patient taking venlafaxine 75mg for 2 years, who had severe dizziness, electric shocks in the head, and panic attacks, after forgetting to take the tablets for a week while on holiday, would score 8 points (high risk) from Table 2.11:

- 2 points for long-term use
- 4 points for venlafaxine
- 0 point for the minimum dose employed clinically
- 2 points for previous severe withdrawal symptoms

Based on this, the initial recommendation would be to reduce the dose according to the slower regime, based on reductions of about 2.5 percentage point of SERT occupancy i.e. to 55mg of venlafaxine (see also the venlafaxine section).

As explained earlier, doses of antidepressant between available tablet doses may require prescription for the liquid version, or forms suitable for making up smaller doses. For example, venlafaxine liquid is available as a liquid in the UK. There are more details of available preparations of medications available around the world in the individual drug sections.

Step 2: Monitoring the withdrawal effects from the initial reduction

- A baseline measure of symptoms, before commencing tapering, can allow any withdrawal symptoms to be more easily separated from adverse medication effects, or other symptoms unrelated to the drug.
- Following the reduction in dose, withdrawal symptoms should be monitored for 2–4 weeks, or until symptoms have resolved. This period of monitoring is recommended because although most withdrawal symptoms emerge in a week, symptom onset can be delayed and it may take time for symptoms to peak.[7] This monitoring period prevents cumulative withdrawal effects accruing from subsequent reductions.
- Monitoring can take different forms. When patients have recognised characteristic withdrawal symptoms it is possible to either monitor 3 or 4 key symptoms, or 'overall symptoms'. The severity of these individual and aggregate symptoms can be rated out of 10 (0 = nil, 10 = severe). For other patients, a guide such as the Discontinuation Emergent Signs and Symptoms (DESS)[4] may be used or Table 2.4. Daily monitoring is useful, but twice weekly or weekly may be more acceptable, and still informative. Patients may use a diary, spreadsheet, or other means to record these symptoms. An example of such a record is given in Figure 2.10.
- Withdrawal symptom monitoring can be visually represented by plotting time after reduction against severity of withdrawal (averaged out of 10). This can be helpful to track the withdrawal process. It is typical for withdrawal effects to be delayed for a few days after a small reduction, to worsen, reach a peak (often around 10 days post reduction), before slowly resolving to or near baseline over a few days (see example in Figure 2.11). This graph can also offer the patient reassurance by demonstrating the quick onset and transience of any withdrawal symptoms, distinguishing them from a return of the underlying condition (which would not resolve in the same manner). This is especially helpful when the nature of the symptoms makes it difficult to distinguish from an underlying condition.

| Miss Y, Citalopram, April 2021. | | | | | |
Day	Dose (mg)	Anxiety /10	Dizziness /10	Insomnia /10	Overall symptom /10
1	20	1	0	0	1
2	20	1	0	0	1
3	20	1	0	0	1
4	20	1	0	0	1
5	15	1	0	0	1
6	15	1	0	0	1
7	15	2	1	1	2
8	15	2	1	2	2
9	15	2	1	2	2
10	15	3	2	2	3
11	15	3	2	3	3
12	15	4	3	3	4
13	15	4	3	4	4
14	15	4	3	4	4
15	15	4	4	3	4
16	15	4	4	3	4
17	15	3	3	2	3
18	15	3	3	2	3
19	15	3	3	2	3
20	15	2	2	2	2
21	15	2	2	2	2
22	15	2	2	1	1
23	15	1	1	1	1
24	15	1	1	1	1
25	15	1	1	1	1

Figure 2.10 Example monitoring form for a patient reducing from 20mg of citalopram to 15mg. From past experience the patient knows their typical withdrawal symptoms are anxiety, insomnia and dizziness.

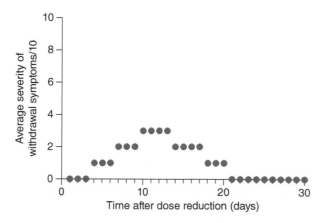

Figure 2.11 Graphical representation of withdrawal symptoms following a dose reduction of citalopram. These probably constitute mild symptoms. The y-axis shows the average patient-rated severity of withdrawal symptoms. Note the delayed onset of significant symptoms after drug reduction, probably related to drug elimination; followed by a peak and then easing of symptoms, probably related to re-adaptation of the system to a new homeostatic 'set-point' (similarly to Figure 2.5b and 2.5c).

Step 3: Determining further dose reductions

Further reductions should be made when withdrawal symptoms from the previous reduction have largely resolved. The size of the next reduction should be adjusted based on the experience of the previous reduction:

- If the initial reduction was tolerable (in the patient's judgement), for example, the maximum severity of withdrawal symptoms was ≤4/10 (as in Figure 2.11), and symptoms resolved within 2 to 4 weeks, then future reductions could be made at the same rate. For example, if a reduction made on the moderate regimen for citalopram (see drug-specific chapters) was tolerable when made every 4 weeks, then the next reduction could also be made according to this regimen.
- If symptoms were moderately severe e.g. 5–8/10 (Figure 2.12), then it may be prudent to wait longer for symptom resolution, before proceeding at a slower reduction rate, perhaps half (or moving to the next slowest reduction regimen in the drug-specific chapters). For example, if a reduction according to the fast regimen for citalopram (see drug-specific chapters) caused moderately severe withdrawal effects, a 6-week pause could be made to allow symptom resolution, before the next dose reduction is made, now following the moderate reduction regimen.
- It might be preferable for some patients to increase their dose either part way, or all the way back to the dose at which they were previously stable (or even higher) to terminate unpleasant withdrawal symptoms. Subsequent reductions should then be made at a slower pace.

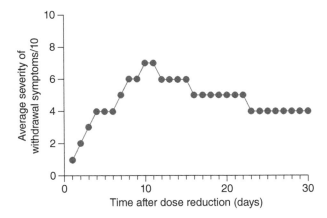

Figure 2.12 Graphical representation of withdrawal symptoms following antidepressant reduction. These constitute moderate symptoms, reaching a maximum of 7 out of 10, and not resolved 30 days after the reduction.

- If the symptoms were severe, e.g. >8/10 (Figure 2.13) then it is advisable to increase the dose back to that before the reduction, wait for symptoms to resolve, then make a considerably smaller reduction, perhaps one-half or one-quarter of the original reduction (e.g. dropping down two steps on the suggested drug-specific regimens). Ideally such a circumstance is avoided (by choosing a conservative starting rate) because it can be very distressing for a patient and deter them from trying to reduce again in future. 'White knuckling' through these symptoms is generally not wise.

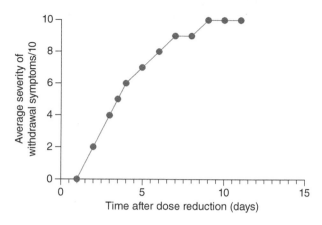

Figure 2.13 Graphical representation of withdrawal symptoms following antidepressant dose reduction. These constitute severe withdrawal symptoms, reaching a maximum of 10 out of 10, and should prompt re-instatement of the previous dose of medication to resolve the symptoms.

What constitutes mild, moderate or severe symptoms is subjective to the patient and some might consider 4 out of 10 symptoms to be unacceptably unpleasant or disruptive, while others will be determined to persevere through more severe symptoms. This depends both on personality as well as social and professional responsibilities. As there is a risk that severe withdrawal symptoms might indicate an increased risk of protracted withdrawal symptoms, it is generally advisable to reduce at a rate that restricts withdrawal symptoms to moderate levels.

Step 4: Continuing tapering by adjusting the rate to be tolerable to the patient

- Subsequent reductions should be made by repeating Steps 2 and 3, with monitoring of symptoms following each reduction, and subsequent reductions adjusted to the experience of the process for the patient.
- Reductions should be made in a hyperbolic manner, so that the reductions become smaller and smaller as total dose gets lower, which can be achieved by reducing the dose according to the receptor occupancy of the drug (see Figure 2.4, and drug-specific sections following).
- After two or three iterations of the above process, it is usually possible to determine a rate of tapering that is tolerable for an individual patient. For example, one patient may be able to tolerate a reduction approximately equivalent to 2 percentage points of SERT occupancy every 4 weeks (i.e. the 'slower' taper trajectories found in the drug-specific section), while another may be able to tolerate a reduction equivalent to 10 percentage points of SERT occupancy every 4 weeks (i.e. the 'fast' taper trajectories in the drug-specific chapters). Patients may need to be seen more often during the first two or three reductions to titrate the rate more carefully. They are likely to require less support once they determine a tolerable rate of tapering.

CHAPTER 2

CHAPTER 2

- The dose can be brought to zero when this final reduction will not cause a greater reduction in receptor occupancy than that caused by previously tolerable reductions. For example, if a patient can taper at a rate equivalent to a reduction of 5 percentage points of SERT occupancy every 4 weeks, then they can reduce their dose to zero when they reach a dose less than or equal to 5 percentage points of SERT occupancy. This final step down will not cause a greater reduction in terms of effect on target receptors than previously tolerated reductions. For some people, this will involve going down to very low doses of antidepressant, such as 1mg, or even less, before completely stopping. These dose regimens are outlined in the drug-specific sections.
- Sometimes underlying issues, which were suppressed by medication, re-surface. Specialised deprescribing services report issues arising related to past abuse, or other traumatic experiences.[5] In these cases counselling or specific psychological interventions may be needed. If underlying mental health conditions arise, patients may wish to trial non-pharmacological treatments, or some may choose to re-commence antidepressants or trial other psychiatric medications.

References

1. National Institute of Health and Social Care (NICE). Depression in adults: treatment and management | Guidance | NICE. 2022; published online June. https://www.nice.org.uk/guidance/ng222 (accessed 16 July 2022).
2. National Institute of Health and Social Care (NICE). Medicines associated with dependence or withdrawal symptoms: Safe prescribing and withdrawal management for adults | Guidance | NICE. 2022. https://www.nice.org.uk/guidance/ng215/chapter/Recommendations (accessed 27 June 2022).
3. Inner Compass Initiative. The Withdrawal Project. 2021. https://withdrawal.theinnercompass.org / (accessed 18 January 2023).
4. Horowitz MA, Taylor D. Distinguishing relapse from antidepressant withdrawal: Clinical practice and antidepressant discontinuation studies. *BJPsych Advances* 2022; 28: 297–311.
5. Framer A. What I have learnt from helping thousands of people taper off psychotropic medications. *Ther Adv Psychopharmacol* 2021; 11: 204512532199127.
6. Rosenbaum JF, Fava M, Hoog SL, Ascroft RC, Krebs WB. Selective serotonin reuptake inhibitor discontinuation syndrome: a randomized clinical trial. *Biol Psychiatry* 1998; 44: 77–87.
7. Cooper RE, Ashman M, Lomani J, et al. 'Stabilise-reduce, stabilise-reduce': a survey of the common practices of deprescribing services and recommendations for future services. PLoS One 2023; 18: e0282988.

Managing complications of antidepressant discontinuation

Troubleshooting

If withdrawal symptoms become intolerable at any point, it is worth repeating that the best approach is to either hold the current dose for longer to allow them to resolve, or to increase the dose to the last dose at which the symptoms were tolerable, remaining there until symptoms resolve. Sometimes patients will need to increase their dose further in order to stabilise after severe withdrawal effects.

After this stabilisation, further tapering will need to be more gradual: with smaller reductions and/or longer periods between reductions. Some patients find they cannot reduce at a rate quicker than that equivalent to 1 percentage point of receptor occupancy every 4 weeks (equivalent to approximately 5–10% dose reductions every 4 weeks), or sometimes by even smaller reductions. Most people can find a rate that is tolerable to them. It is important to remember that if a patient experiences distressing withdrawal symptoms, this does not necessarily indicate that they cannot stop antidepressants, but that they might need to taper more slowly. If complete cessation is too difficult, being on a smaller dose may be a worthwhile goal as patients will be exposed to less adverse effects.

It is not advisable to use other medications that can themselves cause physical dependence and withdrawal in order to manage withdrawal symptoms from antidepressants.[1] These medications include benzodiazepines, other antidepressants, gabapentinoids, opioids and antipsychotics.[2] Use of these medications to manage withdrawal will generally lead to switching from one drug to another. It is better to slow down a taper to produce tolerable withdrawal effects than substitute a different medication.

Switching to fluoxetine

Some deprescribing advice recommends switching antidepressants to fluoxetine, then ceasing this fairly quickly (on the premise that its long elimination half-life makes it at least partially self-tapering).[3,4] However, this approach may be limited in value and authoritative guidance such as NICE does not recommend it.[1] Switching from one antidepressant to another can be an involved process and may induce withdrawal effects, more so when there are large differences between the receptor affinities of the medications being switched (which can even apply when switching between members of a drug class like SSRIs).[5] Withdrawal symptoms from fluoxetine are also more common than perhaps thought, affecting around half of patients who stop the drug.[6] Furthermore, protracted withdrawal syndromes from fluoxetine have been observed.[7] Therefore, fluoxetine, despite its long half-life, generally requires tapering as for other antidepressants. Some commentators have suggested that treatment with both the original antidepressant and fluoxetine should be performed simultaneously for 2 to 4 weeks to achieve a steady state of fluoxetine before the other antidepressant is stopped, but this approach has not been tested empirically.[8,9] If patients, after information about these uncertainties, have a clear preference for this method of discontinuation, or other strategies are not viable, this strategy is an option,[8] but there is a lack of evidence to recommend it widely.

CHAPTER 2

Approach to withdrawal akathisia

One of the worst outcomes of antidepressant withdrawal, generally when it is performed too rapidly, is akathisia.[10–13] Although this has been more often associated with an adverse effect of antipsychotic exposure, it can be induced by antidepressant withdrawal.[10–13] Gradual tapering is thought to minimise the risk of this event, but there have been no trials looking specifically at this topic. As people can be agitated and quite disordered in their behaviour (pacing, restless, grimacing, etc.), it is often mis-diagnosed as mania, psychosis or agitated depression,[12,14,15] and can lead to outcomes like suicide in extreme cases.[7,16] Once a patient is in such a state it is very difficult to treat. This state can be prolonged in some patients.[14]

Although there has been little in the way of research on withdrawal akathisia, the most commonly successful approach in clinical practice is re-instatement of the original antidepressant at the dose at which the patient had been previously stable. As the response to re-introduction of an antidepressant can be somewhat unpredictable when patients are in this state, it is wise for re-introduction to be cautious. Many psychotropic medications recommended to treat this state can themselves exacerbate symptoms for some patients, as reported by patient groups advocating for wider awareness of this syndrome.[16] Medications which can exacerbate akathisia according to patients include benzodiazepines, antipsychotics and antidepressants, such as mirtazapine.[16] The drugs most commonly reported to be useful are beta-blockers like propranolol, cyproheptadine, anti-histamines and benzodiazepines (e.g. clonazepam and diazepam).[14] However, given much uncertainty in response to these medications a cautious approach to treatment is recommended involving exposure to one medication at a time for a short period, with close observation to decide whether it is helpful, and cessation if it is not, before trialling an additional medication.[14,16] Some patient advocacy groups suggest that the best management may be conservative, allowing symptoms to resolve over time with minimal intervention, although this can be difficult for patients to tolerate.[16] Exercise is widely found to be helpful by patients, who often find that pacing somewhat lessens unpleasant sensations, with a cycling intervention supported by a case study.[17]

Management of protracted withdrawal syndrome

Protracted withdrawal, also known as PAWS, occurs in an unknown proportion of patients after stopping antidepressants.[7,11,18] Its risk is thought to be minimised by gradual tapering, but there is a lack of research.[19,20] Some patients may present for assistance in protracted withdrawal from too rapid previous withdrawal experiences. There is limited research on the best management approach. In an analysis of 69 patients with protracted withdrawal from a peer-support community, protracted symptoms lasted for 5 to 166 months, with a median of 26 months.[7] Re-instatement of the original antidepressant resolved the condition in 9 out of the 19 people who attempted this. This re-instatement was undertaken 5 to 60 months into protracted withdrawal, with a median time of 9 months.[7]

In this group, 33 people trialled treatment with drugs other than the original antidepressant ceased, with four reporting some benefit, and two reporting substantial benefit.

For example, one subject reported that escitalopram in month 12 of protracted withdrawal from venlafaxine resolved their symptoms, and another found pregabalin helpful in month 55.[7] Other subjects reported that sporadic use of benzodiazepines, trazodone, propranolol and cannabidiol oil was helpful for transitory symptomatic relief, usually of insomnia or anxiety, without having a significant effect on resolution of protracted withdrawal symptoms. Otherwise, four people reported natural recovery without re-instatement or drug treatment, 12 reported improvement short of full recovery and two people died by suicide. More than a third were lost to follow-up so their outcome was unknown.[7] It is presumed that these cases must represent cases that are more severe than the average due to self-selection.

From this limited data and clinical experience the management of protracted withdrawal can be approach conservatively – that is, without addition of further medication – in the expectation that people recover spontaneously, albeit over sometimes long periods.[21] There are cases of improvement following the introduction of various medications,[21] although it is not clear whether this approach is widely applicable because of a lack of research. There are also reports of symptoms worsening following administration of new psychiatric medications, perhaps because of further perturbation to a disturbed system.[2, 21]

Another option is re-instatement of the original medication, which seems to improve some patients' status.[7] Although re-instatement of an antidepressant soon after cessation almost inevitably leads to resolution of withdrawal symptoms (often in a few days) re-instatement longer periods after cessation has more unpredictable effects. For example, there are reports of patients who experience a paradoxical worsening in response to re-instatement of the original medication, generally long periods after stopping.[21] These paradoxical responses have been linked to a process called kindling, involving sensitisation to the ceased medication.[21] This process is analogous to the kindling effect recognised in repeated cycles of exposure to and cessation of several psychoactive substances, especially alcohol.[21, 23] It is not known how commonly paradoxical reactions occur to re-instatement in the context of protracted withdrawal.[21] One way to mitigate the possibility of negative outcomes whilst trialling re-instatement is to re-instate a very small dose of the original medication, for example 1mg of citalopram, 5% of the usual minimum dose prescribed.[21] This provides a test dose to monitor response.[7, 21] If this test dose has positive effects, an increase in dose may be cautiously trialled.[21]

Management of PSSD

PSSD is a protracted state that persists in an unknown proportion of people after stopping antidepressants that may be related to other protracted withdrawal syndromes, and can cause significant distress.[24] There are no proven treatments for PSSD. Various drugs affecting dopamine and serotonin receptors have been trialled, as have phosphodiesterase inhibitors but none have reliably reduced symptoms.[25] There is no clear consensus on the treatment of PSSD and current approaches have included lifestyle recommendations (e.g. smoking cessation, dietary recommendations, physical activity), supplements, use of phosphodiesterase inhibitors for erectile dysfunction and sex and couples counselling, but none have been evaluated in clinical trials.[26]

CHAPTER 2

Sensitivity to other substances during withdrawal

Patients can become highly sensitive to neuro-active substances in the process of withdrawal, thought to be related to an increased sensitivity to stimuli secondary to the de-stabilisation produced by the drug withdrawal process,[21,27,28] though the mechanism is not fully understood. People can respond to a wide variety of substances with activation or other paradoxical effects, including alcohol, neurologically active antibiotics,[29] caffeine, St John's Wort, and sometimes even specific foods, supplements and herbs.[21,30] This is in addition to other sensitivities to light and sound, more generally recognised.[2] Exposure to these substances can exacerbate withdrawal symptoms, and in this case it can be useful to restrict exposure during the withdrawal process.[21] These sensitivities often resolve or improve markedly when the patient recovers from withdrawal.[21] It is not possible to give blanket advice to avoid all such medications during the withdrawal process, and this will be determined by individual circumstances, including the risks of exacerbating withdrawal, the risks of the condition to be treated and alternative treatments available.

References

1. National Institute of Health and Social Care (NICE). Depression in adults: Treatment and management | Guidance | NICE. 2022; published online June. https://www.nice.org.uk/guidance/ng222 (accessed July 16, 2022).

2. Cosci F, Chouinard G. Acute and persistent withdrawal syndromes following discontinuation of psychotropic medications. *Psychother Psychosom* 2020; 89: 283–306.

3. Jha MK, Rush AJ, Trivedi MH. When discontinuing SSRI antidepressants Is a challenge: Management tips. *Am J Psychiatry* 2018; 175: 1176–84.

4. Wilson E, Lader M. A review of the management of antidepressant discontinuation symptoms. *Ther Adv Psychopharmacol* 2015; 5: 357–68.

5. Haddad PM, Anderson IM. Recognising and managing antidepressant discontinuation symptoms. *Advances in Psychiatric Treatment* 2007; 13: 447–57.

6. Horowitz MA, Taylor D. Distinguishing relapse from antidepressant withdrawal: Clinical practice and antidepressant discontinuation studies. *BJPsych Advances* 2022; 28: 297–311.

7. Hengartner MP, Schulthess L, Sørensen A, Framer A. Protracted withdrawal syndrome after stopping antidepressants: A descriptive quantitative analysis of consumer narratives from a large internet forum. *Ther Adv Psychopharmacol* 2020; 10: 2045125320980573.

8. Ruhe H, Horikx A, van Avendonk M, Groeneweg B, Woutersen-Koch H. Multidisciplinary recommednations for discontinuation of SSRIs and SNRIs. *Lancet Psychiatry* 2019.

9. Shapiro B. Switching to fluoxetine to taper off SSRIs (in preparation).

10. Hirose S. Restlessness related to SSRI withdrawal. *Psychiatry Clin Neurosci* 2001; 55: 79–80.

11. Guy A, Brown M, Lewis S, Horowitz MA. The 'patient voice' – patients who experience antidepressant withdrawal symptoms are often dismissed, or mis-diagnosed with relapse, or onset of a new medical condition. *Ther Adv Psychopharmacol* 2020; 10: 204512532096718.

12. Narayan V, Haddad PM. Antidepressant discontinuation manic states: A critical review of the literature and suggested diagnostic criteria. *J Psychopharmacol* 2010; 25: 306–13.

13. Sathananthan GL, Gershon S. Imipramine withdrawal: an akathisia-like syndrome. *Am J Psychiatry* 1973; 130: 1286–7.

14. Tachere RO, Modirrousta M. Beyond anxiety and agitation: A clinical approach to akathisia. *Aust Fam Physician* 2017; 46: 296–8.

15. Lohr JB, Eidt CA, Abdulrazzaq Alfaraj A, Soliman MA. The clinical challenges of akathisia. *CNS Spectr* 2015; 20 Suppl 1: 1–14; quiz 15–6.

16. Akathisia Alliance for education and research. Akathisia Alliance for education and research. https://akathisiaalliance.org/about-akathisia/ (accessed 17 September 2022).

17. Taubert M, Back I. The akathisic cyclist – an unusual symptomatic treatment. 2007. https://orca.cardiff.ac.uk/id/eprint/117286/ (accessed 24 September 2022).

18. Davies J, Read J. A systematic review into the incidence, severity and duration of antidepressant withdrawal effects: Are guidelines evidence-based? *Addict Behav* 2019; 97: 111–21.

19. Moncrieff J, Read J, Horowitz M. The nature and impact of antidepressant withdrawal symptoms and development of the Discriminatory Antidepressant Withdrawal Symptoms Scale (DAWSS) (in preparation).

20. Horowitz M, Flanigan R, Cooper R, Moncrieff J. The determinants of outcome from antidepressant withdrawal in a large survey of patients (in preparation).

21. Framer A. What I have learnt from helping thousands of people taper off psychotropic medications. *Ther Adv Psychopharmacol* 2021; 11: 204512532199127.

22. Becker HC. Kindling in alcohol withdrawal. *Alcohol Health Res World* 1998; 22: 25–33.

23. Flemenbaum A. Postsynaptic supersensitivity and kindling: Further evidence of similarities. *Am J Drug Alcohol Abuse* 1978; 5: 247–54.

24. Reisman Y. Post-SSRI sexual dysfunction. *BMJ* 2020; 368. doi:10.1136/bmj.m754.

25. Healy D, Le Noury J, Mangin D. Enduring sexual dysfunction after treatment with antidepressants, 5α-reductase inhibitors and isotretinoin: 300 cases. *Int J Risk Saf Med* 2018; 29: 125–34.

26. Reisman Y, Pfaus JG, Lowenstein L. Post-SSRI Sexual dysfunction (PSSD). In: Reisman Y, Lowenstein L, Tripodi F, eds. *Textbook of Rare Sexual Medicine Conditions.* Springer International Publishing, 2022: 51–63.

27. Otis HG, King JH. Unanticipated psychotropic medication reactions. *J Ment Health Couns* 2006; 28: 218–40.

28. Smith SW, Hauben M, Aronson JK. Paradoxical and bidirectional drug effects. *Drug Saf* 2012; 35: 173–89.

29. Bangert MK, Hasbun R. Neurological and psychiatric adverse effects of Antimicrobials. *CNS Drugs* 2019; 33: 727–53.

30. Parker G. Psychotropic Drug intolerance. *J Nerv Ment Dis* 2018; 206: 223–5.

CHAPTER 2

Tapering Guidance for Specific Antidepressants

The following sections include guides to tapering the most commonly used antidepressants. Where neuroimaging of these drugs has been conducted, receptor occupancy was derived from these studies. These data were available for 22 of the 25 drugs. For the three drugs for which there was no nuclear imaging, regimens were based on the common pattern for other drugs in the class. Pharmacologically rational regimens were then calculated from these equations and are presented as 'faster', 'moderate' and 'slower' regimens.

There is little research to determine which of these three regimens is most suitable for a given patient. Some guidance is provided in Tables 2.11, 2.12 and 2.22 on estimating risk of withdrawal for a particular patient which can guide selection of one of these regimens. However, the response of the patient to initial reductions is the best guide to the appropriate pace and the patient's experience should be prioritised over what an algorithm suggests.

These guides include a summary of formulations available around the world for each drug. Licensed and 'off-label' options to enable tapering are presented for all drugs. The guidance presented here is consistent with the UK NICE guidelines on how to safely stop antidepressants,[1,2] and with guidance from RCPsych,[3] but offers more detail in order to allow implementation of deprescribing in clinical practice.

Although there are many uncertainties in the field of deprescribing, the aim of this book is to provide some structure to the process of stopping these drugs, acknowledging that clinical judgement will have to be used to modify the regimens to fit the particular circumstances of individual patients. The key feature of these suggested regimens is that they represent a framework around which deviation can take place according to patient experience. The aim is not necessarily to encourage deprescribing but to assure it is undertaken in a manner that optimises patient experience and outcome.

References

1. National Institute of Health and Social Care (NICE). Medicines associated with dependence or withdrawal symptoms: safe prescribing and withdrawal management for adults | Guidance | NICE. 2022. https://www.nice.org.uk/guidance/ng215/chapter/Recommendations (accessed 27 June 2022).
2. National Institute for Health and Care Excellence (NICE). Depression in adults: treatment and management | Guidance | NICE. 2022; published online June. https://www.nice.org.uk/guidance/ng222 (accessed 16 July 2022).
3. Burn W, Horowitz M, Roycroft G, Taylor D. Stopping antidepressants. Stopping antidepressants. 2020. https://www.rcpsych.ac.uk/mental-health/treatments-and-wellbeing/stopping-antidepressants (accessed 18 February 2023).

Agomelatine

Trade names: Valdoxan, Thymanax.

Description: Agomelatine is a melatonergic agonist, acting on MT_1 and MT_2 receptors, as well as an antagonist at $5\text{-}HT_{2C}$ receptors.[1] Agomelatine has no effect on monoamine uptake and no affinity for adrenergic, histaminergic, cholinergic or dopaminergic receptors.[1]

Withdrawal effects: After 12 weeks of treatment with agomelatine, no withdrawal effects were demonstrated,[2] although there are informal reports of patients experiencing withdrawal effects from the drug.[3]

Peak plasma: 1–2 hours.[1]

Half-life: Approximately 2.3 hours. The manufacturer recommends it be taken once daily at bedtime.[1]

Receptor occupancy: The relationship between dose of agomelatine and occupancy of its target receptors, including its major targets the melatonin receptors MT_1 and MT_2, is hyperbolic, dictated by the law of mass action.[4] Antidepressants also show a hyperbolic pattern between dose and clinical effects,[5] which may be relevant to withdrawal effects from agomelatine. However, there has been no neuroimaging conducted to determine agomelatine's receptor occupancy, and data to derive this relationship is lacking. Here we provide a pharmacologically informed reduction schedule based on the average trajectory for other antidepressants. Linear dose reductions will cause increasingly large reductions in pharmacological effect which may cause increasingly severe withdrawal effects (Figure 2.14a). To produce equal-sized reductions in effect on receptor occupancy will require hyperbolically reducing doses (Figure 2.14b), which informs the reductions presented.

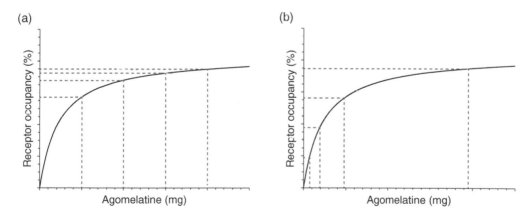

Figure 2.14 (a) Linear reductions of dose cause increasingly large reductions in effect on receptor targets, possibly associated with more withdrawal effects. (b) Even reductions of effect at target receptors requires hyperbolic dose reductions. The final dose before stopping will need to be very small so that this step down is not larger (in terms of effect on receptor occupancy) than previous reductions.

CHAPTER 2

Available formulations: Agomelatine is available in tablets.

Tablets

Dosage	UK	Europe	USA	Australia	Canada
25mg	✓	✓	–	✓	–

Off-label options: Agomelatine's coating has little effect on disintegration and absorption so, although not recommended by the manufacturer, tablets may be split or crushed. Agomelatine is poorly soluble in water.[6] A 1mg/mL suspension could be made by adding water to a 25mg tablet to make up 25mL. The tablet can be crushed with a spoon or pestle and mortar to speed up disintegration. Vigorous shaking of this suspension before administration will ensure that the active drug is equally distributed throughout the liquid. As its stability cannot be assured it should be consumed immediately, and any unused suspension discarded. For example, 1mL of this suspension could be taken to provide 1mg of agomelatine. It may be possible to have a liquid version compounded or smaller formulations of tablets made, e.g. 'tapering strips'.[7]

Worked example: To illustrate how the volumes were calculated in the regimens given below we provide a worked example. To make up 2mg of agomelatine a 1mg/mL suspension can be used, made up as outlined above. The volume of 1mg/mL liquid required to give a dose of 2mg of agomelatine is 2/1 = 2mL.

Deprescribing notes: Initial reductions can be estimated from Tables 2.11 and 2.22, although patient preference should be taken into account. Sometimes an even smaller reduction to start with may be advisable to boost a patient's confidence that they can taper if performed carefully. Each reduction should be made when the withdrawal symptoms from the previous reduction have largely resolved so that subsequent reductions do not lead to cumulative withdrawal symptoms. Withdrawal symptoms should be tolerable and last at most a couple of weeks (see Figure 2.9). Allowing for a sufficient observation period, reductions can therefore be made about every 2 to 4 weeks. If withdrawal symptoms are moderately severe or take longer than a couple of weeks to resolve, dose reductions should be postponed until symptoms resolve and then made more gradual by choosing a slower tapering rate. If severe withdrawal symptoms occur, then the patient should return to a higher dose, wait until symptoms resolve and thereafter taper at a slower rate.

Suggested taper schedules for agomelatine

A. A faster taper with five steps based on average trajectories for other antidepressants (approximate length: 2–3 months). Patients who have been on the medication for only a few weeks will probably be able to taper more quickly and might follow every second or third step of this regimen, and make reductions every few days or so. For people who have only taken an antidepressant for a few weeks, the duration of the taper should not be longer than the period that the patient has been on the drug. For example, if agomelatine is taken for 3 weeks the taper should be less than 3 weeks.

B. A moderate taper with 10 steps based on average trajectories for other antidepressants (approximate length: 5–10 months).

C. A slower taper with 20 steps based on average trajectories for other antidepressants (approximate length: 10–20 months).

D. Some patients will be unable to taper at the slowest rates shown here and will need to taper by even smaller decrements, thus lengthening the overall period of tapering. Such a regimen could be constructed by placing intermediate steps in regimen C. For example, 3mg, 2mg, 1mg, 0mg could be modified to be 3mg, 2.5mg, 2mg, 1.5mg, 1mg, 0.5mg, 0mg. Further intermediate steps could also be added. Microtapering (tapering by a small amount each day, rather than by larger reductions every 2–4 weeks) is another possible approach (see benzodiazepines chapter for further details).

Please note that none of these regimens should be seen as prescriptive – that is, that patients must strictly adhere to them. They are given as example regimens and are not 'set and forget' but should be modified in order to ensure that withdrawal symptoms are tolerable throughout a taper – for example intermediate steps halfway between the doses listed could be added to make a more gradual taper.

A. **Faster taper** with 5 steps – with reductions made every 2–4 weeks.*

Step	Dose (mg)	Tablets
1	50	Use tablets
2	25	Use tablets
3	12.5	Use ½ tablet**
4	6.25	Use ¼ tablet**
5	0	0

*For longer term users, the time between each decrease may be shortened to 1 week if the patient is able to make the first couple of reductions with no withdrawal symptoms. The interval between reductions should never be less than 1 week because this might increase the risk of relapse, even in the absence of withdrawal effects.[8,9]
**Alternatively, could be administered using a liquid formulation.

B. **A moderate taper** with 10 steps – with reductions made every 2–4 weeks.

Step	Dose (mg)	Volume	Step	Dose (mg)	Volume
1	50	Use tablets	6	1.9	1.9mL
2	25	Use tablets	7	1.2	1.2mL
3	12.5	Use ½ tablets*	8	0.8	0.8mL
4	6.25	Use ¼ tablets	9	0.4	0.4mL
Switch to agomelatine **1mg/mL suspension**			10	0	0
5	3.3	3.3mL			
See further steps in the right-hand column					

*Alternatively, could be administered using a liquid formulation.

CHAPTER 2

C. A slower taper with 19 steps – with reductions made every 2–4 weeks.

Step	Dose (mg)	Volume	Step	Dose (mg)	Volume
1	50	Use tablets	10	2.5	2.5mL
2	37.5	Use ½ tablets*	11	1.9	1.9mL
3	25	Use tablets	12	1.5	1.5mL
4	18.75	Use ¾ tablets*	13	1.2	1.2mL
5	12.5	Use ½ tablets*	14	1	1mL
Switch to agomelatine **1mg/mL suspension**			15	0.8	0.8mL
6	9	9mL	16	0.6	0.6mL
7	6.25	6.25mL**	17	0.4	0.4mL
8	4.6	4.6mL	18	0.2	0.2mL
9	3.3	3.3mL	19	0	0
See further steps in the right-hand column					

*Alternatively, could be administered as a liquid formulation
**Alternatively, could be administered as a ¼ tablet.

References

1. Servier. Agomelatine – Summary of product characteristics. https://www.medicines.org.uk/emc/medicine/21830#gref (accessed 8 October 2022).
2. Montgomery SA, Kennedy SH, Burrows GD, Lejoyeux M, Hindmarch I. Absence of discontinuation symptoms with agomelatine and occurrence of discontinuation symptoms with paroxetine: a randomized, double-blind, placebo-controlled discontinuation study. *Int Clin Psychopharmacol* 2004; 19: 271–80.
3. Framer A. What I have learnt from helping thousands of people taper off psychotropic medications. *Ther Adv Psychopharmacol* 2021; 11: 204512532199127.
4. Holford N. Pharmacodynamic principles and the time course of delayed and cumulative drug effects. *Translational and Clinical Pharmacology* 2018; 26: 56.
5. Furukawa TA, Cipriani A, Cowen PJ, Leucht S, Egger M, Salanti G. Optimal dose of selective serotonin reuptake inhibitors, venlafaxine, and mirtazapine in major depression: a systematic review and dose-response meta-analysis. *The Lancet Psychiatry* 2019; 6: 601–9.
6. NPS. Agomelatine – NPS medicine wise. https://www.nps.org.au/medicine-finder/valdoxan-tablets#full-pi (accessed 8 October 2022).
7. Groot PC, van Os J. How user knowledge of psychotropic drug withdrawal resulted in the development of person-specific tapering medication. *Ther Adv Psychopharmacol* 2020; 10: 204512532093245.
8. Baldessarini RJ, Tondo L, Ghiani C, Lepri B. Illness risk following rapid versus gradual discontinuation of antidepressants. *Am J Psychiatry* 2010; 167: 934–41.
9. Gøtzsche PC, Demasi M. Interventions to help patients withdraw from depression drugs: A systematic review. *Int J Risk Saf Med.* 2023 September 13. doi: 10.3233/JRS-230011. Epub ahead of print.

Amitriptyline

Trade names: Elavil, Endep.

Description: Amitriptyline is a tricyclic antidepressant that blocks SERT and NET.[1] It also has strong binding affinities for alpha-adrenergic, histamine (H_1) and muscarinic (M_1) receptors.[1]

Withdrawal effects: In a structured analysis tricyclic antidepressants were placed in a high-risk category for withdrawal effects,[2] with one placebo-controlled double-blind study demonstrating that when amitriptyline was tapered over 6 months 80% of patients experienced withdrawal effects.[3] Amitriptyline was responsible for about the same number of calls regarding issues with withdrawal to a medication helpline (normalised to prescription numbers) for most SSRIs.[4] In an analysis of withdrawal effects in neonates to the World Health Organization (WHO) adverse effect database, tricyclic antidepressants came up with the strongest signal, with amitriptyline the lowest in the group, similar to rates of reporting for SSRIs.[5]

Peak plasma: 1–12 hours.[1]

Half-life: About 25 hours (18 to 28 hours). The manufacturer recommends twice daily dosing, with the highest dose being close to bedtime because of its sedative effect, although it is often taken once at night.[6,7] Every-other-day dosing is not recommended for tapering because of the substantial reductions in plasma concentrations this would produce, possibly giving rise to withdrawal effects.

Receptor occupancy: The relationship between dose of amitriptyline and occupancy of its target receptors SERT and NET is hyperbolic, according to the law of mass action.[8] This also applies to its activity on the alpha-adrenergic, H_1 histamine and M_1 muscarinic receptors.[8] Antidepressants show a hyperbolic pattern between dose and clinical effects,[9] which may be relevant to withdrawal effects from amitriptyline. However, there has been no neuroimaging conducted to determine amitriptyline's receptor occupancy, and data to derive this relationship is lacking. Here we provide a pharmacologically informed reduction schedule based on the average trajectory for other antidepressants. Linear dose reductions will cause increasingly large reductions in pharmacological effect, which may cause increasingly severe withdrawal effects (Figure 2.15a). To produce equal-sized reductions in effect on receptor occupancy will require hyperbolically reducing doses (Figure 2.15b),[10] which informs the reductions presented.

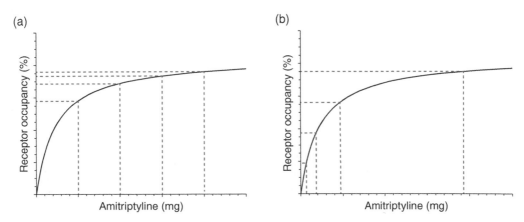

Figure 2.15 (a) Linear reductions of dose cause increasingly large reductions in effect on receptor targets, possibly associated with more withdrawal effects. (b) Even reductions of effect at target receptors requires hyperbolic dose reductions. The final dose before stopping will need to be very small so that this step down is not larger (in terms of effect on receptor occupancy) than previous reductions.

Available formulations: Amitriptyline is available as amitriptyline hydrochloride in tablets, sustained-release capsules and liquid form.

Tablets

Dosage	UK	Europe	USA	Australia	Canada
10mg	✓	✓	✓	✓	✓
25mg	✓	✓	✓	✓	✓
50mg	✓	✓	✓	✓	✓
75mg	–	–	✓	–	✓
100mg	–	–	✓	–	–
150mg	–	–	✓	–	–

Sustained-release capsules

Dosage	UK	Europe	USA	Australia	Canada
25mg	–	✓	–	–	–
50mg	–	✓	–	–	–

Liquid

Dosage	UK	Europe	USA	Australia	Canada
10mg/5mL (2mg/mL)	✓	✓	–	–	✓
25mg/5mL (5mg/mL)	✓	✓	–	–	–
50mg/5mL (10mg/mL)	✓	✓	–	–	–

Dilutions: To make up smaller doses for tapering a dilution of the solution will be required. As amitriptyline is already dissolved in an aqueous solution[11] further dilution in water should be acceptable in terms of solubility. Stability cannot be assured and so dilutions should be consumed immediately following preparation.

Dilutions	Solution required	How to prepare solution
Doses ≥0.4mg	10mg/5mL (2mg/mL)*	Original solution
Doses < 0.4mg	0.2mg/mL	Add 1mL of original solution (10mg/5mL) to 9mL of water**

*Other solutions can also be used.
**Different dilutions will be needed for other starting solutions.

Worked example: To illustrate how the volumes were calculated in the regimens given below we provide a worked example. To make up 4mg of amitriptyline the 2mg/mL solution can be used. The volume of 2mg/mL liquid required to give a dose of 4mg of amitriptyline is 4/2 = 2mL.

Off-label options: Guidelines for people who cannot swallow tablets (e.g. the NEWT guidelines in the UK) suggest that amitriptyline tablets can be crushed and dispersed in water for administration as an off-label use.[12] Crushed tablets have a bitter taste, and produce a local anaesthetic effect on the mouth.[12,13] A 2mg/mL suspension could be made by adding water to a 50mg tablet to make up 25mL. The tablet may be crushed with a spoon or pestle and mortar before mixing with water to speed up this process. The suspension should be shaken vigorously before use. As its stability cannot be assured, it should be consumed immediately, and any unused suspension discarded. Other options to make up small doses include compounding smaller dose tablets, including the option of 'tapering strips'.[14]

Deprescribing notes: Initial reductions can be estimated from Tables 2.11 and 2.22, although patient preference should be taken into account. Sometimes an even smaller reduction to start with may be advisable to boost a patient's confidence that they can taper if performed carefully. Each reduction should be made when the withdrawal symptoms from the previous reduction have largely resolved so that subsequent reductions do not lead to cumulative withdrawal symptoms. Withdrawal symptoms should be tolerable and last at most a couple of weeks (see Figure 2.9). Allowing for a sufficient observation period, reductions can therefore be made about every 2 to 4 weeks. If withdrawal symptoms are moderately severe or take longer than a couple of weeks to resolve, dose reductions should be postponed until symptoms resolve and then made more gradual by choosing a slower tapering rate. If severe withdrawal symptoms occur, then the patient should return to a higher dose, wait until symptoms resolve and thereafter taper at a slower rate.

Suggested taper schedules for amitriptyline

A. A faster taper with 10 steps based on average trajectory for other antidepressants (approximate length: 5–10 months). Patients who have been on the medication for only a few weeks will probably be able to taper more quickly and might follow every second or third step of this regimen, and make reductions every few days or so. For people who have only taken an antidepressant for a few weeks, the duration of the taper should not be longer than the period that the patient has been on the drug. For example, if amitriptyline is taken for 3 weeks the taper should be less than 3 weeks.

B. A moderate taper with 20 steps based on average trajectory for other antidepressants (approximate length: 10–20 months).

C. A slower taper with 40 steps based on average trajectory for other antidepressants (approximate length: 20–40 months).

D. Some patients will be unable to taper at the slowest rates shown here and will need to taper by even smaller decrements, thus lengthening the overall period of tapering. Such a regimen could be constructed by placing intermediate steps in regimen C. For example, 3mg, 2mg, 1mg, 0mg could be modified to be 3mg, 2.5mg, 2mg, 1.5mg, 1mg, 0.5mg, 0mg. Further intermediate steps could also be added. Microtapering (tapering by a small amount each day, rather than by larger reductions every 2–4 weeks) is another possible approach (see benzodiazepines chapter for further details).

Please note that none of these regimens should be seen as prescriptive – that is, it is not suggested that patient must strictly adhere to them. They are given as example regimens and are not 'set and forget' but should be modified in order to ensure that withdrawal symptoms are tolerable throughout a taper – for example intermediate steps halfway between the doses listed could be added to make a more gradual taper.

A. Faster taper with 10 steps – with reductions made every 2–4 weeks.*

Step	Dose (mg)	Volume	Step	Dose (mg)	Volume
1	100	Use tablets	Switch to amitriptyline **2mg/mL solution**		
2	50	Use tablets	7	3	1.5mL
3	25	Use tablets	8	1.6	0.8mL
4	12.5	Use ½ tablets**	9	0.8	0.4mL
5	7.5	Use ¾ tablets**	10	0	0
6	5	Use ½ tablets**			
See further steps in the right-hand column					

*For longer term users, the time between each decrease may be shortened to 1 week if the patient is able to make the first couple of reductions with no withdrawal symptoms. The interval between reductions should never be less than 1 week because this might increase the risk of relapse, even in the absence of withdrawal effects.[15,16]
**Alternatively, there could be a switch to a liquid version sooner if preferred.

B. A moderate taper with 20 steps – with reductions made every 2–4 weeks.

Step	Dose (mg)	Volume	Step	Dose (mg)	Volume
1	100	Use tablets	11	5	2.5mL*
2	70	Use tablets	12	4	2mL
3	50	Use tablets	13	3	1.5mL
4	35	Use tablets	14	2.5	1.25mL
5	25	Use tablets	15	2	1mL
6	17.5	Use ¾ tablets*	16	1.5	0.75mL
7	12.5	Use ½ or ¼ tablets*	17	1	0.5mL
8	10	Use tablets	18	0.6	0.3mL
9	7.5	Use ¾ tablets*	19	0.3	0.15mL
Switch to amitriptyline **2mg/mL solution**			20	0	0
10	6	3mL			
See further steps in the right-hand column					

*Alternatively, these doses could be made up by use of an amitriptyline solution.
**Alternatively, this dose could be made up with a half tablet.

C. **A slower taper** with 39 steps based on average trajectory for other antidepressants – with reductions made every 2–4 weeks.

Step	Dose (mg)	Volume	Step	Dose (mg)	Volume	Step	Dose (mg)	Volume
1	100	Use tablets	14	12.5	6.25mL*	28	2.75	1.38mL
2	85	Use tablets	15	11.25	5.63mL*	29	2.5	1.25mL
3	70	Use tablets	16	10	5mL*	30	2.25	1.13mL
4	60	Use tablets	17	9	4.5mL	31	2	1mL
5	50	Use tablets	18	8	4mL	32	1.75	0.88mL
6	42.5	Use ¼ tablets	19	7	3.5mL	33	1.5	0.75mL
7	35	Use tablets	20	6.5	3.25mL	34	1.25	0.63mL
8	30	Use tablets	21	6	3mL	35	1	0.5
9	25	Use tablet	22	5.5	2.75	36	0.75	0.38mL
Switch to amitriptyline **2mg/mL solution**			23	5	2.5mL*	37	0.5	0.25mL
10	22.5	11.25mL*	24	4.5	2.25mL	Switch to amitriptyline **0.2mg/mL dilution**		
11	20	10mL*	25	4	2mL	38	0.25	1.25mL
12	17.5	8.75mL*	26	3.5	1.75mL	39	0	0
13	15	7.5mL*	27	3	1.5mL			
See further steps in the middle column			**See further steps in the right-hand column**					

*Alternatively, these doses could be made up with tablets, half tablets or quarter tablets.

References

1. Marsh W. Amitriptyline. In: *xPharm: The Comprehensive Pharmacology Reference*. StatPearls Publishing, 2007: 1–6.
2. Henssler J, Heinz A, Brandt L, Bschor T. Antidepressant withdrawal and rebound phenomena. *Dtsch Arztebl Int* 2019; 116: 355–61.
3. Giller E Jr, Bialos D, Harkness L, Jatlow P, Waldo M. Long-term amitriptyline in chronic depression. *Hillside J Clin Psychiatry* 1985; 7: 16–33.
4. Taylor D, Stewart S, Connolly A. Antidepressant withdrawal symptoms – telephone calls to a national medication helpline. *J Affect Disord* 2006; 95: 129–33.
5. Gastaldon C, Arzenton E, Raschi E, et al. Neonatal withdrawal syndrome following in utero exposure to antidepressants: a disproportionality analysis of VigiBase, the WHO spontaneous reporting database. *Psychol Med* 2022: 1–9.
6. Brown & Burk UK. Amitriptyline – summary of product characteristics. 2022. https://www.medicines.org.uk/emc/product/10849/smpc#gref (accessed 12 October 2022).
7. FDA. Amitriptyline – highlights of prescribing information. 2014.
8. Holford N. Pharmacodynamic principles and the time course of delayed and cumulative drug effects. *Transl Clin* 2018; 26: 56.
9. Furukawa TA, Cipriani A, Cowen PJ, Leucht S, Egger M, Salanti G. Optimal dose of selective serotonin reuptake inhibitors, venlafaxine, and mirtazapine in major depression: a systematic review and dose-response meta-analysis. *The Lancet Psychiatry* 2019; 6: 601–9.
10. Horowitz MA, Taylor D. Tapering of SSRI treatment to mitigate withdrawal symptoms. *The Lancet Psychiatry* 2019; 6: 538–46.
11. Thame Laboratories. Amitriptyline hydrochloride 10mg/5ml Oral Solution. https://www.medicines.org.uk/emc/product/2457/smpc (accessed 14 October 2022).
12. Smyth J. The NEWT Guidelines for administration of medication to patients with enteral feeding tubes or swallowing difficulties website. The NEWT Guidelines. 2011. https://www.newtguidelines.com/index.html (accessed 7 September 2022).
13. Bostwick JR, Demehri A. Pills to powder: an updated clinician's reference for crushable psychotropics. *Curr Psychiatr* 2017; 16: 46–9.
14. Groot PC, van Os J. How user knowledge of psychotropic drug withdrawal resulted in the development of person-specific tapering medication. *Ther Adv Psychopharmacol* 2020; 10: 204512532093245.
15. Baldessarini RJ, Tondo L, Ghiani C, Lepri B. Illness risk following rapid versus gradual discontinuation of antidepressants. *Am J Psychiatry* 2010; 167: 934–41.
16. Gøtzsche PC, Demasi M. Interventions to help patients withdraw from depression drugs: A systematic review. *Int J Risk Saf Med.* 2023 September 13. doi: 10.3233/JRS-230011. Epub ahead of print.

CHAPTER 2

CHAPTER 2

Bupropion

Trade names: Wellburtin, Aplenzin, Elontril, Forfivo.

Description: Bupropion is chemically an aminoketone – a substituted amphetamine. Pharmacologically, it is a noradrenaline-dopamine reuptake inhibitor, although its effects on dopamine are relatively weak, and a nicotinic receptor antagonist.[1] Bupropion also acts to a lesser degree on serotonergic receptors.[1]

Withdrawal effects: Bupropion has not been extensively examined for withdrawal effects, with a recent structured review designating it of 'unclear' risk[2]. In an analysis of the WHO adverse effect database bupropion was found to be in the lower risk category for antidepressants.[3] In a recent analysis of an adverse effect reporting database, the incidence of withdrawal effects in neonates born to mothers taking bupropion was uncertain.[4] Withdrawal effects have been described in published case studies.[5]

Peak plasma: About 6 hours.[6]

Half-life: There are three buproprion formulations with varying effective plasma half-lives and therefore durations of action. Immediate-release (IR) tablets, with a half-life of approximately 14 hours, are recommended by the manufacturer to be taken three times a day.[7] Sustained-release (SR) tablets with a half-life of approximately 21 hours are recommended to be taken twice a day.[8] Extended-release (XR or XL) tablets, with a half-life of approximately 21 hours require once-a-day dosing.[9] Every-other-day dosing is not recommended for tapering because of the substantial reductions in plasma concentrations this would produce, possibly giving rise to withdrawal effects.

Receptor occupancy: The relationship between the dose of bupropion and occupancy of its target receptors NET and DAT is hyperbolic, dictated by the law of mass action;[10] this will also apply to its occupancy of other receptors. Antidepressants show a hyperbolic pattern between dose and clinical effects,[11] which may be relevant to withdrawal effects from bupropion. However, there has been no neuroimaging conducted to determine bupropion's receptor occupancy, and data to derive this relationship is lacking. Pharmacologically informed reduction schedules have been derived from an average trajectory for other antidepressants. Linear dose reductions will cause increasingly large reductions in pharmacological effect, which may cause increasingly severe withdrawal effects (Figure 2.16a).

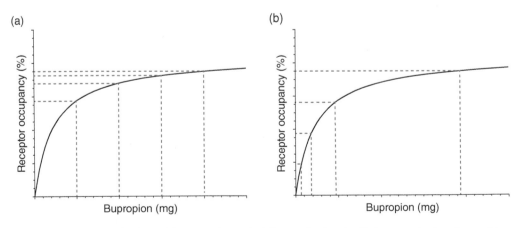

Figure 2.16 (a) Linear reductions of dose cause increasingly large reductions in effect on receptor targets, possibly associated with more withdrawal effects. (b) Even reductions of effect at target receptors requires hyperbolic dose reductions. The final dose before stopping will need to be very small so that this step down is not larger (in terms of effect on receptor occupancy) than previous reductions.

To produce equal-sized reductions in receptor occupancy will require hyperbolically reducing doses (Figure 2.16b),[12] which informs the reductions presented.

Available formulations: Bupropion is available as bupropion hydrochloride in immediate-, sustained- and extended-release tablets. These formulations are all bio-equivalent (both rate and extent of absorption) for bupropion and its three quantitatively important metabolites, and differ only in their elimination half-lives.[13] Bupropion is also available as bupropion hydrobromide in extended-release tablets.

Immediate-release tablets

Dosage	UK	Europe	USA	Australia	Canada
75mg	–	–	✓	–	–
100mg	–	–	✓	–	–

Sustained-release tablets

Dosage	UK	Europe	USA	Australia	Canada
100mg	–	–	✓	–	✓
150mg	✓	✓	✓	✓	✓
200mg	–	–	✓	–	–

Extended-release tablets

Dosage	UK	Europe	USA	Australia	Canada
150mg	–	–	✓	–	✓
300mg	–	–	✓	–	✓
450mg	–	–	✓	–	–

Extended-release tablets

Dosage	UK	Europe	USA	Australia	Canada
174mg*	–	–	✓	–	–
348mg**	–	–	✓	–	–
522mg***	–	–	✓	–	–

*174mg of bupropion hydrobromide is equivalent to 150mg bupropion hydrochloride.
**348mg of bupropion hydrobromide is equivalent to 300mg bupropion hydrochloride.
***522mg of bupropion hydrobromide is equivalent to 450mg bupropion hydrochloride.

Off-label options: Immediate-release bupropion can be split or crushed and mixed with water or a suspending vehicle like Ora-Plus as an off-label use for making small doses to facilitate tapering.[14] Bupropion is highly soluble in water (312mg/mL), but has a bitter taste and produces local anaesthesia of the oral mucosa.[7] A 1mg/mL solution could be made by adding water to a 100mg tablet to make up 100mL. Crushing the tablet with a spoon or pestle and mortar may speed up dispersion and aid dissolution. The solution should be shaken vigorously before use. As its stability cannot be assured it should be consumed immediately, and any unused solution discarded. The label advises that the slow release form of bupropion should not be crushed as this may lead to an increased risk of adverse effects, including seizures.[15] Other options include instructing a compounding pharmacy to make up a liquid or smaller formulations of tablets, for example, 'tapering strips'.[16]

Worked example: To illustrate how the volumes were calculated in the regimens given below we provide a worked example. To make up 5mg of bupropion the 1mg/mL solution can be used, prepared as above. The volume of 1mg/mL liquid required to give a dose of 5mg of bupropion is 5/1 = 5mL.

Deprescribing notes: Initial reductions can be estimated from Tables 2.11 and 2.22, although patient preference should be taken into account. Sometimes an even smaller reduction to start with may be advisable to boost a patient's confidence that they can taper if performed carefully. Each reduction should be made when the withdrawal symptoms from the previous reduction have largely resolved so that subsequent reductions do not lead to cumulative withdrawal symptoms. Withdrawal symptoms should be tolerable and last at most a couple of weeks (see Figure 2.9). Allowing for a sufficient observation period, reductions can therefore be made about every 2 to 4 weeks. If withdrawal symptoms are moderately severe or take longer than a couple of weeks to resolve, dose reductions should be postponed until symptoms resolve and then made more gradual by choosing a slower tapering rate. If severe withdrawal symptoms occur then the patient should return to a higher dose, wait until symptoms resolve and thereafter taper at a slower rate.

Suggested taper schedules for bupropion

A. A faster taper with 11 steps based on average trajectory for other antidepressants (approximate length: 5–10 months). Patients who have been on the medication for only a few weeks will probably be able to taper more quickly and might follow every second or third step of this regimen, and make reductions every few days or so. For people who have only taken an antidepressant for a few weeks, the duration of the taper should not be longer than the period that the patient has been on the drug. For example, if bupropion is taken for 3 weeks the taper should be less than 3 weeks.

B. A moderate taper with 21 steps based on average trajectory for other antidepressants (approximate length: 10–20 months).

C. A slower taper with 41 steps based on average trajectory for other antidepressants (approximate length: 20–40 months).

D. Some patients will be unable to taper at the slowest rates shown here and will need to taper by even smaller decrements, thus lengthening the overall period of tapering. Such a regimen could be constructed by placing intermediate steps in regimen C. For example, 3mg, 2mg, 1mg, 0mg could be modified to be 3mg, 2.5mg, 2mg, 1.5mg, 1mg, 0.5mg, 0mg. Further intermediate steps could also be added. Microtapering (tapering by a small amount each day, rather than by larger reductions every 2–4 weeks) is another possible approach (see benzodiazepines chapter for further details).

Please note that none of these regimens should be seen as prescriptive – that is, it is not suggested that patient must strictly adhere to them. They are given as example regimens and are not 'set and forget' but should be modified in order to ensure that withdrawal symptoms are tolerable throughout a taper – for example intermediate steps halfway between the doses listed could be added to make a more gradual taper.

A. Faster taper with 11 steps – with reductions made every 2–4 weeks.*

Step	Dose (mg)	Volume	Step	Dose (mg)	Volume
1	450	Use SR/XR tablets	6	22.5	11.25mL (twice daily)
2	300	Use SR/XR tablets	7	15	7.5mL (twice daily)
3	150	Use SR/XR tablets	8	10	5mL (twice daily)
4	75	Use ½ IR tablets (twice daily)**	9	5	2.5mL (twice daily)
5	37.5	Use ¼ IR tablets (twice daily)**	10	2.5	1.25mL (twice daily)
Switch to bupropion **solution (1mg/mL)***			11	0	0
See further steps in the right-hand column					

*For longer term users, the time between each decrease may be shortened to 1 week if the patient is able to make the first couple of reductions with no withdrawal symptoms. The interval between reductions should never be less than 1 week because this might increase the risk of relapse, even in the absence of withdrawal effects.[17,18]
**Alternatively, a 1mg/mL solution, made as outlined above, dosed twice daily, could be used to make up these doses.
***This solution can be made up as outlined above as an off-label option.
Note: IR tablets can also be dosed three times a day.

B. A moderate taper with 21 steps – with reductions made every 2–4 weeks.

Step	Dose (mg)	Volume	Step	Dose (mg)	Volume
1	450	Use SR/XR tablets	11	22.5	11.25mL (twice daily)
2	375	Use SR/XR tablets + 75mg IR	12	18.5	9.25mL (twice daily)
3	300	Use SR/XR tablets	13	15	7.5mL (twice daily)
4	200	Use SR tablets	14	12	6mL (twice daily)
5	150	Use SR/XR tablets	15	9	4.5mL (twice daily)
6	112.5	75mg IR tab mane, ½ IR 75mg tablet nocte	16	7	3.5mL (twice daily)
7	75	Use ½ 75mg IR tablets (twice daily)*	17	5	2.5mL (twice daily)
8	50	Use ¼ 100mg IR tablets (twice daily)*	18	3.5	1.75mL (twice daily)
9	37.5	Use ¼ 75mg IR tablets (twice daily)*	19	2.5	1.25mL (twice daily)
Switch to bupropion **solution (1mg/mL)***			20	1.2	0.6mL (twice daily)
10	30	15mL (twice daily)	21	0	0
See further steps in the right-hand column					

*Alternatively, a 1mg/mL solution, made as outlined above, dosed twice daily, could be used to make up these doses.
**This solution can be made up as outlined above as an off-label option.
Note: IR tablets can also be dosed three times a day.

CHAPTER 2

C. **A slower taper** with 41 steps based on average trajectory for other antidepressants – with reductions made every 2–4 weeks.

Step	Dose (mg)	Volume	Step	Dose (mg)	Volume
1	450	Use SR/XR tablets	21	22.5	11.25mL (twice daily)
2	406.25	Use 350mg SR/XR tabs + ¾ 75mg IR tab	22	20.3	10.15mL (twice daily)
3	375	Use SR/XR tablets +75mg IR tablet	23	18.4	9.2mL (twice daily)
4	337.5	Use SR/XR tablets + ½ 75mg IR tablets	24	16.6	8.3mL (twice daily)
5	300	Use SR/XR tablets	25	15	7.5mL (twice daily)
6	250	Use SR/XR tablets	26	13.4	6.7mL (twice daily)
Switch to bupropion **solution (1mg/mL)***			27	12.0	6.0mL (twice daily)
7	210	105mL (twice daily)	28	10.6	5.3mL (twice daily)
8	180	90mL (twice daily)	29	9.2	4.6mL (twice daily)
9	150	75mL (twice daily)**	30	8.0	4.0mL (twice daily)
10	125	62.5mL (twice daily)	31	6.8	3.4mL (twice daily)
11	105	52.5mL (twice daily)	32	5.8	2.9mL (twice daily)
12	90	45mL (twice daily)	33	4.8	2.4mL (twice daily)
13	75	37.5mL (twice daily)**	34	4.0	2.0mL (twice daily)
14	63	31.5mL (twice daily)	35	3.2	1.6mL (twice daily)
15	53	26.5mL (twice daily)	36	2.4	1.2mL (twice daily)
16	44.6	22.3mL (twice daily)	37	1.8	0.9mL (twice daily)
17	37.5	18.75mL (twice daily)**	38	1.2	0.6mL (twice daily)
18	33	16.5mL (twice daily)	39	0.8	0.4mL (twice daily)
19	29	14.5mL (twice daily)	40	0.4	0.2mL (twice daily)
20	25.6	12.8mL (twice daily)	41	0	0
See further steps in the right-hand column					

*This solution can be made up as outlined above as an off-label option.

**Alternatively, a 1mg/mL solution, made as outlined above, dosed twice daily, could be used to make up these doses.

Note: IR tablets can also be dosed three times a day.

References

1. Moser P. Bupropion. In: *xPharm: The Comprehensive Pharmacology Reference*. StatPearls Publishing, 2008: 1–4.
2. Henssler J, Heinz A, Brandt L, Bschor T. Antidepressant withdrawal and rebound phenomena. *Dtsch Arztebl Int* 2019; 116: 355–61.
3. Gastaldon C, Schoretsanitis G, Arzenton E, et al. Withdrawal syndrome following discontinuation of 28 antidepressants: pharmacovigilance analysis of 31,688 reports from the WHO spontaneous reporting database. *Drug Saf* 2022; 45: 1539–49.
4. Gastaldon C, Arzenton E, Raschi E, et al. Neonatal withdrawal syndrome following in utero exposure to antidepressants: a disproportionality analysis of VigiBase, the WHO spontaneous reporting database. *Psychol Med* 2022: 1–9.
5. Berigan TR. Bupropion-associated withdrawal symptoms revisited: a case report. *Prim Care Companion J Clin Psychiatry* 2002; 4: 78.
6. GlaxoSmithKline UK. Bupropion prolonged release tablets – summary of product characteristics. 2022. https://www.medicines.org.uk/emc/product/3827/smpc#gref (accessed 8 October 2022).
7. FDA. Bupropion hydrochloride immediate-release tablets – highlights of prescribing information. 2009.
8. FDA. Bupropion hydrochloride sustained-release tablets – highlights of prescribing information. 2001.
9. FDA. Bupropion hydrochloride extended-release tablets – highlights of prescribing information. 2009.
10. Holford N. Pharmacodynamic principles and the time course of delayed and cumulative drug effects. *Transl Clin* 2018; 26: 56.
11. Furukawa TA, Cipriani A, Cowen PJ, Leucht S, Egger M, Salanti G. Optimal dose of selective serotonin reuptake inhibitors, venlafaxine, and mirtazapine in major depression: a systematic review and dose–response meta-analysis. *The Lancet Psychiatry* 2019; 6: 601–9.
12. Horowitz MA, Taylor D. Tapering of SSRI treatment to mitigate withdrawal symptoms. *The Lancet Psychiatry* 2019; 6: 538–46.
13. Fava M, Rush AJ, Thase ME, et al. 15 years of clinical experience with bupropion HCl: from bupropion to bupropion SR to bupropion XL. *Prim Care Companion J Clin Psychiatry* 2005; 7: 106–13.
14. Bostwick JR, Demehri A. Pills to powder: An updated clinician's reference for crushable psychotropics. *Curr Psychiatr* 2017; 16: 46–9.
15. GlaxoSmithKline. Wellbutrin (bupropion hydrochloride) tablets label. 2017. https://www.accessdata.fda.gov/drugsatfda_docs/label/2017/018644s052lbl.pdf.
16. Groot PC, van Os J. How user knowledge of psychotropic drug withdrawal resulted in the development of person – specific tapering medication. *Ther Adv Psychopharmacol* 2020; 10: 204512532093245.
17. Baldessarini RJ, Tondo L, Ghiani C, Lepri B. Illness risk following rapid versus gradual discontinuation of antidepressants. *Am J Psychiatry* 2010; 167: 934–41.
18. Gøtzsche PC, Demasi M. Interventions to help patients withdraw from depression drugs: A systematic review. *Int J Risk Saf Med.* 2023 September 13. doi: 10.3233/JRS-230011. Epub ahead of print.

CHAPTER 2

Citalopram

Trade names: Celexa, Cipramil.

Description: Citalopram is an SSRI, with SERT as its major target.[1] It has minimal effect on noradrenaline, dopamine and GABA uptake and no or very low affinity for serotonergic, dopaminergic, adrenergic, and cholinergic receptors.[2]

Withdrawal effects: In a double-blind randomised controlled trial of citalopram discontinuation in people who had used the drug for more than 3 months, 70% of patients met criteria for a withdrawal syndrome (four or more withdrawal symptoms), although this study did not measure severity or duration of these symptoms.[3] In an analysis of the WHO adverse effect database, citalopram emerged as a moderate risk for withdrawal effects compared to other antidepressants.[4]

Peak plasma: 3–4 hours.[1]

Half-life: About 35 hours.[1] Every-other-day dosing is not recommended for tapering because of the substantial reductions in plasma concentrations this would produce, possibly giving rise to withdrawal effects.

Receptor occupancy: The relationship between dose of citalopram and occupancy of its major target SERT is hyperbolic.[5] This applies to other receptor targets as well because this relationship is dictated by the law of mass action.[6] Antidepressants also show a hyperbolic pattern between dose and clinical effects,[7] which may be relevant to withdrawal effects from citalopram. Dose reductions made by linear amounts (e.g. 20mg, 15mg, 10mg, 5mg, 0mg) will cause increasingly large reductions in effect which may cause increasingly severe withdrawal effects (Figure 2.17a). To produce equal-sized reductions in effect on serotonin transporter occupancy will require hyperbolically reducing doses (Figure 2.17b),[8] which informs the reductions presented.

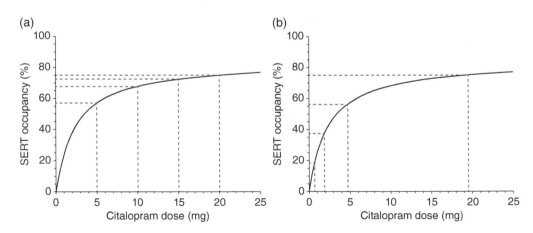

Figure 2.17 (a) Linear reductions of dose cause increasingly large reductions in effect on receptor targets, possibly associated with more withdrawal effects. (b) Even reductions of effect at target receptors requires hyperbolic dose reductions. The final dose before stopping will need to be very small so that this step down is not larger (in terms of effect on receptor occupancy) than previous reductions.

Available formulations: As tablets and liquid.

Tablets
As citalopram hydrobromide.

Dosage	UK	Europe	USA	Australia	Canada
10mg	✓	✓	✓	–	✓
20mg	✓	✓	✓	✓	✓
40mg	✓	✓	✓	✓	✓

Liquid

Concentration	UK	Europe	USA	Australia	Canada
40mg/mL	✓ (15mL)*	–	–	–	–
10mg/5mL (2mg/mL)	–	–	✓ (240mL)**	–	–

*In the UK, the concentrated solution of citalopram hydrochloride (40mg/mL) is 25% more bioavailable than the tablet (hydrobromide) form because of the different salt involved (i.e. 8mg of solution is equivalent to 10mg in tablet form).[1] There are no specific storage instructions for this product.[8]
**In the USA, the liquid form is citalopram hydrobromide, and has equal bioequivalence to tablet form (they are the same salt). Store at 20°–25°C (68°–77°F); excursions permitted to 15°–30°C (59°–86°F).[9]

Dilutions: Dilutions will be required to make the concentrated oral drops into a usable form for many of the doses suggested below. The solution is provided with a dropper mechanism, which provides 2mg of citalopram per drop but does not allow half drops. As this method does not permit many of the regimens outlined below, the dropper mechanism can be removed by hand to allow insertion of a syringe for more precise measurement. According to the manufacturer's instructions, citalopram solution may be mixed with water or juice.[1] The manufacturer recommends consuming this dilution 'immediately', which could be considered meaning within an hour of preparation.[1] Another option is to put one drop of the liquid in some water, mix well and take a portion of the liquid. For example, 1 drop (2mg) could be put into 20mL of water and mixed. Every 10mL of this solution will contain 1mg of citalopram.

UK dilutions*	Solution required	How to prepare solution
Doses ≥ 10mg**	40mg/mL	Original solution
Doses ≥ 1mg**, <10mg**	4mg/mL	Mix 0.5mL of original oral drops solution with 4.5mL of water
Doses < 1mg**	0.4mg/mL	Mix 0.5mL of original oral drops solution with 49.5mL of water

*Note: these drops come as citalopram hydrochloride which are 25% more bioavailable than citalopram hydrobromide (the tablet form) i.e. 8mg in liquid version is equivalent to 10mg in tablet form because of the different salts.[8]
**All these doses refer to tablet equivalent doses.

Worked example: To illustrate how the volumes were calculated in the regimens given below we provide a worked example. To make up a dose equivalent to 3mg of citalopram HBr (tablet form): first, the liquid is more bioavailable than the tablet (8mg of citalopram HCl liquid = 10mg of citalopram HBr tablet) so 0.8 × 3mg of citalopram HCl is required, which is 2.4mg. This can be given with the 4mg/mL solution, prepared as above. The volume of 4mg/mL liquid required to give a dose of 2.4mg of citalopram HCl is 2.4/4 = 0.6mL.

US dilutions*	Solution required	How to prepare solution
Doses ≥ 0.4mg	2mg/mL	Original solution
Doses < 0.4mg	0.2mg/mL	Mix 0.5mL of original solution with 4.5mL of water

*Note: these drops come as citalopram hydrobromide which have the same bioavailability as the tablet form.[9]

Off-label options: Guidelines for people who cannot swallow tablets (e.g. the NEWT guidelines[10] and NHS pharmaceutical guidance[11] in the UK and similar US guidance[12]) suggest that citalopram tablets can be crushed and mixed with water for administration, as an off-label use. Citalopram is poorly soluble and the suspension may taste unpleasant.[10] A 1mg/mL suspension could be made by adding water to a 20mg tablet to make up 20mL. The tablet may be crushed with a spoon or mortar and pestle before mixing with water to speed up this process. This should be shaken vigorously before administration. As its stability cannot be assured it should be consumed immediately, and any unused suspension discarded. Other options to make up small doses include compounding smaller dose tablets, including 'tapering strips'.[13]

Deprescribing notes: Initial reductions can be estimated from Tables 2.11 and 2.22, although patient preference should be taken into account. Sometimes an even smaller reduction to start with may be advisable to boost a patient's confidence that they can taper if performed carefully. Each reduction should be made when the withdrawal symptoms from the previous reduction have largely resolved so that subsequent reductions do not lead to cumulative withdrawal symptoms. Withdrawal symptoms should be tolerable and last at most a couple of weeks (see Figure 2.9). Allowing for a sufficient observation period, reductions can therefore be made about every 2 to 4 weeks. If withdrawal symptoms are moderately severe or take longer than a couple of weeks to resolve, dose reductions should be postponed until symptoms resolve and then made more gradual by choosing a slower tapering rate. If severe withdrawal symptoms occur then the patient should return to a higher dose, wait until symptoms resolve and thereafter taper at a slower rate.

Suggested taper schedules for citalopram

A. A faster taper with up to 11 percentage points of SERT occupancy between each step (approximate length: 4–9 months). Patients who have been on the medication for only a few weeks will probably be able to taper more quickly and might follow every second or third step of this regimen, and make reductions every few days or so. For people who have only taken an antidepressant for a few weeks, the duration of the taper should not be longer than the period that the patient has been on the drug. For example, if citalopram is taken for 3 weeks the taper should be less than 3 weeks.

B. A moderate taper with up to 5 percentage points of SERT occupancy between each step (approximate length: 10–20 months).

C. A slower taper with up to 2.7 percentage points of SERT occupancy between each step (approximate length: 20–40 months).

D. Some patients will be unable to taper at the slowest rates shown here and will need to taper by even smaller decrements, thus lengthening the overall period of tapering. Such a regimen could be constructed by placing intermediate steps in regimen C. For example, 3mg, 2mg, 1mg, 0mg could be modified to be 3mg, 2.5mg, 2mg, 1.5mg, 1mg, 0.5mg, 0mg. Further intermediate steps could also be added. Microtapering (tapering by a small amount each day, rather than by larger reductions every 2–4 weeks) is another possible approach (see benzodiazepines chapter for further details).

Please note that none of these regimens should be seen as prescriptive – that is, it is not suggested that patient must strictly adhere to them. They are given as example regimens and are not 'set and forget' but should be modified in order to ensure that withdrawal symptoms are tolerable throughout a taper – for example intermediate steps halfway between the doses listed could be added to make a more gradual taper.

UK regimens

A. **Faster taper** with up to 11 percentage points of SERT between each step – with reductions made every 2–4 weeks.*

Step	RO (%)	Dose (mg)	Volume**	Step	RO (%)	Dose (mg)	Volume**
1	79	40	Use tablets	6	37	2	0.4mL**
2	75	20	Use tablets	7	27	1.2	0.24mL**
3	68	10	Use tablets	Switch to citalopram **0.4mg/mL dilution****			
4	57	5	Use ½ tablets	8	17	0.7	1.4mL**
Switch to citalopram **4mg/mL dilution****				9	7	0.3	0.6mL**
5	47	3	0.6mL**	10	0	0	0
See further steps in the right-hand column							

RO = receptor occupancy
*For longer term users, the time between each decrease may be shortened to 1 week if the patient is able to make the first couple of reductions with no withdrawal symptoms. The interval between reductions should never be less than 1 week because this might increase the risk of relapse, even in the absence of withdrawal effects.[14,15]
**Note: citalopram drops come as citalopram hydrochloride which are 25% more bioavailable than citalopram hydrobromide (the tablet form) i.e. 8mg in liquid version is equivalent to 10mg in tablet form because they come as different salts.[1] Therefore the volume required is multiplied by 0.8 to get the required value.

B. **Moderate taper** with up to 5 percentage points of SERT between each step – with reductions made every 2–4 weeks.

Step	RO (%)	Dose (mg)	Volume*	Step	RO (%)	Dose (mg)	Volume*
1	79	40	Use tablets	11	38	2	0.4mL*
2	75	20	Use tablets	12	34	1.6	0.32mL*
3	70	15	Use ½ tablets**	13	30	1.3	0.26mL*
4	68	10	Use tablets	14	26	1	0.2mL*
5	64	7.5	Use ¾ tablets**	Switch to citalopram **0.4mg/mL dilution***		
Switch to citalopram **4mg/mL dilution***				15	21	0.8	1.6mL*
6	60	5.5	1.1mL*	16	17	0.6	1.2mL*
7	55	4.5	0.9mL*	17	13	0.4	0.8mL*
8	51	3.6	0.72mL*	18	8.5	0.25	0.5mL*
9	47	2.9	0.58mL*	19	4.3	0.1	0.2mL*
10	43	2.4	0.48mL*	20	0	0	0
See further steps in the right-hand column							

RO = receptor occupancy

*Note: citalopram drops come as citalopram hydrochloride which are 25% more bioavailable than citalopram hydrobromide (the tablet form) i.e. 8mg in liquid version is equivalent to 10mg in tablet form because they come as different salts.[1] Therefore the volume required is multiplied by 0.8 to get the required value.

**Alternatively, this dose could be made up with a liquid preparation.

C. **Slower taper** with up to 2.7 percentage points of SERT occupancy between each step – with reductions made every 2–4 weeks.

Step	RO (%)	Dose (mg)	Volume*	Step	RO (%)	Dose (mg)	Volume*	Step	RO (%)	Dose (mg)	Volume*
1	79.4	40	Use tablets	14	53.7	4.1	0.82mL*	Switch to citalopram **0.4mg/mL dilution***			
2	77.9	30	Use tablets	15	51.6	3.7	0.74mL*	28	24.8	0.97	1.94mL*
3	75.2	20	Use tablets	16	49.5	3.3	0.66mL*	29	22.7	0.86	1.72mL*
4	74.1	17.5	Use ¾ tablets**	17	47.5	3	0.6mL*	30	20.6	0.76	1.52mL*
5	72.7	15	Use ½ tablets**	18	45.4	2.7	0.54mL*	31	18.6	0.66	1.32mL*
6	70.8	12.5	Use ¼ tablets**	19	43.3	2.45	0.49mL*	32	16.5	0.57	1.14mL*
7	68.1	10	Use tablets	20	41.3	2.25	0.45mL*	33	14.4	0.48	0.96mL*
Switch to citalopram **4mg/mL dilution***				21	39.2	2.05	0.41mL*	34	12.4	0.4	0.8mL*
8	66	8.6	1.72mL*	22	37.2	1.85	0.37mL*	35	10.3	0.33	0.66mL*
9	64	7.5	1.5mL*	23	35.1	1.65	0.33mL*	36	8.3	0.26	0.52mL*
10	61.9	6.5	1.3mL*	24	33	1.5	0.3mL*	37	6.2	0.19	0.38mL*
11	59.9	5.8	1.16mL*	25	31	1.35	0.27mL*	38	4.1	0.12	0.24mL*
12	57.8	5.1	1.02mL*	26	28.9	1.2	0.24mL*	39	2.1	0.06	0.12mL*
13	55.7	4.6	0.92mL*	27	26.8	1.08	0.22mL*	40	0	0	0
See further steps in the middle column				**See further steps in the right-hand column**							

RO = receptor occupancy
*Note: citalopram drops come as citalopram hydrochloride which are 25% more bioavailable than citalopram hydrobromide (the tablet form) i.e. 8mg in liquid version is equivalent to 10mg in tablet form because they come as different salts.[12,13] Therefore the volume required is multiplied by 0.8 to get the required value.
**Alternatively, these doses could be made up with a liquid preparation.

CHAPTER 2

US regimens

A. **Faster taper** with up to 11 percentage points of SERT between each step – with reductions made every 2–4 weeks.*

Step	RO (%)	Dose (mg)	Volume**	Step	RO (%)	Dose (mg)	Volume**
1	79	40	Use tablets	6	37	2	1mL
2	75	20	Use tablets	7	27	1.2	0.6mL
3	68	10	Use tablets	8	17	0.7	0.35mL
4	57	5	Use ½ tablets***	Switch to citalopram **0.2mg/mL dilution**		
Switch to citalopram **2mg/mL liquid**				9	7	0.3	1.5mL
5	47	3	1.5mL	10	0	0	0
See further steps in the right-hand column							

RO = receptor occupancy
*For longer term users, the time between each decrease may be shortened to 1 week if the patient is able to make the first couple of reductions with no withdrawal symptoms. The interval between reductions should never be less than 1 week because this might increase the risk of relapse, even in the absence of withdrawal effects.[14,15]
**Note: these drops come as citalopram hydrobromide which have the same bioavailability as the tablet form.[9]
***Alternatively, these doses could be made up with a liquid preparation.

B. **Moderate taper** with up to 5 percentage points of SERT between each step – with reductions made every 2–4 weeks.

Step	RO (%)	Dose (mg)	Volume*	Step	RO (%)	Dose (mg)	Volume*
1	79	40	Use tablets	11	38	2	1mL
2	75	20	Use tablets	12	34	1.6	0.8mL
3	70	15	Use ½ tablets**	13	30	1.3	0.65mL
4	68	10	Use tablets	14	26	1	0.5mL
5	64	7.5	Use ¾ tablets**	15	21	0.8	0.4mL
Switch to citalopram **2mg/mL liquid**				16	17	0.6	0.3mL
6	60	5.5	2.75mL	17	13	0.4	0.2mL
7	55	4.5	2.25mL	Switch to citalopram **0.2mg/mL dilution**		
8	51	3.6	1.8mL	18	8.5	0.25	1.25mL
9	47	2.9	1.45mL	19	4.3	0.1	0.5mL
10	43	2.4	1.2mL	20	0	0	0
See further steps in the right-hand column							

RO = receptor occupancy
*Note: these drops come as citalopram hydrobromide which have the same bioavailability as the tablet form.[9]
**Alternatively, these doses could be made up with a liquid preparation.

C. **Slower taper** with up to 2.7 percentage points of SERT occupancy between each step – with reductions made every 2–4 weeks.

Step	RO (%)	Dose (mg)	Volume*	Step	RO (%)	Dose (mg)	Volume*	Step	RO (%)	Dose (mg)	Volume*
1	79.4	40	Use tablets	14	53.7	4.1	2.05mL	28	24.8	0.97	0.49mL
2	77.9	30	Use tablets	15	51.6	3.7	1.85mL	29	22.7	0.86	0.43mL
3	75.2	20	Use tablets	16	49.5	3.3	1.65mL	30	20.6	0.76	0.38mL
4	74.1	17.5	Use ¾ tablets**	17	47.5	3	1.5mL	31	18.6	0.66	0.33mL
5	72.7	15	Use ½ tablets**	18	45.4	2.7	1.35mL	32	16.5	0.57	0.29mL
6	70.8	12.5	Use ¼ tablets **	19	43.3	2.45	1.23mL	33	14.4	0.48	0.24mL
7	68.1	10	Use tablets	20	41.3	2.25	1.13mL	34	12.4	0.4	0.2mL
Switch to citalopram 2mg/mL liquid*				21	39.2	2.05	1.03mL	Switch to citalopram 0.2mg/mL dilution*			
8	66	8.6	4.3mL	22	37 2	1.85	0.93mL	35	10.3	0.33	1.65mL
9	64	7.5	3.75mL	23	35.1	1.65	0.83mL	36	8.3	0.26	1.3mL
10	61.9	6.5	3.25mL	24	33	1.5	0.75mL	37	6.2	0.19	0.95mL
11	59.9	5.8	2.9mL	25	31	1.35	0.68mL	38	4.1	0.12	0.6mL
12	57.8	5.1	2.55mL	26	28.9	1.2	0.6mL	39	2.1	0.06	0.3mL
13	55.7	4.6	2.3mL	27	26.8	1.08	0.54mL	40	0	0	0
See further steps in the middle column				See further steps in the right-hand column							

RO = receptor occupancy
*Note: these drops come as citalopram hydrobromide which have the same bioavailability as the tablet form.[9]
**Alternatively, these doses could be made up with a liquid preparation.

References

1. Advanz Pharma. Citalopram 40mg/ml Oral drops, solution. https://www.medicines.org.uk/emc/product/3349/smpc (accessed 25 August 2022).

2. Zentiva. Citalopram 20mg tablets – summary of product characteristics (SmPC). https://www.medicines.org.uk/emc/product/5160/smpc#gref (accessed 29 July 2023).

3. Hindmarch I, Kimber S, Cockle SM. Abrupt and brief discontinuation of antidepressant treatment: Effects on cognitive function and psychomotor performance. *Int Clin Psychopharmacol* 2000; 15: 305–18.

4. Gastaldon C, Schoretsanitis G, Arzenton E, et al. Withdrawal syndrome following discontinuation of 28 antidepressants: pharmacovigilance analysis of 31,688 reports from the WHO spontaneous reporting database. *Drug Saf* 2022; 45: 1539–49.

5. Sørensen A, Ruhé HG, Munkholm K. The relationship between dose and serotonin transporter occupancy of antidepressants – a systematic review. *Mol Psychiatry* 2022; 27: 192–201.

6. Holford N. Pharmacodynamic principles and the time course of delayed and cumulative drug effects. *Transl Clin* 2018; 26: 56.

7. Furukawa TA, Cipriani A, Cowen PJ, Leucht S, Egger M, Salanti G. Optimal dose of selective serotonin reuptake inhibitors, venlafaxine, and mirtazapine in major depression: a systematic review and dose-response meta-analysis. *The Lancet Psychiatry* 2019; 6: 601–9.

8. Horowitz MA, Taylor D. Tapering of SSRI treatment to mitigate withdrawal symptoms. *The Lancet Psychiatry* 2019; 6: 538–46.

9. FDA. Celexa (Citalopram hydrobromide) 10mg/5mL oral solution. www.accessdata.fda.gov. 2012; published online March. https://www.accessdata.fda.gov/drugsatfda_docs/nda/2012/021046Orig1s019.pdf (accessed 10 September 2022).

10. Smyth J. The NEWT guidelines for administration of medication to patients with enteral feeding tubes or swallowing difficulties website. The NEWT Guidelines. 2011. https://www.newtguidelines.com/index.html (accessed 7 September 2022).

11. Brennan K. Selective serotonin reuptake inhibitor (SSRI) formulations suggested for adults with swallowing difficulties. SPS – Specialist Pharmacy Service. 2021; published online 1 July. https://www.sps.nhs.uk/articles/selective-serotonin-reuptake-inhibitor-ssri-formulations-suggested-for-adults-with-swallowing-difficulties/ (accessed 19 September 2022).

12. Bostwick JR, Pharm D, Demehri A. Pills to powder: an updated clinician's reference for crushable psychotropics. *Curr Psychiatr* 2017; 16: 46–9.

13. Groot PC, van Os J. How user knowledge of psychotropic drug withdrawal resulted in the development of person-specific tapering medication. *Ther Adv Psychopharmacol* 2020; 10: 204512532093245.

14. Baldessarini RJ, Tondo L, Ghiani C, Lepri B. Illness risk following rapid versus gradual discontinuation of antidepressants. *Am J Psychiatry* 2010; 167: 934–41.

15. Gøtzsche PC, Demasi M. Interventions to help patients withdraw from depression drugs: A systematic review. *Int J Risk Saf Med.* 2023 September 13. doi: 10.3233/JRS-230011. Epub ahead of print.

Clomipramine

Trade name: Anafranil.

Description: Clomipramine is a tricyclic antidepressant,[1] and inhibits the neuronal re-uptake of serotonin by blocking SERT, and of noradrenaline by blocking NET. It also has anti-adrenergic, anticholinergic, antihistamine, anti-dopaminergic and anti-serotonergic properties.[2]

Withdrawal effects: Clomipramine withdrawal effects are recognised,[3] and it was responsible for about as many calls for withdrawal problems as SSRIs (normalised to prescription numbers) to a medication helpline in one study.[4] In an analysis of the WHO adverse effect database clomipramine emerged as at moderate risk for withdrawal effects compared to other antidepressants.[5] Clomipramine was found to have one of the highest reporting odds ratio for withdrawal effects amongst neonates in a WHO database (14-fold increase) compared to other drugs, more pronounced than for SSRIs.[6]

Peak plasma: 2–6 hours (mean 4.7 hours).[1]

Half-life: 21 (range 12–36) hours. According to the manufacturer clomipramine should be taken once or twice per day.[2] Every-other-day dosing is not recommended for tapering because the large reductions in plasma levels might give rise to significant withdrawal symptoms.

Receptor occupancy: The relationship between dose of clomipramine and occupancy of its target, NET, is hyperbolic.[7] Antidepressants also show a hyperbolic pattern between dose and clinical effects,[8] which may be relevant to withdrawal effects from clomipramine. Dose reductions made by linear amounts (e.g. 100mg, 75mg, 50mg, 25mg, 0mg) will cause increasingly large reductions in effect which may cause increasingly severe withdrawal effects (Figure 2.18a). To produce equal-sized reductions in effect on NET occupancy will require hyperbolically reducing doses (Figure 2.18b),[9] which informs the reductions presented below. This hyperbolic

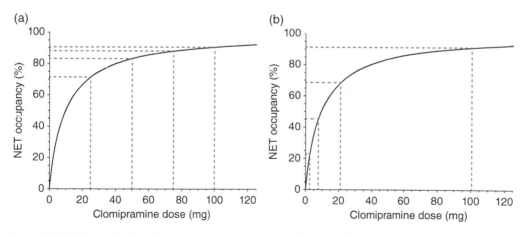

Figure 2.18 (a) Linear reductions of dose cause increasingly large reductions in effect on receptor targets, possibly associated with more withdrawal effects. (b) Even reductions of effect at target receptors requires hyperbolic dose reductions. The final dose before stopping will need to be very small so that this step down is not larger (in terms of effect on receptor occupancy) than previous reductions.

CHAPTER 2

pattern of effect also applies to its occupancy of its other receptor targets as well, because these relationships are dictated by the law of mass action.[10] There may be some differences in the precise dose-related activity between receptor targets but the hyperbolic relationship remains. Consequently, the regimens given below (based on NET occupancy) will be broadly suitable for other receptor occupancies, such as for SERT or cholinergic occupancy.

Available formulations: Clomipramine is available as capsules.

Capsules*

Dosage	UK	Europe	USA	Australia	Canada
10mg	✓	–	✓	–	✓
25mg	✓	✓	✓	✓	✓
50mg	✓	✓	✓	–	✓
75mg	–	✓	–	–	–

*As clomipramine hydrochloride

Off-label options: Clomipramine is available as capsules and is freely soluble in water.[1] Guidelines for people who cannot swallow tablets (e.g. the NEWT guidelines in the UK) suggest that clomipramine capsules can be opened and dispersed in water for administration, as an off-label use.[11] A 1mg/mL solution could be made by adding water to the contents of a 25mg capsule to make up 25mL. This should be shaken vigorously before use. As its stability cannot be assured it should be consumed immediately, and any unused solution discarded. Other options to make up small doses include compounding smaller dose tablets, including 'tapering strips'.[12]

Worked example: To illustrate how the volumes were calculated in the regimens given below we provide a worked example. To make up 3mg of clomipramine the 1mg/mL solution can be used, prepared as above. The volume of 1mg/mL liquid required to give a dose of 3mg of clomipramine is 3/1 = 3mL.

Deprescribing notes: Initial reductions can be estimated from Tables 2.11 and 2.22, although patient preference should be taken into account. Sometimes an even smaller reduction to start with may be advisable to boost a patient's confidence that they can taper if performed carefully. Each reduction should be made when the withdrawal symptoms from the previous reduction have largely resolved so that subsequent reductions do not lead to cumulative withdrawal symptoms. Withdrawal symptoms should be tolerable and last at most a couple of weeks (see Figure 2.9). Allowing for a sufficient observation period, reductions can therefore be made about every 2 to 4 weeks. If withdrawal symptoms are moderately severe or take longer than a couple of weeks to resolve, dose reductions should be postponed until symptoms resolve and then made more gradual by choosing a slower tapering rate. If severe withdrawal symptoms occur then the patient should return to a higher dose, wait until symptoms resolve and thereafter taper at a slower rate.

Suggested taper schedules for Clomipramine

A. A faster taper with up to 14 percentage points of NET occupancy between each step (approximate length: 5–10 months). Patients who have been on the medication for only a few weeks will probably be able to taper more quickly and might follow every second or third step of this regimen, and make reductions every few days or so. For people who have only taken an antidepressant for a few weeks, the duration of the taper should not be longer than the period that the patient has been on the drug. For example, if clomipramine is only taken for 3 weeks the taper should be less than 3 weeks.

B. A moderate taper with 6 percentage points of NET occupancy between each step (approximate length: 10–20 months).

C. A slower taper with up to 3 percentage points of NET occupancy between each step (approximate length: 20–40 months).

D. Some patients will be unable to taper at the slowest rates shown here and will need to taper by even smaller decrements, thus lengthening the overall period of tapering. Such a regimen could be constructed by placing intermediate steps in regimen C. For example, 3mg, 2mg, 1mg, 0mg could be modified to be 3mg, 2.5mg, 2mg, 1.5mg, 1mg, 0.5mg, 0mg. Further intermediate steps could also be added. Microtapering (tapering by a small amount each day, rather than by larger reductions every 2–4 weeks) is another possible approach (see benzodiazepines chapter for further details).

Please note that none of these regimens should be seen as prescriptive – that is, it is not suggested that patient must strictly adhere to them. They are given as example regimens and are not 'set and forget' but should be modified in order to ensure that withdrawal symptoms are tolerable throughout a taper – for example intermediate steps halfway between the doses listed could be added to make a more gradual taper.

A. **Faster taper** with up to 14 percentage points of NET occupancy between each step – with reductions made every 2–4 weeks.*

Step	RO (%)	Dose (mg)	Volume	Step	RO (%)	Dose (mg)	Volume
1	96	250	Use capsules	Switch to clomipramine **1mg/mL solution**			
2	95	200	Use capsules	8	56	12.5	12.5mL
3	94	150	Use capsules	9	42	7	7mL
4	91	100	Use capsules	10	28	4	4mL
5	88	75	Use capsules	11	14	2	2mL
6	83	50	Use capsules	12	0	0	0
7	70	25	Use capsules				
See further steps in the right-hand column							

RO = receptor occupancy
*For longer term users, the time between each decrease may be shortened to 1 week if the patient is able to make the first couple of reductions with no withdrawal symptoms. The interval between reductions should never be less than 1 week because this might increase the risk of relapse, even in the absence of withdrawal effects.[13,14]

B. **Moderate taper** with up to 6 percentage points of NET occupancy between each step – with reductions made every 2–4 weeks.

Step	RO (%)	Dose (mg)	Volume	Step	RO (%)	Dose (mg)	Volume
1	96	250	Use capsules	11	54	11.5	11.5mL
2	95	200	Use capsules	12	48	9	9mL
3	94	150	Use capsules	13	42	7	7mL
4	91	100	Use capsules	14	36	5.5	5.5mL
5	88	75	Use capsules	15	30	4.2	4.2mL
6	83	50	Use capsules	16	24	3.1	3.1mL
Switch to clomipramine **1mg/mL solution**				17	18	2.2	2.2mL
7	77	34	34mL	18	12	1.3	1.3mL
8	72	25	25mL*	19	6	0.6	0.6mL
9	66	19	19mL	20	0	0	0
10	60	14.5	14.5mL				
See further steps in the right-hand column							

RO = receptor occupancy
*Alternatively, this could be administered as a capsule.

C. **Slower taper** with up to 3 percentage points of NET occupancy between each step – with reductions made every 2–4 weeks.

Step	RO (%)	Dose (mg)	Volume	Step	RO (%)	Dose (mg)	Volume	Step	RO (%)	Dose (mg)	Volume
1	96.2	250	Use capsules	14	72.3	25	25mL*	28	33.4	5	5mL
2	95.3	200	Use capsules	15	69.5	22.5	22.5mL	29	30.6	4.4	4.4mL
3	94.6	175	Use capsules	16	66.7	20	20mL*	30	27.8	3.8	3.8mL
4	93.8	150	Use capsules	17	64	17.5	17.5mL	31	25	3.3	3.3mL
5	92.6	125	Use capsules	18	61.2	15.5	15.5mL	32	22.2	2.8	2.8mL
6	91	100	Use capsules	19	58.4	14	14mL	33	19.5	2.4	2.4mL
7	89.5	85	Use capsules	20	55.6	12.5	12.5mL	34	16.7	2	2mL
8	87.6	70	Use capsules	21	52.8	11.1	11.1mL	35	13.9	1.6	1.6mL
9	85.8	60	Use capsules	22	50.1	10	10mL*	36	11.1	1.2	1.2mL
10	83.4	50	Use capsules	23	47.3	8.9	8.9mL	37	8.3	0.9	0.9mL
Switch to clomipramine **1mg/mL solution**				24	44.5	8	8mL	38	5.6	0.6	0.6mL
11	80.6	41.5	41.5mL	25	41.7	7.1	7.1mL	39	2.8	0.3	0.3mL
12	77.9	35	35mL*	26	38.9	6.3	6.3mL	40	0	0	0
13	75.1	30	30mL*	27	36.2	5.6	5.6mL				
See further steps in the middle column				**See further steps in the right-hand column**							

RO = receptor occupancy
*Alternatively, could be made up by capsules.

References

1. FDA. Clomipramine Highlights of prescribing information. 2019.
2. Mylan. Clomipramine – summary of product characteristics. 2020. https://www.medicines.org.uk/emc/product/2552/smpc#gref (accessed 28 September 2022).
3. Martínez-Rodríguez JE, Iranzo A, Santamaría J, et al. Status cataplecticus induced by abrupt withdrawal of clomipramine. *Neurologia* 2002; 17: 113–6.
4. Taylor D, Stewart S, Connolly A. Antidepressant withdrawal symptoms – telephone calls to a national medication helpline. *J Affect Disord* 2006; 95: 129–33.
5. Gastaldon C, Schoretsanitis G, Arzenton E, et al. Withdrawal syndrome following discontinuation of 28 antidepressants: pharmacovigilance analysis of 31,688 reports from the WHO spontaneous peporting Database. *Drug Saf* 2022; 45: 1539–49.
6. Gastaldon C, Arzenton E, Raschi E, et al. Neonatal withdrawal syndrome following in utero exposure to antidepressants: a disproportionality analysis of VigiBase, the WHO spontaneous reporting database. *Psychol Med* 2022: 1–9.
7. Suhara T, Takano A, Sudo Y, et al. High levels of serotonin transporter occupancy with low-dose clomipramine in comparative occupancy study with fluvoxamine using positron emission tomography. *Arch Gen Psychiatry* 2003; 60: 386–91.
8. Furukawa TA, Cipriani A, Cowen PJ, Leucht S, Egger M, Salanti G. Optimal dose of selective serotonin reuptake inhibitors, venlafaxine, and mirtazapine in major depression: a systematic review and dose-response meta-analysis. *The Lancet Psychiatry* 2019; 6: 601–9.
9. Horowitz MA, Taylor D. Tapering of SSRI treatment to mitigate withdrawal symptoms. *The Lancet Psychiatry* 2019; 6: 538–46.
10. Holford N. Pharmacodynamic principles and the time course of delayed and cumulative drug effects. *Transl Clin* 2018; 26: 56.
11. Smyth J. The NEWT guidelines for administration of medication to patients with enteral feeding tubes or swallowing difficulties. 2011. https://www.newtguidelines.com/index.html (accessed 18 February, 2023).
12. Groot PC, van Os J. How user knowledge of psychotropic drug withdrawal resulted in the development of person-specific tapering medication. *Ther Adv Psychopharmacol* 2020; 10: 204512532093245.
13. Baldessarini RJ, Tondo L, Ghiani C, Lepri B. Illness risk following rapid versus gradual discontinuation of antidepressants. *Am J Psychiatry* 2010; 167: 934–41.
14. Gøtzsche PC, Demasi M. Interventions to help patients withdraw from depression drugs: A systematic review. *Int J Risk Saf Med.* 2023 September 13. doi: 10.3233/JRS-230011. Epub ahead of print.

CHAPTER 2

Desvenlafaxine

Trade names: Pristiq, Khedezla.

Description: Desvenlafaxine is an SNRI with SERT and NET as its major targets. Desvenlafaxine (O-desmethylvenlafaxine) is the major active metabolite of venlafaxine.[1]

Withdrawal effects: In prospective open-label studies, the incidence of withdrawal effects on discontinuation of desvenlafaxine after 10 months of treatment was 42%[2] and after 12 months of treatment was 52%.[3] Severity and duration of symptoms were not measured in these studies. The most common withdrawal symptoms in both studies were dizziness, nausea and headache.[2,3] In an analysis of the WHO adverse effect database desvenlafaxine emerged as high risk for withdrawal effects compared to other antidepressants, and had a stronger signal for risk of withdrawal than the opioid buprenorphine.[4]

Peak plasma: 7.5 hours.[1]

Half-life: Ranges from 9 to 13 hours (mean of 11 hours). The monolithic matrix extended-release formulation allows for once daily dosing by extending the effective period of drug action to over 24 hours.[1] Every-other-day dosing is not recommended for tapering because of the substantial reductions in plasma concentrations this would produce, possibly giving rise to withdrawal effects.

Receptor occupancy: The relationship between dose of desvenlafaxine and the occupancy of its major target SERT is hyperbolic.[5] Antidepressants also show a hyperbolic pattern between dose and clinical effects,[6] which may be relevant to withdrawal effects from desvenlafaxine. Dose reductions made by linear amounts (e.g. 100mg, 75mg, 50mg, 25mg, 0mg) will cause increasingly large reductions in effect which may cause increasingly severe withdrawal effects (Figure 2.19a). To produce equal-sized reductions in receptor occupancy will require hyperbolically reducing doses (Figure 2.19b),[7] which informs the reductions presented. This hyperbolic pattern of effect also applies to its occupancy of the NET[8] and other receptor targets as well, because these relationships are dictated by the law of mass action.[9] There may be some differences in the

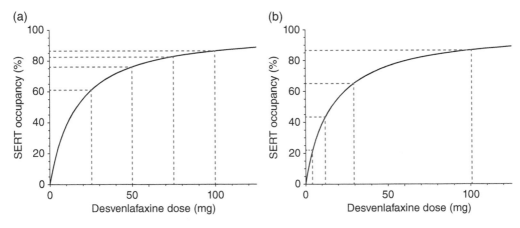

Figure 2.19 (a) Linear reductions of dose cause increasingly large reductions in effect on receptor targets, possibly associated with more withdrawal effects. (b) Even reductions of effect at target receptors requires hyperbolic dose reductions. The final dose before stopping will need to be very small so that this step down is not larger (in terms of effect on receptor occupancy) than previous reductions.

precise dose-related activity between receptor targets but the hyperbolic relationship remains. Consequently, the regimens given below (based on SERT occupancy) will be broadly suitable for other receptor occupancies, such as for NET occupancy.

Available formulations: Desvenlafaxine is only available as extended-release tablets.

Tablets*

Dosage	UK	Europe	USA	Australia	Canada
25mg	–	–	✓	–	–
50mg	–	✓	✓	✓	✓
100mg	–	✓	✓	✓	✓

*As desvenlafaxine succinate[10]

Off-label options: Each desvenlafaxine tablet contains desvenlafaxine succinate held in a monolithic matrix designed to release the equivalent of 25mg, 50mg or 100mg of desvenlafaxine over a day.[1] The extended-release properties are produced by the glue that holds the tablet together, not in the coating (which is only protective).[1] The manufacturer advises against dividing, crushing, chewing or dissolving the tablet,[1] as this will affect the extended-release properties provided by the matrix. An alternative approach is to consider divided tablets as lacking extended-release properties: they could then be regarded as instant release and given the short half-life (11 hours) should be dosed twice daily. The tablet cannot be dissolved in a diluent as it will form a gel that cannot be easily manipulated. Some compounding pharmacies can make up either compounded smaller doses[11] or a liquid version of desvenlafaxine. Switching to venlafaxine may be the easiest approach to tapering.

Switching: Desvenlafaxine (O-desmethylvenlafaxine) is the major active metabolite of venlafaxine. Switching from desvenlafaxine to venlafaxine for tapering is a reasonable option because of the similarities in the pharmacology of these antidepressants. Switching may be necessary because venlafaxine is available in formulations which more easily enable tapering to small doses. Although there is no exact established equivalency, it has been suggested that 50mg of desvenlafaxine is equivalent to 75mg of venlafaxine.[12] This estimate is supported by the similar SERT occupancies produced by these doses.[5]

It may be best to taper doses of desvenlafaxine until tapering is no longer possible with existing formulations and then switch to venlafaxine. This can be performed at 50mg or 100mg of desvenlafaxine, switching to 75mg or 150mg of venlafaxine, respectively. This switch can be made from one day to the next because of the similarity of these two drugs.[13] Switching to another drug like fluoxetine with much greater differences in receptor affinity is likely to be more problematic than a switch to venlafaxine, and this is generally not recommended.

Deprescribing notes: Initial reductions can be estimated from Tables 2.11 and 2.22, although patient preference should be taken into account. Sometimes an even smaller reduction to start with may be advisable to boost a patient's confidence that they can taper if performed carefully. Each reduction should be made when the withdrawal symptoms from the previous reduction have largely resolved so that subsequent reductions do not lead to cumulative withdrawal symptoms. Withdrawal symptoms should be tolerable and last at most a couple of weeks (see Figure 2.9). Allowing for a sufficient observation period, reductions can therefore be made about every 2 to 4 weeks. If withdrawal symptoms are moderately severe or take longer than a couple of weeks to resolve, dose reductions should be postponed until symptoms resolve and then made more gradual by choosing a slower tapering rate. If severe withdrawal symptoms occur then the patient should return to a higher dose, wait until symptoms resolve and thereafter taper at a slower rate.

Suggested taper schedules for desvenlafaxine

A. A faster taper with up to 11 percentage points of SERT between each step with reductions made every 2–4 weeks (approximate length: 5–10 months). Patients who have been on the medication for only a few weeks will probably be able to taper more quickly and might follow every second or third step of this regimen and make reductions every few days or so. For people who have only taken an antidepressant for a few weeks, the duration of the taper should not be longer than the period that the patient has been on the drug. For example, if desvenlafaxine is taken for 3 weeks the taper should be less than 3 weeks.

B. A moderate taper with up to 5 percentage points of SERT between each step with reductions made every 2–4 weeks (approximate length: 10–20 months).

C. A slower taper with up to 2.5 percentage points of SERT between each step with reductions made every 2–4 weeks (approximate length: 20–40 months).

D. Some patients will be unable to taper at the slowest rates shown here and will need to taper by even smaller decrements, thus lengthening the overall period of tapering. Such a regimen could be constructed by placing intermediate steps in regimen C. For example, 3mg, 2mg, 1mg, 0mg could be modified to be 3mg, 2.5mg, 2mg, 1.5mg, 1mg, 0.5mg, 0mg. Further intermediate steps could also be added. Microtapering (tapering by a small amount each day, rather than by larger reductions every 2–4 weeks) is another possible approach (see benzodiazepines chapter for further details).

Please note that none of these regimens should be seen as prescriptive – that is, it is not suggested that patient must strictly adhere to them. They are given as example regimens and are not 'set and forget' but should be modified in order to ensure that withdrawal symptoms are tolerable throughout a taper – for example intermediate steps halfway between the doses listed could be added to make a more gradual taper.

A. **Faster taper** with up to 11 percentage points of SERT between each step – with reductions made every 2–4 weeks.

Step	Receptor occupancy (%)	Dose (mg)
1	92.7	200
2	86.3	100
3	75.8	50
Switch to 75mg of venlafaxine* (see venlafaxine section to continue tapering)		

*50mg of desvenlafaxine is thought to be equivalent to 75mg of venlafaxine. It is possible that further steps could be made with desvenlafaxine using halved or quartered tablets on the understanding that these fragments might have lost their extended-release properties and should be dosed twice daily.

B. **Moderate taper** with up to 5 percentage points of SERT between each step – with reductions made every 2–4 weeks.

Step	Receptor occupancy (%)	Dose (mg)
1	92.7	200
2	90.5	150
3	86.3	100
Switch to 150mg of venlafaxine* (see venlafaxine section to continue tapering)		

*100mg of desvenlafaxine is thought to be equivalent to 150mg of venlafaxine. It is possible that further steps could be made with desvenlafaxine using halved or quartered tablets on the understanding that these fragments might have lost their extended-release properties and should be dosed twice daily.

C. **Slower taper** with up to 2.5 percentage points of SERT occupancy between each step with reductions made every 2–4 weeks.

Step	Receptor occupancy (%)	Dose (mg)
1	92.7	200
2	90.5	150
3	88.8	125*
4	86.3	100
Switch to 150mg of venlafaxine** (see venlafaxine section to continue tapering)		

*If the 25mg presentation is not available, cutting a desvenlafaxine tablet would be necessary (and dosing performed twice daily) before switching to venlafaxine. Alternatively, the switch to venlafaxine can be made at a desvenlafaxine dose of 200mg (to 300mg of venlafaxine) or at 150mg (to 225mg of venlafaxine)

**100mg of desvenlafaxine is thought to be equivalent to 150mg of venlafaxine. It is possible that further steps could be made with desvenlafaxine using halved or quartered tablets on the understanding that these fragments might have lost their extended-release properties and should be dosed twice daily.

References

1. FDA. Desvenlafaxine – highlights of prescribing information. 2011.
2. Tourian KA, Pitrosky B, Padmanabhan SK, Rosas GR. A 10-month, open-label evaluation of desvenlafaxine in outpatients with major depressive disorder. *Prim Care Companion CNS Disord* 2011; 13. doi:10.4088/PCC.10m00977blu.
3. Ferguson JM, Tourian KA, Rosas GR. High-dose desvenlafaxine in outpatients with major depressive disorder. *CNS Spectr* 2012; 17: 121–30.
4. Gastaldon C, Schoretsanitis G, Arzenton E, et al. Withdrawal syndrome following discontinuation of 28 antidepressants: Pharmacovigilance analysis of 31,688 reports from the WHO spontaneous reporting database. *Drug Saf* 2022; 45: 1539–49.
5. Sørensen A, Ruhé HG, Munkholm K. The relationship between dose and serotonin transporter occupancy of antidepressants – a systematic review. *Mol Psychiatry* 2021; 1–10.
6. Furukawa TA, Cipriani A, Cowen PJ, Leucht S, Egger M, Salanti G. Optimal dose of selective serotonin reuptake inhibitors, venlafaxine, and mirtazapine in major depression: a systematic review and dose-response meta-analysis. *The Lancet Psychiatry* 2019; 6: 601–9.
7. Horowitz MA, Taylor D. Tapering of SSRI treatment to mitigate withdrawal symptoms. *The Lancet Psychiatry* 2019; 6: 538–46.
8. Moriguchi S, Takamiya A, Noda Y, et al. Glutamatergic neurometabolite levels in major depressive disorder: a systematic review and meta-analysis of proton magnetic resonance spectroscopy studies. *Mol Psychiatry* 2019; 24: 952–64.
9. Holford N. Pharmacodynamic principles and the time course of delayed and cumulative drug effects. *Transl Clin* 2018; 26: 56.
10. TGA. Desvenlafaxine – Australian Product Information.
11. Groot PC, van Os J. How user knowledge of psychotropic drug withdrawal resulted in the development of person-specific tapering medication. *Ther Adv Psychopharmacol* 2020; 10: 204512532093245.
12. Schwartz TL. Metabolites: Novel therapeutics or 'me-too' drugs? Using desvenlafaxine as an example. *CNS Spectrums* 2000; 17: 103–6.
13. Taylor DM, Barnes TRE, Young AH. *The Maudsley Prescribing Guidelines in Psychiatry*, 14th edn. Hoboken, NJ: Wiley-Blackwell, 2021. doi:10.1002/9781119870203.

Dosulepin

Trade name: Prothiaden.

Description: Dosulepin, also known as dothiepin, is a tricyclic antidepressant that has strong affinity for histamine (H_1) receptors but also blocks both SERT and NET. It also has strong binding affinities for alpha 1-adrenergic, $5HT_{1A}$, $5HT_{2A}$, and muscarinic (M_1) receptors.[1,2] It is highly toxic in overdose and in the UK the NHS recommends that, where possible, dosulepin should be gradually withdrawn and stopped if no longer clinically indicated.[2]

Withdrawal effects: There is limited research on the withdrawal effects of dosulepin, with some structured analyses placing it in a high-risk category,[3] but analysis of calls regarding withdrawal to a phone line (normalised to prescription numbers) suggests a lower risk.[4]

Peak plasma: 2.2 hours.[5]

Half-life: About 20.4 hours. The manufacture recommends once or twice per day dosing (or three times a day for high doses).[2] Every-other-day dosing is not recommended for tapering because of the substantial reductions in plasma concentrations this would produce, possibly giving rise to withdrawal effects.

Receptor occupancy: The pharmacology of dosulepin is complex and not fully understood. The relationship between dose of dosulepin and occupancy of histamine H_1 receptors is hyperbolic.[1] This also applies to its activity on other receptor targets according to the law of mass action.[6] Antidepressants show a hyperbolic pattern between dose and clinical effects,[7] which may be relevant to withdrawal effects from dosulepin. Dose reductions made by linear amounts (e.g. 100mg, 75mg, 50mg, 25mg, 0mg) will cause increasingly large reductions in effect on receptor occupancy, which may cause increasingly severe withdrawal effects (Figure 2.20a). To produce equal-sized reductions in receptor occupancy will require hyperbolically reducing doses (Figure 2.20b), which informs the reductions presented.

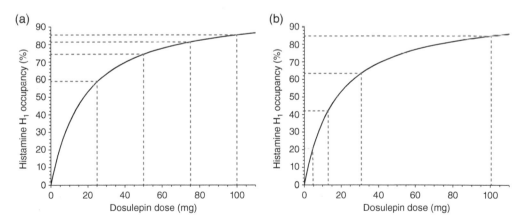

Figure 2.20 (a) Linear reductions of dose cause increasingly large reductions in effect on receptor targets, possibly associated with more withdrawal effects. (b) Even reductions of effect at target receptors requires hyperbolic dose reductions. The final dose before stopping will need to be very small so that this step down is not larger (in terms of effect on receptor occupancy) than previous reductions.

Available formulations: Dosulepin is available in tablets and capsules.

Tablets

Dosage	UK	Europe	USA	Australia	Canada
75mg	✓	–	–	✓	–

Capsules

Dosage	UK	Europe	USA	Australia	Canada
25mg	✓	–	–	✓	–

Off-label options: Dosulepin is available as a solution and a suspension as a 'Special' in the UK. Guidelines for people who cannot swallow tablets (e.g. the NEWT guidelines in the UK) mention that tablets have been crushed, however this is not recommended as the tablets are very hard and many brands are coated.[8] Capsules can be emptied and the powder dispersed in water, noting that the powder has a local anaesthetic action.[8] For example, a 25mg capsule could be emptied and mixed with water to make up 25mL to prepare a 1mg/mL suspension. 1mL of this suspension will provide 1mg of dosulepin. This should be shaken vigorously before use. As its stability cannot be assured, the measured dose should be consumed immediately, and any unused suspension discarded. Where available, smaller doses might be made up by compounding pharmacies.

Worked example: To illustrate how the volumes were calculated in the regimens given below we provide a worked example. To make up 2mg of dosulepin a 1mg/mL suspension can be used, made up as outlined above. The volume of 1mg/mL liquid required to give a dose of 2mg of dosulepin is 2/1 = 2mL.

Deprescribing notes: Initial reductions can be estimated from Tables 2.11 and 2.22, although patient preference should be taken into account. Sometimes an even smaller reduction to start with may be advisable to boost a patient's confidence that they can taper if performed carefully. Each reduction should be made when the withdrawal symptoms from the previous reduction have largely resolved so that subsequent reductions do not lead to cumulative withdrawal symptoms. Withdrawal symptoms should be tolerable and last at most a couple of weeks (see Figure 2.9). Allowing for a sufficient observation period, reductions can therefore be made about every 2 to 4 weeks. If withdrawal symptoms are moderately severe or take longer than a couple of weeks to resolve, dose reductions should be postponed until symptoms resolve and then made more gradual by choosing a slower tapering rate. If severe withdrawal symptoms occur then the patient should return to a higher dose, wait until symptoms resolve and thereafter taper at a slower rate. NHS guidance recommends that for patients who have been taking dosulepin for longer than 1 year more gradual tapering 'in the region of at least 6 months' is recommended.[2]

Suggested taper schedules for dosulepin

A. A faster taper with up to 10 percentage points of histamine H_1 receptor occupancy between each step (approximate length: 5–10 months). Patients who have been on the medication for only a few weeks will probably be able to taper more quickly and might follow every second or third step of this regimen, and make reductions every few days or so. For people who have only taken an antidepressant for a few weeks, the duration of the taper should not be longer than the period that the patient has been on the drug. For example, if dosulepin is taken for 3 weeks the taper should be less than 3 weeks.

B. A moderate taper with up to 6 percentage points of histamine H_1 receptor occupancy between each step (approximate length: 10–20 months).

C. A slower taper with up to 2.5 percentage points of histamine H_1 receptor occupancy between each step (approximate length: 20–40 months).

D. Some patients will be unable to taper at the slowest rates shown here and will need to taper by even smaller decrements, thus lengthening the overall period of tapering. Such a regimen could be constructed by placing intermediate steps between regimen C. For example, 3mg, 2mg, 1mg, 0mg could be modified to be 3mg, 2.5mg, 2mg, 1.5mg, 1mg, 0.5mg, 0mg. Further intermediate steps could also be added. Microtapering (tapering by a small amount each day, rather than by larger reductions every 2–4 weeks) is another possible approach (see benzodiazepines chapter for further details).

Please note that none of these regimens should be seen as prescriptive – that is, it is not suggested that patient must strictly adhere to them. They are given as example regimens and are not 'set and forget' but should be modified in order to ensure that withdrawal symptoms are tolerable throughout a taper – for example intermediate steps halfway between the doses listed could be added to make a more gradual taper.

A. **Faster taper** with up to 10 percentage points of histamine H_1 receptor occupancy between each step – with reductions made every 2–4 weeks.*

Step	RO (%)	Dose (mg)	Volume	Step	RO (%)	Dose (mg)	Volume
1	89	150	Use tabs or caps	6	49	17	17mL
2	81	75	Use tabs or caps	7	39	11	11mL
3	76	56.25	Use ¾ tablet**	8	29	7.3	7.3mL
4	68	37.5	Use ½ tablet**	9	19	4.3	4.3mL
5	58	25	Use capsules	10	9.7	1.9	1.9mL
Switch to dosulepin **1mg/mL suspension**				11	0	0	0
See further steps in the right-hand column							

RO = receptor occupancy, caps = capsules, tabs = tablets

*For longer term users, the time between each decrease may be shortened to 1 week if the patient is able to make the first couple of reductions with no withdrawal symptoms. The interval between reductions should never be less than 1 week because this might increase the risk of relapse, even in the absence of withdrawal effects.[9,10]

**Alternatively, this could be administered as a liquid preparation.

B. **A moderate taper** with up to 6 percentage points of histamine H_1 receptor occupancy between each step – with reductions made every 2–4 weeks.

Step	RO (%)	Dose (mg)	Volume	Step	RO (%)	Dose (mg)	Volume
1	89	150	Use tabs or caps	11	46	15	15mL
2	86	112.5	Use ½ tablets*	12	40	12	12mL
3	84	93.75	Use ¼ tablets*	13	35	9.7	9.7mL
4	81	75	Use tabs or caps	14	30	7.7	7.7mL
5	76	56.25	Use ¾ tablets*	15	25	6	6mL
Switch to dosulepin **1mg/mL suspension**				16	20	4.5	4.5mL
6	71	43	43mL	17	15	3.2	3.2mL
7	66	34	34mL	18	10	2	2mL
8	61	27	27mL	19	5.1	0.9	0.9mL
9	56	22	22mL	20	0	0	0
10	51	18	18mL				
See further steps in the right-hand column							

RO = receptor occupancy, caps = capsules, tabs = tablets
**Alternatively, this could be administered as a liquid preparation.

C. **A slower taper** with up to 2.5 percentage points of histamine H_1 receptor occupancy between each step – with reductions made every 2–4 weeks.

Step	RO (%)	Dose (mg)	Volume	Step	RO (%)	Dose (mg)	Volume	Step	RO (%)	Dose (mg)	Volume
1	89.5	150	Use tabs or caps	14	59.6	26.1	26.1mL	28	27.5	6.7	6.7mL
Switch to dosulepin **1mg/mL suspension**				15	57.3	23.8	23.8mL	29	25.2	6.0	6.0mL
2	87.2	120	120mL	16	55.1	21.6	21.6mL	30	22.9	5.3	5.3mL
3	84.9	100	100mL	17	52.8	19.7	19.7mL	31	20.6	4.6	4.6mL
4	82.6	83.8	83.8mL	18	50.5	18	18mL	32	18.4	4	4mL
5	80.3	72	72mL	19	48.2	16.4	16.4mL	33	16.1	3.4	3.4mL
6	78	62.6	62.6mL	20	45.9	15	15mL	34	13.8	2.8	2.8mL
7	75.7	55.1	55.1mL	21	43.6	13.7	13.7mL	35	11.5	2.3	2.3mL
8	73.4	48.8	48.8mL	22	41.3	12.4	12.4mL	36	9.2	1.8	1.8mL
9	71.1	43.5	43.5mL	23	39	11.3	11.3mL	37	6.9	1.3	1.3mL
10	68.8	39	39mL	24	36.7	10.2	10.2mL	38	4.6	0.85	0.85mL
11	66.5	35.1	35.1mL	25	34.4	9.3	9.3mL	39	2.3	0.4	0.4mL
12	64.2	31.7	31.7mL	26	32.1	8.4	8.4mL	40	0	0	0
13	61.9	28.8	28.8mL	27	29.8	7.5	7.5mL				
See further steps in the middle column				**See further steps in the right-hand column**							

RO = receptor occupancy, caps = capsules, tabs = tablets

References

1. DrugBank. Dosulepin: uses, interactions, mechanism of action I DrugBank Online. 2021. https://go.drugbank.com/drugs/DB09167 (accessed 13 October 2022).
2. South West London and St George's Mental Health Trust Drugs and Therapeutics Committee. Dosulepin (Prothiaden®): guidance on withdrawal. South West London and St George's Mental Health Trust. https://www.swlstg.nhs.uk/documents/related-documents/health-professionals/723-dosulepin-withdrawal-guidance-patient-leaflet (accessed 15 October 2022).
3. Henssler J, Heinz A, Brandt L, Bschor T. Antidepressant withdrawal and rebound phenomena. *Dtsch Arztebl Int* 2019; 116: 355–61.
4. Taylor D, Stewart S, Connolly A. Antidepressant withdrawal symptoms – telephone calls to a national medication helpline. *J Affect Disord* 2006; 95: 129–33.
5. New Zealand Data Sheet. DOSULEPIN VIATRIS. 2021.
6. Holford N. Pharmacodynamic principles and the time course of delayed and cumulative drug effects. *Ther Adv Psychopharmacol* 2018; 26: 56.
7. Furukawa TA, Cipriani A, Cowen PJ, Leucht S, Egger M, Salanti G. Optimal dose of selective serotonin reuptake inhibitors, venlafaxine, and mirtazapine in major depression: a systematic review and dose-response meta-analysis. *The Lancet Psychiatry* 2019; 6: 601–9.
8. Smyth J. The NEWT guidelines for administration of medication to patients with enteral feeding tubes or swallowing difficulties. 2011. https://www.newtguidelines.com/index.html (accessed 18 February 2023).
9. Baldessarini RJ, Tondo L, Ghiani C, Lepri B. Illness risk following rapid versus gradual discontinuation of antidepressants. *Am J Psychiatry* 2010; 167: 934–41.
10. Gøtzsche PC, Demasi M. Interventions to help patients withdraw from depression drugs: A systematic review. *Int J Risk Saf Med.* 2023 September 13. doi: 10.3233/JRS-230011. Epub ahead of print.

CHAPTER 2

Doxepin

Trade names: Adapin, Sinequan.

Description: Doxepin is a tricyclic antidepressant that acts by blocking both SERT and NET.[1] Its strongest affinity is for H_1 histaminergic receptors and it also has strong binding affinities for alpha-adrenergic and muscarinic (M_1) receptors.[1]

Withdrawal effects: Tricyclic antidepressants were classified as high risk for withdrawal in a structured analysis of antidepressant withdrawal effects.[2] In an analysis of withdrawal effects in neonates from a WHO adverse effect database, doxepin had amongst the strongest signals for withdrawal effects amongst all antidepressants examined.[3]

Peak plasma: 3.5 hours.[4]

Half-life: Approximately 15 hours.[1] The manufacturer recommends once or twice daily dosing.[4] Every-other-day dosing is not recommended for tapering because of the substantial reductions in plasma concentrations this would produce, possibly giving rise to withdrawal effects.

Receptor occupancy: The relationship between dose of doxepin and its occupancy of H_1 histaminergic receptors is hyperbolic.[5] Antidepressants show a hyperbolic pattern between dose and clinical effects,[6] which may be relevant to withdrawal effects from doxepin. Dose reductions made by linear amounts (e.g. 200mg, 150mg, 100mg, 50mg, 0mg) will cause increasingly large reductions in effect, which may cause increasingly severe withdrawal effects (Figure 2.21a). To produce equal-sized reductions in effect on receptor occupancy will require hyperbolically reducing doses (Figure 2.21b),[7] which informs the reductions presented. This hyperbolic pattern also applies to its occupancy of its other target receptors because these relationships are dictated by the law of mass action.[8] Consequently, there may be some differences in the precise dose-related activity between receptors but the hyperbolic relationship remains. The regimens given below (based on H_1 histaminergic occupancy) will therefore be broadly suitable for other receptor occupancies, such as for the NET or SERT.

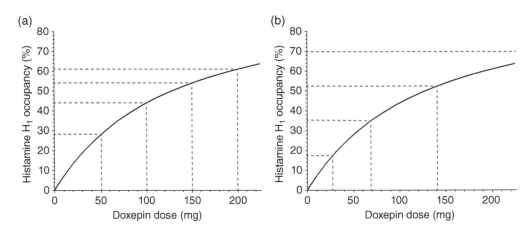

Figure 2.21 (a) Linear reductions of dose cause increasingly large reductions in effect on receptor targets, possibly associated with more withdrawal effects. (b) Even reductions of effect at target receptors requires hyperbolic dose reductions. The final dose before stopping will need to be very small so that this step down is not larger (in terms of effect on receptor occupancy) than previous reductions.

How supplied: Doxepin is available as doxepin hydrochloride in capsules, tablets and as a liquid.

Capsules

Dosage	UK	Europe	USA	Australia	Canada
10mg	✓	–	✓	✓	✓
25mg	✓	✓	✓	✓	✓
50mg	✓	✓	✓	✓	✓
75mg	–	–	✓	–	✓
100mg	–	–	✓	–	✓
150mg	–	–	✓	–	✓

Tablets

Dosage	UK	Europe	USA	Australia	Canada
3mg	–	–	✓	–	✓
6mg	–	–	✓	–	✓

Liquid

Dosage	UK	Europe	USA	Australia	Canada
10mg/mL	–	–	✓(120mL)	–	–

Dilutions: With smaller doses a dilution of the solution will be required. The manufacturer instructs that the oral solution can be mixed with water, whole or skimmed milk or orange, grapefruit, tomato, prune or pineapple juice.[9]

Dilutions	Solution required	How to prepare solution
Doses ≥2mg	10mg/mL	Original solution
Doses < 2mg	2mg/mL	Add 1mL of original solution (10mg/mL) to 4mL of water

Available formulations: To illustrate how the volumes were calculated in the regimens given below we provide a worked example. To make up 1mg of doxepin the 2mg/mL dilution can be used, prepared as above. The volume of 2mg/mL liquid required to give a dose of 1mg clomipramine is 1/2 = 0.5mL.

Off-label options: Guidelines for people who cannot swallow tablets (e.g. the NEWT guidelines in the UK) suggest that doxepin capsules can be opened and the contents dispersed in water as an off-label use.[10] The powder has a bitter taste.[10] A 1mg/mL suspension could be made by adding water to the contents of a 50mg capsule to make up a 50mL suspension. This should be shaken vigorously before use. As its stability cannot be assured it should be consumed immediately, and any unused suspension discarded. Compounding pharmacies may also be able to make up smaller doses to assist the tapering process.

Deprescribing notes: Initial reductions can be estimated from Tables 2.11 and 2.22, although patient preference should be taken into account. Sometimes an even smaller reduction to start with may be advisable to boost a patient's confidence that they can taper if performed carefully. Each reduction should be made when the withdrawal symptoms from the previous reduction have largely resolved so that subsequent reductions do not lead to cumulative withdrawal symptoms. Withdrawal symptoms should be tolerable and last at most a couple of weeks (see Figure 2.9). Allowing for a sufficient observation period, reductions can therefore be made about every 2 to 4 weeks. If withdrawal symptoms are moderately severe or take longer than a couple of weeks to resolve, dose reductions should be postponed until symptoms resolve and then made more gradual by choosing a slower tapering rate. If severe withdrawal symptoms occur then the patient should return to a higher dose, wait until symptoms resolve and thereafter taper at a slower rate.

Suggested taper schedules for doxepin

A. A faster taper with up to 9 percentage points of H_1 occupancy between each step (approximate length: 5–10 months). Patients who have been on the medication for only a few weeks will probably be able to taper more quickly and might follow every second or third step of this regimen, and make reductions every few days or so. For people who have only taken an antidepressant for a few weeks, the duration of the taper should not be longer than the period that the patient has been on the drug. For example, if doxepin is taken for 3 weeks the taper should be less than 3 weeks.
B. A moderate taper with up to 4 percentage points of H_1 occupancy between each step (approximate length: 10–20 months).
C. A slower taper with up to 2.1 percentage points of H_1 occupancy between each step (approximate length: 20–40 months).
D. Some patients will be unable to taper at the slowest rates shown here and will need to taper by even smaller decrements, thus lengthening the overall period of tapering. Such a regimen could be constructed by placing intermediate steps between regimen C. For example, 3mg, 2mg, 1mg, 0mg could be modified to be 3mg, 2.5mg, 2mg, 1.5mg, 1mg, 0.5mg, 0mg. Further intermediate steps could also be added. Microtapering (tapering by a small amount each day, rather than by larger reductions every 2–4 weeks) is another possible approach (see benzodiazepines chapter for further details).

Please note that none of these regimens should be seen as prescriptive – that is, it is not suggested that patient must strictly adhere to them. They are given as example regimens and are not 'set and forget' but should be modified in order to ensure that withdrawal symptoms are tolerable throughout a taper – for example intermediate steps halfway between the doses listed could be added to make a more gradual taper.

A. **Faster taper** with up to 9 percentage points of H_1 occupancy between each step – with reductions made every 2–4 weeks.*

Step	RO (%)	Dose (mg)	Volume	Step	RO (%)	Dose (mg)	Volume
1	70	300	Use capsules	7	29	50	Use capsules
2	61	200	Use capsules	8	22	35**	Use capsules
3	54	150	Use capsules	9	15	20**	Use capsules
4	50	125	Use capsules	10	7.3	10**	Use capsules
5	44	100	Use capsules	11	0	0	Use capsules
6	37	75	Use capsules				
See further steps in the right-hand column							

RO = receptor occupancy

*For longer term users, the time between each decrease may be shortened to 1 week if the patient is able to make the first couple of reductions with no withdrawal symptoms. The interval between reductions should never be less than 1 week because this might increase the risk of relapse, even in the absence of withdrawal effects.[11,12]

**Alternatively, where 10mg capsules are not available, a suspension made from an opened capsule can be used off-label, as outlined above.

B. **A moderate taper** with up to 4 percentage points of H_1 occupancy between each step – with reductions made every 2–4 weeks.

Step	RO (%)	Dose (mg)	Volume	Step	RO (%)	Dose (mg)	Volume
1	70.2	300	Use capsules	15	28.2	50	Use capsules
2	66.3	250	Use capsules	16	26.1	45*	Use capsules
3	63.9	225	Use capsules	17	23.9	40*	Use capsules
4	61.1	200	Use capsules	18	21.6	35*	Use capsules
5	57.9	175	Use capsules	19	19.1	30*	Use capsules
6	54.1	150	Use capsules	20	16.4	25	Use capsules
7	51.5	135*	Use capsules	21	13.6	20*	Use capsules
8	48.5	120*	Use capsules	Switch to doxepin **10mg/mL solution****			
9	45.2	105*	Use capsules	22	10.9	16	1.6mL
10	41.4	90*	Use capsules	23	8.2	12	1.2mL
11	38.6	80*	Use capsules	24	5.4	8	0.8mL
12	35.5	70*	Use capsules	25	2.7	4	0.4mL
13	32.1	60*	Use capsules	26	0	0	0
14	30.2	55*	Use capsules				
See further steps in the right-hand column							

RO = receptor occupancy

*Alternatively, where 10mg capsules are not available, a suspension from an opened capsule can be made up, as an off-label use, as outlined above.

**Alternatively, where the manufacturer's solution is not available, this could be made up as a suspension from an opened capsule, as an off-label use, as outlined above.

C. A slower taper with up to 2.1 percentage points of H_1 occupancy between each step – with reductions made every 2–4 weeks.

Step	RO (%)	Dose (mg)	Volume	Step	RO (%)	Dose (mg)	Volume*	Step	RO (%)	Dose (mg)	Volume*
1	70.2	300	Use capsules	18	46.4	110*	Use capsules	34	22.4	36.8	3.68mL
2	68.4	275	Use capsules	19	45.2	105*	Use capsules	35	20.8	33.5	3.35mL
3	66.3	250	Use capsules	20	44	100	Use capsules	36	19.2	30.3	3.03mL
4	64.9	235*	Use capsules	21	42.8	95*	Use capsules	37	17.6	27.2	2.72mL
5	63.4	220*	Use capsules	22	41.4	90*	Use capsules	38	16	24.3	2.43mL
6	62.3	210*	Use capsules	23	40.1	85*	Use capsules	39	14.4	21.4	2.14mL
7	61.1	200	Use capsules	24	38.6	80*	Use capsules	40	12.8	18.7	1.87mL
8	59.9	190*	Use capsules	25	37.1	75	Use capsules	41	11.2	16.1	1.61mL
9	58.6	180*	Use capsules	26	35.5	70*	Use capsules	42	9.6	13.5	1.35mL
10	57.2	170*	Use capsules	27	33.8	65*	Use capsules	43	8.0	11.1	1.11mL
11	55.7	160*	Use capsules	28	32.1	60*	Use capsules	44	6.4	8.7	0.87mL
12	54.1	150	Use capsules	Switch to doxepin **10mg/mL solution****			43	4.8	6.3	0.63mL
13	52.4	140*	Use capsules	29	30.5	55.7	5.57mL	46	3.2	4.2	0.42mL
14	50.5	130*	Use capsules	30	28.8	51.6	5.16mL	47	1.6	2.1	0.21mL
15	49.6	125	Use capsules	31	27.2	47.6	4.76mL	48	0	0	0
16	48.5	120*	Use capsules	32	25.6	43.9	4.39mL				
17	47.5	115*	Use capsules	33	24.0	40.3	4.03mL				
	See further steps in the middle column				**See further steps in the right-hand column**						

RO = receptor occupancy

*Alternatively, where 10mg capsules are not available, a suspension from an opened capsule can be made up, as an off-label use.

**Alternatively, where the manufacturer's solution is not available, this could be made up as a suspension from an opened capsule, as an off-label use.

References

1. Marsh W. Doxepin. In: *xPharm: The Comprehensive Pharmacology Reference*. StatPearls Publishing, 2007: 1–5.
2. Henssler J, Heinz A, Brandt L, Bschor T. Antidepressant withdrawal and rebound phenomena. *Dtsch Arztebl Int* 2019; 116: 355–61.
3. Gastaldon C, Arzenton E, Raschi E, et al. Neonatal withdrawal syndrome following in utero exposure to antidepressants: a disproportionality analysis of VigiBase, the WHO spontaneous reporting database. *Psychol Med* 2022: 1–9.
4. Marlborough Pharmaceuticals. Doxepin- Summary of product characteristics. 2021. https://www.medicines.org.uk/emc/product/5850/smpc#gref (accessed 13 October 2022).
5. Derijks HJ, Heerdink ER, Janknegt R, et al. Visualizing pharmacological activities of antidepressants: a novel approach. *Open Pharmacol J* 2008; 2: 54–62.
6. Furukawa TA, Cipriani A, Cowen PJ, Leucht S, Egger M, Salanti G. Optimal dose of selective serotonin reuptake inhibitors, venlafaxine, and mirtazapine in major depression: a systematic review and dose-response meta-analysis. *The Lancet Psychiatry* 2019; 6: 601–9.
7. Horowitz MA, Taylor D. Tapering of SSRI treatment to mitigate withdrawal symptoms. *The Lancet Psychiatry* 2019; 6: 538–46.
8. Holford N. Pharmacodynamic principles and the time course of delayed and cumulative drug effects. *Transl Clin* 2018; 26: 56.
9. FDA. Doxepin. 2014.
10. Smyth J. The NEWT guidelines for administration of medication to patients with enteral feeding tubes or swallowing difficulties. 2011. https://www.newtguidelines.com/index.html (accessed 23 February 2023).
11. Baldessarini RJ, Tondo L, Ghiani C, Lepri B. Illness risk following rapid versus gradual discontinuation of antidepressants. *Am J Psychiatry* 2010; 167: 934–41.
12. Gøtzsche PC, Demasi M. Interventions to help patients withdraw from depression drugs: A systematic review. *Int J Risk Saf Med*. 2023 September 13. doi: 10.3233/JRS-230011. Epub ahead of print.

Duloxetine

Trade name: Cymbalta.

Description: Duloxetine is an SNRI with major targets the SERT and NET. It weakly inhibits dopamine reuptake, and has no significant affinity for histaminergic, dopaminergic, cholinergic and adrenergic receptors.[1]

Withdrawal effects: In a double-blind randomised controlled trial, 31% of people taking duloxetine for 9 weeks had withdrawal effects on stopping. Dizziness, headache, insomnia, nausea and paraesthesia were the most common withdrawal symptoms.[2] Severity and duration of symptoms were not measured in this study. Longer-term treatment is likely to increase the incidence and severity of withdrawal symptoms.[3] In an analysis of the WHO adverse effect database duloxetine emerged as high risk for withdrawal effects compared to other antidepressants, and had a stronger signal for risk of withdrawal than the opioid buprenorphine.[4] In a self-selected survey of patients on long-term duloxetine conducted by RCPsych 69% reported withdrawal effects.[5]

Peak plasma: 6 hours.[1]

Half-life: Ranges from 8 to 17 hours (mean of 12 hours).[1] The manufacturer advises that the medication should be taken once daily.[1] Every-other-day dosing is not recommended for tapering because of the substantial reductions in plasma concentrations this would produce, possibly giving rise to withdrawal effects.

Receptor occupancy: The relationship between dose of duloxetine and occupancy of one of its targets, SERT, is hyperbolic.[6] Antidepressants also show a hyperbolic pattern between dose and clinical effects,[7] which may be relevant to withdrawal effects from duloxetine. Dose reductions made by linear amounts (e.g. 40mg, 30mg, 20mg, 10mg, 0mg) will cause increasingly large reductions in effect which may cause increasingly severe withdrawal effects (Figure 2.22a). To produce equal-sized reductions in effect on receptor occupancy will require hyperbolically reducing doses (Figure 2.22b),[8] which

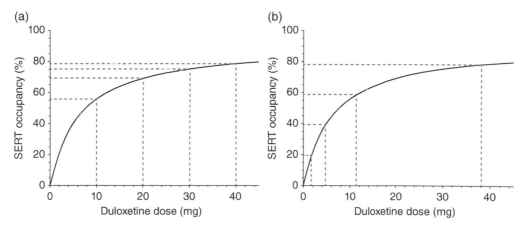

Figure 2.22 (a) Linear reductions of dose cause increasingly large reductions in effect on receptor targets, possibly associated with more withdrawal effects. (b) Even reductions of effect at target receptors requires hyperbolic dose reductions. The final dose before stopping will need to be very small so that this step down is not larger (in terms of effect on receptor occupancy) than previous reductions.

CHAPTER 2

informs the reductions presented. This hyperbolic pattern of effect also applies to its occupancy of NET[9] and other receptor targets as well, because these relationships are dictated by the law of mass action.[10] There may be some differences in the precise dose-related activity between receptor targets but the hyperbolic relationship remains. Consequently, the regimens given (based on SERT occupancy) will be broadly suitable for other receptor occupancies, such as for NET occupancy.

Available formulations: Duloxetine is only available as gastro-resistant capsules.

Capsules*

Dosage	UK	Europe	USA	Australia	Canada
20mg	✓	✓	✓	–	–
30mg	✓	✓	✓	✓	✓
40mg	✓	✓	✓	–	–
60mg	✓	✓	✓	✓	✓
90mg	–	✓	–	–	–
120mg	–	✓	–	–	–

*As duloxetine hydrochloride.[1]

Off-label options: Most duloxetine capsules contain small beads covered with an enteric coating. The enteric coating is employed because duloxetine hydrochloride is an acid-labile substance and the coating prevents degradation of the active drug in the acidic environment of the stomach.[11] Duloxetine cannot be crushed or liquefied because the enteric coating on the beads must remain intact for drug absorption to take place.[11]

Guidelines for people who cannot swallow tablets (e.g. the NEWT guidelines in the UK) suggest that duloxetine capsules can be opened and the beads administered as an off-label use.[12] The official drug label advises against sprinkling contents onto food or mixing with liquids because these actions might affect its enteric coating.[11] However, a formal analysis conducted by the manufacturer, Eli Lilly, concluded that duloxetine beads were stable and that their absorption profile was not altered by opening the capsule and mixing the beads with apple juice or apple sauce (but not chocolate pudding).[13] The Institute for Safe Medication Practices in the USA also advises that the contents of a capsule can be safely added to apple sauce or apple juice.[14,15]

Small doses of duloxetine can be obtained but the process is complicated. It involves first emptying out a capsule. The beads from the capsule can be weighed or counted. This should be done with clean and dry hands (or using an instrument like a ruler or pair of tweezers). The number of beads to be taken will need to be placed back into the original capsule or another gelatine capsule bought from a pharmacy or online. The beads should not be swallowed without a capsule as there are some reports of throat irritation occurring.[16]

Each capsule contains the same weight of drug but, because the beads vary in size, they may have differing numbers of beads. The regimens given below (in mg) can then be converted into the number of beads required. For example, if a 30mg capsule contains, on average, 250 beads, then to achieve a dose of 5mg 42 beads are needed (rounded to the nearest bead). There are various tools to help with these calculations available online. Beads can be kept in a suitable container for a couple of days as their enteric coating is stable in air.[17]

Some capsules contain 'mini-tablets' (4 to 12 in number) of duloxetine, each containing 5mg of duloxetine, which may be used to taper at higher doses. These cannot be split or dissolved in water. Compounding pharmacies may also be able to make up smaller doses of duloxetine.

Deprescribing notes: Initial reductions can be estimated from Tables 2.11 and 2.22, although patient preference should be taken into account. Sometimes an even smaller reduction to start with may be advisable to boost a patient's confidence that they can taper if performed carefully. Each reduction should be made when the withdrawal symptoms from the previous reduction have largely resolved so that subsequent reductions do not lead to cumulative withdrawal symptoms. Withdrawal symptoms should be tolerable and last at most a couple of weeks (see Figure 2.9). Allowing for a sufficient observation period, reductions can therefore be made about every 2 to 4 weeks. If withdrawal symptoms are moderately severe or take longer than a couple of weeks to resolve, dose reductions should be postponed until symptoms resolve and then made more gradual by choosing a slower tapering rate. If severe withdrawal symptoms occur then the patient should return to a higher dose, wait until symptoms resolve and thereafter taper at a slower rate.

Suggested taper schedules for duloxetine

A. A faster taper with up to 10 percentage points of SERT between each step with reductions made every 2–4 weeks (approximate length: 5–10 months). Patients who have been on the medication for only a few weeks will probably be able to taper more quickly and might follow every second or third step of this regimen, and make reductions every few days or so. For people who have only taken an antidepressant for a few weeks, the duration of the taper should not be longer than the period that the patient has been on the drug. For example, if duloxetine is taken for 3 weeks the taper should be less than 3 weeks.

B. A moderate taper with up to 6 percentage points of SERT between each step with reductions made every 2–4 weeks (approximate length: 10–20 months).

C. A slower taper with up to 2.5 percentage points of SERT between each step with reductions made every 2–4 weeks (approximate length: 20–40 months).

D. Some patients will be unable to taper at the slowest rates shown here and will need to taper by even smaller decrements, thus lengthening the overall period of tapering. Such a regimen could be constructed by placing intermediate steps in regimen C. For example, 3mg, 2mg, 1mg, 0mg could be modified to be 3mg, 2.5mg, 2mg, 1.5mg, 1mg, 0.5mg, 0mg. Further intermediate steps could also be added. Microtapering (tapering by a small amount each day, rather than by larger reductions every 2–4 weeks) is another possible approach (see benzodiazepines chapter for further details).

Please note that none of these regimens should be seen as prescriptive – that is, it is not suggested that patient must strictly adhere to them. They are given as example regimens and are not 'set and forget' but should be modified in order to ensure that withdrawal symptoms are tolerable throughout a taper – for example intermediate steps halfway between the doses listed could be added to make a more gradual taper.

A. **Faster taper** with up to 10 percentage points of SERT between each step – with reductions made every 2–4 weeks.*

Step	Receptor occupancy (%)	Dose (mg)	Step	Receptor occupancy (%)	Dose (mg)
1	82	60	7	39	4.8**
2	78	40	8	30	3**
3	75	30	9	20	1.7**
4	69	20	10	10	0.8**
5	59	12**	11	0	0
6	49	7.5**			
See further steps in the right-hand column					

*For longer term users, the time between each decrease may be shortened to 1 week if the patient is able to make the first couple of reductions with no withdrawal symptoms. The interval between reductions should never be less than 1 week because this might increase the risk of relapse, even in the absence of withdrawal effects.[18,19]
**Doses will require off-label options, as outlined above.

B. **Moderate taper** with up to 6 percentage points of SERT between each step – with reductions made every 2–4 weeks.

Step	Receptor occupancy (%)	Dose (mg)	Step	Receptor occupancy (%)	Dose (mg)
1	82	60	11	39	4.7*
2	78	40	12	35	3.9*
3	75	30	13	30	3.1*
4	69	20	14	26	2.5*
5	65	16*	15	22	2*
6	60	13*	16	17	1.5*
7	56	10*	17	13	1*
8	52	8.3*	18	9	0.65*
9	47	6.9*	19	4	0.3*
10	43	5.7*	20	0	0
See further steps in the right-hand column					

*Doses will require off-label options, as outlined above.

C. **Slower taper** with up to 2.5 percentage points of SERT occupancy between each step – with reductions made every 2–4 weeks.

Step	RO (%)	Dose (mg)	Step	RO (%)	Dose (mg)	Step	RO (%)	Dose (mg)
1	82.2	60	15	54	9.2*	29	23.7	2.2*
2	80.6	50	16	51.8	8.3*	30	21.6	1.9*
3	78.5	40	17	49.7	7.6*	31	19.4	1.65*
4	77.0	35*	18	47.5	6.9*	32	17.3	1.4*
5	75.1	30	19	45.3	6.3*	33	15.1	1.2*
6	72.6	25*	20	43.2	5.7*	34	13	1*
7	70.6	22*	21	41	5.2*	35	10.8	0.85*
8	69.1	20	22	38.9	4.7*	36	8.6	0.6*
9	66.9	18*	23	36.7	4.3*	37	6.5	0.45*
10	64.8	16*	24	34.5	3.9*	38	4.3	0.3*
11	62 6	14*	25	32.4	3.5*	39	2.2	0.15*
12	60.5	12*	26	30.2	3.1*	40	0	0
13	58.3	11*	27	28.1	2.8*			
14	56.1	10*	28	25.9	2.5*			
See further steps in the middle column			**See further steps in the right-hand column**					

RO = receptor occupancy
*Doses will require off-label options, as outlined above.

References

1. Eli Lilly. Duloxetine summary of product characteristics. https://www.medicines.org.uk/emc/product/3880/smpc#PHARMACOLOGICAL_PROPS (accessed 8 September 2022).

2. Koponen H, Allgulander C, Erickson J, et al. Efficacy of duloxetine for the treatment of generalized anxiety disorder: implications for primary care physicians. *Prim Care Companion J Clin Psychiatry* 2007; 9: 100–7.

3. Horowitz MA, Framer A, Hengartner MP, Sørensen A, Taylor D. Estimating risk of antidepressant withdrawal from a review of published data. *CNS Drugs* 2022; published online 14 December. doi:10.1007/s40263-022-00960-y.

4. Gastaldon C, Schoretsanitis G, Arzenton E, et al. Withdrawal syndrome following discontinuation of 28 antidepressants: pharmacovigilance analysis of 31,688 reports from the WHO spontaneous reporting database. *Drug Saf* 2022; 45: 1539–49.

5. Davies J, Read J. A systematic review into the incidence, severity and duration of antidepressant withdrawal effects: are guidelines evidence-based? *Addict Behav* 2019; 97: 111–21.

6. Sørensen A, Ruhé HG, Munkholm K. The relationship between dose and serotonin transporter occupancy of antidepressants – a systematic review. *Mol Psychiatry* 2022; 27: 192–201.

7. Furukawa TA, Cipriani A, Cowen PJ, Leucht S, Egger M, Salanti G. Optimal dose of selective serotonin reuptake inhibitors, venlafaxine, and mirtazapine in major depression: a systematic review and dose-response meta-analysis. *The Lancet Psychiatry* 2019; 6: 601–9.

8. Horowitz MA, Taylor D. Tapering of SSRI treatment to mitigate withdrawal symptoms. *The Lancet Psychiatry* 2019; 6: 538–46.

9. Moriguchi S, Takamiya A, Noda Y, et al. Glutamatergic neurometabolite levels in major depressive disorder: a systematic review and meta-analysis of proton magnetic resonance spectroscopy studies. *Mol Psychiatry* 2019; 24: 952–64.

10. Holford N. Pharmacodynamic principles and the time course of delayed and cumulative drug effects. *Transl Clin* 2018; 26: 56.

11. Eli Lilly. Drug label: Cymbalta. 2020.

12. Smyth J. The NEWT guidelines for administration of medication to patients with enteral feeding tubes or swallowing difficulties. 2011. https://www.newtguidelines.com/index.html (accessed 23 February 2023).

13. Wells KA, Losin WG. In vitro stability, potency, and dissolution of duloxetine enteric-coated pellets after exposure to applesauce, apple juice, and chocolate pudding. *Clin Ther* 2008; 30: 1300–8.

14. Bostwick JR, Demehri A. Pills to powder: an updated clinician's reference for crushable psychotropics. *Curr Psychiatr* 2017; 16: 46–9.

15. Institute for Safe Medication Practices. https://www.ismp.org/ (accessed October 10, 2022).

16. FDA. Memorandum: DMETS medication error postmarketing safety review: Cymbalta. Fda.gov. 2007; published online 8 March. www.fda.gov/media/74134/download (accessed September 9, 2022).

17. Kuang C, Sun Y, Li B, et al. Preparation and evaluation of duloxetine hydrochloride enteric-coated pellets with different enteric polymers. *Asian J Pharm Sci* 2017; 12: 216–26.

18. Baldessarini RJ, Tondo L, Ghiani C, Lepri B. Illness risk following rapid versus gradual discontinuation of antidepressants. *Am J Psychiatry* 2010; 167: 934–41.

19. Gøtzsche PC, Demasi M. Interventions to help patients withdraw from depression drugs: A systematic review. *Int J Risk Saf Med.* 2023 September 13. doi: 10.3233/JRS-230011. Epub ahead of print.

Escitalopram

Trade names: Lexapro, Cipralex.

Description: Escitalopram is an SSRI with SERT as its major target.[1]

Withdrawal effects: After 24 weeks of treatment with escitalopram at doses from 5mg to 20mg, 15–22% of patients experienced a withdrawal syndrome (four or more withdrawal symptoms as captured by the DESS).[2,3] Severity and duration of withdrawal symptoms were not measured in this trial. Longer treatment with antidepressants is associated with a higher incidence of withdrawal effects, and with greater severity.[4] In a self-selected survey of people on long-term antidepressants conducted by RCPsych 75% of those who stopped escitalopram reported withdrawal effects.[5]

Peak plasma: 4 hours.[1]

Half-life: About 30 hours.[1] Every-other-day dosing is not recommended for tapering because the large reductions in plasma levels could give rise to significant withdrawal symptoms.

Receptor occupancy: The relationship between dose of escitalopram and occupancy of its major target SERT is hyperbolic.[6] This applies to other receptor targets as well, because this relationship is dictated by the law of mass action.[7] Antidepressants also show a hyperbolic pattern between dose and clinical effects, which may be relevant to withdrawal effects from escitalopram.[8] Dose reductions made by linear amounts (e.g. 20mg, 15mg, 10mg, 5mg, 0mg) will cause increasingly large reductions in effect which may cause increasingly severe withdrawal effects (Figure 2.23a). To produce equal-sized reductions in effect on SERT, occupancy will require hyperbolically reducing doses (Figure 2.23b),[9] which informs the reductions presented.

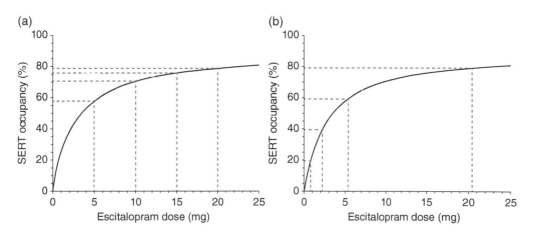

Figure 2.23 (a) Linear reductions of dose cause increasingly large reductions in effect on receptor targets, possibly associated with more withdrawal effects. (b) Even reductions of effect at target receptors requires hyperbolic dose reductions. The final dose before stopping will need to be very small so that this step down is not larger (in terms of effect on receptor occupancy) than previous reductions.

Available formulations: As tablets and liquid.

Tablets*

Dosage	UK	Europe	USA	Australia	Canada
5mg	✓	✓	✓	✓	✓
10mg	✓	✓	✓	✓	✓
15mg	–	✓	–	✓	✓
20mg	✓	✓	✓	✓	✓

*As escitalopram oxalate

Liquid

Dosage	UK	Europe	USA	Australia	Canada
20mg/mL	✓ (15mL)*	✓ (15mL)*	–	✓ (15mL)*	–
5mg/5mL (1mg/mL)	–	–	✓ (240mL)**	–	–

*In the UK, Europe and Australia the concentrated solution of escitalopram oxalate (20mg/mL) is bioequivalent to the tablet form. After opening store at 25°C (77°F).[1,10]
**In the USA, liquid form is escitalopram oxalate, and has equal bioequivalence to tablet form. Store at 25°C (77°F); excursions permitted to 15°–30°C (59°–86°F).[11]

Dilutions: In the UK, Europe and Australia, to make the concentrated oral drops into a usable form for many doses suggested for tapering, dilutions will be required. According to the manufacturer's instructions, this solution may be mixed with water or juice.[10] As its stability cannot be assured it should be consumed immediately, and any unused suspension discarded. The manufacturer recommends using the drops within 8 weeks after opening them. Please note that in order to prepare solutions using a small syringe (e.g. 1mL) the dropper mechanism must be removed by hand. Another option is to dilute using the dropper mechanism. 1 drop (1mg) can be put in 20mL of water, mixed well, and 5mL consumed to take, for example, 0.25mg of drug.

UK/Europe/Australia dilutions	Solution required	How to prepare solution
Doses ≥ 4mg	20mg/mL	Original solution
Doses ≥ 0.4mg, <4mg	2mg/mL	Mix 0.5mL of original oral solution with 4.5mL of water
Doses <0.4mg	0.2mg/mL	Mix 0.5mL of original oral solution with 49.5mL of water

Worked example: To illustrate how the volumes were calculated in the regimens given below we provide a worked example. To make up 3mg of escitalopram the 2mg/mL dilution can be used, prepared as above. The volume of 2mg/mL liquid required to give a dose of 3mg escitalopram is 3/2 = 1.5mL.

US dilutions*	Solution required	How to prepare solution
Doses ≥ 0.2mg	1mg/mL*	Original solution
Doses <0.2mg	0.2mg/mL	Mix 1mL of original oral solution with 4mL of water

*Note: the original solution is 5mg/5mL which is 1mg/mL.

Off-label options: Guidelines for people who cannot swallow tablets (e.g. the NEWT guidelines in the UK, NHS pharmaceutical guidance[12] and similar guidance in the USA) suggest that escitalopram tablets can be crushed and/or dispersed in water for administration.[13,14] Escitalopram tablets disperse quickly, have an unpleasant taste and are poorly soluble in water.[13] A 1mg/mL suspension could be made by adding water to a 10mg tablet to make up 10mL. The tablet may be crushed with a spoon or pestle and mortar before mixing with water to speed up this process. The suspension should be shaken vigorously before use. As its stability cannot be assured it should be consumed immediately, and any unused suspension discarded. Other options include a compounding pharmacy making up a liquid or smaller formulations of tablets, for example, 'tapering strips'.[15]

Deprescribing notes: Initial reductions can be estimated from Tables 2.11 and 2.22, although patient preference should be taken into account. Sometimes an even smaller reduction to start with may be advisable to boost a patient's confidence that they can taper if performed carefully. Each reduction should be made when the withdrawal symptoms from the previous reduction have largely resolved so that subsequent reductions do not lead to cumulative withdrawal symptoms. Withdrawal symptoms should be tolerable and last at most a couple of weeks (see Figure 2.9). Allowing for a sufficient observation period, reductions can therefore be made about every 2 to 4 weeks. If withdrawal symptoms are moderately severe or take longer than a couple of weeks to resolve, dose reductions should be postponed until symptoms resolve and then made more gradual by choosing a slower tapering rate. If severe withdrawal symptoms occur, then the patient should return to a higher dose, wait until symptoms resolve and thereafter taper at a slower rate.

Suggested taper schedules for escitalopram

A. A faster taper with up to 9 percentage points of SERT between each step with reductions made every 2–4 weeks (approximate length: 5–10 months). Patients who have been on the medication for only a few weeks will probably be able to taper more quickly and might follow every second or third step of this regimen, and make reductions every few days or so. For people who have only taken an antidepressant for a few weeks, the duration of the taper should not be longer than the period that the patient has been on the drug. For example, if escitalopram is taken for 3 weeks the taper should take less than 3 weeks.

B. A moderate taper with up to 5 percentage points of SERT between each step with reductions made every 2–4 weeks (approximate length: 10–20 months).

C. A slower taper with up to 3 percentage points of SERT between each step with reductions made every 2–4 weeks (approximate length: 20–40 months).

D. Some patients will be unable to taper at the slowest rates shown here and will need to taper by even smaller decrements, thus lengthening the overall period of tapering. Such a regimen could be constructed by placing intermediate steps in regimen C. For example, 3mg, 2mg, 1mg, 0mg could be modified to be 3mg, 2.5mg, 2mg, 1.5mg, 1mg, 0.5mg, 0mg. Further intermediate steps could also be added. Microtapering (tapering by a small amount each day, rather than by larger reductions every 2–4 weeks) is another possible approach (see benzodiazepines chapter for further details).

Please note that none of these regimens should be seen as prescriptive – that is, it is not suggested that patient must strictly adhere to them. They are given as example regimens and are not 'set and forget' but should be modified in order to ensure that withdrawal symptoms are tolerable throughout a taper – for example intermediate steps halfway between the doses listed could be added to make a more gradual taper.

UK/Europe/Australia regimens

A. **Faster taper** with up to 9 percentage points of SERT between each step – with reductions made every 2–4 weeks.*

Step	RO (%)	Dose (mg)	Volume	Step	RO (%)	Dose (mg)	Volume
1	79	20	Use tablets	7	33	1.6	0.8mL
2	70	10	Use tablets	8	25	1.0	0.5mL
3	66	7.5	Use ½ tablets**	9	17	0.6	0.3mL
4	58	5	Use tablets	Switch to escitalopram **0.2mg/mL dilution**			
Switch to escitalopram **2mg/mL dilution**				10	8.3	0.3	1.5mL
5	50	3.4	1.7mL	11	0	0	0
6	41	2.3	1.15mL				
See further steps in the right-hand column							

RO = receptor occupancy

*For longer term users, the time between each decrease may be shortened to 1 week if the patient is able to make the first couple of reductions with no withdrawal symptoms. The interval between reductions should never be less than 1 week because this might increase the risk of relapse, even in the absence of withdrawal effects.[16,17]

**Alternatively, these doses could be made up with a liquid version.

B. **Moderate taper** with up to 5 percentage points of SERT between each step – with reductions made every 2-4 weeks.

Step	RO (%)	Dose (mg)	Volume	Step	RO (%)	Dose (mg)	Volume
1	79	20	Use tablets	12	37	2.0	1.0mL
2	76	15	Use tablets	13	33	1.6	0.8mL
3	74	12.5	Use ½ tablets*	14	29	1.3	0.65mL
4	70	10	Use tablets	15	25	1.05	0.53mL
5	66	7.5	Use ½ tablets*	16	21	0.8	0.4mL
6	62	6.25	Use ¼ tablets*	17	17	0.6	0.3mL
7	58	5	Use tablets	18	12	0.45	0.23mL
Switch to escitalopram **2mg/mL dilution**				Switch to escitalopram **0.2mg/mL dilution**			
8	54	4.1	2.05mL	19	8.3	0.3	1.5mL
9	50	3.4	1.7mL	20	4.2	0.15	0.75mL
10	46	2.8	1.4mL	21	0	0	0
11	42	2.4	1.2mL				
See further steps in the right-hand column							

RO = receptor occupancy

*Alternatively, these doses could be made up with a liquid version.

C. **Slower taper** with 3 percentage points of SERT occupancy between each step – with reductions made every 2–4 weeks.

Step	RO (%)	Dose (mg)	Volume	Step	RO (%)	Dose (mg)	Volume	Step	RO (%)	Dose (mg)	Volume
1	79	20	Use tablets	14	55	4.4	2.2mL	28	26	1.08	0.54mL
2	78	17.5	Use ½ tablets*	15	53	4	2mL	29	23	0.96	0.48mL
3	76	15	Use tablets	16	51	3.6	1.8mL	30	21	0.85	0.43mL
4	75	13.75	Use ¾ tablets*	17	49	3.3	1.65mL	31	19	0.74	0.37mL
5	74	12.5	Use ½ tablets*	18	47	3	1.5mL	32	17	0.64	0.32mL
6	72	11.25	Use ¼ tablets*	19	45	2.72	1.36mL	33	15	0.54	0.27mL
7	70	10	Use tablets	20	43	2.48	1.24mL	34	13	0.45	0.23mL
	Switch to escitalopram 2mg/mL dilution			21	41	2.24	1.12mL		**Switch to escitalopram 0.2mg/mL** dilution		
8	68	8.7	4.35mL	22	38	2.04	1.02mL	35	11	0.37	1.85mL
9	66	7.7	3.85mL	23	36	1.86	0.93mL	36	8.5	0.29	1.45mL
10	64	6.8	3.4mL	24	34	1.68	0.84mL	37	6.4	0.21	1.05mL
11	62	6.1	3.05mL	25	32	1.52	0.76mL	38	4.3	0.14	0.7mL
12	60	5.4	2.7mL	26	30	1.36	0.68mL	39	2.1	0.07	0.35mL
13	58	4.9	2.45mL	27	28	1.22	0.61mL	40	0	0	0
	See further steps in the middle column				**See further steps in the right-hand column**						

RO = receptor occupancy
*Alternatively, these doses could be made up with a liquid version.

US regimens

A. **Faster taper** with up to 9 percentage points of SERT between each step – with reductions made every 2–4 weeks.*

Step	RO (%)	Dose (mg)	Volume	Step	RO (%)	Dose (mg)	Volume
1	79	20	Use tablets	7	33	1.6	1.6mL
2	70	10	Use tablets	8	25	1.0	1.0mL
3	66	7.5	Use ½ tablets**	9	17	0.6	0.6mL
4	58	5	Use tablets		**Switch to escitalopram 0.2mg/mL dilution**		
	Switch to escitalopram 1mg/mL dilution			10	8.3	0.3	1.5mL
5	50	3.4	3.4mL	11	0	0	0
6	41	2.3	2.3mL				
See further steps in the right-hand column							

RO = receptor occupancy
*For longer term users, the time between each decrease may be shortened to 1 week if the patient is able to make the first couple of reductions with no withdrawal symptoms. The interval between reductions should never be less than 1 week because this might increase the risk of relapse, even in the absence of withdrawal effects.[16,17]
**Alternatively, these doses could be made up with a liquid version.

B. **Moderate taper** with up to 5 percentage points of SERT between each step – with reductions made every 2–4 weeks.

Step	RO (%)	Dose (mg)	Volume	Step	RO (%)	Dose (mg)	Volume
1	79	20	Use tablets	12	37	2.0	2.0mL
2	76	15	Use tablets	13	33	1.6	1.6mL
3	74	12.5	Use ½ tablets*	14	29	1.3	1.3mL
4	70	10	Use tablets	15	25	1.05	1.05mL
5	66	7.5	Use ½ tablets*	16	21	0.8	0.8mL
6	62	6.25	Use ¼ tablets*	17	17	0.6	0.6mL
7	58	5	Use tablets	18	12	0.45	0.45mL
Switch to escitalopram **1mg/mL dilution**				Switch to escitalopram **0.2mg/mL dilution**			
8	54	4.1	4.1mL	19	8.3	0.3	1.5mL
9	50	3.4	3.4mL	20	4.2	0.15	0.75mL
10	46	2.8	2.8mL	21	0	0	0
11	42	2.4	2.4mL				
See further steps in the right-hand column							

RO = receptor occupancy
*Alternatively, these doses could be made up with a liquid version.

C. **Slower taper** with up to 3 percentage points of SERT occupancy between each step – with reductions made every 2–4 weeks.

Step	RO (%)	Dose (mg)	Volume	Step	RO (%)	Dose (mg)	Volume	Step	RO (%)	Dose (mg)	Volume
1	79	20	Use tablets	14	55	4.4	4.4mL	28	26	1.08	1.08mL
2	78	17.5	Use ½ tablets*	15	53	4	4mL	29	23	0.96	0.96mL
3	76	15	Use tablets	16	51	3.6	3.6mL	30	21	0.85	0.85mL
4	75	13.75	Use ¾ tablets*	17	49	3.3	3.3mL	31	19	0.74	0.74mL
5	74	12.5	Use ½ tablets*	18	47	3	3mL	32	17	0.64	0.64mL
6	72	11.25	Use ¼ tablets*	19	45	2.72	2.72mL	33	15	0.54	0.54mL
7	70	10	Use tablets	20	43	2.48	2.48mL	34	13	0.45	0.45mL
Switch to escitalopram **1mg/mL dilution**				21	41	2.24	2.24mL	Switch to escitalopram **0.2mg/mL dilution**			
8	68	8.7	8.7mL	22	38	2.04	2.04mL	35	11	0.37	1.85mL
9	66	7.7	7.7mL	23	36	1.86	1.86mL	36	8.5	0.29	1.45mL
10	64	6.8	6.8mL	24	34	1.68	1.68mL	37	6.4	0.21	1.05mL
11	62	6.1	6.1mL	25	32	1.52	1.52mL	38	4.3	0.14	0.7mL
12	60	5.4	5.4mL	26	30	1.36	1.36mL	39	2.1	0.07	0.35mL
13	58	4.9	4.9mL	27	28	1.22	1.22mL	40	0	0	0
See further steps in the middle column				**See further steps in the right-hand column**							

RO = receptor occupancy
*Alternatively, these doses could be made up with a liquid version.

References

1. Aurobindo Pharma – Milpharm. Escitalopram 20mg tablets SmPC. https://www.medicines.org.uk/emc/product/7059/smpc#gref (accessed 7 September 2022).

2. Baldwin DS, Montgomery SA, Nil R, Lader M. Discontinuation symptoms in depression and anxiety disorders. *Int J Neuropsychopharmacol* 2007; 10: 73–84.

3. Lader M, Stender K, Bürger V, Nil R. Efficacy and tolerability of escitalopram in 12- and 24-week treatment of social anxiety disorder: randomised, double-blind, placebo-controlled, fixed-dose study. *Depress Anxiety* 2004; 19: 241–8.

4. Horowitz MA, Framer A, Hengartner MP, Sørensen A, Taylor D. Estimating risk of antidepressant withdrawal from a review of published data. *CNS Drugs* 2022; published online 14 December. doi:10.1007/s40263-022-00960-y.

5. Davies J, Read J. A systematic review into the incidence, severity and duration of antidepressant withdrawal effects: are guidelines evidence-based? *Addict Behav* 2019; 97: 111–21.

6. Sørensen A, Ruhé HG, Munkholm K. The relationship between dose and serotonin transporter occupancy of antidepressants-a systematic review. *Mol Psychiatry* 2022; 27: 192–201.

7. Holford N. Pharmacodynamic principles and the time course of delayed and cumulative drug effects. *Ther Adv Psychopharmacol* 2018; 26: 56.

8. Furukawa TA, Cipriani A, Cowen PJ, Leucht S, Egger M, Salanti G. Optimal dose of selective serotonin reuptake inhibitors, venlafaxine, and mirtazapine in major depression: a systematic review and dose-response meta-analysis. *The Lancet Psychiatry* 2019; 6: 601–9.

9. Horowitz MA, Taylor D. Tapering of SSRI treatment to mitigate withdrawal symptoms. *The Lancet Psychiatry* 2019; 6: 538–46.

10. Lundbeck. Cipralex oral drops solution, 20mg/mL – summary of product characteristics (SmPC) – (emc). https://www.medicines.org.uk/emc/product/4306/smpc#gref (accessed 29 July 23).

11. FDA. Lexapro (escitalopram oxalate). www.accessdata.fda.gov. 2017; published online January https://www.accessdata.fda.gov/drugsatfda_docs/label/2017/021323s047lbl.pdf (accessed 10 September 2022).

12. Brennan K. Selective serotonin reuptake inhibitor (SSRI) formulations suggested for adults with swallowing difficulties. SPS – Specialist Pharmacy Service. 2021; published online 1 July. https://www.sps.nhs.uk/articles/selective-serotonin-reuptake-inhibitor-ssri-formulations-suggested-for-adults-with-swallowing-difficulties/ (accessed 19 September 2022).

13. Smyth J. The NEWT guidelines for administration of medication to patients with enteral feeding tubes or swallowing difficulties website. The NEWT Guidelines. 2011. https://www.newtguidelines.com/index.html (accessed 7 September 2022).

14. Bostwick JR, Demehri A. Pills to powder: an updated clinician's reference for crushable psychotropics. *Curr Psychiatr* 2017; 16: 46–9.

15. Groot PC, van Os J. How user knowledge of psychotropic drug withdrawal resulted in the development of person-specific tapering medication. *Ther Adv Psychopharmacol* 2020; 10: 204512532093245.

16. Baldessarini RJ, Tondo L, Ghiani C, Lepri B. Illness risk following rapid versus gradual discontinuation of antidepressants. *Am J Psychiatry* 2010; 167: 934–41.

17. Gøtzsche PC, Demasi M. Interventions to help patients withdraw from depression drugs: A systematic review. *Int J Risk Saf Med.* 2023 September 13. doi: 10.3233/JRS-230011. Epub ahead of print.

Fluoxetine

Trade names: Prozac, Olena, Oxactin, Sarafem.

Description: Fluoxetine is an SSRI with SERT as its major target. Fluoxetine has practically no affinity for adrenergic, serotonergic, dopaminergic, histaminergic, muscarinic and GABA receptors.[1]

Withdrawal effects: In double-blind randomised controlled trials of fluoxetine discontinuation 50% of people on average experienced withdrawal effects,[2] although these studies did not measure severity or duration of these symptoms. Fluoxetine withdrawal effects can be delayed by weeks after stopping because of the long elimination half-life of its active metabolite norfluoxetine.[3] The frequency of its withdrawal effects may therefore have been underestimated. In an analysis of the WHO adverse effect database, fluoxetine emerged as disproportionately associated with withdrawal compared to medications as a whole but low risk compared to other antidepressants.[4]

Peak plasma: 6 to 8 hours.[1]

Half-life: 4 to 6 days for fluoxetine and 4 to 16 days for norfluoxetine, its active metabolite.[1] Due to its long half-life it is reasonable to dose every other day or at even greater intervals to facilitate tapering.

Receptor occupancy: The relationship between dose of fluoxetine and occupancy of its major target SERT is hyperbolic.[5] Antidepressants also show a hyperbolic pattern between dose and clinical effects,[6] which may be relevant to withdrawal effects from fluoxetine. Dose reductions made by linear amounts (e.g. 20mg, 15mg, 10mg, 5mg, 0mg) will cause increasingly large reductions in effect which may cause increasingly severe withdrawal effects (Figure 2.24a). To produce equal-sized reductions in effect on serotonin transporter occupancy will require hyperbolically reducing doses (Figure 2.24b),[7] which informs the reductions presented.

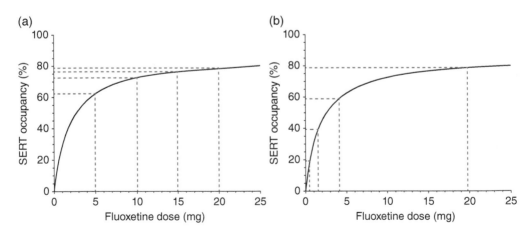

Figure 2.24 (a) Linear reductions of dose cause increasingly large reductions in effect on receptor targets, possibly associated with more withdrawal effects. (b) Even reductions of effect at target receptors requires hyperbolic dose reductions. The final dose before stopping will need to be very small so that this step down is not larger (in terms of effect on receptor occupancy) than previous reductions.

Available formulations: As tablets, capsules and liquid.

Tablets*

Dosage	UK	Europe	USA	Australia	Canada
10mg	✓	–	✓	–	–
20mg	✓**	–	✓	–	–
30mg	–	–	–	–	–
40mg	–	–	–	–	–
60mg	–	–	✓	–	–

*As fluoxetine hydrochloride
**Dispersible tablet

Capsules*

Dosage	UK	Europe	USA	Australia	Canada
10mg	✓	–	✓	–	✓
20mg	✓	✓	✓	✓	✓
30mg	✓	–	–	–	–
40mg	✓	–	✓	–	✓
60mg	✓	–	–	–	–
90mg (weekly DR)	–	–	✓	–	–

*As fluoxetine hydrochloride

Liquid*

Dosage	UK	Europe	USA	Australia	Canada
20mg/5mL (4mg/mL)	✓	✓	✓	–	✓

*The solution of fluoxetine hydrochloride 20mg/5mL is bioequivalent to tablet form.[8] Store at controlled room temperature, 15° to 30°C (59° to 86°F).[8]

Dilutions: To make up some of the small doses outlined below, dilution of the liquid available from the manufacturer will be required. Adding water to the original solution may have the effect of precipitating fluoxetine and so a suspension might be formed.[9] All dilutions need therefore to be shaken thoroughly. Drug stability cannot be assured and so dilutions should be taken immediately after preparation (and any remainder should be discarded).

UK/USA/Europe dilutions	Solution required	How to prepare solution
Doses ≥ 0.8 mg	20mg/5mL (4mg/mL)	Original solution
Doses > 0.08mg to 0.8mg	0.4mg/mL	Mix 0.5mL of original solution with 4.5mL of water
Doses ≤ 0.08mg	0.04mg/mL	Mix 0.5mL of the original solution with 49.5mL of water

CHAPTER 2

Worked example: To illustrate how the volumes were calculated in the regimens given below we provide a worked example. To make up 0.5mg of fluoxetine the 0.4mg/mL dilution can be used, prepared as above. The volume of 0.4mg/mL liquid required to give a dose of 0.5mg fluoxetine is 0.5/0.4 = 1.25mL.

Off-label options: Guidelines for people who cannot swallow tablets (e.g. the NEWT guidelines in the UK,[10] the NHS[11] and similar US guidance[12]) suggest that capsules of fluoxetine can be opened and dispersed in water.[10,11] Dispersion takes about 5 minutes.[10,11] As its stability cannot be assured it should be consumed immediately, and any unused solution discarded.

According to NPS MedicineWise 20mg dispersible fluoxetine tablets can also be dissolved in 100mL of water,[8] making up a 0.2mg/mL solution of fluoxetine (it is soluble in water up to 14mg/mL).[13] Tablets may be crushed with a spoon or pestle and mortar before mixing with water to speed up this process. This should be shaken vigorously before administration. As its stability cannot be assured it should be consumed immediately, and any unused solution discarded. Other options to make up small doses include compounding smaller dose tablets, including 'tapering strips'.[14]

Deprescribing notes: Initial reductions can be estimated from Tables 2.11 and 2.22, although patient preference should be taken into account. Sometimes an even smaller reduction to start with may be advisable to boost a patient's confidence that they can taper if performed carefully. Each reduction should be made when the withdrawal symptoms from the previous reduction have largely resolved so that subsequent reductions do not lead to cumulative withdrawal symptoms. Withdrawal symptoms should be tolerable and last at most a couple of weeks (see Figure 2.9). As the elimination half-life of fluoxetine is about 1 week, this may delay the onset of withdrawal symptoms and represent a partial 'self-tapering' effect. Therefore it may be advisable to make every second reduction in the regimens suggested below at spacing of 6 to 8 weeks rather than each step at intervals of 2 to 4 weeks as for most other antidepressants. If withdrawal symptoms are moderately severe or take longer than a couple of weeks to resolve, dose reductions should be postponed until symptoms resolve and then made more gradual by choosing a slower tapering rate. If severe withdrawal symptoms occur then the patient should return to a higher dose, wait until symptoms resolve and thereafter taper at a slower rate.

Suggested taper schedules for fluoxetine

A. A faster taper with up to 11 percentage points of SERT occupancy between each step (approximate length: 4–9 months). Patients who have been on the medication for only a few weeks will probably be able to taper more quickly and might follow every second or third step of this regimen, and make reductions every few days or so. For people who have only taken an antidepressant for a few weeks, the duration of the taper should not be longer than the period that the patient has been on the drug. For example, if fluoxetine is taken for 3 weeks the taper should be less than 3 weeks.

B. A moderate taper with 5 percentage points of SERT between each step (approximate length: 9–18 months).

C. A slower taper with 3 percentage points of SERT between each step (approximate length: 18–34 months).

D. Some patients will be unable to taper at the slowest rates shown here and will need to taper by even smaller decrements, thus lengthening the overall period of tapering. Such a regimen could be constructed by placing intermediate steps in regimen C. For example, 3mg, 2mg, 1mg, 0mg could be modified to be 3mg, 2.5mg, 2mg, 1.5mg, 1mg, 0.5mg, 0mg. Further intermediate steps could also be added. Microtapering (tapering by a small amount each day, rather than by larger reductions every 2–4 weeks) is another possible approach (see benzodiazepines chapter for further details).

Please note that none of these regimens should be seen as prescriptive – that is, it is not suggested that patient must strictly adhere to them. They are given as example regimens and are not 'set and forget' but should be modified in order to ensure that withdrawal symptoms are tolerable throughout a taper – for example intermediate steps halfway between the doses listed could be added to make a more gradual taper.

Less than once a day dosing: As fluoxetine and its active metabolite norfluoxetine have half-lives of 4–6 days and 4–16 days,[1] respectively, dosing up to once every 8–10 days is reasonable for this drug as plasma levels will not drop greatly during this time. This allows some of the doses suggested below to be made up using tablets, (or halves or quarters of tablets) where these are available (UK and USA), administered up to every 8th or 10th day as long as the patient has a good way of remembering this dosing.

A. **Faster taper** with up to 11 percentage points of SERT between each step – with reductions made every 2–4 weeks.*

Step	RO (%)	Dose (mg)	Volume	Alternative approach**
1	82	40	Use tablets/capsules	Use tablets/capsules
2	79	20	Use tablets/capsules	Use tablets/capsules
3	72	10	Use tablets/capsules***	Use tablets/capsules
4	62	5	Use ½ tablets***	Use ½ tablets
Switch to fluoxetine **20mg/5mL (4mg/mL) liquid**				
5	53	3	0.75mL	10mg tablet every 3rd day
6	42	1.8	0.45mL	10mg tablet every 5th day
7	32	1.1	0.28mL	5mg (½ tablet) every 5th day
Switch to fluoxetine **0.4mg/mL dilution**				
8	21	0.6	1.5mL	2.5mg (¼ tablet) every 4th day
9	11	0.26	0.65mL	2.5 mg (¼ tablet) every 10th day****
10	0	0	0	0

RO = receptor occupancy

*Alternatively, it may be reasonable to make every second reduction in this regime at intervals of 6–8 weeks in order to give time for delayed onset withdrawal effects to arise due to the long elimination half-life (and taking advantage of its partial 'self-tapering' properties).

**This approach allows reductions to be made using only tablets, if 10mg tablets are available (UK and USA).

***Where tablets/capsules of this dose are not available, liquids could be used instead.

****May risk withdrawal symptoms in some patients – caution suggested. Switch to liquid may be advisable at this point.

B. **A moderate taper** with up to 5 percentage points of SERT between each step – with reductions made every 2–4 weeks.*

Step	RO (%)	Dose (mg)	Volume	Step	RO (%)	Dose (mg)	Volume
1	82	40	Use tablets/capsules	11	38	1.52	0.38mL
2	79	20	Use tablets/capsules	12	34	1.2	0.3mL
3	76	15	Use ½ tablets**	13	29	0.96	0.24mL
4	72	10	Use tablets/capsules**	Switch to fluoxetine **0.4mg/mL dilution**			
Switch to fluoxetine **20mg/5mL (4mg/mL) liquid**				14	24	0.72	1.8mL
5	68	7	1.75mL	15	19	0.56	1.4mL
6	62	5	1.25mL***	16	14	0.4	1.0mL
7	58	3.8	0.95mL	17	10	0.24	0.6mL
8	53	3	0.75mL	18	5	0.12	0.3mL
9	48	2.4	0.6mL	19	0	0	0
10	43	1.92	0.48mL				
See further steps in the right-hand column							

RO = receptor occupancy

*Alternatively, it may be reasonable to make every second reduction in this regime at intervals of 6–8 weeks in order to give time for delayed onset withdrawal effects to arise due to the long elimination half-life (and taking advantage of its partial 'self-tapering' properties).

**Where tablets/capsules of this dose are not available, liquids could be used.

***Alternatively, half a 10mg tablet could be used where this is available.

C. **A slower taper** with up to 3 percentage points of SERT occupancy between each step – with reductions made every 2–4 weeks.*

Step	RO (%)	Dose (mg)	Volume	Step	RO (%)	Dose (mg)	Volume	Step	RO (%)	Dose (mg)	Volume
1	82	40	Use tablets/capsules	13	55	3.32	0.83mL	25	25	0.77	1.93mL
2	81	30	Use tablets/capsules	14	52	2.96	0.74mL	26	22	0.67	1.68mL
3	79	20	Use tablets/capsules	15	50	2.6	0.65mL	27	20	0.57	1.43mL
4	76	15	Use ½ tablets**	16	47	2.32	0.58mL	28	17	0.48	1.2mL
Switch to fluoxetine **20mg/5mL liquid (4mg/mL)**				17	45	2.08	0.52mL	29	15	0.4	1mL
5	75	12.5	3.1mL	18	42	1.84	0.46mL	30	12	0.32	0.8mL
6	72	10	2.5mL***	19	40	1.64	0.41mL	31	10	0.25	0.63mL
7	70	8.2	2.1mL	20	37	1.44	0.36mL	32	7	0.18	0.45mL
8	67	6.8	1.7mL	21	35	1.28	0.32mL	33	5	0.12	0.3mL
9	65	5.8	1.45mL	22	32	1.14	0.29mL	Switch to fluoxetine **0.04mg/mL dilution**			
10	62	5	1.25mL***	23	30	1	0.25mL	34	2	0.06	1.5mL
11	60	4.32	1.08mL	24	27	0.88	0.22mL	35	0	0	0
12	57	3.8	0.95mL	Switch to fluoxetine **0.4mg/mL dilution**							
See further steps in the middle column				**See further steps in the right-hand column**							

RO = receptor occupancy

*Alternatively, it may be reasonable to make every second reduction in this regimen at intervals of 6–8 weeks in order to give time for delayed onset withdrawal effects to arise due to the long elimination half-life (and taking advantage of its partial 'self-tapering' properties).

**Where tablets are not available a liquid version could be used.

***Alternatively, a 10mg tablet or half of this tablet could be used where this is available.

References

1. Fluoxetine 20 mg Capsules. https://www.medicines.org.uk/emc/medicine/25737 (accessed 12 October 2022).
2. Horowitz MA, Framer A, Hengartner MP, Sørensen A, Taylor D. Estimating risk of antidepressant withdrawal from a review of published data. *CNS Drugs* 2022; published online 14 December. doi:10.1007/s40263-022-00960-y.
3. Fava GA, Gatti A, Belaise C, Guidi J, Offidani E. Withdrawal symptoms after selective serotonin reuptake inhibitor discontinuation: a systematic review. *Psychother Psychosom* 2015; 84: 72–81.
4. Gastaldon C, Schoretsanitis G, Arzenton E, et al. Withdrawal syndrome following discontinuation of 28 antidepressants: pharmacovigilance analysis of 31,688 reports from the WHO spontaneous reporting database. *Drug Saf* 2022; 45: 1539–49.
5. Sørensen A, Ruhé HG, Munkholm K. The relationship between dose and serotonin transporter occupancy of antidepressants – a systematic review. *Mol Psychiatry* 2022; 27: 192–201.
6. Furukawa TA, Cipriani A, Cowen PJ, Leucht S, Egger M, Salanti G. Optimal dose of selective serotonin reuptake inhibitors, venlafaxine, and mirtazapine in major depression: a systematic review and dose-response meta-analysis. *The Lancet Psychiatry* 2019; 6: 601–9.
7. Horowitz MA, Taylor D. Tapering of SSRI treatment to mitigate withdrawal symptoms. *The Lancet Psychiatry* 2019; 6: 538–46.
8. FDA. Label for Prozac (fluoxetine). FDA. 2017. https://www.accessdata.fda.gov/drugsatfda_docs/label/2017/018936s108lbl.pdf (accessed 12 October 2022).
9. Pinewood Healthcare. Fluoxetine 20mg/5ml oral solution. https://www.medicines.org.uk/emc/product/4564/smpc#gref (accessed 29 July 23).
10. Smyth J. The NEWT guidelines for administration of medication to patients with enteral feeding tubes or swallowing difficulties website. The NEWT Guidelines. 2011. https://www.newtguidelines.com/index.html (accessed 7 September 2022).
11. Brennan K. Selective serotonin reuptake inhibitor (SSRI) formulations suggested for adults with swallowing difficulties. SPS – Specialist Pharmacy Service. 2021; published online 1 July. https://www.sps.nhs.uk/articles/selective-serotonin-reuptake-inhibitor-ssri-formulations-suggested-for-adults-with-swallowing-difficulties/ (accessed 19 September 2022).
12. Bostwick JR, Demehri A. Pills to powder: an updated clinician's reference for crushable psychotropics. *Curr Psychiatr* 2017; 16: 46–9.
13. Prozac. NPS MedicineWise. https://www.nps.org.au/medicine-finder/prozac-dispersible-tablets (accessed 12 October 2022).
14. Groot PC, van Os J. How user knowledge of psychotropic drug withdrawal resulted in the development of person-specific tapering medication. *Ther Adv Psychopharmacol* 2020; 10: 204512532093245.

Fluvoxamine

Trade names: Luvox, Faverin.

Description: Fluvoxamine is an SSRI with SERT as its major target. Apart from its activity on SERT, fluvoxamine also acts as a sigma-1 receptor agonist. It has minimal binding capacity for alpha-adrenergic, beta-adrenergic, histaminergic, muscarinic, dopaminergic or serotonergic receptors.[1]

Withdrawal effects: In one open-label study patients stopping fluvoxamine experienced withdrawal symptoms in 85.7% of cases,[2] after 8 months of treatment, although severity was not measured. Based on calls regarding withdrawal to a help line (normalised to prescription numbers) fluvoxamine was responsible for more calls than any other SSRI except paroxetine.[3] In an analysis of the WHO adverse effect database fluvoxamine emerged as disproportionately associated with withdrawal compared to medications as a whole but low risk compared to other antidepressants.[4]

Peak plasma: 3–8 hours.[1]

Half-life: 13–15 hours after a single dose and slightly longer (17–22 hours) during repeated dosing. Every-other-day dosing is not recommended for tapering because of the substantial reductions in plasma concentrations this would produce, possibly giving rise to withdrawal effects.

Receptor occupancy: The relationship between the dose of fluvoxamine and occupancy of its major target the serotonin transporter is hyperbolic,[5] and this also applies to other receptor targets.[6] Antidepressants also show a hyperbolic pattern between dose and clinical effects,[7] which may be relevant to withdrawal effects from fluvoxamine. Dose reductions made by linear amounts (e.g. 100mg, 75mg, 50mg, 25mg, 0mg) will cause increasingly large reductions in receptor occupancy, which may cause increasingly severe withdrawal effects (Figure 2.25a). To produce equal-sized reductions in effect on SERT occupancy will require hyperbolically reducing doses (Figure 2.25b),[8] which informs the reductions presented.

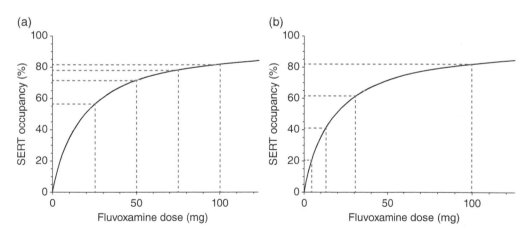

Figure 2.25 (a) Linear reductions of dose cause increasingly large reductions in effect on receptor targets, possibly associated with more withdrawal effects. (b) Even reductions of effect at target receptors require hyperbolic dose reductions. The final dose before stopping will need to be very small so that this step down is not larger (in terms of effect on receptor occupancy) than previous reductions.

CHAPTER 2

Available formulations: Fluvoxamine is available as tablets.

Tablets*

Dosage	UK	Europe	USA	Australia	Canada
25mg	–	–	✓	–	–
50mg	✓	✓	✓	✓	✓
100mg	✓	✓	✓	✓	✓

*As fluvoxamine maleate

Off-label options: Guidelines for people who cannot swallow tablets (e.g. the NEWT guidelines in the UK,[9] based on local hospital policies and information direct from the manufacturer and similar US guidance)[10] suggest that immediate-release fluvoxamine tablets can be crushed and dispersed in water for administration, for off-label use.[9] A 1mg/mL suspension could be made by adding water to a 50mg tablet to make up a 50mL. The tablet may be crushed with a spoon or pestle and mortar before mixing with water to speed up this process. The suspension should be shaken vigorously before use, as fluvoxamine is poorly soluble in water. As its stability cannot be assured it should be consumed immediately, and any unused suspension discarded. Other options to make up small doses include compounding smaller dose tablets, including 'tapering strips'.[11]

Worked example: To illustrate how the volumes were calculated in the regimens given below we provide a worked example. To make up 2mg of fluvoxamine the 1mg/mL suspension can be used, prepared as above. The volume of 1mg/mL liquid required to give a dose of 2mg fluvoxamine is 2/1 = 2mL.

Deprescribing notes: Initial reductions can be estimated from Tables 2.11 and 2.22, although patient preference should be taken into account. Sometimes an even smaller reduction to start with may be advisable to boost a patient's confidence that they can taper if performed carefully. Each reduction should be made when the withdrawal symptoms from the previous reduction have largely resolved so that subsequent reductions do not lead to cumulative withdrawal symptoms. Withdrawal symptoms should be tolerable and last at most a couple of weeks (see Figure 2.9). Allowing for a sufficient observation period, reductions can therefore be made about every 2 to 4 weeks. If withdrawal symptoms are moderately severe or take longer than a couple of weeks to resolve, dose reductions should be postponed until symptoms resolve and then made more gradual by choosing a slower tapering rate. If severe withdrawal symptoms occur then the patient should return to a higher dose, wait until symptoms resolve and thereafter taper at a slower rate.

Suggested taper schedules for fluvoxamine

A. A faster taper with up to 11 percentage points of SERT between each step with reductions made every 2–4 weeks (approximate length: 5–10 months). Patients who have been on the medication for only a few weeks will probably be able to taper more quickly and might follow every second or third step of this regimen and make reductions every few days or so. For people who have only taken an antidepressant for a few weeks, the duration of the taper should not be longer than the period that the patient has been on the drug. For example, if fluvoxamine is taken for 3 weeks the taper should be less than 3 weeks.

B. A moderate taper with up to 5 percentage points of SERT between each step with reductions made every 2–4 weeks (approximate length: 10–20 months).

C. A slower taper with up to 3 percentage points of SERT between each step with reductions made every 2–4 weeks (approximate length: 20–40 months).

D. Some patients will be unable to taper at the slowest rates shown here and will need to taper by even smaller decrements, thus lengthening the overall period of tapering. Such a regimen could be constructed by placing intermediate steps in regimen C. For example, 3mg, 2mg, 1mg, 0mg could be modified to be 3mg, 2.5mg, 2mg, 1.5mg, 1mg, 0.5mg, 0mg. Further intermediate steps could also be added. Microtapering (tapering by a small amount each day, rather than by larger reductions every 2–4 weeks) is another possible approach (see benzodiazepines chapter for further details).

Please note that none of these regimens should be seen as prescriptive – that is, it is not suggested that patient must strictly adhere to them. They are given as example regimens and are not 'set and forget' but should be modified in order to ensure that withdrawal symptoms are tolerable throughout a taper – for example intermediate steps halfway between the doses listed could be added to make a more gradual taper.

Metabolic note: Fluvoxamine is both a metabolic substrate and a potent inhibitor of CYP P450 1A2.[12] As the dose is reduced this will lead to reduced inhibition (i.e. induction) of its metabolism thereby leading to a more rapid drop in plasma levels. This may present a rationale to slow the rate of reduction even further, and to consider twice daily dosing, at lower doses.

A. **Faster taper** with up to 11 percentage points of SERT between each step – with reductions made every 2–4 weeks.*

Step	RO (%)	Dose (mg)	Volume	Step	RO (%)	Dose (mg)	Volume
1	82	100	Use tablets	6	41	12.5	6.25mL***
2	78	75	Use tablets	7	31	8	4mL
3	71	50	Use tablets	8	20	4.5	2.25mL
Switch to fluvoxamine **2mg/mL suspension****				9	10	2	1mL
4	61	30	15mL	10	0	0	0
5	51	20	10mL				
See further steps in the right-hand column							

RO = receptor occupancy

*For longer term users, the time between each decrease may be shortened to 1 week if the patient is able to make the first couple of reductions with no withdrawal symptoms. The interval between reductions should never be less than 1 week because this might increase the risk of relapse, even in the absence of withdrawal effects.[13,14]

**This can be prepared as above.

***Could be made up by a portion of a tablet.

CHAPTER 2

B. **Moderate taper** with 5 percentage points of SERT between each step – with reductions made every 2–4 weeks.

Step	RO (%)	Dose (mg)	Volume	Step	RO (%)	Dose (mg)	Volume
1	82	100	Use tablets	11	40	12	6mL
2	78	75	Use tablets	12	36	10	5mL
3	75	62.5	Use ½ or ¼ tablets*	13	31	8.4	4.2mL
4	71	50	Use tablets	14	27	6.7	3.35mL
Switch to fluvoxamine **2mg/mL suspension****				15	22	5.3	2.65mL
5	67	40	20mL	16	18	4	2mL
6	63	32	16mL	17	13	2.8	1.4mL
7	58	26	13mL	18	8.9	1.8	0.9mL
8	54	22	11mL	19	4.5	0.9	0.45mL
9	49	18	9mL	20	0	0	0
10	45	15	7.5mL				
See further steps in the right-hand column							

*Alternatively, could be administered as a suspension.
**This can be prepared as above.

C. **Slower taper** with 3 percentage points of SERT occupancy between each step – with reductions made every 2–4 weeks.

Step	RO (%)	Dose (mg)	Volume	Step	RO (%)	Dose (mg)	Volume	Step	RO (%)	Dose (mg)	Volume
1	82	100	Use tablets	14	56	24	12mL	28	26	6.4	3.2mL
Switch to fluvoxamine **2mg/mL suspension***				15	54	22	11mL	29	24	5.7	2.85mL
2	80	88	44mL	16	52	20	10mL	30	22	5	2.5mL
3	78	75	37.5mL**	17	50	18.5	9.25mL	31	19	4.4	2.2mL
4	76	65	32.5mL	18	48	17	8.5mL	32	17	3.8	1.9mL
5	75	60	30mL	19	45	15.5	7.75mL	33	15	3.2	1.6mL
6	73	55	27.5mL	20	43	14	7mL	34	13	2.7	1.35mL
7	71	50	25mL**	21	41	13	6.5mL	35	11	2.2	1.1mL
8	69	45	22.5mL	22	39	12	6mL	36	8.7	1.7	0.85mL
9	67	40	20mL	23	37	11	5.5mL	37	6.5	1.2	0.6mL
10	65	36	18mL	24	35	10	5mL	38	4.3	0.8	0.4mL
11	63	33	16.5mL	25	32	9	4.5mL	39	2.2	0.4	0.2mL
12	61	30	15mL	26	30	8	4mL	40	0	0	0
13	58	27	13.5mL	27	28	7.2	3.6mL				
See further steps in the middle column				**See further steps in the right-hand column**							

RO = receptor occupancy
*This can be prepared as above.
**Alternatively, could be administered as a tablet or fraction of a tablet.

References

1. Mylan. Fluvoxamine-summary of product characteristics (SmPC) – (emc). https://www.medicines.org.uk/emc/product/1169/smpc#gref (accessed 13 September 2022).

2. Black DW, Wesner R, Gabel J. The abrupt discontinuation of fluvoxamine in patients with panic disorder. *J Clin Psychiatry* 1993; 54: 146–9.

3. Taylor D, Stewart S, Connolly A. Antidepressant withdrawal symptoms – telephone calls to a national medication helpline. *J Affect Disord* 2006; 95: 129–33.

4. Gastaldon C, Schoretsanitis G, Arzenton E, et al. Withdrawal syndrome following discontinuation of 28 antidepressants: pharmacovigilance analysis of 31,688 reports from the WHO spontaneous reporting database. *Drug Saf* 2022; 45: 1539–49.

5. Sørensen A, Ruhé HG, Munkholm K. The relationship between dose and serotonin transporter occupancy of antidepressants – a systematic review. *Mol Psychiatry* 2022; 27: 192–201.

6. Holford N. Pharmacodynamic principles and the time course of delayed and cumulative drug effects. *Ther Adv Psychopharmacol* 2018; 26: 56.

7. Furukawa TA, Cipriani A, Cowen PJ, Leucht S, Egger M, Salanti G. Optimal dose of selective serotonin reuptake inhibitors, venlafaxine, and mirtazapine in major depression: a systematic review and dose-response meta-analysis. *The Lancet Psychiatry* 2019; 6: 601–9.

8. Horowitz MA, Taylor D. Tapering of SSRI treatment to mitigate withdrawal symptoms. *The Lancet Psychiatry* 2019; 6: 538–46.

9. Smyth J. The NEWT guidelines for administration of medication to patients with enteral feeding tubes or swallowing difficulties website. The NEWT Guidelines. 2011. https://www.newtguidelines.com/index.html (accessed 7 September 2022).

10. Bostwick JR, Demehri A. Pills to powder: an updated clinician's reference for crushable psychotropics. *Curr Psychiatr* 2017; 16: 46–9.

11. Groot PC, van Os J. How user knowledge of psychotropic drug withdrawal resulted in the development of person-specific tapering medication. *Ther Adv Psychopharmacol* 2020; 10: 204512532093245.

12. Spina E, Santoro V, D'Arrigo C. Clinically relevant pharmacokinetic drug interactions with second-generation antidepressants: an update. *Clin Ther* 2008; 30: 1206–27.

13. Baldessarini RJ, Tondo L, Ghiani C, Lepri B. Illness risk following rapid versus gradual discontinuation of antidepressants. *Am J Psychiatry* 2010; 167: 934–41.

14. Gøtzsche PC, Demasi M. Interventions to help patients withdraw from depression drugs: A systematic review. *Int J Risk Saf Med.* 2023 September 13. doi: 10.3233/JRS-230011. Epub ahead of print.

CHAPTER 2

Imipramine

Trade name: Tofranil.

Description: Imipramine is a tricyclic antidepressant that acts by blocking SERT and NET.[1] It also has strong binding affinities for alpha-1 and -2 adrenergic receptors, histamine (H_1), serotonin, dopamine (D_2) and muscarinic (M_1) receptors.[1,2]

Withdrawal effects: In a structured analysis of antidepressant withdrawal, tricyclics were designated a high-risk category, with some withdrawal symptoms characteristic of cholinergic rebound.[3] Imipramine was responsible for approximately the same rate of calls to a helpline related to withdrawal problems (normalised to prescription numbers) as common SSRIs.[4,5] In an analysis of the WHO adverse effect database, imipramine emerged as disproportionately associated with withdrawal compared to medications as a whole and moderate risk compared to other antidepressants.[6]

Peak plasma: 1–2 hours.[7]

Half-life: 19 hours. The manufacturer recommends up to 3 times a day dosing.[1] Every-other-day dosing is not recommended for tapering because of the substantial reductions in plasma concentrations this would produce, possibly giving rise to withdrawal effects.

Receptor occupancy: The relationship between the dose of imipramine and occupancy of one of its major targets, the SERT, is hyperbolic.[8] Antidepressants also show a hyperbolic pattern between dose and clinical effects,[9] which may be relevant to withdrawal effects from imipramine. Dose reductions made by linear amounts (e.g. 100mg, 75mg, 50mg, 25mg, 0mg) will cause increasingly large reductions in effect which may cause increasingly severe withdrawal effects (Figure 2.26a). To produce equal-sized reductions in effect on SERT occupancy will require hyperbolically reducing doses (Figure 2.26b),[10] which informs the reductions presented. This hyperbolic pattern also applies to its occupancy of other receptor targets (including NET, histamine and

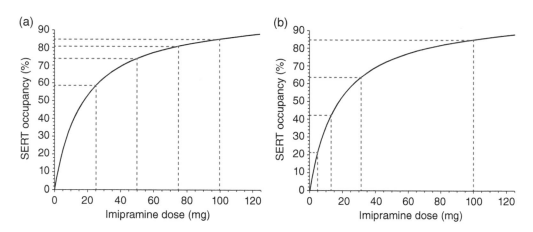

Figure 2.26 (a) Linear reductions of dose cause increasingly large reductions in effect on receptor targets, possibly associated with more withdrawal effects. (b) Even reductions of effect at target receptors requires hyperbolic dose reductions. The final dose before stopping will need to be very small so that this step down is not larger (in terms of effect on receptor occupancy) than previous reductions.

muscarinic acetylcholine receptors) as these relationships are dictated by the law of mass action.[11] There may be some differences in the precise dose-related activity between receptors but the hyperbolic relationship remains. It is expected that the regimens given below (based on SERT occupancy) will be broadly suitable for other receptor occupancies, such as for histamine H_1 and acetylcholine.

Available formulations: Imipramine is available as tablets, capsules and liquids.

Tablets*

Dosage	UK	Europe	USA	Australia	Canada
10mg	✓	✓	✓	✓	✓
25mg	✓	✓	✓	✓	✓
50mg	–	✓	✓	–	✓
75mg	–	–	–	–	✓

*As imipramine hydrochloride

Liquid*

Dosage	UK	Europe	USA	Australia	Canada
25mg/5mL (5mg/mL)	✓	–	–	–	–

*As imipramine hydrochloride. Do not store above 25°C.[12]

Capsules*

Dosage	UK	Europe	USA	Australia	Canada
75mg	–	–	✓	–	–
100mg	–	–	✓	–	–
125mg	–	–	✓	–	–
150mg	–	–	✓	–	–

*As imipramine pamoate

Dilutions: In order to make up smaller doses for tapering dilution of the manufacturer's solution may be required. Adding water to the original solution may have the effect of precipitating imipramine and so a suspension might be formed. All dilutions need therefore to be shaken thoroughly. Drug stability cannot be assured and so dilutions should be taken immediately after preparation (and any remainder should be discarded).

Dilutions	Solution required	How to prepare solution
Doses ≥ 1 mg	5mg/mL	Original solution 25mg/5mL (5mg/mL)
Doses < 1mg	0.5mg/mL	Mix 1mL of original oral solution with 9mL of water

Worked example: To illustrate how the volumes were calculated in the regimens given below, we provide a worked example. To make up 2.5mg of imipramine the 5mg/mL original solution can be used. The volume of 5mg/mL liquid required to give a dose of 2.5mg imipramine is 2.5/5 = 0.5mL.

Off-label options: Guidelines for people who cannot swallow tablets (e.g. the NEWT guidelines in the UK,[13] based on local hospital policies, and information direct from the manufacturer and similar US guidance[14]) suggest that imipramine tablets (in the form of imipramine hydrochloride) can be crushed and mixed in water for administration as an off-label use.[13] However imipramine pamoate (in capsule form) is insoluble in water.[15] A 1mg/mL suspension could be made by adding water to a 20mg tablet to make up 20mL. The tablet may be crushed with a spoon or pestle and mortar before mixing with water to speed up this process. The suspension should be shaken vigorously before use. As its stability cannot be assured it should be consumed immediately, and any unused suspension discarded. Other options to make up small doses include compounding smaller dose tablets, including the option of 'tapering strips'.[16]

Deprescribing notes: Initial reductions can be estimated from Tables 2.11 and 2.22, although patient preference should be taken into account. Sometimes an even smaller reduction to start with may be advisable to boost a patient's confidence that they can taper if performed carefully. Each reduction should be made when the withdrawal symptoms from the previous reduction have largely resolved so that subsequent reductions do not lead to cumulative withdrawal symptoms. Withdrawal symptoms should be tolerable and last at most a couple of weeks (see Figure 2.9). Allowing for a sufficient observation period, reductions can therefore be made about every 2 to 4 weeks. If withdrawal symptoms are moderately severe or take longer than a couple of weeks to resolve, dose reductions should be postponed until symptoms resolve and then made more gradual by choosing a slower tapering rate. If severe withdrawal symptoms occur then the patient should return to a higher dose, wait until symptoms resolve and thereafter taper at a slower rate.

Taper schedules for imipramine

A. A faster taper with up to 11 percentage points of SERT occupancy between each step (approximate length: 5–10 months). Patients who have been on the medication for only a few weeks will probably be able to taper more quickly and might do every second or third step of this regimen, and make reductions every few days or so. For people who have only taken an antidepressant for a few weeks, the duration of the taper should not be longer than the period that the patient has been on the drug. For example, if imipramine is taken for 3 weeks the taper should be less than 3 weeks.

B. A moderate taper with up to 5.5 percentage points of SERT occupancy between each step (approximate length: 10–20 months).

C. A slower taper with up to 2.8 percentage points of SERT occupancy between each step (approximate length: 20–40 months).

D. Some patients will be unable to taper at the slowest rates shown here and will need to taper by even smaller decrements, thus lengthening the overall period of tapering. Such a regimen could be constructed by placing intermediate steps in regimen C. For example, 3mg, 2mg, 1mg, 0mg could be modified to be 3mg, 2.5mg, 2mg, 1.5mg, 1mg, 0.5mg, 0mg. Further intermediate steps could also be added. Microtapering (tapering by a small amount each day, rather than by larger reductions every 2–4 weeks) is another possible approach (see benzodiazepines chapter for further details).

Please note that none of these regimens should be seen as prescriptive – that is, it is not suggested that patient must strictly adhere to them. They are given as example regimens and are not 'set and forget' but should be modified in order to ensure that withdrawal symptoms are tolerable throughout a taper – for example intermediate steps halfway between the doses listed could be added to make a more gradual taper.

A. **Faster taper** with up to 11 percentage points of SERT occupancy between each step – with reductions made every 2–4 weeks.*

Step	RO (%)	Dose (mg)	Volume	Step	RO (%)	Dose (mg)	Volume
1	92	200	Use tablets	7	42	12.5	Use ½ tablets**
2	85	100	Use tablets	8	32	7.5	Use ¾ tablets**
3	81	75	Use tablets	9	21	5	Use ½ tablets**
4	74	50	Use tablets	10	11	2.5	Use ¼ tablets**
5	63	30	Use tablets	11	0	0	0
6	53	20	Use tablets				

RO = receptor occupancy
*For longer term users, the time between each decrease may be shortened to 1 week if the patient is able to make the first couple of reductions with no withdrawal symptoms. The interval between reductions should never be less than 1 week because this might increase the risk of relapse, even in the absence of withdrawal effects.[17,18]
**Alternatively, a liquid version of imipramine could be used to make up these doses.

B. **Moderate taper** with up to 5.5 percentage points of SERT occupancy between each step – with reductions made every 2–4 weeks.

Step	RO (%)	Dose (mg)	Volume	Step	RO (%)	Dose (mg)	Volume
1	91.9	200	Use tablets	13	45.9	15	Use ½ tablets*
2	89.5	150	Use tablets	14	41.4	12.5	Use ½ tablets*
3	85	100	Use tablets	15	36.2	10	Use tablets
4	80.9	75	Use tablets		Switch to imipramine **5mg/mL solution**		
5	77.3	60	Use tablets	16	31.2	8	1.6mL
6	73.9	50	Use tablets	17	26.1	6.25	1.25mL
7	69.4	40	Use tablets	18	21.2	4.75	0.95mL
8	66.5	35	Use tablets	19	16.5	3.5	0.7mL
9	62.9	30	Use tablets	20	11.3	2.25	0.45mL
10	58.6	25	Use tablets	21	6.6	1.25	0.25mL
11	53.1	20	Use tablets	22	2.8	0.5	0.1mL
12	49.8	17.5	Use ½ or ¾ tablets*	23	0	0	0
	See further steps in the right-hand column						

RO = receptor occupancy
*Alternatively, a liquid version of imipramine could be used to make up these doses.

C. **Slower taper** with 2.8 percentage points of SERT occupancy between each step – with reductions made every 2–4 weeks.

Step	RO (%)	Dose (mg)	Volume	Step	RO (%)	Dose (mg)	Volume	Step	RO (%)	Dose (mg)	Volume
1	91.9	200	Use tablets	14	61.3	28	5.6mL	28	28.3	7	1.4mL
2	89.5	150	Use tablets	15	58.9	25.25	5.05mL	29	25.9	6.25	1.25mL
3	87.2	120	Use tablets	16	56.5	23	4.6mL	30	23.6	5.5	1.1mL
4	84.8	97.5	Use ½ tablets*	17	54.2	20.9	4.18mL	31	21.2	4.75	0.95mL
5	82.5	82.5	Use ½ tablets*	18	51.8	19	3.8mL	32	18.8	4	0.8mL
6	80.1	70	Use tablets	19	49.5	17.25	3.45mL	33	16.5	3.5	0.7mL
7	77.8	62.5	Use tablets	20	47.1	15.75	3.15mL	34	14.5	3	0.6mL
8	75.4	55	Use tablets	21	44.8	14.25	2.85mL	35	12.4	2.5	0.5mL
9	73	47.5	Use tablets	22	42.4	13	2.6mL	36	10.2	2.0	0.4mL
10	70.7	42.5	Use tablets	23	40.1	11.75	2.35mL	37	7.8	1.5	0.3mL
Switch to imipramine **5mg/mL solution**				24	37.7	10.75	2.15mL	38	5.4	1	0.2mL
11	68.3	38	7.6mL	25	35.3	9.75	1.95mL	Switch to imipramine **0.5mg/mL solution**			
12	66	34.25	6.85mL	26	33	8.75	1.75mL	39	2.8	0.5	1mL
13	63.6	31	6.2mL	27	30.6	7.75	1.55mL	40	0	0	0
	See further steps in the middle column				**See further steps in the right-hand column**						

RO = receptor occupancy
*Alternatively, a liquid version of imipramine could be used to make up these doses.

References

1. SmPC. Imipramine – summary of product characteristics. 2022. https://www.medicines.org.uk/emc/product/5789/smpc#gref (accessed 12 October 2022).
2. Marsh W. Imipramine. In: *xPharm: The Comprehensive Pharmacology Reference*. StatPearls Publishing, 2007: 1–5.
3. Henssler J, Heinz A, Brandt L, Bschor T. Antidepressant withdrawal and rebound phenomena. *Dtsch Arztebl Int* 2019; 116: 355–61.
4. Taylor D, Stewart S, Connolly A. Antidepressant withdrawal symptoms – telephone calls to a national medication helpline. *J Affect Disord* 2006; 95: 129–33.
5. Horowitz MA, Framer A, Hengartner MP, Sørensen A, Taylor D. Estimating risk of antidepressant withdrawal from a review of published data. *CNS Drugs* 2022; published online 14 December. doi:10.1007/s40263-022-00960-y.
6. Gastaldon C, Schoretsanitis G, Arzenton E, et al. Withdrawal syndrome following discontinuation of 28 antidepressants: pharmacovigilance analysis of 31,688 reports from the WHO spontaneous reporting database. *Drug Saf* 2022; 45: 1539–49.
7. Bentley Suzanne MD MPH, Staros EBMD. Imipramine level: reference range, interpretation, collection and panels. 2014. https://emedicine.medscape.com/article/2090130-overview (accessed 12 October 2022).
8. Brøsen K, Gram LF, Klysner R, Bech P. Steady-state levels of imipramine and its metabolites: significance of dose-dependent kinetics. *Eur J Clin Pharmacol* 1986; 30: 43–9.
9. Furukawa TA, Cipriani A, Cowen PJ, Leucht S, Egger M, Salanti G. Optimal dose of selective serotonin reuptake inhibitors, venlafaxine, and mirtazapine in major depression: a systematic review and dose-response meta-analysis. *The Lancet Psychiatry* 2019; 6: 601–9.
10. Horowitz MA, Taylor D. Tapering of SSRI treatment to mitigate withdrawal symptoms. *The Lancet Psychiatry* 2019; 6: 538–46.
11. Holford N. Pharmacodynamic principles and the time course of delayed and cumulative drug effects. *Ther Adv Psychopharmacol* 2018; 26: 56.
12. Essential Pharma. Imipramine hydrochloride 25mg/5ml Oral Solution. https://www.medicines.org.uk/emc/product/13879/smpc (accessed 22 October 2022).
13. Smyth J. The NEWT guidelines for administration of medication to patients with enteral feeding tubes or swallowing difficulties website. The NEWT Guidelines. 2011. https://www.newtguidelines.com/index.html (accessed 23 February 2023).
14. Bostwick JR, Demehri A. Pills to powder: an updated clinician's reference for crushable psychotropics. *Curr Psychiatr* 2017; 16: 46–9.
15. FDA. Imipramine pamoate – highlights of prescribing information. 2014.
16. Groot PC, van Os J. How user knowledge of psychotropic drug withdrawal resulted in the development of person-specific tapering medication. *Ther Adv Psychopharmacol* 2020; 10: 204512532093245.
17. Baldessarini RJ, Tondo L, Ghiani C, Lepri B. Illness risk following rapid versus gradual discontinuation of antidepressants. *Am J Psychiatry* 2010; 167: 934–41.
18. Gøtzsche PC, Demasi M. Interventions to help patients withdraw from depression drugs: A systematic review. *Int J Risk Saf Med.* 2023 September 13. doi: 10.3233/JRS-230011. Epub ahead of print.

Lofepramine

Trade names: Lomont, Gamanil.

Description: Lofepramine is a tricyclic antidepressant that strongly inhibits noradrenaline reuptake by blockade of NET and moderately inhibits SERT.[1] It is a relatively weak antagonist of muscarinic acetylcholine receptors.[2]

Withdrawal effects: In a structured analysis tricyclic antidepressants were placed in a high-risk category for withdrawal effects.[3] Lofepramine was responsible for about the same number of calls regarding issues with withdrawal to a medication helpline (normalised to prescription numbers) as most SSRIs.[4]

Peak plasma: 1 hour.[1]

Half-life: Lofepramine's half-life is up to 5 hours, and the half-life of its active metabolite, desipramine, is 12–24 hours.[5] The manufacturer recommends twice or three times daily dosing.[1] Every-other-day dosing is not recommended for tapering because of the substantial reductions in plasma concentrations this would produce, possibly giving rise to withdrawal effects.

Receptor occupancy: The relationship between dose of lofepramine (and its active metabolite desipramine) and occupancy of its target, NET, is hyperbolic.[6] Antidepressants show a hyperbolic pattern between dose and clinical effects,[7] which may be relevant to withdrawal effects from lofepramine. Dose reductions made by linear amounts (e.g. 140mg, 105mg, 70mg, 35mg, 0mg) will cause increasingly large reductions in effect which may cause increasingly severe withdrawal effects (Figure 2.27a). To produce equal-sized reductions in effect on NET occupancy will require hyperbolically reducing doses (Figure 2.27b),[8] which informs the reductions presented. This hyperbolic pattern of effect also applies to its occupancy of SERT and its other receptor targets as well, because these relationships are dictated by the law of mass action.[9] There may be some differences in the precise dose-related activity between receptor targets but the hyperbolic relationship remains. Consequently, the

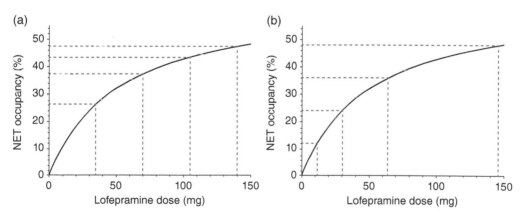

Figure 2.27 (a) Linear reductions of dose cause increasingly large reductions in effect on receptor targets, possibly associated with more withdrawal effects. (b) Even reductions of effect at target receptors requires hyperbolic dose reductions. The final dose before stopping will need to be very small so that this step down is not larger (in terms of effect on receptor occupancy) than previous reductions.

regimens given below (based on NET occupancy) will be broadly suitable for other receptor occupancies, such as for SERT occupancy.

Available formulations: Lofepramine is available as lofepramine hydrochloride in tablet form and an oral suspension.

Tablets

Dosage	UK	Europe	USA	Australia	Canada
70mg	✓	✓	–	–	–

Oral suspension

Dosage	UK	Europe	USA	Australia	Canada
70mg/5mL (14mg/mL)	✓(150mL)	–	–	–	–

Dilution: The NEWT guidelines in the UK recommend against making dilutions of the original suspension because this will de-stabilise the suspension according to correspondence with the manufacturer.[10]

Worked example: To illustrate how the volumes were calculated in the regimens given below we provide a worked example. To make up 5mg of lofepramine the 14mg/mL original solution can be used. The volume of 14mg/mL liquid required to give a dose of 5mg lofepramine is 5/14 = 0.36mL.

Off-label options: Guidelines for people who cannot swallow tablets (e.g. the NEWT guidelines in the UK) recommend that the tablets are not suitable for crushing.[10] Compounding pharmacies may be able to make up smaller doses.

Deprescribing notes: Initial reductions can be estimated from Tables 2.11 and 2.22, although patient preference should be taken into account. Sometimes an even smaller reduction to start with may be advisable to boost a patient's confidence that they can taper if performed carefully. Each reduction should be made when the withdrawal symptoms from the previous reduction have largely resolved so that subsequent reductions do not lead to cumulative withdrawal symptoms. Withdrawal symptoms should be tolerable and last at most a couple of weeks (see Figure 2.9). Allowing for a sufficient observation period, reductions can therefore be made about every 2 to 4 weeks. If withdrawal symptoms are moderately severe or take longer than a couple of weeks to resolve, dose reductions should be postponed until symptoms resolve and then made more gradual by choosing a slower tapering rate. If severe withdrawal symptoms occur then the patient should return to a higher dose, wait until symptoms resolve and thereafter taper at a slower rate.

Taper schedules for lofepramine

A. A faster taper with up to 6.5 percentage points of NET occupancy between each step (approximate length: 5–10 months). Patients who have been on the medication for only a few weeks will probably be able to taper more quickly and might follow every second or third step of this regimen, and make reductions every few days or so. For people who have only taken an antidepressant for a few weeks, the duration of the taper should not be longer than the period that the patient has been on the drug. For example, if lofepramine is taken for 3 weeks the taper should be less than 3 weeks.

B. A moderate taper with up to 3 percentage points of NET occupancy between each step (approximate length: 10–20 months).

C. A slower taper with up to 1.5 percentage points of NET occupancy between each step (approximate length: 20–40 months).

D. Some patients will be unable to taper at the slowest rates shown here and will need to taper by even smaller decrements, thus lengthening the overall period of tapering. Such a regimen could be constructed by placing intermediate steps in regimen C. For example, 3mg, 2mg, 1mg, 0mg could be modified to be 3mg, 2.5mg, 2mg, 1.5mg, 1mg, 0.5mg, 0mg. Further intermediate steps could also be added. Microtapering (tapering by a small amount each day, rather than by larger reductions every 2–4 weeks) is another possible approach (see benzodiazepines chapter for further details).

Please note that none of these regimens should be seen as prescriptive – that is, it is not suggested that patient must strictly adhere to them. They are given as example regimens and are not 'set and forget' but should be modified in order to ensure that withdrawal symptoms are tolerable throughout a taper – for example intermediate steps halfway between the doses listed could be added to make a more gradual taper.

A. **Faster taper** with up to 6.5 percentage points of NET occupancy between each step – with reductions made every 2–4 weeks.*

Step	RO (%)	Dose (mg)	Volume	Step	RO (%)	Dose (mg)	Volume
1	52.2	210	Use tablets	6	31.1	52.5	3.75mL
2	47.5	140	Use tablets	7	24.9	35	2.5mL**
3	43.5	105	Use ½ tablet	8	18.7	17.5	1.25mL
Switch to lofepramine **14mg/mL suspension**				9	12.5	12.3	0.88mL
4	40.8	87.5	6.25mL**	10	6.2	5.5	0.40mL
5	37.4	70	5mL**	11	0	0	0
See further steps in the right-hand column							

RO = receptor occupancy

*For longer term users, the time between each decrease may be shortened to 1 week if the patient is able to make the first couple of reductions with no withdrawal symptoms. The interval between reductions should never be less than 1 week because this might increase the risk of relapse, even in the absence of withdrawal effects.[11,12]

**Alternatively, could be made up by tablets or half tablets.

B. **Moderate taper** with up to 3 percentage points of NET occupancy between each step – with reductions made every 2–4 weeks.

Step	RO (%)	Dose (mg)	Volume	Step	RO (%)	Dose (mg)	Volume
1	52.2	210	Use tablets	11	26.3	35.2	2.5mL*
2	50.2	175	Use ½ tablets	12	23.3	29.1	2.1mL
3	47.5	140	Use tablets	13	20.4	23.8	1.7mL
Switch to lofepramine **14mg/mL suspension**				14	17.5	19.1	1.36mL
4	45.7	122.5	8.75mL	15	14.6	15	1.07mL
5	43.5	105	7.5mL*	16	11.7	11.4	0.8mL
6	40.8	87.5	6.25mL*	17	8.8	8.1	0.6mL
7	37.9	72.6	5.2mL	18	5.8	5.1	0.36mL
8	35	60.5	4.3mL	19	2.9	2.4	0.17mL
9	32.1	50.6	3.6mL	20	0	0	0
10	29.2	42.2	3mL				
See further steps in the right-hand column							

RO = receptor occupancy
*Alternatively, could be made up with halved or quartered tablets.

C. **Slower taper** with up to 1.5 percentage points of NET occupancy between each step – with reductions made every 2–4 weeks.

Step	RO (%)	Dose (mg)	Volume	Step	RO (%)	Dose (mg)	Volume
1	52.2	210	Use tablets	21	25.8	34.1	2.44mL
Switch to lofepramine **14mg/mL suspension**				22	24.4	31.3	2.24mL
2	51.3	192.5	13.8mL	23	23.1	28.6	2.04mL
3	50.2	175	12.5mL*	24	21.7	26	1.86mL
4	49	157.5	11.3mL	25	20.4	23.7	1.69mL
5	47.5	140	10mL*	26	19	21.5	1.54mL
6	46.1	126	9mL	27	17.6	19.4	1.39mL
7	44.8	114	8.14mL	28	16.3	17.4	1.24mL
8	43.4	104	7.43mL	29	14.9	15.5	1.11mL
9	42.1	94.9	6.78mL	30	13.6	13.7	0.98mL
10	40.7	86.7	6.19mL	31	12.2	12	0.86mL
11	39.3	79.4	5.67mL	32	10.9	10.4	0.74mL
12	38	72.9	5.21mL	33	9.5	8.9	0.64mL
13	36.6	66.9	4.78mL	34	8.14	7.4	0.53mL
14	35.3	61.5	4.39mL	35	6.78	6.0	0.43mL
15	33.9	56.6	4.04mL	36	5.43	4.7	0.34mL
16	32.6	52.1	3.72mL	37	4.07	3.5	0.25mL
17	31.2	47.9	3.42mL	38	2.71	2.3	0.16mL
18	29.9	44.1	3.15mL	39	1.36	1.1	0.08mL
19	28.5	40.5	2.89mL	40	0	0	0
20	27.1	37.2	2.66mL				
See further steps in the right-hand column							

RO = receptor occupancy
*Alternatively, these doses could be made up with tablets or half tablets.

References

1. Zentiva. Lofepramine – summary of product characteristics. 2020. https://www.medicines.org.uk/emc/product/13706/smpc (accessed 29 July 23).
2. PDSP Database – UNC. https://pdsp.unc.edu/databases/pdsp.php?receptorDD=&receptor=&speciesDD=&species=&sourcesDD=&source=&hotLigandDD=&hotLigand=&testLigandDD=&testFreeRadio=testFreeRadio&testLigand=Lofepramine&referenceDD=&reference=&Ki Greater=&KiLess=&kiAllRadio=all&doQuery=Submit+Query (accessed 23 October 2022).
3. Henssler J, Heinz A, Brandt L, Bschor T. Antidepressant withdrawal and rebound phenomena. *Dtsch Arztebl Int* 2019; 116: 355–61.
4. Taylor D, Stewart S, Connolly A. Antidepressant withdrawal symptoms – telephone calls to a national medication helpline. *J Affect Disord* 2006; 95: 129–33.
5. Lancaster SG, Gonzalez JP. Lofepramine. *Drugs* 1989; 37: 123–40.
6. Plym Forshell G, Siwers B, Tuck JR. Pharmacokinetics of lofepramine in man: relationship to inhibition of noradrenaline uptake. *Eur J Clin Pharmacol* 1976; 9: 291–8.
7. Furukawa TA, Cipriani A, Cowen PJ, Leucht S, Egger M, Salanti G. Optimal dose of selective serotonin reuptake inhibitors, venlafaxine, and mirtazapine in major depression: a systematic review and dose-response meta-analysis. *The Lancet Psychiatry* 2019; 6: 601–9.
8. Horowitz MA, Taylor D. Tapering of SSRI treatment to mitigate withdrawal symptoms. *The Lancet Psychiatry* 2019; 6: 538–46.
9. Holford N. Pharmacodynamic principles and the time course of delayed and cumulative drug effects. *Transl Clin* 2018; 26: 56.
10. Smyth J. The NEWT guidelines for administration of medication to patients with enteral feeding tubes or swallowing difficulties. 2011. https://www.newtguidelines.com/index.html (accessed 23 February 2023).
11. Baldessarini RJ, Tondo L, Ghiani C, Lepri B. Illness risk following rapid versus gradual discontinuation of antidepressants. *Am J Psychiatry* 2010; 167: 934–41.
12. Gøtzsche PC, Demasi M. Interventions to help patients withdraw from depression drugs: A systematic review. *Int J Risk Saf Med.* 2023 September 13. doi: 10.3233/JRS-230011. Epub ahead of print.

CHAPTER 2

Mirtazapine

Trade names: Remeron, Avanza, Zispin Soltab.

Description: Mirtazapine is a centrally active presynaptic alpha-2 adrenoreceptor antagonist and H_1 histaminergic inverse agonist.[1] It is also an antagonist to 5-HT_1, 5-HT_2 and 5-HT_3 serotonergic receptors.[1]

Withdrawal effects: Mirtazapine led to more calls to a helpline for withdrawal effects (normalised to national prescription rates) than any SSRI except paroxetine and fluvoxamine.[2] According to the WHO spontaneous adverse drug reaction database mirtazapine had a similar rate of reports for withdrawal reactions in neonates as other antidepressants, including paroxetine, venlafaxine and sertraline.[3] It is reported by patients to frequently cause withdrawal effects[4] but it has not been investigated in controlled trials.[5]

Peak plasma: approximately 2 hours.[1]

Half-life: Ranges from 20 to 40 hours.[6] Every-other-day dosing is not recommended for tapering because the large reductions in plasma levels can give rise to significant withdrawal symptoms.[7]

Receptor occupancy: The relationship between dose of mirtazapine and the occupancy of its major target α-2 adrenoreceptors is hyperbolic.[8] Mirtazapine and other antidepressants demonstrate a hyperbolic relationship between dose and clinical effects,[9] which may be relevant to withdrawal effects from mirtazapine. Dose reductions made by linear amounts (e.g. 15mg, 11.25mg, 7.5mg, 3.75mg, 0mg) will cause increasingly large reductions in effect which may cause increasingly severe withdrawal effects (Figure 2.28a). To produce equal-sized reductions in effect on receptor occupancy will require hyperbolically reducing doses (Figure 2.28b),[10] which informs the reductions presented. This hyperbolic pattern of effect also applies to its occupancy of its other receptor targets as well, because these relationships are dictated by the law of mass action.[11] There may be some differences in the precise dose-related activity between receptor targets but the hyperbolic relationship remains. Consequently, the regimens given below (based on α-2 adrenoreceptor occupancy) will be broadly suitable for other receptor occupancies.

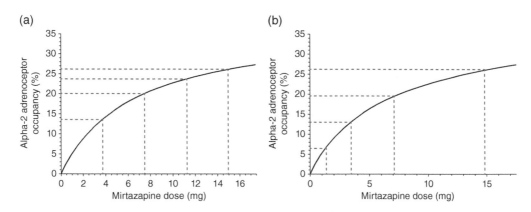

Figure 2.28 (a) Linear reductions of dose cause increasingly large reductions in effect on receptor targets, possibly associated with more withdrawal effects. (b) Even reductions of effect at target receptors requires hyperbolic dose reductions. The final dose before stopping will need to be very small so that this step down is not larger (in terms of effect on receptor occupancy) than previous reductions.

Available formulations: Mirtazapine is available as tablets, orodispersible tablets and liquid.

Tablets and orodispersible tablets

Dosage	UK	Europe	USA	Australia	Canada
7.5mg	–	–	✓*	–	–
15mg	✓	✓	✓	✓	✓
30mg	✓	✓	✓	✓	✓
45mg	✓	✓	✓	✓	✓

*Only available as a film-coated tablets. All other formulations are available as both film-coated tablets and orodispersible tablets.

Liquid*

Dosage	UK	Europe	USA	Australia
15mg/mL	✓(66mL)	✓(66mL)	–	–

*Do not store above 25°C.[12]

Dilutions: To make up smaller doses a dilution of the manufacturer's solution will be required. The manufacturer instructs that the oral solution can be mixed with water.[12]

Dilutions	Solution/ suspension required	How to prepare solution
Doses ≥ 0.4mg	2mg/mL	Mix 1mL of original solution with 6.5mL of water
Doses < 0.4mg	0.5mg/mL	Mix 1mL of original oral solution with 29mL of water

Worked example: To illustrate how the volumes were calculated in the regimens given below we provide a worked example. To make up 1mg of mirtazapine a 2mg/mL dilution can be used, made up as outlined above. The volume of 2mg/mL liquid required to give a dose of 1mg mirtazapine is 1/2 = 0.5mL.

Off-label options: Guidelines for people who cannot swallow tablets (e.g. the NEWT guidelines in the UK,[13] based on local hospital policies, and information direct from the manufacturer and similar US guidance[14]) suggest that mirtazapine tablets or orodispersible tablets can be dispersed in water for administration.[13] This is an off-label use.[13] Water could be added to a 15mg tablet to make up a 30mL suspension (concentration 0.5mg/mL). Dispersal and suspension of the tablet may take some time. The tablet may be crushed with a spoon or pestle and mortar before mixing with water to speed up this process. The suspension should be shaken vigorously before administration. The suspension will have a bitter taste and a local anaesthetic effect on the mouth.[13] As its stability cannot be assured it should be consumed immediately, and any unused suspension discarded. Other options to make up small doses include compounding smaller dose tablets, including 'tapering strips'.[15]

Deprescribing notes: Initial reductions can be estimated from Tables 2.11 and 2.22, although patient preference should be taken into account. Sometimes an even smaller reduction to start with may be advisable to boost a patient's confidence that they can taper if performed carefully. Each reduction should be made when the withdrawal symptoms from the previous reduction have largely resolved so that subsequent reductions do not lead to cumulative withdrawal symptoms. Withdrawal symptoms should be tolerable and last at most a couple of weeks (see Figure 2.9). Allowing for a sufficient observation period, reductions can therefore be made about every 2 to 4 weeks. If withdrawal symptoms are moderately severe or take longer than a couple of weeks to resolve, dose reductions should be postponed until symptoms resolve and then made more gradual by choosing a slower tapering rate. If severe withdrawal symptoms occur then the patient should return to a higher dose, wait until symptoms resolve and thereafter taper at a slower rate.

Suggested taper schedules for mirtazapine

A. A faster taper with up to 4 percentage points of α-2 occupancy between each step with reductions made every 2–4 weeks (approximate length: 5–10 months). Patients who have been on the medication for only a few weeks will probably be able to taper more quickly and might follow every second or third step of this regimen and make reductions every few days or so. Normally the duration of the taper should not be longer than the period that the patient has been on the drug for people who have only taken it for a few weeks. For example, if mirtazapine is taken for 3 weeks the taper should be less than 3 weeks.

B. A moderate taper with up to 2 percentage points of α-2 occupancy between each step with reductions made every 2–4 weeks (approximate length: 10–20 months).

C. A slower taper with up to 1 percentage points of α-2 occupancy between each step with reductions made every 2–4 weeks (approximate length: 20–40 months).

D. Some patients will be unable to taper at the slowest rates shown here and will need to taper by even smaller decrements, thus lengthening the overall period of tapering. Such a regimen could be constructed by placing intermediate steps in regimen C. For example, 3mg, 2mg, 1mg, 0mg could be modified to be 3mg, 2.5mg, 2mg, 1.5mg, 1mg, 0.5mg, 0mg. Further intermediate steps could also be added. Microtapering (tapering by a small amount each day, rather than by larger reductions every 2–4 weeks) is another possible approach (see benzodiazepines chapter for further details).

Please note that none of these regimens should be seen as prescriptive – that is, it is not suggested that patient must strictly adhere to them. They are given as example regimens and are not 'set and forget' but should be modified in order to ensure that withdrawal symptoms are tolerable throughout a taper – for example intermediate steps halfway between the doses listed could be added to make a more gradual taper.

A. **Faster taper** with up to 4 percentage points of α-2 occupancy between each step – with reductions made every 2–4 weeks.*

Step	RO (%)	Dose (mg)	Volume	Step	RO (%)	Dose (mg)	Volume
1	32.8	45	Use tablets	Switch to mirtazapine **2mg/mL solution****			
2	30.8	30	Use tablets	7	16	5	2.5mL
3	29.1	22.5	Use ½ tablets	8	12	3.1	1.55mL
4	26.1	15	Use tablets	9	8	1.8	0.9mL
5	23.7	11.25	Use ¾ tablets	10	4	0.8	0.4mL
6	20	7.5	Use tablets	11	0	0	0
See further steps in the right-hand column							

RO = receptor occupancy
*For longer term users, the time between each decrease may be shortened to 1 week if the patient is able to make the first couple of reductions with no withdrawal symptoms. The interval between reductions should never be less than 1 week because this might increase the risk of relapse, even in the absence of withdrawal effects.[16,17]
**Where a liquid preparation is not available a suspension can be made up as outlined above.

B. **Moderate taper** with up to 2 percentage points of α-2 occupancy between each step – with reductions made every 2–4 weeks.

Step	RO (%)	Dose (mg)	Volume	Step	RO (%)	Dose (mg)	Volume
1	32.8	45	Use tablets	11	15.8	4.8	2.4mL
2	30.8	30	Use tablets	12	14.2	4.0	2.0mL
3	29.1	22.5	Use ½ tablets	13	12.2	3.2	1.6mL
4	27.8	18.75	Use ¼ tablet	14	10.4	2.6	1.3mL
5	26.1	15	Use tablets	15	8.7	2	1mL
6	24.4	11.25	Use ¾ tablets	16	6.96	1.5	0.75mL
Switch to mirtazapine **2mg/mL solution***				17	5.22	1.1	0.55mL
7	22.5	9.8	4.9mL	18	3.48	0.7	0.35mL
8	21.1	8.4	4.2mL	Switch to mirtazapine **0.5mg/mL dilution***			
9	19.6	7.2	3.6mL	19	1.74	0.3	0.6mL
10	17.6	6.0	3.0mL	20	0	0	0
See further steps in the right-hand column							

RO = receptor occupancy
*Where a liquid preparation is not available a suspension can be made up as outlined above.

CHAPTER 2

CHAPTER 2

C. **Slower taper** with up to 1 percentage points of α-2 occupancy between each step – with reductions made every 2–4 weeks.

Step	RO (%)	Dose (mg)	Volume	Step	RO (%)	Dose (mg)	Volume	Step	RO (%)	Dose (mg)	Volume
1	32.8	45	Use tablets	14	22.3	9.6	4.8mL	28	10.3	2.5	1.25mL
2	32	37.5	Use ½ tablets	15	21.4	8.7	4.35mL	29	9.42	2.2	1.1mL
3	31.4	33.75	Use ¼ tablets	16	20.5	8	4mL	Switch to mirtazapine **0.5mg/mL dilution***		
4	30.8	30	Use tablets	17	19.7	7.3	3.65mL	30	8.56	1.95	3.9mL
Switch to mirtazapine **2mg/mL solution***				18	18.8	6.6	3.3mL	31	7.7	1.7	3.4mL
5	30.2	27	13.5mL	19	18	6	3mL	32	6.85	1.47	2.94mL
6	29.5	24	12mL	20	17.1	5.5	2.75mL	33	5.99	1.25	2.5mL
7	28.6	21	10.5mL	21	16.3	5	2.5mL	34	5.14	1.04	2.08mL
8	27.6	18.2	9.1mL	22	15.4	4.6	2.3mL	35	4.28	0.85	1.7mL
9	26.6	16.0	8.0mL	23	14.6	4.2	2.1mL	36	3.42	0.66	1.32mL
10	25.7	14.2	7.1mL	24	13.7	3.8	1.9mL	37	2.57	0.48	0.96mL
11	24.8	12.8	6.4mL	25	12.8	3.4	1.7mL	38	1.71	0.31	0.62mL
12	24	11.6	5.8mL	26	12	3.1	1.55mL	39	0.9	0.15	0.3mL
13	23.1	10.5	5.25mL	27	11.1	2.8	1.4mL	40	0	0	0
See further steps in the middle column				**See further steps in the right-hand column**							

RO = receptor occupancy
*Where a liquid preparation is not available a suspension can be made up as outlined above.

References

1. Aurobindo Pharma – Milpharm. Mirtazapine – summary of product characteristics. 2021. https://www.medicines.org.uk/emc/product/531/smpc#gref (accessed 26 September 2022).
2. Taylor D, Stewart S, Connolly A. Antidepressant withdrawal symptoms – telephone calls to a national medication helpline. *J Affect Disord* 2006; 95: 129–33.
3. Gastaldon C, Arzenton E, Raschi E, et al. G. Neonatal withdrawal syndrome following in utero exposure to antidepressants: a disproportionality analysis of VigiBase, the WHO spontaneous reporting database. *Psychol Med* 2022: 1–9. doi:10.1017/S0033291722002859
4. White E, Read J, Julo S. The role of Facebook groups in the management and raising of awareness of antidepressant withdrawal: Is social media filling the void left by health services? *Ther Adv Psychopharmacol* 2021; 11: 2045125320981174.
5. Horowitz MA, Framer A, Hengartner MP, Sørensen A, Taylor D. Estimating risk of antidepressant withdrawal from a review of published data. *CNS Drugs* 2022; published online 14 December. doi:10.1007/s40263-022-00960-y.
6. FDA. Mirtazapine – highlights of prescribing information. 2020.
7. Framer A. What I have learnt from helping thousands of people taper off psychotropic medications. *Ther Adv Psychopharmacol* 2021; 11: 204512532199127.
8. Smith DF, Stork BS, Wegener G, et al. Receptor occupancy of mirtazapine determined by PET in healthy volunteers. *Psychopharmacology* 2007; 195: 131–8.
9. Furukawa TA, Cipriani A, Cowen PJ, Leucht S, Egger M, Salanti G. Optimal dose of selective serotonin reuptake inhibitors, venlafaxine, and mirtazapine in major depression: a systematic review and dose-response meta-analysis. *The Lancet Psychiatry* 2019; 6: 601–9.
10. Horowitz MA, Taylor D. Tapering of SSRI treatment to mitigate withdrawal symptoms. *The Lancet Psychiatry* 2019; 6: 538–46.
11. Holford N. Pharmacodynamic principles and the time course of delayed and cumulative drug effects. *Transl Clin* 2018; 26: 56.
12. Rosemont Pharmaceuticals. Mirtazapine 15 mg/ml oral solution. https://www.medicines.org.uk/emc/product/2023/smpc (accessed 12 October 2022).
13. Smyth J. The NEWT guidelines for administration of medication to patients with enteral feeding tubes or swallowing difficulties website. The NEWT Guidelines. 2011. https://www.newtguidelines.com/index.html (accessed 23 February 2023).
14. Bostwick JR, Demehri A. Pills to powder: an updated clinician's reference for crushable psychotropics. *Curr Psychiatr* 2017; 16: 46–9.
15. Groot PC, van Os J. How user knowledge of psychotropic drug withdrawal resulted in the development of person-specific tapering medication. *Ther Adv Psychopharmacol* 2020; 10: 204512532093245.
16. Baldessarini RJ, Tondo L, Ghiani C, Lepri B. Illness risk following rapid versus gradual discontinuation of antidepressants. *Am J Psychiatry* 2010; 167: 934–41.
17. Gøtzsche PC, Demasi M. Interventions to help patients withdraw from depression drugs: A systematic review. *Int J Risk Saf Med.* 2023 September 13. doi: 10.3233/JRS-230011. Epub ahead of print.

Moclobemide

Trade names: Aurorix, Manerix.

Description: Moclobemide is a reversible inhibitor of monoamine oxidase (MAO), primarily type A (RIMA). This action reduces the rate of neuronal breakdown of noradrenaline, dopamine and serotonin.[1]

Withdrawal effects: Moclobemide withdrawal has not been evaluated in a randomised controlled trial, but an analysis of calls regarding withdrawal problems to a helpline (normalised to number of prescriptions) places it in a high-risk category.[2,3]

Peak plasma: 1 hour.[1]

Half-life 1–4 hours; this increases with higher doses due to saturation of the metabolic pathways.[1] Despite its short plasma half-life the pharmacodynamic action of a single dose persists for approximately 16 hours.[4] The manufacturer recommends dosing two or three times a day, after meals.[1] Once a day or every-other-day dosing is not recommended for tapering because the large reductions in plasma levels could give rise to withdrawal effects.

Receptor occupancy: The relationship between dose of moclobemide and the occupancy of monoamine oxidase (MAO-A) is hyperbolic.[5] This applies to its occupancy of other receptors because these relationships are dictated by the law of mass action.[6] Antidepressants show a hyperbolic pattern between dose and clinical effects,[7] which may be relevant to withdrawal effects from moclobemide. Dose reductions made by linear amounts (e.g. 300 mg, 225mg, 150mg, 75mg, 0mg) will cause increasingly large reductions in effect which may cause increasingly severe withdrawal effects (Figure 2.29a). To produce equal-sized reductions in receptor occupancy will require hyperbolically reducing doses (Figure 2.29b),[8] which informs the reductions presented.

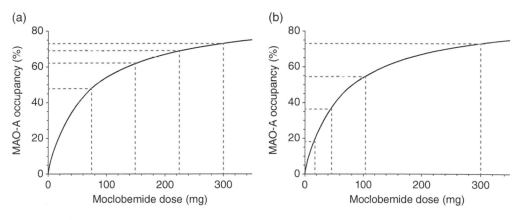

Figure 2.29 (a) Linear reductions of dose cause increasingly large reductions in effect on receptor targets, possibly associated with more withdrawal effects. (b) Even reductions of effect at target receptors requires hyperbolic dose reductions. The final dose before stopping will need to be very small so that this step down is not larger (in terms of effect on receptor occupancy) than previous reductions.

CHAPTER 2

Available formulations: Moclobemide is available as tablets.

Tablets

Dosage	UK	Europe	USA	Australia	Canada
100mg	–	–	–	–	✓
150mg	✓	✓	–	✓	✓
300mg	✓	✓	–	✓	✓

Off-label options Guidelines for people who cannot swallow tablets (e.g. the NEWT guidelines in the UK) suggest that moclobemide tablets can be crushed and dispersed in water for administration as an off-label use.[9] A 1mg/mL suspension could be made by adding water to a 150mg tablet to make up 150mL. The process of dispersion can be made easier by crushing the tablet with a spoon or a pestle and mortar. The suspension should be shaken vigorously before use. When evenly dispersed, 1mL of this suspension will contain 1mg of the drug. As the stability of the suspension cannot be assured it should be consumed immediately, and any unused suspension discarded. Other options to make up smaller doses include compounding liquids or smaller formulations of tablets, such as 'tapering strips'.[10]

Worked example: To illustrate how the volumes were calculated in the regimens given below we provide a worked example. To make up 2mg of moclobemide a 1mg/mL suspension can be used, made up as outlined above. The volume of 1mg/mL liquid required to give a dose of 2mg of moclobemide is 2/1 = 2mL.

Deprescribing notes: Initial reductions can be estimated from Tables 2.11 and 2.22, although patient preference should be taken into account. Sometimes an even smaller reduction to start with may be advisable to boost a patient's confidence that they can taper if performed carefully. Each reduction should be made when the withdrawal symptoms from the previous reduction have largely resolved so that subsequent reductions do not lead to cumulative withdrawal symptoms. Withdrawal symptoms should be tolerable and last at most a couple of weeks (see Figure 2.9). Allowing for a sufficient observation period, reductions can therefore be made about every 2 to 4 weeks. If withdrawal symptoms are moderately severe or take longer than a couple of weeks to resolve, dose reductions should be postponed until symptoms resolve and then made more gradual by choosing a slower tapering rate. If severe withdrawal symptoms occur then the patient should return to a higher dose, wait until symptoms resolve and thereafter taper at a slower rate.

Suggested taper schedules for moclobemide

A. A faster taper with up to 8 percentage points of MAO-A occupancy between each step (approximate length: 5–10 months). Patients who have been on the medication for only a few weeks will probably be able to taper more quickly and might follow every second or third step of this regimen, and make reductions every few days or so. For people who have only taken an antidepressant for a few weeks, the duration of the taper should not be longer than the period that the patient has been on the drug. For example, if moclobemide is taken for 3 weeks the taper should be less than 3 weeks.

B. A moderate taper with up to 4.6 percentage points of MAO-A occupancy between each step (approximate length: 10–20 months).
C. A slower taper with up to 2.2 percentage points of MAO-A occupancy between each step (approximate length: 20–40 months).
D. Some patients will be unable to taper at the slowest rates shown here and will need to taper by even smaller decrements, thus lengthening the overall period of tapering. Such a regimen could be constructed by placing intermediate steps in regimen C. For example, 3mg, 2mg, 1mg, 0mg could be modified to be 3mg, 2.5mg, 2mg, 1.5mg, 1mg, 0.5mg, 0mg. Further intermediate steps could also be added. Microtapering (tapering by a small amount each day, rather than by larger reductions every 2–4 weeks) is another possible approach (see benzodiazepines chapter for further details).

Please note that none of these regimens should be seen as prescriptive – that is, it is not suggested that patient must strictly adhere to them. They are given as example regimens and are not 'set and forget' but should be modified in order to ensure that withdrawal symptoms are tolerable throughout a taper – for example intermediate steps halfway between the doses listed could be added to make a more gradual taper.

A. **Faster taper** with up to 8 percentage points of MAO-A occupancy between each step – with reductions made every 2– 4 weeks.*

Step	RO (%)	Dose (mg)	Volume	Step	RO (%)	Dose (mg)	Volume
1	80	600	Use tablets	6	39	50	25mL twice daily
2	73	300	Use tablets	7	31	35	17.5mL twice daily
3	62	150	Use tablets	8	23	23	11.5mL twice daily
Switch to moclobemide **1mg/mL suspension**				9	16	14	7mL twice daily
4	54	100	50mL twice daily	10	7.8	6	3mL twice daily
5	47	70	35mL twice daily	11	0	0	0
See further steps in the right-hand column							

RO = receptor occupancy
*For longer term users, the time between each decrease may be shortened to 1 week if the patient is able to make the first couple of reductions with no withdrawal symptoms. The interval between reductions should never be less than 1 week because this might increase the risk of relapse, even in the absence of withdrawal effects.[11,12]

CHAPTER 2

B. **Moderate taper** with up to 4.6 percentage points of MAO-A occupancy between each step – with reductions made every 2–4 weeks.

Step	RO (%)	Dose (mg)	Volume	Step	RO (%)	Dose (mg)	Volume
1	80.1	600	Use tablets	11	44.3	65	32.5mL twice daily
2	77.6	450	Use tablets	12	39.9	55	27.5mL twice daily
Switch to moclobemide **1mg/mL suspension**				13	35.4	45	22.5mL twice daily
3	75.7	370	185mL twice daily	14	31	35	17.5mL twice daily
4	73	300	150mL twice daily*	15	26.6	28	14mL twice daily
5	68.9	230	115mL twice daily*	16	22.1	21	10.5mL twice daily
6	64.8	180	90mL twice daily	17	17.7	16	8mL twice daily
7	62	150	75mL twice daily*	18	13.3	11	5.5mL twice daily
8	57.6	120	60mL twice daily	19	8.7	7	3.5mL twice daily
9	53.1	95	47.5mL twice daily	20	4.4	3.5	1.75mL twice daily
10	48.7	80	40mL twice daily	21	0	0	0
See further steps in the right-hand column							

RO = receptor occupancy
*Alternatively, could be made up by using tablets or ½ tablets

C. **Slower taper** with up to 2.2 percentage points of MAO-A occupancy between each step – with reductions made every 2–4 weeks.

Step	RO (%)	Dose (mg)	Volume	Step	RO (%)	Dose (mg)	Volume	Step	RO (%)	Dose (mg)	Volume
1	80.1	600	Use tablets	14	57.3	118	59mL BD	28	26.6	28	14mL BD
Switch to moclobemide **1mg/mL suspension**				15	55.3	107	53.5 BD	29	24.4	24	12mL BD
2	78.1	475	237.5mL BD	16	53.1	97	48.5mL BD	30	22.1	21	10.5mL BD
3	76.4	400	200mL BD	17	50.9	87	43.5mL BD	31	19.9	18	9mL BD
4	74.9	350	175mL BD	18	48.7	79	39.5mL BD	32	17.7	15.5	7.75mL BD
5	73	300	150mL BD*	19	46.5	71	35.5mL BD	33	15.5	13	6.5mL BD
6	71.8	275	137.5mL BD	20	44.3	64	32mL BD	34	13.3	11	5.5mL BD
7	70.5	250	125mL BD	21	42.1	58	29mL BD	35	11.1	9	4.5mL BD
8	68.9	225	112.5mL BD*	22	39.9	53	26.5mL BD	36	8.9	7.2	3.6mL BD
9	67.1	200	100mL BD	23	37.6	48	24mL BD	37	6.6	5.4	2.7mL BD
10	64.8	175	87.5mL BD	24	35.4	43	21.5mL BD	38	4.4	3.6	1.8mL BD
11	63.5	160	80mL BD	25	33.2	39	19.5mL BD	39	2.2	1.8	0.9mL BD
12	61.4	145	72.5mL BD	26	31	35	17.5mL BD	40	0	0	0
13	59.3	130	65mL BD	27	28.8	31	15.5mL BD				
See further steps in the middle column				**See further steps in the right-hand column**							

RO = receptor occupancy
*Alternatively, could be made up by using tablets or ½ tablets

References

1. Sandoz. Moclobemide – summary of product characteristics. 2020. https://www.medicines.org.uk/emc/product/7296/smpc#PHARMACODYNAMIC_PROPS (accessed 12 October 2022).
2. Taylor D, Stewart S, Connolly A. Antidepressant withdrawal symptoms – telephone calls to a national medication helpline. *J Affect Disord* 2006; 95: 129–33.
3. Horowitz MA, Framer A, Hengartner MP, Sørensen A, Taylor D. Estimating risk of antidepressant withdrawal from a review of published data. *CNS Drugs* 2022; published online 14 December. doi:10.1007/s40263-022-00960-y.
4. Buschmann H, Holenz J, Párraga A, Torrens A, Vela JM, Díaz JL. *Antidepressants, Antipsychotics, Anxiolytics From Chemistry and Pharmacology to Clinical Application*. Wiley, 2007 https://books.google.co.uk/books?id=APcYEAAAQBAJ (accessed 18 February 2023)
5. Chiuccariello L, Cooke RG, Miler L, et al. Monoamine oxidase-A occupancy by moclobemide and phenelzine: implications for the development of monoamine oxidase inhibitors. *Int J Neuropsychopharmacol* 2015; 19. doi:10.1093/ijnp/pyv078.
6. Holford N. Pharmacodynamic principles and the time course of delayed and cumulative drug effects. *Transl Clin* 2018; 26: 56.
7. Furukawa TA, Cipriani A, Cowen PJ, Leucht S, Egger M, Salanti G. Optimal dose of selective serotonin reuptake inhibitors, venlafaxine, and mirtazapine in major depression: a systematic review and dose-response meta-analysis. *The Lancet Psychiatry* 2019; 6: 601–9.
8. Horowitz MA, Taylor D. Tapering of SSRI treatment to mitigate withdrawal symptoms. *The Lancet Psychiatry* 2019; 6: 538–46.
9. Smyth J. The NEWT guidelines for administration of medication to patients with enteral feeding tubes or swallowing difficulties. 2011. https://www.newtguidelines.com/index.html (accessed 18 February 2023)
10. Groot PC, van Os J. How user knowledge of psychotropic drug withdrawal resulted in the development of person-specific tapering medication. *Ther Adv Psychopharmacol* 2020; 10: 204512532093245.
11. Baldessarini RJ, Tondo L, Ghiani C, Lepri B. Illness risk following rapid versus gradual discontinuation of antidepressants. *Am J Psychiatry* 2010; 167: 934–41.
12. Gøtzsche PC, Demasi M. Interventions to help patients withdraw from depression drugs: A systematic review. *Int J Risk Saf Med.* 2023 September 13. doi: 10.3233/JRS-230011. Epub ahead of print.

Nortriptyline

Trade names: Pamelor, Allegron, Avently.

Description: Nortriptyline is a tricyclic antidepressant and the principal active metabolite of amitriptyline.[1] Nortriptyline strongly inhibits NET and moderately inhibits SERT.[2] It also inhibits the activity of histamine, 5-hydroxytryptamine and acetylcholine.[2]

Withdrawal effects: In a structured analysis tricyclic antidepressants were placed in a high risk category for withdrawal effects.[3] Nortriptyline was responsible for about the same number of calls regarding issues with withdrawal to a medication helpline (normalised to prescription numbers) as most SSRIs.[4]

Peak plasma: 7 to 8.5 hours.[2]

Half-life: Approximately 26 hours. According to the manufacturer nortriptyline should be taken 3 to 4 times per day, however they do mention the possibility of once per day dosing.[5] Every-other-day dosing is not recommended for tapering because of large reductions in plasma levels caused by such a regimen, which might lead to withdrawal effects.

Receptor occupancy: The relationship between dose of nortriptyline and the occupancy of one of its principal targets the norepinephrine transporter (NET) is hyperbolic.[6] Antidepressants also show a hyperbolic pattern between dose and clinical effects,[7] which may be relevant to withdrawal effects from nortriptyline. Dose reductions made by linear amounts (e.g. 100mg, 75mg, 50mg, 25mg, 0mg) will cause increasingly large reductions in effect which may cause increasingly severe withdrawal effects (Figure 2.30a). To produce equal-sized reductions in effect on NET occupancy will require hyperbolically reducing doses (Figure 2.30b),[8] which informs the reductions presented. This hyperbolic pattern of effect also applies to its occupancy of its other receptor targets as well, because these relationships are dictated by the law of mass action.[9] There may be some differences in the precise dose-related activity between receptor targets but the hyperbolic relationship remains. Consequently, the regimens given below (based on NET occupancy) will be broadly suitable for other receptor occupancies.

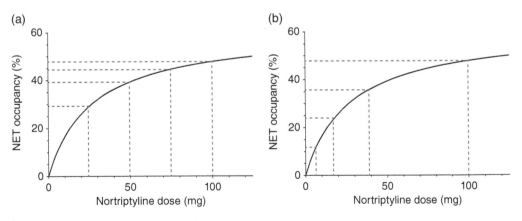

Figure 2.30 (a) Linear reductions of dose cause increasingly large reductions in effect on receptor targets, possibly associated with more withdrawal effects. (b) Even reductions of effect at target receptors requires hyperbolic dose reductions. The final dose before stopping will need to be very small so that this step down is not larger (in terms of effect on receptor occupancy) than previous reductions.

Available formulations: Nortriptyline is available as tablets, capsules and in liquid form as nortriptyline hydrochloride.

Tablets

Dosage	UK	Europe	USA	Australia	Canada
10mg	✓	✓	–	✓	–
25mg	✓	✓	–	✓	–
50mg	✓	✓	–	–	–

Capsules

Dosage	UK	Europe	USA	Australia	Canada
10mg	–	–	✓	–	✓
25mg	–	–	✓	–	✓
50mg	–	–	✓	–	–
75mg	–	–	✓	–	–

Liquid

Dosage	UK	Europe	USA	Australia	Canada
25mg/5mL (5mg/mL)	✓(250mL)	✓(250mL)	–	–	–
10mg/5mL (2mg/mL)	✓(250mL)	✓(250mL)	✓(473mL)	–	–

Worked example: To illustrate how the volumes were calculated in the regimens given below we provide a worked example. To make up 2mg of nortriptyline the 2mg/mL original solution can be used. The volume of 2mg/mL liquid required to give a dose of 2mg of nortriptyline is 2/2 = 1mL.

Off-label options: Guidelines for people who cannot swallow tablets (e.g. the NEWT guidelines in the UK) suggest that nortriptyline tablets can be dispersed in water for administration as an off-label use, and that tablets take about 1–2 minutes to disperse.[10] A 1mg/mL suspension could be made by adding water to a 50mg tablet to make up a 50mL suspension. The suspension should be shaken vigorously before use. As its stability cannot be assured, it should be consumed immediately, and any unused suspension discarded. Other options to make up small doses include compounding smaller dose tablets, including 'tapering strips'.[11]

Deprescribing notes: Initial reductions can be estimated from Tables 2.11 and 2.22, although patient preference should be taken into account. Sometimes an even smaller reduction to start with may be advisable to boost a patient's confidence that they can taper if performed carefully. Each reduction should be made when the withdrawal symptoms from the previous reduction have largely resolved so that subsequent reductions do not lead to cumulative withdrawal symptoms. Withdrawal symptoms should be tolerable and last at most a couple of weeks (see Figure 2.9). Allowing for a sufficient observation period, reductions can therefore be made about every 2 to 4 weeks. If withdrawal symptoms are moderately severe or take longer than a couple of weeks to resolve, dose reductions should be postponed until symptoms resolve and then made more gradual by choosing a slower tapering rate. If severe withdrawal symptoms occur then the patient should return to a higher dose, wait until symptoms resolve and thereafter taper at a slower rate.

Suggested taper schedules for nortriptyline

A. A faster taper with up to 5.2 percentage points of NET occupancy between each step (approximate length: 5–10 months). Patients who have been on the medication for only a few weeks will probably be able to taper more quickly and might follow every second or third step of this regimen, and make reductions every few days or so. Normally the duration of the taper should not be longer than the period that the patient has been on the drug for people who have only taken it for a few weeks. For example, if nortriptyline is taken for 3 weeks the taper should be less than 3 weeks.

B. A moderate taper with 3 percentage points of NET occupancy between each step (approximate length: 10–20 months).

C. A slower taper with 1.5 percentage points of NET occupancy between each step (approximate length: 20–40 months).

D. Some patients will be unable to taper at the slowest rates shown here and will need to taper by even smaller decrements, thus lengthening the overall period of tapering. Such a regimen could be constructed by placing intermediate steps in regimen C. For example, 3mg, 2mg, 1mg, 0mg could be modified to be 3mg, 2.5mg, 2mg, 1.5mg, 1mg, 0.5mg, 0mg. Further intermediate steps could also be added. Microtapering (tapering by a small amount each day, rather than by larger reductions every 2–4 weeks) is another possible approach (see benzodiazepines chapter for further details).

Please note that none of these regimens should be seen as prescriptive – that is, it is not suggested that patient must strictly adhere to them. They are given as example regimens and are not 'set and forget' but should be modified in order to ensure that withdrawal symptoms are tolerable throughout a taper – for example intermediate steps halfway between the doses listed could be added to make a more gradual taper.

A. **Faster taper** with up to 5.2 percentage points of NET occupancy between each step – with reductions made every 2–4 weeks.*

Step	RO (%)	Dose (mg)	Volume	Step	RO (%)	Dose (mg)	Volume
1	51.4	150	Use tablets	7	24.6	17.5	8.75mL
2	47.7	100	Use tablets	8	19.7	12.5	6.25mL
3	44.6	75	Use tablets	9	14.8	8.5	4.25mL
4	39.4	50	Use tablets	10	9.8	5	2.5mL
Switch to nortriptyline **2mg/mL solution**				11	4.9	2.5	1.25mL
5	34.4	35	17.5mL**	12	0	0	0
6	29.5	25	12.5mL**				
See further steps in the right-hand column							

RO = receptor occupancy
*For longer term users, the time between each decrease may be shortened to 1 week if the patient is able to make the first couple of reductions with no withdrawal symptoms. The interval between reductions should never be less than 1 week because this might increase the risk of relapse, even in the absence of withdrawal effects.[12,13]
**Alternatively, fractions of tablets could be used to make up these doses.

B. Moderate taper with up to 3 percentage points of NET occupancy between each step – with reductions made every 2–4 weeks.

Step	RO (%)	Dose (mg)	Volume	Step	RO (%)	Dose (mg)	Volume
1	51.4	150	Use tablets	11	26.5	21	10.5mL
2	49.8	125	Use tablets	12	23.9	17.5	8.75mL
3	47.7	100	Use tablets	13	21.2	14.5	7.25mL
4	45.1	80	Use tablets	14	18.6	12	6mL
5	42.4	62.5	Use ¼ tablets*	15	15.9	9.5	4.75mL
6	39.8	50	Use tablets	16	13.3	7.5	3.75mL
7	37.1	42.5	Use ¼ tablets*	17	10.6	5.7	2.85mL
8	34.5	35	Use tablets	18	7.95	4.1	2.05mL
9	31.8	30	Use tablets	19	5.3	2.6	1.3mL
10	29.2	25	Use tablets	20	2.65	1.2	0.6mL
Switch to nortriptyline **2mg/mL solution**				21	0	0	0
See further steps in the right-hand column							

RO = receptor occupancy
*Alternatively, doses can also be achieved using the liquid form (10mg/5mL) of the drug.

C. Slower taper with up to 1.5 percentage points of NET occupancy between each step – with reductions made every 2–4 weeks.

Step	RO (%)	Dose (mg)	Volume	Step	RO (%)	Dose (mg)	Volume	Step	RO (%)	Dose (mg)	Volume
1	51.4	150	Use tablets	15	33.8	34	17mL	30	15	8.9	4.45mL
2	50.1	130	Use tablets	16	32.6	31	15.5mL	31	13.8	7.9	3.95mL
3	48.8	112.5	Use ½ tablets*	17	31.3	28.5	14.25mL	32	12.5	7.0	3.5mL
4	47.6	100	Use tablets	18	30.1	26.5	13.25mL	33	11.3	6.1	3.05mL
Switch to nortriptyline **2mg/mL solution**				19	28.8	24.5	12.25mL	34	10.0	5.3	2.65mL
5	46.3	87.5	43.75mL	20	27.6	22.5	11.25mL	35	8.77	4.5	2.25mL
6	45.1	77.5	38.75mL	21	26.3	20.5	10.25mL	36	7.52	3.8	1.9mL
7	43.8	70.5	35.25mL	22	25.1	19	9.5mL	37	6.26	3.1	1.55mL
8	42.6	64	32mL	23	23.8	17.5	8.75mL	38	5.01	2.4	1.2mL
9	41.3	58	29mL	24	22.5	16	8mL	39	3.76	1.8	0.9mL
10	40.1	53	26.5mL	25	21.3	14.5	7.25mL	40	2.51	1.2	0.6mL
11	38.8	48	24mL	26	20	13.3	6.65mL	41	1.25	0.6	0.3mL
12	37.6	44	22mL	27	18.8	12.1	6.05mL	42	0	0	0
13	36.3	40	20mL	28	17.5	11	5.5mL				
14	35.1	37	18.5mL	29	16.3	9.9	4.95mL				
See further steps in the middle column				**See further steps in the right-hand column**							

RO = receptor occupancy
*Alternatively, doses can also be achieved using the liquid form (10mg/5mL) of the drug.

CHAPTER 2

References

1. Advanz Pharma. Nortriptyline – summary of product characteristics. 2022. https://www.medicines.org.uk/emc/product/2423/smpc#gref (accessed 29 September 2022).

2. Marsh W. Nortriptyline. In: *xPharm: The Comprehensive Pharmacology Reference*. StatPearls Publishing, 2007: 1–6.

3. Henssler J, Heinz A, Brandt L, Bschor T. Antidepressant withdrawal and rebound phenomena. *Dtsch Arztebl Int* 2019; 116: 355–61.

4. Taylor D, Stewart S, Connolly A. Antidepressant withdrawal symptoms- telephone calls to a national medication helpline. *J Affect Disord* 2006; 95: 129–33.

5. FDA. Nortriptyline – highlights of prescribing information. 2012.

6. Takano H, Arakawa R, Nogami T, et al. Norepinephrine transporter occupancy by nortriptyline in patients with depression: a positron emission tomography study with (S,S)-[18F]FMeNER-D2. *Int. J. Neuropsychopharmacol* 2014; 17: 553–60.

7. Furukawa TA, Cipriani A, Cowen PJ, Leucht S, Egger M, Salanti G. Optimal dose of selective serotonin reuptake inhibitors, venlafaxine, and mirtazapine in major depression: a systematic review and dose-response meta-analysis. *The Lancet Psychiatry* 2019; 6: 601–9.

8. Horowitz MA, Taylor D. Tapering of SSRI treatment to mitigate withdrawal symptoms. *The Lancet Psychiatry* 2019; 6: 538–46.

9. Holford N. Pharmacodynamic principles and the time course of delayed and cumulative drug effects. *Transl Clin* 2018; 26: 56.

10. Smyth J. The NEWT guidelines for administration of medication to patients with enteral feeding tubes or swallowing difficulties. 2011. https://www.newtguidelines.com/index.html (accessed 23 February 2023).

11. Groot PC, van Os J. How user knowledge of psychotropic drug withdrawal resulted in the development of person-specific tapering medication. *Ther Adv Psychopharmacol* 2020; 10: 204512532093245.

12. Baldessarini RJ, Tondo L, Ghiani C, Lepri B. Illness risk following rapid versus gradual discontinuation of antidepressants. *Am J Psychiatry* 2010; 167: 934–41.

13. Gøtzsche PC, Demasi M. Interventions to help patients withdraw from depression drugs: A systematic review. *Int J Risk Saf Med.* 2023 September 13. doi: 10.3233/JRS-230011. Epub ahead of print.

Paroxetine

Trade names: Paxil, Seroxat, Brisdelle, Pexeva.

Description: Paroxetine is a potent and one of the most specific inhibitors of SERT.[1,2] It also has mild action as a noradrenaline reuptake inhibitor targeting NET, as well as some affinity for muscarinic cholinergic receptors.[1] It has little affinity for alpha-1, alpha-2 and beta-adrenoceptors, dopamine (D_2), 5-HT$_1$-like, 5-HT$_2$ and histamine (H_1) receptors.[1]

Withdrawal effects: Paroxetine is the antidepressant perhaps most implicated in withdrawal effects – in double-blind randomised controlled trials discontinuation produced a withdrawal syndrome (defined as four or more withdrawal symptoms) in 66%[3] and 100%[4] of patients, with a mean of 7.8 and 10.1 withdrawal symptoms per patient, respectively. The severity and duration of these symptoms were not measured in these studies.[3-5] In an analysis of the WHO adverse effect database paroxetine emerged as high risk for withdrawal effects compared to other antidepressants, and had a stronger signal for risk of withdrawal than the opioid buprenorphine.[6]

Peak plasma: 6.4 hours.[7]

Half-life: 21 hours for the regular tablet,[7] 15–20 hours for extended release[8] (which controls the disintegration rate over 4 to 5 hours). The manufacturer recommends that paroxetine is administered once a day.[1] Every-other-day dosing is not recommended for tapering because of the substantial reductions in plasma concentrations this would produce, possibly giving rise to withdrawal effects.

Receptor occupancy: The relationship between dose of paroxetine and occupancy of its major target SERT is hyperbolic.[9] Antidepressants also show a hyperbolic pattern between dose and clinical effects,[10] which may be relevant to withdrawal effects from paroxetine. Dose reductions made by linear amounts (e.g. 40mg, 30mg, 20mg, 10mg, 0mg) will cause increasingly large reductions in effect which may cause increasingly severe withdrawal effects (Figure 2.31a). To produce equally sized reductions in effect on SERT occupancy will require hyperbolically reducing doses (Figure 2.31b),[11] which informs the reductions presented. This hyperbolic pattern of effect also applies to its occupancy of its other receptor targets as well, because these relationships are dictated

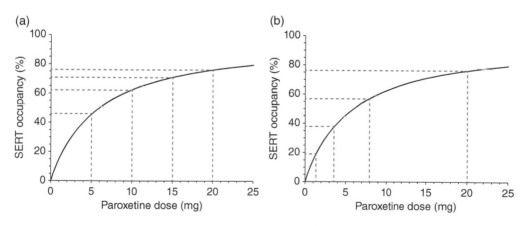

Figure 2.31 (a) Linear reductions of dose cause increasingly large reductions in effect on receptor targets, possibly associated with more withdrawal effects. (b) Even reductions of effect at target receptors requires hyperbolic dose reductions. The final dose before stopping will need to be very small so that this step down is not larger (in terms of effect on receptor occupancy) than previous reductions.

by the law of mass action.[12] There may be some differences in the precise dose-related activity between receptor targets but the hyperbolic relationship remains. Consequently, the regimens given below (based on SERT occupancy) will be broadly suitable for other receptor occupancies, such as for NET occupancy.

Available formulations: As tablets, extended-release tablets and liquid.

Tablets*

Dosage	UK	Europe	USA	Australia	Canada
10mg	✓	✓	✓	–	✓
20mg	✓	✓	✓	✓	✓
30mg	✓	✓	✓	–	✓
40mg	✓	✓	✓	–	–

*As paroxetine hydrochloride

Extended-release tablets*

Dosage	UK	Europe	USA	Australia	Canada
12.5mg	–	–	✓	–	✓
25mg	–	–	✓	–	✓
37.5mg	–	–	✓	–	✓

*As paroxetine hydrochloride

Liquid

Dosage	UK	Europe	USA	Australia	Canada
20mg/10mL (2mg/mL)	✓(150mL)*	–		–	–
10mg/5mL (2mg/mL)	–	–	✓ (250mL)	–	–

*Note that although GSK has stopped producing Seroxat (paroxetine) in liquid form, paroxetine liquid is available in the UK through compounding pharmacies. Please check the concentration of these liquids before using the guides below.

Dilutions: In order to make up smaller doses for tapering dilution of the solution will be required. Paroxetine is soluble in water (about 5mg/mL). Dilution of the stock solution should therefore be acceptable, although stability cannot be guaranteed.[7,13]

USA/UK dilutions*	Suspension required	How to prepare suspension
Doses ≥ 0.4mg	2mg/mL	Original suspension
Doses <0.4mg	0.2mg/mL	Mix 1mL of original oral suspension with 9mL of water

*Note: these solutions come as paroxetine hydrochloride, which is approximately bioequivalent to tablet form.

Worked example: To illustrate how the volumes were calculated in the regimens given below we provide a worked example. To make up 0.3mg of paroxetine a 0.2mg/mL dilution can be used, made up as outlined above. The volume of 0.2mg/mL liquid required to give a dose of 0.3mg of paroxetine is 0.3/0.2 = 1.5mL.

Off-label options: Guidelines for people who cannot swallow tablets (e.g. the NEWT guidelines in the UK,[14] NHS pharmaceutical guidance[15] and similar US guidance[16]) suggest that immediate release forms of paroxetine tablets can be dispersed in water for administration.[14] This is an off-label use.[14] Water could be added to a 20mg tablet to make up a 40mL suspension (concentration 0.5mg/mL). Dispersal and suspension of the tablet may take some time. Suspended particles are probably tablet excipients as paroxetine should fully dissolve at this concentration. The tablet may be crushed with a spoon or pestle and mortar before mixing with water to speed up this process.[14,16] The suspension will have a bitter taste and a local anaesthetic effect on the mouth.[14] The suspension should be shaken vigorously before use. As its stability cannot be assured it should be consumed immediately, and any unused suspension discarded. If the controlled-release form is crushed it will lose its controlled-release properties and should therefore be treated as an immediate release preparation.[16] Other options to make up small doses include compounding smaller dose tablets, including 'tapering strips'.[17]

Deprescribing notes: Initial reductions can be estimated from Tables 2.11 and 2.22 although patient preference should be respected. Sometimes an even smaller reduction to start with may be advisable to boost a patient's confidence that they can taper if performed carefully. Each reduction should be made when the withdrawal symptoms from the previous reduction have largely resolved so that subsequent reductions do not lead to cumulative withdrawal symptoms. Withdrawal symptoms should be tolerable and last at most a couple of weeks (see Figure 2.9). Allowing for a sufficient observation period, reductions can therefore be made about every 2 to 4 weeks. If withdrawal symptoms are moderately severe or take longer than a couple of weeks to resolve, dose reductions should be postponed until symptoms resolve and then made more gradual by choosing a slower tapering rate. If severe withdrawal symptoms occur then the patient should return to a higher dose, wait until symptoms resolve and thereafter taper at a slower rate.

Suggested taper schedules for paroxetine

A. A faster taper with up to 9 percentage points of SERT occupancy between each step (approximate length: 5–10 months). Patients who have been on the medication for only a few weeks will probably be able to taper more quickly and might follow every second or third step of this regimen, and make reductions every few days or so. For people who have only taken an antidepressant for a few weeks, the duration of the taper should not be longer than the period that the patient has been on the drug. For example, if paroxetine is taken for three weeks the taper should be less than 3 weeks.
B. A moderate taper with up to 5.1 percentage points of SERT occupancy between each step (approximate length: 10–20 months).
C. A slower taper with up to 2.8 percentage points of SERT occupancy between each step (approximate length: 20–40 months).
D. Some patients will be unable to taper at the slowest rates shown here and will need to taper by even smaller decrements, thus lengthening the overall period of tapering. Such a regimen could be constructed by placing intermediate steps in regimen C. For example, 3mg, 2mg, 1mg, 0mg could be modified to be 3mg, 2.5mg, 2mg, 1.5mg, 1mg, 0.5mg, 0mg. Further intermediate steps could also be added. Microtapering (tapering by a small amount each day, rather than by larger reductions every 2–4 weeks) is another possible approach (see benzodiazepines chapter for further details).

Please note that none of these regimens should be seen as prescriptive – that is, it is not suggested that patient must strictly adhere to them. They are given as example regimens and are not 'set and forget' but should be modified in order to ensure that withdrawal symptoms are tolerable throughout a taper – for example intermediate steps halfway between the doses listed could be added to make a more gradual taper.

Metabolic note Paroxetine is both a metabolic substrate and a potent inhibitor of CYP P450 2D6.[18] As the dose is reduced this will lead to reduced inhibition (i.e. induction) of its metabolism thereby leading to a more rapid drop in plasma levels. This may be one reason that paroxetine withdrawal is especially severe and may present a rationale to slow rate of reduction even further, and to consider twice daily dosing at lower doses.[19]

A. **A faster taper** with up to 9 percentage points of SERT between each step – with reductions made every 2–4 weeks.

Step	RO (%)	Dose (mg)	Volume	Step	RO (%)	Dose (mg)	Volume
1	85	40	Use tablets	7	39	3.5	1.75mL
2	76	20	Use tablets	8	31	2.5	1.25mL**
3	71	15	Use ½ tablets*	9	23	1.8	0.9mL
4	62	10	Use tablets	10	16	1.1	0.55mL
Switch to paroxetine **2mg/mL liquid**				11	7.8	0.5	0.25mL
5	54	7	3.5mL	12	0	0	0
6	47	5	2.5mL**				
See further steps in the right-hand column							

RO = receptor occupancy
*Alternatively, a liquid version of the drug could be used to make up these doses.
**Alternatively, a portion of a tablet may be used.

B. **A moderate taper** with up to 5.1 percentage points of SERT between each step – with reductions made every 2–4 weeks.

Step	RO (%)	Dose (mg)	Volume	Step	RO (%)	Dose (mg)	Volume
1	85.2	40	Use tablets	12	45.5	5	2.5mL
2	81.9	30	Use tablets	13	40.4	4	2mL
3	79.3	25	Use ½ tablets*	14	35.4	3.2	1.6mL
4	75.9	20	Use tablets	15	30.3	2.5	1.25mL**
5	73.6	17.5	Use ¾ tablets	16	25.3	2	1mL
6	70.7	15	Use ½ tablets*	17	20.2	1.5	0.75mL
Switch to paroxetine **2mg/mL liquid**				18	15.2	1	0.5mL
7	66.9	12.5	6.25mL	19	10.1	0.64	0.32mL
8	62.3	10	5mL**	Switch to paroxetine **0.2mg/mL dilution**			
9	58.6	8.5	4.25mL	20	5.1	0.3	1.5mL
10	55.6	7.5	3.75mL*	21	0	0	0
11	50.6	6.1	3.05mL				
See further steps in the right-hand column							

RO = receptor occupancy
*Alternatively, a liquid version of the drug could be used to make up these doses.
**Alternatively, a tablet or portion of a tablet may be used.

C. **A slower taper** with up to 2.8 percentage points of SERT occupancy between each step – with reductions made every 2–4 weeks.

Step	RO (%)	Dose (mg)	Volume	Step	RO (%)	Dose (mg)	Volume	Step	RO (%)	Dose (mg)	Volume
1	85.2	40	Use tablets	14	62.3	10	5mL**	28	27.4	2.2	1.1mL
2	83.7	35	Use ½ tablets*	15	59.9	9	4.5mL	29	24.6	1.9	0.95mL
3	81.9	30	Use tablets	16	57.4	8.1	4.05mL	30	22.6	1.7	0.85mL
4	79.4	25	Use ½ tablets*	17	55	7.3	3.65mL	31	20.5	1.5	0.75mL
Switch to paroxetine **2mg/mL liquid**				18	52.2	6.5	3.25mL	32	18.3	1.3	0.65mL
5	77.8	22	11mL	19	49.8	5.9	2.95mL	33	15.9	1.1	0.55mL
6	75.9	20	10mL**	20	47.2	5.3	2.65mL	34	13.5	0.9	0.45mL
7	74.1	18	9mL	21	44.8	4.8	2.4mL	35	10.8	0.7	0.35mL
8	72	16	8mL	22	42.2	4.3	2.15mL	36	8.7	0.55	0.28mL
9	70.7	15	7.5mL	23	39.9	3.9	1.95mL	37	6.5	0.4	0.2mL
10	69.4	14	7mL	24	37.4	3.5	1.75mL	Switch to paroxetine **0.2mg/mL dilution**			
11	67.9	13	6.5mL	25	34.6	3.1	1.55mL	38	4.2	0.25	1.25mL
12	66.2	12	6mL	26	32.4	2.8	1.4mL	39	1.7	0.1	0.5mL
13	64.4	11	5.5mL	27	30	2.5	1.25mL	40	0	0	0
See further steps in the middle column				**See further steps in the right-hand column**							

RO = receptor occupancy
*Alternatively, a liquid version of the drug could be used to make up these doses.
**Alternatively, a tablet or portion of a tablet may be used.

CHAPTER 2

References

1. Aurobindo Pharma – Milpharm Ltd. Paroxetine – summary of product characteristics. 2021. https://www.medicines.org.uk/emc/medicine/23046/SPC/Paroxetine+20mg+Tablets/ (accessed 23 September 2022).
2. Mellerup ET, Plenge P. High affinity binding of 3H-paroxetine and 3H-imipramine to rat neuronal membranes. *Psychopharmacology* 1986; 89: 436–9.
3. Rosenbaum JF, Fava M, Hoog SL, Ascroft RC, Krebs WB. Selective serotonin reuptake inhibitor discontinuation syndrome: a randomized clinical trial. *Biol Psychiatry* 1998; 44: 77–87.
4. Hindmarch I, Kimber S, Cockle SM. Abrupt and brief discontinuation of antidepressant treatment – effects on cognitive function and psychomotor performance. 2000; 15: 305–18.
5. Horowitz MA, Framer A, Hengartner MP, Sørensen A, Taylor D. Estimating risk of antidepressant withdrawal from a review of published data. *CNS Drugs* 2023; 37: 143–57.
6. Gastaldon C, Schoretsanitis G, Arzenton E, et al. Withdrawal syndrome following discontinuation of 28 antidepressants: pharmacovigilance analysis of 31,688 reports from the WHO spontaneous reporting database. *Drug Saf* 2022; 45: 1539–49.
7. FDA. Paroxetine – highlights of prescribing information. 2021. https://www.accessdata.fda.gov/drugsatfda_docs/label/2021/020031s077lbl.pdf (accessed 23 September 2022).
8. FDA. Paroxetine extended-release tablets – highlights of prescribing information. 2019. https://www.accessdata.fda.gov/drugsatfda_docs/label/2019/020936s047lbl.pdf (accessed 23 September 2022).
9. Sørensen A, Ruhé HG, Munkholm K. The relationship between dose and serotonin transporter occupancy of antidepressants – a systematic review. *Mol Psychiatry* 2022; 27: 192–201.
10. Furukawa TA, Cipriani A, Cowen PJ, Leucht S, Egger M, Salanti G. Optimal dose of selective serotonin reuptake inhibitors, venlafaxine, and mirtazapine in major depression: a systematic review and dose-response meta-analysis. *The Lancet Psychiatry* 2019; 6: 601–9.
11. Horowitz MA, Taylor D. Tapering of SSRI treatment to mitigate withdrawal symptoms. *The Lancet Psychiatry* 2019; 6: 538–46.
12. Holford N. Pharmacodynamic principles and the time course of delayed and cumulative drug effects. *Transl Clin* 2018; 26: 56.
13. Seroxat 20mg/10ml oral suspension. https://www.medicines.org.uk/emc/product/7594/smpc (accessed 19 October 2022).
14. Smyth J. The NEWT guidelines for administration of medication to patients with enteral feeding tubes or swallowing difficulties website. The NEWT Guidelines. 2011. https://www.newtguidelines.com/index.html (accessed 18 February 2023).
15. Brennan K. Selective serotonin reuptake inhibitor (SSRI) formulations suggested for adults with swallowing difficulties. SPS – Specialist Pharmacy Service. 2021; published online 1 July. https://www.sps.nhs.uk/articles/selective-serotonin-reuptake-inhibitor-ssri-formulations-suggested-for-adults-with-swallowing-difficulties/ (accessed September 19, 2022).
16. Bostwick JR, Demehri A. Pills to powder: an updated clinician's reference for crushable psychotropics. *Curr Psychiatr* 2017; 16: 46–9.
17. Groot PC, van Os J. How user knowledge of psychotropic drug withdrawal resulted in the development of person-specific tapering medication. *Ther Adv Psychopharmacol* 2020; 10: 204512532093245.
18. Harvey BH, Slabbert FN. New insights on the antidepressant discontinuation syndrome. *Hum Psychopharmacol* 2014; 29: 503–16.
19. Framer A. What I have learnt from helping thousands of people taper off psychotropic medications. *Ther Adv Psychopharmacol* 2021; 11: 204512532199127.

Phenelzine

Trade name: Nardil.

Description: Phenelzine is a non-selective and irreversible monoamine oxidase-A (MAO-A) and-B (MAO-B) inhibitor (MAO-I) with slight preference for MAO-A.[1]

Withdrawal effects: In a structured analysis of withdrawal risk for antidepressants phenelzine was designated as 'very high risk'.[2] In an analysis of calls to a helpline for withdrawal effects from drugs (normalised to prescription numbers) phenelzine also emerged as one of the antidepressants most commonly causing withdrawal effects.[3]

Peak plasma: 43 minutes.[4]

Half-life: 11–12 hours. The manufacturer recommends up to three times per day dosing, but also suggests every-other-day dosing is reasonable.[5] As phenelzine irreversibly inhibits MAO (and this enzyme needs to be regenerated) its pharmacodynamic half-life may be as long as one week (or perhaps longer), similar to that estimated for tranylcypromine.[6] Every-other-day dosing or dosing at even greater intervals may be reasonable because of this long pharmacodynamic half-life.

Receptor occupancy: The relationship between dose of phenelzine and the occupancy of MAO-A is hyperbolic.[7,8] This pattern also applies to its occupancy of other receptor targets such as MAO-B, as dictated by the law of mass action.[9] Antidepressants also show a hyperbolic pattern between dose and clinical effects,[10] which may be relevant to withdrawal effects from phenelzine. Dose reductions made by linear amounts (e.g. 30 mg, 22.5mg, 15mg, 7.5mg, 0mg) will cause increasingly large reductions in receptor occupancy which may cause increasingly severe withdrawal effects (Figure 2.32a). To produce equal-sized reductions in effect on MAO-A occupancy will require hyperbolically reducing doses (Figure 2.32b),[11] which informs the reductions presented.

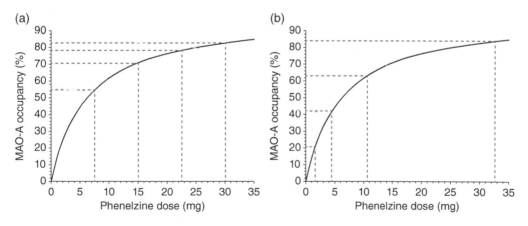

Figure 2.32 (a) Linear reductions of dose cause increasingly large reductions in effect on receptor targets, possibly associated with more withdrawal effects. (b) Even reductions of effect at target receptors requires hyperbolic dose reductions. The final dose before stopping will need to be very small so that this step down is not larger (in terms of effect on receptor occupancy) than previous reductions.

Available formulations: Phenelzine is available as tablets.

Tablets

Dosage	UK	Europe	USA	Australia	Canada
15mg	✓	✓	✓	✓	✓

Off-label options: Guidelines for people who cannot swallow tablets (e.g. the NEWT guidelines in the UK,[12] based on local hospital policies and information direct from the manufacturer and similar USA guidance)[13] suggest that phenelzine tablets can be crushed[13] and mixed in water for administration as an off-label use. A 1mg/mL suspension could be made by adding water to a 15mg tablet to make up 15mL. The tablet may be crushed with a spoon or pestle and mortar before mixing with water to speed up this process. This should be shaken vigorously before administration. Phenelzine is unstable in water, so administration should be immediate,[12] and any unused suspension discarded.

Worked example: To illustrate how the volumes were calculated in the regimens given below we provide a worked example. To make up 2mg of phenelzine a 1mg/mL suspension can be used, made up as outlined above. The volume of 1mg/mL liquid required to give a dose of 2mg phenelzine is 2/1 = 2mL.

Deprescribing notes: Initial reductions can be estimated from Tables 2.11 and 2.22, although patient preference should be respected. Each reduction should be made when the withdrawal symptoms from the previous reduction have largely resolved so that subsequent reductions do not lead to cumulative withdrawal symptoms. Withdrawal symptoms should be tolerable and last at most a couple of weeks (see Figure 2.9). As the pharmacodynamic half-life of phenelzine is about 1 week, this may delay the onset of withdrawal symptoms and represent a partial 'self-tapering' effect. Therefore it may be best to make every second reduction in the regimens suggested below at spacing of 6 to 8 weeks rather than each step at intervals of 2 to 4 weeks as for most other antidepressants. If withdrawal symptoms are moderately severe or take longer than a couple of weeks to resolve, dose reductions should be postponed until symptoms resolve and then made more gradual by choosing a slower tapering rate. If severe withdrawal symptoms occur then the patient should return to a higher dose, wait until symptoms resolve and thereafter taper at a slower rate.

Taper schedules for phenelzine

A. A faster taper with up to 10.1 percentage points of MAO-A occupancy between each step (approximate length: 5–10 months). Patients who have been on the medication for only a few weeks will probably be able to taper more quickly and might follow every second or third step of this regimen, and make reductions every few days or so. For people who have only taken an antidepressant for a few weeks, the duration of the taper should not be longer than the period that the patient has been on the drug. For example, if phenelzine is taken for 3 weeks the taper should be less than 3 weeks.

B. A moderate taper with up to 5 percentage points of MAO-A occupancy between each step (approximate length: 10–20 months).

C. A slower taper with up to 2.5 percentage points of MAO-A occupancy between each step (approximate length: 20–40 months).

D. Some patients will be unable to taper at the slowest rates shown here and will need to taper by even smaller decrements, thus lengthening the overall period of tapering. Such a regimen could be constructed by placing intermediate steps in regimen C. For example, 3mg, 2mg, 1mg, 0mg could be modified to be 3mg, 2.5mg, 2mg, 1.5mg, 1mg, 0.5mg, 0mg. Further intermediate steps could also be added. Microtapering (tapering by a small amount each day, rather than by larger reductions every 2–4 weeks) is another possible approach (see benzodiazepines chapter for further details).

Please note that none of these regimens should be seen as prescriptive – that is, it is not suggested that patient must strictly adhere to them. They are given as example regimens and are not 'set and forget' but should be modified in order to ensure that withdrawal symptoms are tolerable throughout a taper – for example intermediate steps halfway between the doses listed could be added to make a more gradual taper.

A. **Faster taper** with up to 10.1 percentage points of MAO-A occupancy between each step – with reductions made every 2–4 weeks.*,**

Step	RO (%)	Dose (mg)	Volume	Alternative approach using tablets
1	90.6	60	Use tablets	Use tablets
2	82.9	30	Use tablets	Use tablets
Switch to **1mg/mL suspension**				–
3	78.4	22.5	22.5mL***	Use ½ tablet
4	70.7	15	15mL***	Use tablets
5	60.6	10	10mL	1 tablet and ½ tablet alternating days
6	50.5	6.3	6.3mL	Tablets 3 times/week (e.g. Mon, Wed, Fri)
7	40.4	4.2	4.2mL	Tablets 2 times/week (e.g. Mon, Thurs)
8	30.3	2.7	2.7mL	¼ tablet 5 times/week (e.g. weekdays)
9	20.2	1.6	1.6mL	¼ tablet 3 times/week
10	10.1	0.7	0.7mL	¼ tablet, once every 5 days
11	0	0	0	0

RO = receptor occupancy
*For longer term users, the time between each decrease may be shortened to 1 week if the patient is able to make the first couple of reductions with no withdrawal symptoms. The interval between reductions should never be less than 1 week because this might increase the risk of relapse, even in the absence of withdrawal effects.[14,15]
**Because of the long pharmacodynamic half-life of phenelzine, a reasonable approach would be to make every second reduction outlined here at intervals of 6–8 weeks in case of delayed onset withdrawal effects (and taking into account its 'self-tapering' properties).
***Alternatively, a tablet or ½ tablet could be administered.

B. **Moderate taper** with up to 5 percentage points of MAO-A occupancy between each step – with reductions made every 2–4 weeks.*

Step	RO (%)	Dose (mg)	Volume	Step	RO (%)	Dose (mg)	Volume
1	90.6	60	Use tablets	11	44.1	4.9	4.9mL
2	87.9	45	Use tablets	12	39.2	4	4mL
3	82.9	30	Use tablets	13	34.3	3.2	3.2mL
4	78.4	22.5	Use ½ tablets	14	29.4	2.6	2.6mL
	Switch to **1mg/mL suspension**			15	24.5	2	2mL
5	73.5	17	17mL	16	19.6	1.5	1.5mL
6	68.6	14	14mL	17	14.7	1.05	1.05mL
7	63.7	11	11mL	18	9.8	0.66	0.66mL
8	58.8	8.9	8.9mL	19	4.9	0.32	0.32mL
9	53.9	7.3	7.3mL	20	0	0	0
10	49	6	6mL				
	See further steps in the right-hand column						

RO = receptor occupancy
*Because of the long pharmacodynamic half-life of phenelzine, a reasonable approach would be to make every second reduction outlined here at intervals of 6–8 weeks in case of delayed onset withdrawal effects (and taking into account its 'self-tapering' properties).

C. **Slower taper** with 2.5 percentage points of MAO-A occupancy between each step – with reductions made every 2–4 weeks.*

Step	RO (%)	Dose (mg)	Volume	Step	RO (%)	Dose (mg)	Volume	Step	RO (%)	Dose (mg)	Volume
1	90.6	60	Use tablets	14	63.7	10.9	10.9mL	28	29.4	2.58	2.58mL
2	89.4	52.5	Use ½ tablets**	15	61.2	9.81	9.81mL	29	26.9	2.29	2.29mL
3	87.9	45	Use tablets	16	58.8	8.85	8.85mL	30	24.5	2.01	2.01mL
4	85.8	37.5	Use ½ tablets**	17	56.3	8.01	8.01mL	31	22	1.76	1.76mL
5	84.5	33.75	Use ¼ tablets**	18	53.9	7.25	7.25mL	32	19.6	1.51	1.51mL
6	82.9	30	Use tablets	19	51.4	6.58	6.58mL	33	17.1	1.28	1.28mL
	Switch to **1mg/mL suspension**			20	49	5.96	5.96mL	34	14.7	1.05	1.05mL
7	80.9	26.25	26.25mL***	21	46.5	5.4	5.4mL	35	12.2	0.84	0.84mL
8	78.4	22.5	22.5mL***	22	44.1	4.9	4.9mL	36	9.8	0.65	0.65mL
9	75.9	19.6	19.6mL	23	41.6	4.43	4.43mL	37	7.35	0.49	0.49mL
10	73.5	17.2	17.2mL	24	39.2	4	4mL	38	4.9	0.32	0.32mL
11	71	15.2	15.2mL	25	36.7	3.61	3.61mL		Switch to **0.1mg/mL suspension**		
12	68.6	13.6	13.6mL	26	34.3	3.24	3.24mL	39	2.45	0.16	1.6mL
13	66.1	12.1	12.1mL	27	31.8	2.9	2.9mL	40	0	0	0
	See further steps in the middle column				**See further steps in the right-hand column**						

RO = receptor occupancy
*Because of the long pharmacodynamic half-life of phenelzine, a reasonable approach would be to make every second reduction outlined here at intervals of 6–8 weeks in case of delayed onset withdrawal effects (and taking into account its 'self-tapering' properties).
**Alternatively, this could be made up with liquid.
***Alternatively, this could be made up with fractions of tablets.

References

1. Happe K. Phenelzine. In: *xPharm: The Comprehensive Pharmacology Reference*. StatPearls Publishing, 2011: 1–1.

2. Henssler J, Heinz A, Brandt L, Bschor T. Antidepressant withdrawal and rebound phenomena. *Dtsch Arztebl Int* 2019; 116: 355–61.

3. Taylor D, Stewart S, Connolly A. Antidepressant withdrawal symptoms – telephone calls to a national medication helpline. *J Affect Disord* 2006; 95: 129–33.

4. FDA. Phenelzine sulfate – highlights of prescribing information. 2007.

5. Neon Healthcare Phenelzine – summary of product characteristics. 2022. https://www.medicines.org.uk/emc/product/228/smpc#gref (accessed 12 October 2022).

6. Ulrich S, Ricken R, Adli M. Tranylcypromine in mind (Part I): review of pharmacology. *Eur Neuropsychopharmacol* 2017; 27: 697–713.

7. Chiuccariello L, Cooke RG, Miler L, et al. Monoamine oxidase-A occupancy by moclobemide and phenelzine: implications for the development of monoamine oxidase inhibitors. *Int J Neuropsychopharmacol* 2015; 19. doi:10.1093/ijnp/pyv078.

8. Thentu JB, Bhyrapuneni G, Padala NP, Chunduru P, Pantangi HR, Nirogi R. Evaluation of monoamine oxidase A and B type enzyme occupancy using non-radiolabelled tracers in rat brain. *Neurochem Int* 2021; 145: 105006.

9. Holford N. Pharmacodynamic principles and the time course of delayed and cumulative drug effects. *Transl Clin* 2018; 26: 56.

10. Furukawa TA, Cipriani A, Cowen PJ, Leucht S, Egger M, Salanti G. Optimal dose of selective serotonin reuptake inhibitors, venlafaxine, and mirtazapine in major depression: a systematic review and dose-response meta-analysis. *The Lancet Psychiatry* 2019; 6: 601–9.

11. Horowitz MA, Taylor D. Tapering of SSRI treatment to mitigate withdrawal symptoms. *The Lancet Psychiatry* 2019; 6: 538–46.

12. Smyth J. The NEWT Guidelines for administration of medication to patients with enteral feeding tubes or swallowing difficulties website. The NEWT Guidelines. 2011. https://www.newtguidelines.com/index.html (accessed 18 February 2023).

13. Bostwick JR, Demehri A. Pills to powder: an updated clinician's reference for crushable psychotropics. *Curr Psychiatr* 2017; 16: 46–9.

14. Baldessarini RJ, Tondo L, Ghiani C, Lepri B. Illness risk following rapid versus gradual discontinuation of antidepressants. *Am J Psychiatry* 2010; 167: 934–41.

15. Gøtzsche PC, Demasi M. Interventions to help patients withdraw from depression drugs: A systematic review. *Int J Risk Saf Med*. 2023 September 13. doi: 10.3233/JRS-230011. Epub ahead of print.

Sertraline

Trade names: Zoloft, Lustral.

Description: Sertraline is an SSRI with SERT as its major target. It has only very weak effects on noradrenaline and dopamine reuptake.[1] It has no affinity for muscarinic, serotonergic, dopaminergic, adrenergic, or histaminergic receptors.[1]

Withdrawal effects: In a double-blind randomised controlled trial of sertraline discontinuation in people who had used the drug for more than 3 months, 59% of patients met criteria for a withdrawal syndrome (four or more withdrawal symptoms), although this study did not measure severity or duration of these symptoms.[2] Two other double-blind randomised controlled trials found that sertraline withdrawal was experienced by 58% and 60% of patients.[3,4] After 8 weeks of treatment 34.3% of patients were observed to have at least moderately severe withdrawal effects when the medication was stopped.[4] Longer term treatment is associated with increased incidence of withdrawal symptoms of greater severity.[5] In an analysis of the WHO adverse effect database sertraline emerged as at moderate risk for withdrawal effects compared to other antidepressants.[6]

Peak plasma: 4.5 to 8.4 hours.[1]

Half-life: About 26 hours.[1] Every-other-day dosing is not recommended for tapering because of the substantial reductions in plasma concentrations this would produce, possibly giving rise to withdrawal effects.

Receptor occupancy: The relationship between dose of sertraline and occupancy of its major target SERT is hyperbolic.[7] This applies to other receptor targets as well because this relationship is dictated by the law of mass action.[8] Antidepressants also show a hyperbolic pattern between dose and clinical effects,[9] which may be relevant to withdrawal effects from sertraline. Dose reductions made by linear amounts (e.g. 100mg, 75mg, 50mg, 25mg, 0mg) will cause increasingly large reductions in effect which may cause increasingly severe withdrawal effects (Figure 2.33a). To produce equal-sized reductions in effect on SERT occupancy will require hyperbolically reducing doses (Figure 2.33b),[10] which informs the reductions presented.

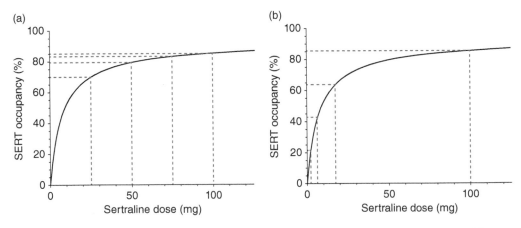

Figure 2.33 (a) Linear reductions of dose cause increasingly large reductions in effect on receptor targets, possibly associated with more withdrawal effects. (b) Even reductions of effect at target receptors requires hyperbolic dose reductions. The final dose before stopping will need to be very small so that this step down is not larger (in terms of effect on receptor occupancy) than previous reductions.

Available formulations: As tablets, capsules and liquid.

Tablets*

Dosage	UK	Europe	USA	Australia	Canada
25 mg	✓	✓	✓	–	–
50 mg	✓	✓	✓	✓	–
100 mg	✓	✓	✓	✓	–

*As sertraline hydrochloride.

Capsules

Dosage	UK	Europe	USA	Australia	Canada
25 mg	–	–	–	–	✓
50 mg	–	–	–	–	✓
100 mg	–	–	–	–	✓

Liquid

Dosage	UK	Europe	USA	Australia
20mg/mL	–	–	✓ (60mL)**	–
100mg/5mL (20mg/mL)	✓ (60mL)*	–	–	–

*In the UK, a liquid form of sertraline hydrochloride is now licensed and does not require any special storage conditions.[11]
**In the USA, liquid form of sertraline hydrochloride (20mg/mL) is approximately bioequivalent to tablet form. It is recommended to be stored at 20°C to 25°C (68°F to 77°F).[12]

Dilutions: In the UK and USA, the manufacturer advises the solution must be diluted before use.[11,12] It recommends using either water, ginger ale, lemon/lime soda, lemonade or orange juice only. After mixing a slight haze may appear, which is normal.[11,12] The patient can either use the dropper provided or a syringe to be more precise. The FDA and MHRA labels advise the dose to be taken 'immediately' after mixing, which could be considered meaning within an hour of preparation.[11,12]

Dilutions*	Solution required	How to prepare solution
Doses ≥ 4mg	20mg/mL	Original solution
Doses ≥ 0.4mg, <4mg	2mg/mL	Mix 0.5mL of original oral solution with 4.5mL of water or juice
Doses <0.4mg	0.2mg/mL	Mix 0.5mL of original oral solution with 49.5mL of water or juice

*Note: these drops come as sertraline hydrochloride which is approximately bioequivalent to tablet form.[12]

Worked example: To illustrate how the below volumes were calculated in the regimens given we provide a worked example. To make up 3mg of sertraline a 2mg/mL dilution can be used, made up as outlined above. The liquid is bioequivalent to the tablet so 3mg of the drug in liquid form is required. The volume of 2mg/mL liquid required to give a dose of 3mg of sertraline is 3/2 = 1.5mL.

Off-label options: Guidelines for people who cannot swallow tablets (e.g. the NEWT guidelines[13] and NHS pharmaceutical guidance in the UK[14] and similar USA guidance)[15] suggest that sertraline tablets can be dispersed in water for administration.[13] The tablets disperse in 1 to 5 minutes. The resulting suspension may have a bitter taste and an anaesthetic effect on the tongue, so advise caution and take care with hot foods after administration.[13] This represents an off-label use. A 1mg/mL suspension could be made by adding water to a 50mg tablet to make up 50mL. This should be shaken vigorously before use. As its stability cannot be assured it should be consumed immediately, and any unused suspension discarded. Other options to make up small doses include compounding smaller dose tablets, including 'tapering strips'.[16]

Deprescribing notes: Initial reductions can be estimated from Tables 2.11 and 2.22 although patient preference should be taken into account. Sometimes an even smaller reduction to start with may be advisable to boost a patient's confidence that they can taper if performed carefully. Each reduction should be made when the withdrawal symptoms from the previous reduction have largely resolved so that subsequent reductions do not lead to cumulative withdrawal symptoms. Withdrawal symptoms should be tolerable and last at most a couple of weeks (see Figure 2.9). Allowing for a sufficient observation period, reductions can therefore be made about every 2 to 4 weeks. If withdrawal symptoms are moderately severe or take longer than a couple of weeks to resolve, dose reductions should be postponed until symptoms resolve and then made more gradual by choosing a slower tapering rate. If severe withdrawal symptoms occur then the patient should return to a higher dose, wait until symptoms resolve and thereafter taper at a slower rate.

Suggested taper schedules for sertraline

A. A faster taper with up to 10 percentage points of SERT occupancy between each step (approximate length: 5–10 months). Patients who have been on the medication for only a few weeks will probably be able to taper more quickly and might follow every second or third step of this regimen, and make reductions every few days or so. For people who have only taken an antidepressant for a few weeks, the duration of the taper should not be longer than the period that the patient has been on the drug. For example, if sertraline is taken for 3 weeks the taper should be less than 3 weeks.

B. A moderate taper with up to 5 percentage points of SERT occupancy between each step (approximate length: 10–20 months).

C. A slower taper with up to 2.6 percentage points of SERT occupancy between each step (approximate length: 20–40 months).

D. Some patients will be unable to taper at the slowest rates shown here and will need to taper by even smaller decrements, thus lengthening the overall period of tapering. Such a regimen could be constructed by placing intermediate steps in regimen C. For example, 3mg, 2mg, 1mg, 0mg could be modified to be 3mg, 2.5mg, 2mg, 1.5mg, 1mg, 0.5mg, 0mg. Further intermediate steps could also be added. Microtapering (tapering by a small amount each day, rather than by larger reductions every 2–4 weeks) is another possible approach (see benzodiazepines chapter for further details).

Please note that none of these regimens should be seen as prescriptive – that is, it is not suggested that patient must strictly adhere to them. They are given as example regimens and are not 'set and forget' but should be modified in order to ensure that withdrawal symptoms are tolerable throughout a taper – for example intermediate steps halfway between the doses listed could be added to make a more gradual taper.

A. **A faster taper** with up to 10 percentage points of SERT between each step – with reductions made every 2–4 weeks.*

Step	RO (%)	Dose (mg)	Volume	Step	RO (%)	Dose (mg)	Volume
1	89	200	Use tablets	7	40	6	0.3mL
2	85	100	Use tablets	8	30	4	0.2mL
3	80	50	Use tablets	Switch to sertraline **2mg/mL dilution**			
4	70	25	Use tablets	9	20	2	1mL
Switch to sertraline **20mg/mL liquid**				10	10	1	0.5mL
5	60	15	0.75mL	11	0	0	0
6	50	10	0.5mL				
See further steps in the right-hand column							

RO = receptor occupancy

*For longer term users, the time between each decrease may be shortened to 1 week if the patient is able to make the first couple of reductions with no withdrawal symptoms. The interval between reductions should never be less than 1 week because this might increase the risk of relapse, even in the absence of withdrawal effects.[17,18]

CHAPTER 2

B. **A moderate taper** with up to 5 percentage points of SERT between each step – with reductions made every 2–4 weeks.

Step	RO (%)	Dose (mg)	Volume	Step	RO (%)	Dose (mg)	Volume
1	89	200	Use tablets	12	46	8.0	0.4mL
2	85	100	Use tablets	Switch to sertraline **2mg/mL dilution**			
3	83	75	Use tablets	13	42	6.5	3.25mL
4	80	50	Use tablets	14	37	5.3	2.65mL
Switch to sertraline **20mg/mL liquid**				15	33	4.3	2.15mL
5	77	40	2mL	16	28	3.4	1.7mL
6	73	32	1.6mL	17	23	2.6	1.3mL
7	70	25	1.25mL*	18	19	2.0	1mL
8	65	19	0.95mL	19	14	1.4	0.7mL
9	60	15	0.75mL	20	9	0.9	0.45mL
10	56	12	0.6mL	21	5	0.4	0.2mL
11	51	9.8	0.49mL	22	0	0	0
See further steps in the right-hand column							

RO = receptor occupancy
*Alternatively, tablets or fragments of tablets could be used.

C. **A slower taper** with up to 2.6 percentage points of SERT occupancy between each step – with reductions made every 2–4 weeks.

Step	RO (%)	Dose (mg)	Volume	Step	RO (%)	Dose (mg)	Volume	Step	RO (%)	Dose (mg)	Volume
1	88.5	200	Use tablets	15	60.7	15	0.75mL	29	26.7	3.2	1.6mL
2	87.5	150	Use tablets	16	58.2	13.3	0.67mL	30	24.2	2.8	1.4mL
3	85.4	100	Use tablets	17	55.8	12	0.6mL	31	21.8	2.4	1.2mL
4	83.4	75	Use tablets	18	53.4	10.7	0.54mL	32	19.4	2.1	1.05mL
Switch to sertraline **20mg/mL liquid**				19	51.0	9.6	0.48mL	33	17.4	1.8	0.9mL
5	81.5	60	3mL	20	48.5	8.6	0.43mL	34	15.0	1.5	0.75mL
6	79.7	50	2.5mL*	Switch to sertraline **2mg/mL dilution**				35	12.4	1.2	0.6mL
7	78.3	44	2.2mL	21	46.2	7.8	3.9mL	36	10.1	0.95	0.48mL
8	76.4	38	1.9mL	22	43.8	7	3.5mL	Switch to sertraline **0.2mg/mL dilution**			
9	74.5	33	1.65mL	23	41.2	6.3	3.15mL	37	7.6	0.7	3.5mL
10	72.7	29	1.45mL	24	38.8	5.6	2.8mL	38	5.1	0.45	2.25mL
11	70.3	25	1.25mL*	25	36.3	5	2.5mL	39	2.5	0.22	1.1mL
12	67.9	22	1.1mL	26	33.9	4.4	2.2mL	40	0	0	0
13	65.5	19	0.95mL	27	31.5	4	2.0mL				
14	63.3	17	0.85mL	28	29.1	3.6	1.8mL				
See further steps in the middle column				**See further steps in the right-hand column**							

RO = receptor occupancy
*Alternatively, tablets or fragments of tablets could be used.

References

1. Lupin Healthcare. Sertraline 50 mg Tablets. 2020; published online December. https://www.medicines.org.uk/emc/product/7162/smpc (accessed 9 September 2022).

2. Hindmarch I, Kimber S, Cockle SM. Abrupt and brief discontinuation of antidepressant treatment: effects on cognitive function and psychomotor performance. *Int Clin Psychopharmacol* 2000; 15: 305–18.

3. Rosenbaum JF, Fava M, Hoog SL, Ascroft RC, Krebs WB. Selective serotonin reuptake inhibitor discontinuation syndrome: a randomized clinical trial. *Biol Psychiatry* 1998; 44: 77–87.

4. Sir A, D'Souza RF, Uguz S, et al. Randomized trial of sertraline versus venlafaxine XR in major depression: efficacy and discontinuation symptoms. *J Clin Psychiatry* 2005; 66: 1312–20.

5. Horowitz MA, Framer A, Hengartner MP, Sørensen A, Taylor D. Estimating risk of antidepressant withdrawal from a review of published data. *CNS Drugs* 2022; published online 14 December. doi:10.1007/s40263-022-00960-y.

6. Gastaldon C, Schoretsanitis G, Arzenton E, et al. Withdrawal syndrome following discontinuation of 28 antidepressants: pharmacovigilance analysis of 31,688 reports from the WHO spontaneous reporting database. *Drug Saf* 2022; 45: 1539–49.

7. Sørensen A, Ruhé HG, Munkholm K. The relationship between dose and serotonin transporter occupancy of antidepressants – a systematic review. *Mol Psychiatry* 2022; 27: 192–201.

8. Holford N. Pharmacodynamic principles and the time course of delayed and cumulative drug effects. *Transl Clin* 2018; 26: 56.

9. Furukawa TA, Cipriani A, Cowen PJ, Leucht S, Egger M, Salanti G. Optimal dose of selective serotonin reuptake inhibitors, venlafaxine, and mirtazapine in major depression: a systematic review and dose-response meta-analysis. *The Lancet Psychiatry* 2019; 6: 601–9.

10. Horowitz MA, Taylor D. Tapering of SSRI treatment to mitigate withdrawal symptoms. *The Lancet Psychiatry* 2019; 6: 538–46.

11. Thame Laboratories. Sertraline 100mg/5ml Concentrate for Oral Solution. 2023. https://www.medicines.org.uk/emc/product/14703/smpc/print (accessed 18 November 2023)

12. U.S. Food and Drug Administration. Zoloft (sertraline hydrochloride) tablets and oral concentrate. 2009.

13. Smyth J. The NEWT guidelines for administration of medication to patients with enteral feeding tubes or swallowing difficulties website. The NEWT Guidelines, 2011. https://www.newtguidelines.com/index.html (accessed 7 September 2022).

14. Brennan K. Selective serotonin reuptake inhibitor (SSRI) formulations suggested for adults with swallowing difficulties. SPS – Specialist Pharmacy Service. 2021; published online 1 July. https://www.sps.nhs.uk/articles/selective-serotonin-reuptake-inhibitor-ssri-formulations-suggested-for-adults-with-swallowing-difficulties/ (accessed 19 September 2022).

15. Bostwick JR, Demehri A. Pills to powder: an updated clinician's reference for crushable psychotropics. *Curr Psychiatr* 2017; 16: 46–9.

16. Groot PC, van Os J. How user knowledge of psychotropic drug withdrawal resulted in the development of person-specific tapering medication. *Ther Adv Psychopharmacol* 2020; 10: 204512532093245.

17. Baldessarini RJ, Tondo L, Ghiani C, Lepri B. Illness risk following rapid versus gradual discontinuation of antidepressants. *Am J Psychiatry* 2010; 167: 934–41.

18. Gøtzsche PC, Demasi M. Interventions to help patients withdraw from depression drugs: A systematic review. *Int J Risk Saf Med.* 2023 September 13. doi: 10.3233/JRS-230011. Epub ahead of print.

CHAPTER 2

Tranylcypromine

Trade name: Parnate.

Description: Tranylcypromine is a non-selective and irreversible monoamine oxidase A and B inhibitor (MAO-I) with slight preference for MAO-B.[1]

Withdrawal effects: Tranylcypromine is recognised to cause physical dependence, withdrawal and addiction.[2] In a structured analysis of withdrawal risk for antidepressants tranylcypromine was designated 'very high risk'.[3] In an analysis of calls to a helpline for withdrawal effects from drugs (normalised to prescription numbers) tranylcypromine also emerged as one of the antidepressants most commonly causing withdrawal effects.[4]

Peak plasma: 2.5 hours.[5]

Half-life: The elimination half-life is 2 hours. However, as tranylcypromine irreversibly inhibits MAO (and this enzyme needs to be regenerated) the pharmacodynamic half-life has been estimated to be about one week (or perhaps longer).[6] The manufacturer recommends two or three times per day dosing.[1] Every-other-day dosing (or even more seldom dosing) may be reasonable because of the long pharmacodynamic half-life.

Receptor occupancy: The relationship between dose of tranylcypromine and the occupancy of MAO-B is hyperbolic.[7] This hyperbolic pattern also applies to its occupancy of other receptors, including MAO-A, as this relationship is dictated by the law of mass action.[8] Antidepressants also show a hyperbolic pattern between dose and clinical effects,[9] which may be relevant to withdrawal effects from tranylcypromine. Dose reductions made by linear amounts (e.g. 20mg, 15mg, 10mg, 5mg, 0mg) will cause increasingly large reductions in MAO-A receptor occupancy which may cause increasingly severe withdrawal effects (Figure 2.34a). To produce equal-sized reductions in effect on MAO-B occupancy will require hyperbolically reducing doses (Figure 2.34b),[10] which informs the reductions presented.

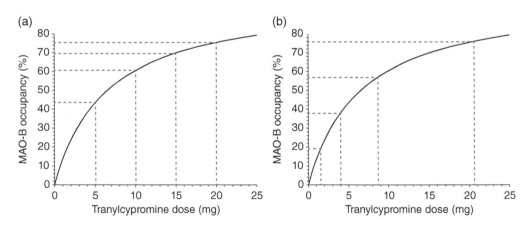

Figure 2.34 (a) Linear reductions of dose cause increasingly large reductions in effect on receptor targets, possibly associated with more withdrawal effects. (b) Even reductions of effect at target receptors requires hyperbolic dose reductions. The final dose before stopping will need to be very small so that this step down is not larger (in terms of effect on receptor occupancy) than previous reductions.

Available formulations: Tranylcypromine is available as tranylcypromine sulfate in tablets.

Tablets

Dosage	UK	Europe	USA	Australia	Canada
10mg	✓	✓	✓	✓	✓

Off-label options: Advice for patients who cannot swallow tablets[11] suggests that tranylcypromine tablets can be crushed and mixed with water for administration. This solution could be used to make up the small doses suggested below. For example, a 1mg/mL solution could be made by adding water to a 10mg tablet to make up 10mL as tranylcypromine is soluble in water (1.49mg/mL).[12] The tablet may be crushed with a spoon or pestle and mortar before mixing with water to speed up this process. The solution should be shaken vigorously before use. As its stability cannot be assured it should be consumed immediately, and any unused solution discarded. Alternatively some compounding pharmacies may be able to make up smaller dose formulations, including 'tapering strips' as an option.[13]

Worked example: To illustrate how the volumes were calculated in the regimens given below we provide a worked example. To make up 2mg of tranylcypromine a 1mg/mL suspension can be used, made up as outlined above. The volume of 1mg/mL liquid required to give a dose of 2mg of tranylcypromine is 2/1 = 2mL.

Deprescribing notes: Initial reductions can be estimated from Tables 2.11 and 2.22, although patient preference should be respected. Sometimes an even smaller reduction to start with may be advisable to boost a patient's confidence that they can taper if performed carefully. Each reduction should be made when the withdrawal symptoms from the previous reduction have largely resolved so that subsequent reductions do not lead to cumulative withdrawal symptoms. Withdrawal symptoms should be tolerable and last at most a couple of weeks (see Figure 2.9). As the pharmacodynamic half-life of tranylcypromine is about one week, this may delay the onset of withdrawal symptoms and represent a partial 'self-tapering' effect. Therefore it may be best to make every second reduction in the regimens suggested below at spacing of 6 to 8 weeks rather than each step at intervals of 2 to 4 weeks as for most other antidepressants. If withdrawal symptoms are moderately severe or take longer than a couple of weeks to resolve, dose reductions should be postponed until symptoms resolve and then made more gradual by choosing a slower tapering rate. If severe withdrawal symptoms occur then the patient should return to a higher dose, wait until symptoms resolve and thereafter taper at a slower rate.

Taper schedules for tranylcypromine

A. A faster taper with up to 10 percentage points of MAO-B occupancy between each step (approximate length: 5–10 months). Patients who have been on the medication for only a few weeks will probably be able to taper more quickly and might do every second or third step of this regimen, and make reductions every few days or so. Normally the duration of the taper should not be longer than the period that the patient has been on the drug for people who have only taken it for a few weeks. For example, if tranylcypromine is taken for 3 weeks the taper should be less than 3 weeks.

B. A moderate taper with up to 5 percentage points of MAO-B occupancy between each step (approximate length: 10–20 months).

C. A slower taper with up to 2.5 percentage points of MAO-B occupancy between each step (approximate length: 20–40 months).

D. Some patients will be unable to taper at the slowest rates shown here and will need to taper by even smaller decrements, thus lengthening the overall period of tapering. Such a regimen could be constructed by placing intermediate steps in regimen C. For example, 3mg, 2mg, 1mg, 0mg could be modified to be 3mg, 2.5mg, 2mg, 1.5mg, 1mg, 0.5mg, 0mg. Further intermediate steps could also be added. Microtapering (tapering by a small amount each day, rather than by larger reductions every 2–4 weeks) is another possible approach (see benzodiazepines chapter for further details).

Please note that none of these regimens should be seen as prescriptive – that is, it is not suggested that patient must strictly adhere to them. They are given as example regimens and are not 'set and forget' but should be modified in order to ensure that withdrawal symptoms are tolerable throughout a taper – for example intermediate steps halfway between the doses listed could be added to make a more gradual taper.

A. **Faster taper** with up to 10 percentage points of MAO-B occupancy between each step – with reductions made every 2–4 weeks.*

Step	RO (%)	Dose (mg)	Volume	Step	RO (%)	Dose (mg)	Volume
1	82	30	Use tablets	6	35	3.5	3.5mL
2	75	20	Use tablets	7	26	2.3	2.3mL
3	60	10	Use tablets	8	17	1.4	1.4mL
Switch to **1mg/mL suspension**				9	8.6	0.6	0.6mL
4	52	7	7mL	10	0	0	0
5	43	5	5mL**				
See further steps in the right-hand column							

RO = receptor occupancy

*Alternatively, it may be advisable to make every second reduction in this regime at intervals of 6–8 weeks in order to give time for delayed onset withdrawal effects to arise due to the long pharmacodynamic half-life.

**Alternatively, could be administered as half tablets.

B. **Moderate taper** with up to 5 percentage points of MAO-B occupancy between each step – with reductions made every 2–4 weeks.*

Step	RO (%)	Dose (mg)	Volume	Step	RO (%)	Dose (mg)	Volume
1	82.1	30	Use tablets	11	39.9	4.3	4.3mL
2	79.2	25	Use ½ tablets	12	35.5	3.6	3.6mL
3	75.3	20	Use tablets	13	31	2.9	2.9mL
Switch to **1mg/mL suspension**				14	26.6	2.4	2.4mL
4	70.9	16	16mL	15	22.2	1.9	1.9mL
5	66.5	13	13mL	16	17.7	1.4	1.4mL
6	62	10.9	10.9mL	17	13.3	1	1mL
7	57.6	8.9	8.9mL	18	8.86	0.65	0.65mL
8	53.2	7.4	7.4mL	19	4.43	0.3	0.3mL
9	48.7	6.2	6.2mL	20	0	0	0
10	44.3	5.2	5.2mL				
See further steps in the right-hand column							

RO = receptor occupancy

*Alternatively it may be advisable to make every second reduction in this regime at intervals of 6–8 weeks in order to give time for delayed onset withdrawal effects to arise due to the long pharmacodynamic half-life.

CHAPTER 2

C. **Slower taper** with 2.5 percentage points of MAO-B occupancy between each step – with reductions made every 2–4 weeks.**

Step	RO (%)	Dose (mg)	Volume	Step	RO (%)	Dose (mg)	Volume	Step	RO (%)	Dose (mg)	Volume
1	82.1	30	Use Tablets	14	54.7	7.9	7.9mL	28	25.3	2.21	2.21mL
Switch to **1mg/mL suspension**				15	52.6	7.3	7.3mL	29	23.2	1.97	1.97mL
2	80	26	26mL	16	50.5	6.7	6.7mL	30	21	1.75	1.75mL
3	77.8	23	23mL	17	48.4	6.1	6.1mL	31	18.9	1.53	1.53mL
4	75.3	20	20mL**	18	46.3	5.6	5.6mL	32	16.8	1.33	1.33mL
5	73.3	18	18mL	19	44.2	5.2	5.2mL	33	14.7	1.13	1.13mL
6	71.5	16	16mL	20	42.1	4.8	4.8mL	34	12.6	0.95	0.95mL
7	68.9	14.5	14.5mL	21	40	4.4	4.4mL	35	10.5	0.77	0.77mL
8	66.5	13	13mL	22	37.9	4	4mL	36	8.42	0.6	0.6mL
9	64.3	11.8	11.8mL	23	35.8	3.6	3.6mL	37	6.31	0.44	0.44mL
10	62.3	10.8	10.8mL	24	33.7	3.3	3.3mL	38	4.21	0.29	0.29mL
11	60.4	10	10mL**	25	31.6	3	3mL	Switch to **0.1mg/mL suspension**			
12	58.4	9.2	9.2mL	26	29.5	2.73	2.73mL	39	2.1	0.14	1.4mL
13	56.8	8.5	8.5mL	27	27.4	2.47	2.47mL	40	0	0	0
See further steps in the middle column				**See further steps in the right-hand column**							

RO = receptor occupancy
*Alternatively it may be advisable to make every second reduction in this regime at intervals of 6–8 weeks in order to give time for delayed onset withdrawal effects to arise due to the long pharmacodynamic half-life.
**Alternatively, these doses could be administered as tablets or half, or three-quarter tablets.

References

1. Advanz Pharma. Tranylcypromine – Summary of Product Characteristics. 2022. https://www.medicines.org.uk/emc/product/2788/smpc#gref (accessed 12 October 2022).
2. Haddad P. Do antidepressants have any potential to cause addiction? *J Psychopharmacol* 1999; 13: 300–7.
3. Henssler J, Heinz A, Brandt L, Bschor T. Antidepressant withdrawal and rebound phenomena. *Dtsch Arztebl Int* 2019; 116: 355–61.
4. Taylor D, Stewart S, Connolly A. Antidepressant withdrawal symptoms – telephone calls to a national medication helpline. *J Affect Disord* 2006; 95: 129–33.
5. FDA. Tranylcypromine – highlights of prescribing information. 2018.
6. Ulrich S, Ricken R, Adli M. Tranylcypromine in mind (Part I): review of pharmacology. *Eur Neuropsychopharmacol* 2017; 27: 697–713.
7. Thentu JB, Bhyrapuneni G, Padala NP, Chunduru P, Pantangi HR, Nirogi R. Evaluation of monoamine oxidase A and B type enzyme occupancy using non-radiolabelled tracers in rat brain. *Neurochem Int* 2021; 145: 105006.
8. Holford N. Pharmacodynamic principles and the time course of delayed and cumulative drug effects. *Transl Clin* 2018; 26: 56.
9. Furukawa TA, Cipriani A, Cowen PJ, Leucht S, Egger M, Salanti G. Optimal dose of selective serotonin reuptake inhibitors, venlafaxine, and mirtazapine in major depression: a systematic review and dose-response meta-analysis. *The Lancet Psychiatry* 2019; 6: 601–9.
10. Horowitz MA, Taylor D. Tapering of SSRI treatment to mitigate withdrawal symptoms. *The Lancet Psychiatry* 2019; 6: 538–46.
11. Bostwick JR, Demehri A. Pills to powder: An updated clinician's reference for crushable psychotropics. *Curr Psychiatr* 2017; 16: 46–9.
12. Tranylcypromine sulfate. https://go.drugbank.com/salts/DBSALT000960 (accessed 25 October 2022).
13. Groot PC, van Os J. How user knowledge of psychotropic drug withdrawal resulted in the development of person-specific tapering medication. *Ther Adv Psychopharmacol* 2020; 10: 204512532093245.

Trazodone

Trade names: Desyrel, Molipaxin.

Description: Trazodone is a triazolopyridine derivative that inhibits SERT, and is an antagonist at serotonin type 2 receptors.[1] It is also an antagonist at histamine and alpha-1 adrenergic receptors, amongst other targets.[1]

Withdrawal effects: There have not been controlled studies of withdrawal effects from trazodone but there are published case studies.[2] Trazodone was classified as lower risk for withdrawal effects based on calls regarding withdrawal to a pharmacy help line (normalised to prescription numbers).[3]

Peak plasma: 1– 2 hours.[1]

Half-life: Ranges from 5–13 hours.[4] According to the manufacturer trazodone should be taken in divided doses during the day. It is often taken at night because of its hypnotic effects. Every-other-day dosing is not recommended for tapering because of its short half-life, as this can lead to substantial reductions in plasma levels which might give rise to withdrawal effects. Extended-release tablets extend the duration of action to 24 hours,[5] allowing for once per day administration.

Receptor occupancy: The relationship between dose of trazodone and occupancy of one of its targets, SERT, is hyperbolic.[6] Antidepressants also show a hyperbolic pattern between dose and clinical effects,[7] which may be relevant to withdrawal effects from trazodone. Dose reductions made by linear amounts (e.g. 150mg, 112.5mg, 75mg, 37.5mg, 0mg) will cause increasingly large reductions in receptor occupancy which may cause increasingly severe withdrawal effects (Figure 2.35a). To produce equal-sized reductions in effect on SERT occupancy will require hyperbolically reducing doses (Figure 2.35b),[8] which informs the reductions presented. This hyperbolic pattern also applies to its occupancy of its other target receptors because of the law of mass action.[9] Consequently, there may be some differences in the precise dose-related activity between receptors but the hyperbolic relationship remains. It is expected that

CHAPTER 2

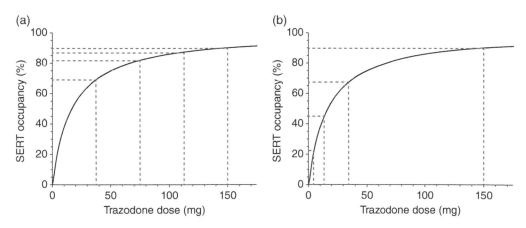

Figure 2.35 (a) Linear reductions of dose cause increasingly large reductions in effect on receptor targets, possibly associated with more withdrawal effects. (b) Even reductions of effect at target receptors requires hyperbolic dose reductions. The final dose before stopping will need to be very small so that this step down is not larger (in terms of effect on receptor occupancy) than previous reductions.

the regimens given below (based on SERT occupancy) will be broadly suitable for other receptor occupancies, such as H_1 histamine.

Available formulations: Trazodone is available as trazodone hydrochloride in capsules, tablets, extended-release tablets and as a liquid.[4,10,11]

Capsules

Dosage	UK	Europe	USA	Australia	Canada
50mg	✓	✓	–	–	–
100mg	✓	✓	–	–	–

Tablets

Dosage	UK	Europe	USA	Australia	Canada
50mg	–	–	✓	–	✓
100mg	–	–	✓	–	✓
150mg	✓	✓	✓	–	✓
300mg	–	–	✓	–	✓

Extended-release tablets

Dosage	UK	Europe	USA	Australia	Canada
50mg	–	–	✓	–	–
100mg	–	–	✓	–	–
150mg	–	–	–	–	✓
300mg	–	–	–	–	✓

Liquid form

Dosage	UK	Europe	USA	Australia	Canada
50mg/5mL (10mg/mL)	✓	–	–	–	–

Dilutions: With smaller doses a dilution of the solution will be required. The manufacturer instructs that the oral solution should not be mixed with fluids other than water.

Dilutions	Solution required	How to prepare solution
Doses ≥2 mg	10mg/mL	Original solution
Doses <2 mg, ≥0.4mg	2mg/mL	Add 1mL of original solution to 4mL of water

Worked example: To illustrate how the volumes were calculated in the regimens given below we provide a worked example. To make up 1mg of trazodone a 2mg/mL dilution can be used, made up as outlined above. The volume of 2mg/mL liquid required to give a dose of 1mg of trazodone is 1/2 = 0.5mL.

Off-label options: Although not recommending it, guidelines for people who cannot swallow tablets (e.g. the NEWT guidelines in the UK)[12] mention the possibility of capsules being opened and diluted in water, as an off-label use.[12] The taste is unpleasant and the drug has a local anaesthetic effect in the mouth. Any cloudiness of the solution is probably a consequence of insoluble capsule excipients. A 2mg/mL suspension could be made by emptying the contents of a 50mg capsule into 25mL of water. This suspension should be shaken vigorously before use. As its stability cannot be assured it should be consumed immediately, and any unused suspension discarded.

Guidance in the USA advises that the tablets can be crushed and mixed with water for administration.[13] Water could be added to a 150mg tablet to make up 75mL, yielding a 2mg/mL suspension.[13] The tablet may be crushed with a spoon or pestle and mortar before mixing with water to speed up this process. This suspension should be shaken vigorously before use. As its stability cannot be assured it should be consumed immediately, and any unused suspension discarded. Other options include a compounding pharmacy making up a liquid or smaller formulations of tablets.

Deprescribing notes: Initial reductions can be estimated from Tables 2.11 and 2.22, although patient preference should be respected. Sometimes an even smaller reduction to start with may be advisable to boost a patient's confidence that they can taper if performed carefully. Each reduction should be made when the withdrawal symptoms from the previous reduction have largely resolved so that subsequent reductions do not lead to cumulative withdrawal symptoms. Withdrawal symptoms should be tolerable and last at most a couple of weeks (see Figure 2.9). Allowing for a sufficient observation period, reductions can therefore be made about every 2 to 4 weeks. If withdrawal symptoms are moderately severe or take longer than a couple of weeks to resolve, dose reductions should be postponed until symptoms resolve and then made more gradual by choosing a slower tapering rate. If severe withdrawal symptoms occur then the patient should return to a higher dose, wait until symptoms resolve and thereafter taper at a slower rate.

Suggested taper schedules for trazodone

A. A faster taper with up to 12.5 percentage points of SERT occupancy between each step with reductions made every 2–4 weeks (approximate length: 5–10 months). Patients who have been on the medication for only a few weeks will probably be able to taper more quickly and might follow every second or third step of this regimen and make reductions every few days or so. For people who have only taken an antidepressant for a few weeks, the duration of the taper should not be longer than the period that the patient has been on the drug.

B. A moderate taper with up to 6 percentage points of SERT occupancy between each step with reductions made every 2–4 weeks (approximate length: 10–20 months).

C. A slower taper with up to 2.5 percentage points of SERT occupancy between each step with reductions made every 2–4 weeks (approximate length: 20–40 months).

D. Some patients will be unable to taper at the slowest rates shown here and will need to taper by even smaller decrements, thus lengthening the overall period of tapering. Such a regimen could be constructed by placing intermediate steps in regimen C. For example, 3mg, 2mg, 1mg, 0mg could be modified to be 3mg, 2.5mg, 2mg, 1.5mg,

1mg, 0.5mg, 0mg. Further intermediate steps could also be added. Microtapering (tapering by a small amount each day, rather than by larger reductions every 2–4 weeks) is another possible approach (see benzodiazepines chapter for further details).

Please note that none of these regimens should be seen as prescriptive – that is, it is not suggested that patient must strictly adhere to them. They are given as example regimens and are not 'set and forget' but should be modified in order to ensure that withdrawal symptoms are tolerable throughout a taper – for example intermediate steps halfway between the doses listed could be added to make a more gradual taper.

A. **Faster taper** with up to 12.5 percentage points of SERT occupancy between each step – with reductions made every 2–4 weeks.*

Step	RO (%)	Dose (mg)	Volume	Step	RO (%)	Dose (mg)	Volume
1	97.3	600	Use tabs or caps	6	62.5	30	3mL
2	94.7	300	Use tabs or caps	7	50	15	1.5mL
3	90	150	Use tabs or caps	8	37.5	10	1mL
4	81.8	75	Use tabs or caps	9	25	5	0.5mL
5	75	50	Use tabs or caps	10	12.5	2.5	0.25mL
Switch to trazodone **10mg/mL solution****				11	0	0	0
See further steps in the right-hand column							

RO = receptor occupancy, caps = capsules, tabs = tablets
*For longer term users, the time between each decrease may be shortened to 1 week if the patient is able to make the first couple of reductions with no withdrawal symptoms. The interval between reductions should never be less than 1 week because this might increase the risk of relapse, even in the absence of withdrawal effects.[14,15]
**When the manufacturer's liquid is not available, a suspension can be made as an off-label option, as outlined above.

B. **Moderate taper** with up to 6 percentage points of SERT occupancy between each step – with reductions made every 2–4 weeks.

Step	RO (%)	Dose (mg)	Volume	Step	RO (%)	Dose (mg)	Volume
1	97.3	600	Use tabs or caps	11	49.4	16	1.6mL
2	94.7	300	Use tabs or caps	12	43.9	13	1.3mL
3	90	150	Use tabs or caps	13	38.4	10	1mL
4	85.7	100	Use tabs or caps	Switch to trazodone **2mg/mL dilution***			
Switch to trazodone **10mg/mL solution***				14	32.9	8.1	4.05mL
5	81.8	70	7mL	15	27.4	6.3	3.15mL
6	76.8	50	5mL**	16	21.9	4.7	2.35mL
7	71.3	40	4mL	17	16.5	3.3	1.65mL
8	65.8	32.5	3.25mL	18	11	2.1	1.05mL
9	60.4	25	2.5mL**	19	5.5	1	0.5mL
10	54.9	20	2mL	20	0	0	0
See further steps in the right-hand column							

RO = receptor occupancy, caps = capsules, tabs = tablets
*When the manufacturer's liquid is not available, a suspension can be made as an off-label option, as outlined above.
**Alternatively, this could be given as a tablet of half tablet.

CHAPTER 2

C. **Slower taper** with up to 2.5 percentage points of SERT occupancy between each step – with reductions made every 2–4 weeks.

Step	RO (%)	Dose (mg)	Volume	Step	RO (%)	Dose (mg)	Volume	Step	RO (%)	Dose (mg)	Volume
1	97.3	600	Use tabs or caps	14	64.9	31	3.1mL	27	32.4	8	4mL
2	94.8	300	Use tabs or caps	15	62.4	28	2.8mL	28	29.9	7.1	3.55mL
3	92.3	200	Use tabs or caps	16	59.9	25	2.5mL**	29	27.4	6.3	3.15mL
4	89.8	150	Use tabs or caps	17	57.4	22	2.2mL	30	24.9	5.5	2.75mL
Switch to trazodone **10mg/mL solution***				18	54.9	20	2mL	31	22.5	4.8	2.4mL
5	87.3	110	11mL	Switch to trazodone **2mg/mL dilution***				32	20	4.1	2.05mL
6	84.8	93	9.3mL	19	52.4	18.3	9.15mL	33	17.5	3.5	1.75mL
7	82.3	78	7.8mL	20	49.9	16.6	8.3mL	34	15	2.9	1.45mL
8	79.8	66	6.6mL	21	47.4	15	7.5mL	35	12.5	2.3	1.15mL
9	77.3	57	5.7mL	22	44.9	13.6	6.8mL	36	10.0	1.8	0.9mL
10	74.8	50	5mL**	23	42.4	12.3	6.15mL	37	7.5	1.3	0.65mL
11	72.4	44	4.4mL	24	39.9	11.1	5.55mL	38	5.0	0.8	0.4mL
12	69.9	39	3.9mL	25	37.4	10	5mL	39	2.5	0.4	0.2mL
13	67.4	34	3.4mL	26	34.9	9	4.5mL	40	0	0	0
See further steps in the middle column				**See further steps in the right-hand column**							

RO = receptor occupancy, caps = capsules, tabs = tablets
*When the manufacturer's liquid is not available, a suspension can be made as an off-label option, as outlined above.
**Alternatively, this could be given as a tablet or half tablet

CHAPTER 2

References

1. Shin JJ, Saadabadi A. *Trazodone*. StatPearls Publishing, 2022 https://www.ncbi.nlm.nih.gov/books/NBK470560/ (accessed 25 March 2023).
2. Montalbetti DJ, Zis AP. Cholinergic rebound following trazodone withdrawal? *J Clin Psychopharmacol* 1988; 8: 73.
3. Taylor D, Stewart S, Connolly A. Antidepressant withdrawal symptoms – telephone calls to a national medication helpline. *J Affect Disord* 2006; 95: 129–33.
4. FDA. Trazodone – highlights of prescribing information. 2017.
5. Reed M, Stezzi TJ, Peart W, Herr JD, Caspi A. Trazodone hydrochloride extended-release tablets – product profiler. 2010.
6. Settimo L, Taylor D. Evaluating the dose-dependent mechanism of action of trazodone by estimation of occupancies for different brain neurotransmitter targets. *J Psychopharmacol* 2018; 32: 96–104.
7. Furukawa TA, Cipriani A, Cowen PJ, Leucht S, Egger M, Salanti G. Optimal dose of selective serotonin reuptake inhibitors, venlafaxine, and mirtazapine in major depression: a systematic review and dose-response meta-analysis. *The Lancet Psychiatry* 2019; 6: 601–9.
8. Horowitz MA, Taylor D. Tapering of SSRI treatment to mitigate withdrawal symptoms. *The Lancet Psychiatry* 2019; 6: 538–46.
9. Holford N. Pharmacodynamic principles and the time course of delayed and cumulative drug effects. *Transl Clin* 2018; 26: 56.
10. FDA. Trazodone – XR highlights of prescribing information. 2014.
11. Advanz pharma. Trazodone summary of product characteristics. 2018. https://www.medicines.org.uk/emc/product/7186/smpc#gref (accessed 29 September 2022).
12. Smyth J. The NEWT guidelines for administration of medication to patients with enteral feeding tubes or swallowing difficulties website. The NEWT Guidelines. 2011. https://www.newtguidelines.com/index.html (accessed 7 September 2022).
13. Bostwick JR, Demehri A. Pills to powder: An updated clinician's reference for crushable psychotropics. *Curr Psychiatr* 2017; 16: 46–9.
14. Baldessarini RJ, Tondo L, Ghiani C, Lepri B. Illness risk following rapid versus gradual discontinuation of antidepressants. *Am J Psychiatry* 2010; 167: 934–41.
15. Gøtzsche PC, Demasi M. Interventions to help patients withdraw from depression drugs: A systematic review. *Int J Risk Saf Med.* 2023 September 13. doi: 10.3233/JRS-230011. Epub ahead of print.

Venlafaxine

Trade names: Effexor, Alventa, Amphero, Depefex, Efexor, Foraven, Majoven, Politid, Sunveniz, Tonpular, Trevilor, Venadex, Venaxx, Vencarm, Venlablue, Venlaclic, Venladex, Venlasoz, Vensir, ViePax.

Description: Venlafaxine is an SNRI with SERT and NET as its major targets.[1] It weakly inhibits dopamine re-uptake and has virtually no affinity for muscarinic, cholinergic, histaminergic and α_1-adrenergic receptors.[1]

Withdrawal effects: Venlafaxine is classified in the high risk category for withdrawal effects in a number of analyses.[2-4] In a randomised controlled trial of venlafaxine given for 8 weeks, 71% (44/62) of patients had withdrawal symptoms after a 2 week taper.[5] After discontinuation following 8 weeks of medication use, 38.7% of patients were judged to have withdrawal symptoms that were moderately severe, 3.2% to be severe and 1.6% to be very severe.[5] Severe effects are likely to be more common after longer-term use.[4] This study only followed up people for 2 weeks after stopping, so overall duration of symptoms was not measured.[5] In an analysis of the WHO adverse effect database venlafaxine emerged as high risk for withdrawal effects compared to other antidepressants, and had a stronger signal for risk of withdrawal than the opioid buprenorphine.[6]

Peak plasma: Venlafaxine is extensively metabolised to O-desmethylvenlafaxine (ODV). After immediate-release venlafaxine administration, the peak plasma concentrations of venlafaxine and ODV occur at 2 and 3 hours, respectively. For the modified-release form of venlafaxine peak plasma concentrations of venlafaxine and ODV are attained within 5.5 hours and 9 hours, respectively.[1]

Half-life: Venlafaxine is extensively metabolised, primarily to the active metabolite, ODV. The elimination half-lives of venlafaxine and ODV are approximately 5 hours and 11 hours, respectively.[1] The half-lives of the immediate-release version and modified-release version are the same but the modified-release spheroids release the drug slowly in the digestive tract, extending the absorption half life to 7.5 to 13.9 hours. Every-other-day dosing is not recommended for tapering because of the substantial reductions in plasma concentrations this would produce, possibly giving rise to withdrawal effects. Patients who take immediate-release formulations of venlafaxine (including liquid versions) may need to take their dose two (or even three) times a day because of the short half-life.

Receptor occupancy: The relationship between dose of venlafaxine and occupancy of one of its major targets, SERT, is hyperbolic.[7] The relationship with occupancy of other receptors will also be hyperbolic according to the law of mass action.[8] Antidepressants also show a hyperbolic pattern between dose and clinical effects,[9] which may be relevant to withdrawal effects from venlafaxine. Dose reductions made by linear amounts (e.g. 150mg, 112.5mg, 75mg, 37.5mg, 0mg) will cause increasingly large reductions in effect which may cause increasingly severe withdrawal effects (Figure 2.36a). To produce an equal-sized reduction in effect on SERT occupancy will require hyperbolically reducing doses (Figure 2.36b),[10] which informs the reductions presented. This hyperbolic pattern also applies to its occupancy of its other target receptors because of the law of mass action.[8] Consequently, there may be some differences in the precise dose-related activity between receptors but the hyperbolic relationship remains. It is expected that the regimens given below (based on SERT occupancy) will be broadly suitable for other receptor occupancies, such as NET.

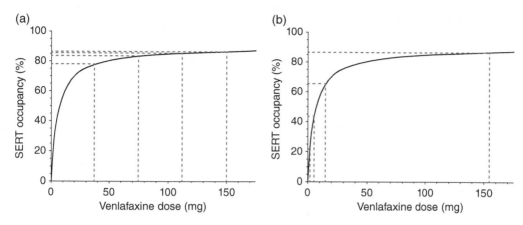

Figure 2.36 (a) Linear reductions of dose cause increasingly large reductions in effect on receptor targets, possibly associated with more withdrawal effects. (b) Even reductions of effect at target receptors requires hyperbolic dose reductions. The final dose before stopping will need to be very small so that this step down is not larger (in terms of effect on receptor occupancy) than previous reductions.

Available formulations: Supplied as tablets in immediate-release and modified-release tablet forms, in capsules as a modified-release form and as a liquid.

Tablets (immediate release)*

Dosage	UK	Europe	USA	Australia	Canada
25mg	–	✓	✓	–	–
37.5mg	✓	✓	✓	✓	✓
50mg	–	✓	✓	–	✓
75mg	✓	✓	✓	✓	✓
150mg	–	–	✓	✓	–
225mg	–	–	✓	–	–

*Tablets supplied as venlafaxine hydrochloride.

Tablets (modified release)*

Dosage	UK	Europe	USA	Australia	Canada
37.5mg	✓	✓	✓	–	–
75mg	✓	✓	✓	–	–
112.5mg	–	–	✓	–	–
150mg	✓	✓	✓	–	–
225mg	✓	✓	✓	–	–
300mg	✓	✓	–	–	–

*Tablets supplied as venlafaxine hydrochloride.

Capsules (modified release)*

Dosage	UK	Europe	USA	Australia	Canada
37.5mg	✓	✓	✓	✓	✓
75mg	✓	✓	✓	✓	✓
150mg	✓	✓	✓	✓	✓
225mg	✓	✓	–	–	–
300mg	✓	–	–	–	–

*Capsules supplied as venlafaxine hydrochloride.

Liquid

Dosage	UK*	Europe	USA	Australia	Canada
37.5mg/5mL (7.5mg/mL)	✓ (150mL)	–	–	–	–
75mg/5mL (15mg/mL)	✓ (150mL)	–	–	–	–

*In UK, liquid form of venlafaxine hydrochloride – is approximately bioequivalent to tablet form. It is recommended that it is not stored at temperatures above 25°C (77°F).[11]

Dilutions: In the UK, to make the solution into a usable form for many doses dilutions will be required. As the liquid solution is dissolved in water and the solubility of venlafaxine hydrochloride is 572mg/mL in water[11] further dilution in water should be acceptable in terms of drug solubility. As its stability cannot be assured it should be consumed immediately, and any unused mixture discarded.

UK dilutions*	Solution required	How to prepare solution
Doses ≥1.5mg	7.5mg/mL	Original solution
Doses ≥0.15mg, <1.5mg	0.75mg/mL	Mix 0.5mL of original solution with 4.5mL of water
Doses <0.15mg	0.075mg/mL	Mix 0.5mL of original solution with 49.5mL of water

*Note: this solution comes as venlafaxine hydrochloride which is approximately bioequivalent to tablet form.

Worked example: To illustrate how the volumes were calculated in the regimens given below we provide a worked example to make up 1mg of venlafaxine. The liquid is bioequivalent to the tablet so 1mg of drug in liquid form is required. This will require a 0.75mg/mL solution, prepared as above. Concentration = mass/volume, so volume = mass/concentration. Therefore, volume = 1/0.75 = 1.33mL (rounded to the nearest 0.01mL). **Off-label options:** Most venlafaxine capsules contain small spheroid beads coated in a membrane that controls diffusion of the drug, and is not pH-dependent.[12] The manufacturer advises that the capsule may be carefully opened and the contents sprinkled on to a spoonful of apple sauce.[12] If the beads are not crushed then their absorption profile is unaffected by this process.[13]

Small doses of venlafaxine can be obtained from these beads but the process is complicated. It involves first emptying out a capsule. The beads from the capsule can be weighed or counted. This should be done with clean and dry hands (or using an instrument like a ruler). The number of beads to be taken will need to be placed back into the original capsule or another gelatine capsule bought from a pharmacy or online. The beads should not be swallowed without a capsule as there are some reports of throat irritation occurring,[14] and should not be chewed as this will remove their extended-release properties.

Each capsule contains the same weight of drug but, because the beads vary in size, they may have different numbers of beads. The regimens given below (in mg) can then be converted into the number of beads required. For example, if a 37.5mg capsule contains, on average, 250 beads, then to achieve a dose of 5mg 33 beads are needed (rounded to the nearest bead). There are various tools to help with these calculations available online.

Alternatively, guidelines for people who cannot swallow tablets (e.g. the NEWT guidelines in the UK,[15] based on local hospital policies and information direct from the manufacturer, and similar USA guidance)[16] suggest that immediate-release tablets of venlafaxine can be crushed and dispersed in water.[15,17] Water could be added to a 37.5mg instant release tablet to make up 37.5mL to yield a 1mg/mL suspension. The tablet may be crushed with a spoon or pestle and mortar before mixing with water to speed up this process. The suspension should be shaken vigorously before use. It should be taken in two divided doses per day because of its short half-life. As its stability cannot be assured it should be consumed immediately, and any unused suspension discarded. Other options to make up small doses include compounding smaller dose tablets, including 'tapering strips'.[18]

Deprescribing notes: Initial reductions can be estimated from Tables 2.11 and 2.22, although patient preference should be taken into account. Sometimes an even smaller reduction to start with may be advisable to boost a patient's confidence that they can taper if performed carefully. Each reduction should be made when the withdrawal symptoms from the previous reduction have largely resolved so that subsequent reductions do not lead to cumulative withdrawal symptoms. Withdrawal symptoms should be tolerable and last at most a couple of weeks (see Figure 2.9). Allowing for a sufficient observation period, reductions can therefore be made about every 2 to 4 weeks. If withdrawal symptoms are moderately severe or take longer than a couple of weeks to resolve, dose reductions should be postponed until symptoms resolve and then made more gradual by choosing a slower tapering rate. If severe withdrawal symptoms occur then the patient should return to a higher dose, wait until symptoms resolve and thereafter taper at a slower rate.

Suggested taper schedules for venlafaxine

A. A faster taper with up to 10 percentage points of SERT between each step (approximate length: 6–10 months). Patients who have been on the medication for only a few weeks will probably be able to taper more quickly and might follow every second or third step of this regimen, and make reductions every few days or so. For people who have only taken an antidepressant for a few weeks, the duration of the taper should not be longer than the period that the patient has been on the drug. For example, if venlafaxine is taken for 3 weeks the taper should be less than 3 weeks.

B. A moderate taper with up to 5 percentage points of SERT between each step (approximate length: 10–20 months).

C. A slower taper with up to 2.5 percentage points of SERT between each step (approximate length: 20–40 months).

D. Some patients will be unable to taper at the slowest rates shown here and will need to taper by even smaller decrements, thus lengthening the overall period of tapering. Such a regimen could be constructed by placing intermediate steps in regimen C. For example, 3mg, 2mg, 1mg, 0mg could be modified to be 3mg, 2.5mg, 2mg, 1.5mg, 1mg, 0.5mg, 0mg. Further intermediate steps could also be added. Microtapering (tapering by a small amount each day, rather than by larger reductions every 2–4 weeks) is another possible approach (see benzodiazepines chapter for further details).

Please note that none of these regimens should be seen as prescriptive – that is, it is not suggested that patient must strictly adhere to them. They are given as example regimens and are not 'set and forget' but should be modified in order to ensure that withdrawal symptoms are tolerable throughout a taper – for example intermediate steps halfway between the doses listed could be added to make a more gradual taper.

A. **Faster taper** with 10 percentage points of SERT between each step – with reductions made every 2–4 weeks.

Step	RO (%)	Dose (mg)	Volume	Step	RO (%)	Dose (mg)	Volume
1	88	300	Use tablets/capsules	7	49	6.9	0.46mL (twice daily)
2	87	150	Use tablets/capsules	8	39	4.5	0.3mL (twice daily)
3	84	75	Use tablets/capsules	Switch to venlafaxine **0.75mg/mL dilution***		
4	78	37.5	Use tablets/capsules	9	29	2.85	1.9mL (twice daily)
Switch to venlafaxine **7.5mg/mL solution***				10	20	1.65	1.1mL (twice daily)
5	68	18	1.2mL (twice daily)**	11	10	0.75	0.50mL (twice daily)
6	59	10.8	0.72mL (twice daily)	12	0	0	Stop Taper
See further steps in the right-hand column							

RO = receptor occupancy
*If a manufacturer's solution is not available, then off-label options for making up small doses including measuring out beads or making a suspension are outlined above.
**Alternatively, one-quarter of a 37.5mg instant release tablet could be taken twice a day.

B. **Moderate taper** with 5 percentage points of SERT between each step – with reductions made every 2–4 weeks.

Step	RO (%)	Dose (mg)	Volume	Step	RO (%)	Dose (mg)	Volume
1	88.4	300	Use tablets/capsules	14	41.1	4.9	0.33mL (twice daily)
2	86.7	150	Use tablets/capsules	15	36.9	4	0.27mL (twice daily)
3	83.6	75	Use tablets/capsules	16	32.8	3.3	0.22mL (twice daily)
Switch to venlafaxine **7.5mg/mL solution**				Switch to venlafaxine **0.75mg/mL dilution**			
4	80.7	50	3.33mL (twice daily)**	17	28.7	2.7	1.80mL (twice daily)
5	78.0	37.5	2.50mL (twice daily)**	18	24.6	2.2	1.47mL (twice daily)
6	73.9	27	1.80mL (twice daily)	19	20.5	1.7	1.13mL (twice daily)
7	69.8	20	1.33mL (twice daily)	20	16.4	1.3	0.87mL (twice daily)
8	65.7	16	1.07mL (twice daily)	21	12.3	0.92	0.61mL (twice daily)
9	61.6	13	0.87mL (twice daily)	22	8.2	0.58	0.39mL (twice daily)
10	57.5	10	0.67mL (twice daily)	Switch to venlafaxine **0.075mg/mL dilution**			
11	53.4	8.4	0.56mL (twice daily)	23	4.1	0.28	1.87mL (twice daily)
12	49.3	7	0.47mL (twice daily)	24	0	0	0
13	45.2	5.8	0.39mL (twice daily)				
See further steps in the right-hand column							

RO = receptor occupancy
*If a manufacturer's solution is not available, then off-label options for making up small doses including measuring out beads or making a suspension are outlined above.
**Alternatively, a capsule or tablet, or portion of a tablet can be used. If this is immediate release then it should be taken twice a day in divided portions.

C. **Slower taper** with 2.5 percentage points of SERT occupancy between each step – with reductions made every 2–4 weeks.

Step	RO (%)	Dose (mg)	Volume	Step	RO (%)	Dose (mg)	Volume
1	88.4	300	Use tablets/capsules	25	41.7	5	0.33mL (twice daily)
2	86.7	150	Use tablets/capsules	26	39.8	4.6	0.31mL (twice daily)
3	85.7	112.5	Use tablets/capsules	27	37.8	4.2	0.28mL (twice daily)
4	83.6	75	Use tablets/capsules	28	35.7	3.8	0.25mL (twice daily)
Switch to venlafaxine **7.5mg/mL solution***				29	33.9	3.5	0.23mL (twice daily)
5	81.5	55	3.67mL (twice daily)	30	32.0	3.2	0.21mL (twice daily)
6	79.8	45	3.00mL (twice daily)	Switch to venlafaxine **0.75mg/mL dilution***			
7	77.6	37.5	2.50mL (twice daily)**	31	30.0	2.9	1.93mL (twice daily)
8	75.7	30.4	2.03mL (twice daily)	32	27.9	2.6	1.73mL (twice daily)
9	73.7	26	1.73mL (twice daily)	33	25.6	2.3	1.53mL (twice daily)
10	71.7	22.6	1.51mL (twice daily)	34	23.5	2.05	1.37mL (twice daily)
11	69.7	19.8	1.32mL (twice daily)	35	21.3	1.8	1.2mL (twice daily)
12	67.7	17.5	1.17mL (twice daily)	36	19.5	1.6	1.07mL (twice daily)
13	65.7	15.6	1.04mL (twice daily)	37	17.5	1.4	0.93mL (twice daily)
14	63.7	14	0.93mL (twice daily)	38	16.0	1.25	0.83mL (twice daily)
15	61.7	12.6	0.84mL (twice daily)	39	14.4	1.1	0.73mL (twice daily)
16	59.7	11.4	0.76mL (twice daily)	40	12.7	0.95	0.63mL (twice daily)
17	57.7	10.4	0.69mL (twice daily)	41	10.9	0.8	0.53mL (twice daily)
18	55.7	9.4	0.63mL (twice daily)	42	9.1	0.65	0.43mL (twice daily)
19	53.8	8.6	0.57mL (twice daily)	43	7.1	0.5	0.33mL (twice daily)
20	51.8	7.8	0.52mL (twice daily)	44	5.1	0.35	0.23mL (twice daily)
21	49.8	7.2	0.48mL (twice daily)	Switch to venlafaxine **0.075mg/mL dilution***			
22	47.8	6.6	0.44mL (twice daily)	45	3.0	0.2	1.33mL (twice daily)
23	45.8	6	0.40mL (twice daily)	46	1.5	0.1	0.67mL (twice daily)
24	43.8	5.5	0.37mL (twice daily)	47	0	0	0
See further steps in the right-hand column							

RO = receptor occupancy

*If a manufacturer's solution is not available, then off-label options for making up small doses including measuring out beads or making a suspension are outlined above.

**Alternatively, a capsule or tablet can be used. If this is instant release then it should be taken twice a day in divided portions.

References

1. Dexcel Pharma. Venlafaxine 37.5 mg tablets. https://www.medicines.org.uk/emc/product/773/smpc (accessed 15 October 2022).
2. Henssler J, Heinz A, Brandt L, Bschor T. Antidepressant withdrawal and rebound phenomena. *Dtsch Arztebl Int* 2019; 116: 355–61.
3. Quilichini J-B, Revet A, Garcia P, et al. Comparative effects of 15 antidepressants on the risk of withdrawal syndrome: a real-world study using the WHO pharmacovigilance database. *J Affect Disord* 2021; 297: 189–93.
4. Horowitz MA, Framer A, Hengartner MP, Sørensen A, Taylor D. Estimating risk of antidepressant withdrawal from a review of published data. *CNS Drugs* 2022; published online 14 December. doi:10.1007/s40263-022-00960-y.
5. Sir A, D'Souza RF, Uguz S, et al. Randomized trial of sertraline versus venlafaxine XR in major depression: efficacy and discontinuation symptoms. *J Clin Psychiatry* 2005; 66: 1312–20.
6. Gastaldon C, Schoretsanitis G, Arzenton E, et al. Withdrawal syndrome following discontinuation of 28 antidepressants: pharmacovigilance analysis of 31,688 reports from the WHO spontaneous reporting database. *Drug Saf* 2022; 45: 1539–49.
7. Sørensen A, Ruhé HG, Munkholm K. The relationship between dose and serotonin transporter occupancy of antidepressants – a systematic review. *Mol Psychiatry* 2022; 27: 192–201.
8. Holford N. Pharmacodynamic principles and the time course of delayed and cumulative drug effects. *Transl Clin* 2018; 26: 56–59.
9. Furukawa TA, Cipriani A, Cowen PJ, Leucht S, Egger M, Salanti G. Optimal dose of selective serotonin reuptake inhibitors, venlafaxine, and mirtazapine in major depression: a systematic review and dose-response meta-analysis. *The Lancet Psychiatry* 2019; 6: 601–9.
10. Horowitz MA, Taylor D. Tapering of SSRI treatment to mitigate withdrawal symptoms. *The Lancet Psychiatry* 2019; 6: 538–46.
11. Rosemont Pharmaceuticals. Venlafaxine 75mg/5ml oral solution. https://www.medicines.org.uk/emc/product/12750/smpc (accessed 15 October 2022).
12. Pfizer. Label for effexor XR (venlafaxine Extended-Release) capsules. 2017. https://www.accessdata.fda.gov/drugsatfda_docs/label/2017/020699s107lbl.pdf (accessed 15 February 2023).
13. Jain RT, Panda J, Srivastava A. Two formulations of venlafaxine are bioequivalent when administered as open capsule mixed with applesauce to healthy subjects. *Indian J Pharm Sci* 2011; 73: 510–6.
14. FDA. Memorandum: DMETS medication error postmarketing safety review: Cymbalta. Fda.gov. 2007; published online 8 March. www.fda.gov/media/74134/download (accessed 9 September 2022).
15. Smyth J. The NEWT guidelines for administration of medication to patients with enteral feeding tubes or swallowing difficulties website. The NEWT Guidelines. 2011. https://www.newtguidelines.com/index.html (accessed 7 September 2022).
16. Bostwick JR, Demehri A. Pills to powder: An updated clinician's reference for crushable psychotropics. *Curr Psychiatr* 2017; 16: 46–9.
17. Brennan K. Selective serotonin reuptake inhibitor (SSRI) formulations suggested for adults with swallowing difficulties. SPS – Specialist Pharmacy Service. 2021; published online 1 July. https://www.sps.nhs.uk/articles/selective-serotonin-reuptake-inhibitor-ssri-formulations-suggested-for-adults-with-swallowing-difficulties/ (accessed 19 September 2022).
18. Groot PC, van Os J. How user knowledge of psychotropic drug withdrawal resulted in the development of person-specific tapering medication. *Ther Adv Psychopharmacol* 2020; 10: 204512532093245.

Vilazodone

Trade name: Viibryd.

Description: Vilazodone binds with high affinity to SERT and is also as a 5-HT$_{1A}$ receptor partial agonist.[1] It has little affinity for noradrenaline or dopamine transporters.[1]

Withdrawal effects: Withdrawal effects from vilazodone have been demonstrated in double-blind placebo-controlled randomised controlled trials after 8 weeks of treatment. Withdrawal effects including nightmares, suicidal ideation, depression, anxiety and abnormal dreams were all more likely in the group of patients stopping vilazodone compared with those stopping placebo.[2] The incidence of a withdrawal syndrome or its severity and duration have not been reported. In an analysis of the WHO adverse effect database, vilazodone emerged as moderate risk for withdrawal effects compared to other antidepressants.[3]

Peak plasma: 4–5 hours.[1]

Half-life: Approximately 25 hours, allowing for once per day administration.[4] Every-other-day dosing is not recommended for tapering because of the substantial reductions in plasma concentrations this would produce, possibly giving rise to withdrawal effects.

Receptor occupancy: The relationship between dose of vilazodone and the occupancy of SERT, for which neuroimaging has been performed, is hyperbolic.[5] This applies to its occupancy of other receptors because of the law of mass action.[6] Antidepressants also show a hyperbolic pattern between dose and clinical effects,[7] which may be relevant to withdrawal effects from vilazodone (Figure 2.37a and b). There may be some differences in the precise dose-related activity between receptor targets but the hyperbolic relationship remains. Consequently, the regimens given below (based on SERT occupancy) will be broadly suitable for other receptor occupancies.

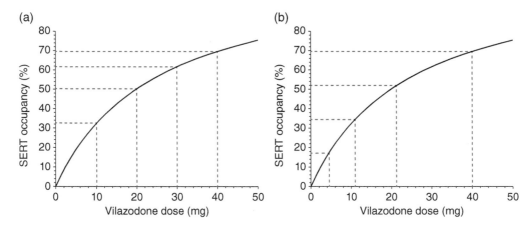

Figure 2.37 (a) Linear reductions of dose cause increasingly large reductions in effect on receptor targets, possibly associated with more withdrawal effects. (b) Even reductions of effect at target receptors requires hyperbolic dose reductions. The final dose before stopping will need to be very small so that this step down is not larger (in terms of effect on receptor occupancy) than previous reductions.

Available formulations: Vilazodone is available as vilazodone hydrochloride in tablets.

Tablets

Dosage	UK	Europe	USA	Australia	Canada
5mg	–	–	✓	–	✓
20mg	–	–	✓	–	✓
40mg	–	–	✓	–	✓

Off-label options: Vilazodone is provided as a standard tablet and so can be split or crushed in order to taper.[8] It has limited solubility in water.[9] A 1mg/mL suspension could be formed by adding water to a 20mg tablet to make up 20mL. This should be shaken vigorously before use. The stability of this suspension cannot be assured and so it should be consumed immediately after preparation and the remnants discarded. Compounding pharmacies may be able to make up liquid versions or compound smaller formulations of tablets, as for 'tapering strips'.[10]

Worked example: To illustrate how the volumes were calculated in the regimens given below we provide a worked example. To make up 2mg of vilazodone a 1mg/mL suspension can be used, made up as outlined above. The volume of 1mg/mL liquid required to give a dose of 2mg of vilazodone is $2/1 = 2mL$.

Deprescribing notes: Initial reductions can be estimated from Tables 2.11 and 2.22, although patient preference should be taken into account. Sometimes an even smaller reduction to start with may be advisable to boost a patient's confidence that they can taper if performed carefully. Each reduction should be made when the withdrawal symptoms from the previous reduction have largely resolved so that subsequent reductions do not lead to cumulative withdrawal symptoms. Withdrawal symptoms should be tolerable and last at most a couple of weeks (see Figure 2.9). Allowing for a sufficient observation period, reductions can therefore be made about every 2 to 4 weeks. If withdrawal symptoms are moderately severe or take longer than a couple of weeks to resolve, dose reductions should be postponed until symptoms resolve and then made more gradual by choosing a slower tapering rate. If severe withdrawal symptoms occur then the patient should return to a higher dose, wait until symptoms resolve and thereafter taper at a slower rate.

Suggested taper schedules for vilazodone

A. A faster taper with up to 10 percentage points of SERT occupancy between each step with reductions made every 2–4 weeks (approximate length: 5–10 months). Patients who have been on the medication for only a few weeks will probably be able to taper more quickly and might follow every second or third step of this regimen and make reductions every few days or so. For people who have only taken an antidepressant for a few weeks, the duration of the taper should not be longer than the period that the patient has been on the drug.

B. A moderate taper with up to 5 percentage points of SERT occupancy between each step with reductions made every 2–4 weeks (approximate length: 10–20 months).

C. A slower taper with up to 2.5 percentage points of SERT occupancy between each step with reductions made every 2–4 weeks (approximate length: 20–40 months).

D. Some patients will be unable to taper at the slowest rates shown here and will need to taper by even smaller decrements, thus lengthening the overall period of tapering.

Such a regimen could be constructed by placing intermediate steps in regimen C. For example, 3mg, 2mg, 1mg, 0mg could be modified to be 3mg, 2.5mg, 2mg, 1.5mg, 1mg, 0.5mg, 0mg. Further intermediate steps could also be added. Microtapering (tapering by a small amount each day, rather than by larger reductions every 2–4 weeks) is another possible approach (see benzodiazepines chapter for further details).

Please note that none of these regimens should be seen as prescriptive – that is, it is not suggested that patient must strictly adhere to them. They are given as example regimens and are not 'set and forget' but should be modified in order to ensure that withdrawal symptoms are tolerable throughout a taper – for example intermediate steps halfway between the doses listed could be added to make a more gradual taper.

A. **Faster taper** with up to 10 percentage points of SERT occupancy between each step – with reductions made every 2–4 weeks.*

Step	RO (%)	Dose (mg)	Volume	Step	RO (%)	Dose (mg)	Volume
1	69.7	40	Use tablets	7	26.4	7.5	Use ½ tablets**
2	61.9	30	Use tablets	8	19.1	5	Use tablets
3	56.8	25	Use tablets	9	10.4	2.5	Use ½ tablets**
4	50.5	20	Use tablets	10	5.5	1.25	Use ¼ tablets**
5	42.7	15	Use tablets	11	0	0	0
6	32.6	10	Use tablets				
See further steps in the right-hand column							

RO = receptor occupancy
*The time between each decrease may be shortened to one week if the patient is able to make the first couple of reductions with no withdrawal symptoms. The interval between reductions should never be less than one week because this might increase the risk of relapse, even in the absence of withdrawal effects.[11,12]
**Alternatively, a liquid or compounded version of vilazodone could be used to make up these doses, as above.

B. **Moderate taper** with up to 5 percentage points of SERT occupancy between each step – with reductions made every 2–4 weeks.

Step	RO (%)	Dose (mg)	Volume	Step	RO (%)	Dose (mg)	Volume
1	69.7	40	Use tablets	12	32.6	10	Use tablets
2	66.1	35	Use tablets	13	29.6	8.75	Use ¾ tablets*
3	61.9	30	Use tablets	14	26.4	7.5	Use ½ tablets*
4	59.5	27.5	Use ½ tablets*	15	22.9	6.25	Use ¼ tablets*
5	56.8	25	Use tablets	16	19.1	5	Use tablets
6	53.8	22.5	Use ½ tablets*	17	14.9	3.75	Use ¾ tablets
7	50.5	20	Use tablets	18	10.4	2.5	Use ½ tablets*
8	46.9	17.5	Use ½ tablets*	19	5.5	1.25	Use ¼ tablets*
9	42.7	15	Use tablets	Switch to vilazodone **1mg/mL suspension**			
10	38	12.5	Use ½ tablets*	20	2.7	0.6	0.6mL
11	35.4	11.25	Use ¼ tablets*	21	0	0	0
See further steps in the right-hand column							

RO = receptor occupancy
*Alternatively, a liquid or compounded version of vilazodone could be used to make up these doses, as above.

C. **Slower taper** with up to 2.5 percentage points of SERT occupancy between each step – with reductions made every 2–4 weeks.

Step	RO (%)	Dose (mg)	Volume	Step	RO (%)	Dose (mg)	Volume	Step	RO (%)	Dose (mg)	Volume
1	69.7	40	Use tabs	14	46.9	17.5	Use ½ tabs*	25	22.9	6.25	6.25mL
2	68	37.5	Use ½ tabs*	15	44.9	16.25	Use ¼ tabs*	26	20.6	5.5	5.5mL
3	66.1	35	Use tabs	16	42.7	15	Use tabs	27	18.3	4.75	4.75mL
4	64.1	32.5	Use ½ tabs*	17	40.4	13.75	Use ¾ tabs*	28	15.8	4	4mL
5	61.9	30	Use tabs	18	38	12.5	Use ½ tabs*	29	14.1	3.5	3.5mL
6	59.5	27.5	Use ½ tabs*	Switch to vilazodone **1mg/mL suspension**			30	12.3	3	3mL
7	58.1	26.25	Use ¼ tabs*	19	35.9	11.5	11.5mL	31	10.4	2.5	2.5mL
8	56.8	25	Use tabs*	20	33.8	10.5	10.5mL	32	8.5	2	2mL
9	55.3	23.75	Use ¾ tabs*	21	31.4	9.5	9.5mL	33	6.5	1.5	1.5mL
10	53.8	22.5	Use ½ tabs*	22	29	8.5	8.5mL	34	4.4	1	1mL
11	52.2	21.25	Use ¼ tabs*	23	27	7.75	7.75mL	35	2.3	0.5	0.5mL
12	50.5	20	Use tabs	24	25	7	7mL	36	0	0	0
13	48.8	18.75	Use ¾ tabs*								
See further steps in the middle column				**See further steps in the right-hand column**							

RO = receptor occupancy, tabs = tablets
*Alternatively, a liquid or compounded version of vilazodone could be used to make up these doses, as above.

References

1. FDA. Vilazodone – highlights of prescribing information. 2021.
2. Kaja H, Oosthuizen F, Michael H, Mensah KB, Bangalee V, Wiafe E. A systematic review of the psychiatric-adverse effects associated with the administration of vilazodone. *Sys Rev Pharm* 2021; 12: 3657–65.
3. Gastaldon C, Schoretsanitis G, Arzenton E, et al. Withdrawal syndrome following discontinuation of 28 antidepressants: Pharmacovigilance analysis of 31,688 reports from the WHO spontaneous reporting database. *Drug Saf* 2022; 45: 1539–49.
4. Cruz MP. Vilazodone HCl (Viibryd): A serotonin partial agonist and reuptake inhibitor for the treatment of major depressive disorder. *P T* 2012; 37: 28–31.
5. Hughes ZA, Starr KR, Langmead CJ, et al. Neurochemical evaluation of the novel 5-HT1A receptor partial agonist/serotonin reuptake inhibitor, vilazodone. *Eur J Pharmacol* 2005; 510: 49–57.
6. Holford N. Pharmacodynamic principles and the time course of delayed and cumulative drug effects. *Transl Clin* 2018; 26: 56.
7. Furukawa TA, Cipriani A, Cowen PJ, Leucht S, Egger M, Salanti G. Optimal dose of selective serotonin reuptake inhibitors, venlafaxine, and mirtazapine in major depression: a systematic review and dose-response meta-analysis. *The Lancet Psychiatry* 2019; 6: 601–9.
8. Bostwick JR, Demehri A. Pills to powder: an updated clinician's reference for crushable psychotropics Jolene. *Curr Psychiatr* 2017; 16: 46–9.
9. Chemical C. Vilazodone (hydrochloride) – product information. Cayman Chemical. 2022. https://cdn.caymanchem.com/cdn/insert/21547.pdf (accessed 15 October 2022).
10. Groot PC, van Os J. How user knowledge of psychotropic drug withdrawal resulted in the development of person-specific tapering medication. *Ther Adv Psychopharmacol* 2020; 10: 204512532093245.
11. Baldessarini RJ, Tondo L, Ghiani C, Lepri B. Illness risk following rapid versus gradual discontinuation of antidepressants. *Am J Psychiatry* 2010; 167: 934–41.
12. Gøtzsche PC, Demasi M. Interventions to help patients withdraw from depression drugs: A systematic review. *Int J Risk Saf Med*. 2023 September 13. doi: 10.3233/JRS-230011. Epub ahead of print.

CHAPTER 2

Vortioxetine

Trade names: Trintellix, Brintellix.

Description: Vortioxetine inhibits SERT.[1] It is also thought to be a 5-HT_3, 5-HT_7 and 5-HT_{1D} receptor antagonist, a 5-HT_{1B} receptor partial agonist, and a 5-HT_{1A} receptor agonist. It is suspected to also have activity in the norepinephrine, dopamine, histamine, acetylcholine, GABA and glutamate systems.[1]

Withdrawal effects: Vortioxetine was classified as of moderate risk of withdrawal effects in a structured analysis,[2] but there is a lack of trials evaluating the incidence, severity and duration of its withdrawal effects.[3]

Peak plasma: 7–11 hours.[1]

Half-life: 66 hours. According to the manufacturer vortioxetine should be taken once daily.[1] Because of its long half-life every-other-day dosing should not produce significant withdrawal effects, although this has not been formally evaluated. Less frequent than every-other-day dosing may precipitate withdrawal effects because of substantial reductions in plasma levels, possibly leading to withdrawal effects.

Receptor occupancy: The relationship between dose of vortioxetine and occupancy of SERT is hyperbolic.[4] This hyperbolic pattern also applies to its occupancy of the other receptors targets because of the law of mass action.[5] Antidepressants also show a hyperbolic pattern between dose and clinical effects,[6] which may be relevant to withdrawal effects from vortioxetine. Dose reductions made by linear amounts (e.g. 20mg, 15mg, 10mg, 5mg, 0mg) will cause increasingly large reductions in effect which may cause increasingly severe withdrawal effects (Figure 2.38a). To produce equal-sized reductions in effect on SERT occupancy will require hyperbolically reducing doses (Figure 2.38b),[7] which informs the reductions presented.

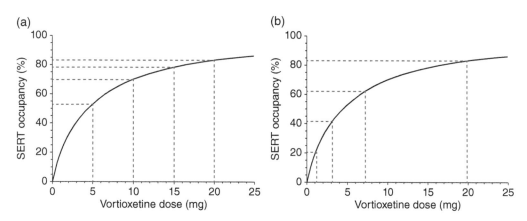

Figure 2.38 (a) Linear reductions of dose cause increasingly large reductions in effect on receptor targets, possibly associated with more withdrawal effects. (b) Even reductions of effect at target receptors requires hyperbolic dose reductions. The final dose before stopping will need to be very small so that this step down is not larger (in terms of effect on receptor occupancy) than previous reductions.

Available formulations: Vortioxetine is available as film-coated tablets.

Tablets

Dosage	UK	Europe	USA	Australia	Canada
5mg	✓	✓	✓	✓	✓
10mg	✓	✓	✓	✓	✓
15mg	–	✓	–	✓	✓
20mg	✓	✓	✓	✓	✓

Off-label options: Vortioxetine comes as a film-coated tablet. Authoritative guidance from the USA for people who cannot swallow tablets advises that vortioxetine can be safely crushed and mixed with water for administration,[8] to facilitate the tapering process. The film coating does not confer any particular properties with respect to absorption. A 1mg/mL suspension could be made by adding water to a 10mg tablet to make up 10mL. The tablet can be crushed with a spoon or pestle and mortar to speed up disintegration. Vigorous shaking of this suspension before administration will ensure that the active drug is equally distributed throughout the liquid. As its stability cannot be assured it should be consumed immediately, and any unused suspension discarded.

Worked example: To illustrate how the volumes were calculated in the regimens given below we provide a worked example. To make up 2mg of vortioxetine a 1mg/mL suspension can be used, made up as outlined above. The volume of 1mg/mL liquid required to give a dose of 2mg of vortioxetine is 2/1 = 2mL.

Deprescribing notes: Initial reductions can be estimated from Tables 2.11 and 2.22, although patient preference should be respected. Sometimes an even smaller reduction to start with may be advisable to boost a patient's confidence that they can taper if performed carefully. Each reduction should be made when the withdrawal symptoms from the previous reduction have largely resolved so that subsequent reductions do not lead to cumulative withdrawal symptoms. Withdrawal symptoms should be tolerable and last at most a couple of weeks (see Figure 2.9). Allowing for a sufficient observation period, reductions can therefore be made about every 2 to 4 weeks. If withdrawal symptoms are moderately severe or take longer than a couple of weeks to resolve, dose reductions should be postponed until symptoms resolve and then made more gradual by choosing a slower tapering rate. If severe withdrawal symptoms occur then the patient should return to a higher dose, wait until symptoms resolve and thereafter taper at a slower rate.

Suggested taper schedules for vortioxetine

A. A faster taper with up to 10 percentage points of SERT occupancy between each step (approximate length: 5–10 months). Patients who have been on the medication for only a few weeks will probably be able to taper more quickly and might follow every second or third step of this regimen, and make reductions every few days or so. For people who have only taken an antidepressant for a few weeks, the duration of the taper should not be longer than the period that the patient has been on the drug. For example, if vortioxetine is taken for 3 weeks the taper should be less than 3 weeks.

B. A moderate taper with 5 percentage points of SERT occupancy between each step (approximate length: 10–20 months).

C. A slower taper with 2.5 percentage points of SERT occupancy between each step (approximate length: 20–40 months).

D. Some patients will be unable to taper at the slowest rates shown here and will need to taper by even smaller decrements, thus lengthening the overall period of tapering. Such a regimen could be constructed by placing intermediate steps in regimen C. For example, 3mg, 2mg, 1mg, 0mg could be modified to be 3mg, 2.5mg, 2mg, 1.5mg, 1mg, 0.5mg, 0mg. Further intermediate steps could also be added. Microtapering (tapering by a small amount each day, rather than by larger reductions every 2–4 weeks) is another possible approach (see benzodiazepines chapter for further details).

Please note that none of these regimens should be seen as prescriptive – that is, it is not suggested that patient must strictly adhere to them. They are given as example regimens and are not 'set and forget' but should be modified in order to ensure that withdrawal symptoms are tolerable throughout a taper – for example intermediate steps halfway between the doses listed could be added to make a more gradual taper.

A. **Faster taper** with up to 10 percentage points of SERT occupancy between each step – with reductions made every 2–4 weeks.*

Step	RO (%)	Dose (mg)	Volume	Step	RO (%)	Dose (mg)	Volume
1	82.9	20	Use tablets	6	43.3	3.5	3.5mL
2	77.9	15	Use tablets	7	34.6	2.4	2.4mL***
3	69.3	10	Use tablets	8	26	1.6	1.6mL
Switch to vortioxetine **1mg/mL suspension**				9	17.3	1	1mL
4	60.6	7	7mL**	10	8.7	0.4	0.4mL
5	52	5	5mL***	11	0	0	0
See further steps in the right-hand column							

RO = receptor occupancy

* For longer term users, the time between each decrease may be shortened to 1 week if the patient is able to make the first couple of reductions with no withdrawal symptoms. The interval between reductions should never be less than 1 week because this might increase the risk of relapse, even in the absence of withdrawal effects.[9,10]

**Alternatively, this could be given as alternating day dosing of vortioxetine (due to its long elimination half-life). E.g. 5mg alternating with 10mg to make approximately 7mg and 5mg every-other-day to make up 2.4mg.

***Alternatively, this could be administered as a tablet or half tablet.

B. **Moderate taper** with 5 percentage points of SERT occupancy between each step – with reductions made every 2–4 weeks.

Step	RO (%)	Dose (mg)	Volume	Step	RO (%)	Dose (mg)	Volume
1	82.9	20	Use tablets	11	41	3.1	3.1mL
2	77.9	15	Use tablets	12	36.9	2.6	2.6mL**
Switch to vortioxetine **1mg/mL suspension**				13	32.8	2.2	2.2mL
3	73.8	12	12mL*	14	28.7	1.8	1.8mL
4	69.7	10	10mL**	15	24.6	1.5	1.5mL
5	65.6	8.5	8.5mL	16	20.5	1.2	1.2mL
6	61.5	7	7mL*	17	16.4	0.9	0.9mL
7	57.4	6	6mL	18	12.3	0.6	0.6mL
8	53.3	5	5mL**	19	8.2	0.4	0.4mL
9	49.2	4.3	4.3mL	20	4.1	0.2	0.2mL
10	45.1	3.7	3.7mL	21	0	0	0
See further steps in the right-hand column							

RO = receptor occupancy
*Alternatively, this could be given as alternating day dosing of vortioxetine (due to its long elimination half-life). E.g. 15mg alternating with 10mg to make approximately 12mg, 5mg alternating with 10mg to make approximately 7mg and 5mg every-other-day to make up 2.6mg approximately.
**Alternatively, could be administered as a tablet or half tablet.

C. **Slower taper** with 2.5 percentage points of SERT occupancy between each step – with reductions made every 2–4 weeks.

Step	RO (%)	Dose (mg)	Volume	Step	RO (%)	Dose (mg)	Volume	Step	RO (%)	Dose (mg)	Volume
1	82.9	20	Use tablets	14	54.8	5.4	5.4mL	28	25.3	1.5	1.5mL
2	80.7	17.5	Use ¾ tablets*	15	52.7	5	5mL**	29	23.2	1.35	1.35mL
3	77.9	15	Use tablets	16	50.5	4.6	4.6mL	30	21.1	1.2	1.2mL
Switch to vortioxetine **1mg/mL suspension**				17	48.4	4.2	4.2mL	31	19	1.05	1.05mL
4	75.8	13.5	13.5mL	18	46.3	3.9	3.9mL	32	16.8	0.9	0.9mL
5	73.7	12	12mL***	19	44.2	3.6	3.6mL	33	14.7	0.75	0.75mL
6	71.6	11	11mL	20	42.1	3.3	3.3mL	34	12.6	0.6	0.6mL
7	69.5	10	10mL**	21	40	3	3mL	35	10.5	0.5	0.5mL
8	67.4	9	9mL	22	37.9	2.7	2.7mL	36	8.42	0.4	0.4mL
9	65.3	8.3	8.3mL	23	35.8	2.5	2.5mL***	37	6.32	0.3	0.3mL
10	63.2	7.6	7.6mL***	24	33.7	2.3	2.3mL	38	4.21	0.2	0.2mL
11	61.1	7	7mL	25	31.6	2.1	2.1mL	Switch to vortioxetine **0.1mg/mL suspension**			
12	59	6.4	6.4mL	26	29.5	1.9	1.9mL	39	2.11	0.1	1mL
13	56.9	5.9	5.9mL	27	27.4	1.7	1.7mL	40	0	0	0
See further steps in the middle column				**See further steps in the right-hand column**							

RO = receptor occupancy
*Alternatively, could be administered as a liquid (17.5mL of a 1mg/mL suspension).
**Alternatively, could be administered as a tablet or half tablet.
***Alternatively, this could be given as alternating day dosing of vortioxetine (due to its long elimination half-life). E.g. 15mg alternating with 10mg to make approximately 12mg and 5mg alternating with 10mg to make approximately 7.6mg.

References

1. Lundbeck. Vortioxetine summary of product characteristics. 2021. https://www.medicines.org.uk/emc/product/7121/smpc#gref (accessed 27 September 2022).
2. Henssler J, Heinz A, Brandt L, Bschor T. Antidepressant withdrawal and rebound phenomena. *Dtsch Arztebl Int* 2019; 116: 355–61.
3. Horowitz MA, Framer A, Hengartner MP, Sørensen A, Taylor D. Estimating risk of antidepressant withdrawal from a review of published data. *CNS Drugs* 2022; published online 14 December. doi:10.1007/s40263-022-00960-y.
4. Sørensen A, Ruhé HG, Munkholm K. The relationship between dose and serotonin transporter occupancy of antidepressants – a systematic review. *Mol Psychiatry* 2022; 27: 192–201.
5. Holford N. Pharmacodynamic principles and the time course of delayed and cumulative drug effects. *Transl Clin* 2018; 26: 56.
6. Furukawa TA, Cipriani A, Cowen PJ, Leucht S, Egger M, Salanti G. Optimal dose of selective serotonin reuptake inhibitors, venlafaxine, and mirtazapine in major depression: a systematic review and dose-response meta-analysis. *The Lancet Psychiatry* 2019; 6: 601–9.
7. Horowitz MA, Taylor D. Tapering of SSRI treatment to mitigate withdrawal symptoms. *The Lancet Psychiatry* 2019; 6: 538–46.
8. Bostwick JR, Demehri A. Pills to powder: an updated clinician's reference for crushable psychotropics. *Curr Psychiatr* 2017; 16: 46–9.
9. Baldessarini RJ, Tondo L, Ghiani C, Lepri B. Illness risk following rapid versus gradual discontinuation of antidepressants. *Am J Psychiatry* 2010; 167: 934–41.
10. Gøtzsche PC, Demasi M. Interventions to help patients withdraw from depression drugs: A systematic review. *Int J Risk Saf Med.* 2023 September 13. doi: 10.3233/JRS-230011. Epub ahead of print.

Safe Deprescribing of Benzodiazepines and Z-drugs

When and Why to Stop Benzodiazepines and Z-drugs

Benzodiazepines and z-drugs are widely used throughout the world for conditions such as anxiety, insomnia, epilepsy, alcohol withdrawal and pre-medication before procedures. They are also used in a wide variety of 'off-label' cases such as restless leg syndrome, tinnitus, dementia and mania. Their benefits in acute syndromes are clear and there is some evidence that efficacy persists when used for a number of weeks.[1,2] Nonetheless, the dangers of long-term prescribing are widely accepted.[3] Longer-term use is associated with a number of physical and cognitive risks, including loss of efficacy, physical dependence, tolerance, memory disturbance,[4] falls and fractures,[5] potentially dementia[6,7] and likely increased mortality.[8] The FDA in the USA has recently re-emphasised the risks of abuse, misuse, addiction, physical dependence and withdrawal with benzodiazepines by requiring a boxed warning (previously called a black box warning), its most prominent warning, for this drug class.[9] Most clinical guidelines recommend that benzodiazepines and z-drugs should be used only for crisis situations, and not for longer than 2–4 weeks.[10–12]

Guidelines often recommend that long-term users should have benzodiazepines deprescribed because of their unfavourable balance of benefits and harms. For example, in the USA, Kaiser Permanente advises that 'all patients should be encouraged to discontinue chronic use of benzodiazepines and Z-drugs' as 'there is no evidence to support the long-term use [longer than 2 weeks] of these drugs for insomnia or any mental health indication'.[10] In the UK, NICE recommends that people on long-term benzodiazepines or z-drugs should be advised to stop, largely because of the risks of tolerance and dependence.[13] NICE recommends that dependence-forming medications like benzodiazepines and z-drugs should be reviewed regularly, with the benefits and harms assessed and support provided for people who wish to stop taking them.[13]

Long-term use remains common in the UK with 300,000 adults taking either a benzodiazepine or z-drug for more than 12 months.[14] In the USA, in 2019, an estimated

92 million benzodiazepine prescriptions were dispensed from US outpatient pharmacies, with alprazolam (38%) being the most common, followed by clonazepam (24%) and then lorazepam (20%).[9] In total, 30.6 million adults in the USA (one in eight adults) used benzodiazepines in 2015/2016.[15] In 2018, an estimated 50% of patients who were dispensed oral benzodiazepines received them for a duration of two months or longer.[9]

It should be noted that this chapter focuses on patients taking benzodiazepines and z-drugs for common mental health conditions such as anxiety and insomnia. People with serious mental illness (bipolar disorder, schizophrenia, etc) are also prescribed benzodiazepines, and while deprescribing may also be warranted in these patients, the risks may be greater (while the benefits are likely similar) and a more cautious approach is generally warranted.

Adverse effects

The dangers of long-term benzodiazepine use are well recognised (Table 3.1). Benzodiazepines impair cognition: long-term use has been associated with deficits in memory, attention, processing speed, and reaction time.[16] They can also cause motor

Table 3.1 Adverse effects of benzodiazepines.

Cognitive*[5,13,17,19]	Reactions which can be mistaken for a psychiatric disorder[44]
■ Deficits in memory ■ Deficits in attention ■ Increased reaction time ■ Motor incoordination ■ Drowsiness ■ Nightmares/intrusive thoughts ■ Impaired judgement ■ Reduced social functioning due to effects on memory, inability to remember new people, appointments, etc ■ Perceptual illusions/hallucinations	■ Agitation ■ Emotional lability ■ Restlessness ■ Inter-dose withdrawal
Physical[16]	**Emotional[13,16]**
■ Motor incoordination/ataxia ■ Dizziness ■ Slurred speech ■ Sensory alterations (e.g. tinnitus, strange tastes, paraesthesia, numbness and burning) ■ Rash ■ Autonomic dysfunction (e.g. tachycardia, bradycardia, diaphoresis, hypotension and hypertension)	■ Depression/dysphoria (new onset or worsening – in some cases this can involve precipitation of suicidality) ■ Emotional blunting/numbness ■ Anxiety/phobias/panic ■ Anger/irritability/mood lability ■ Agoraphobia ■ Reduced coping skills ■ Excitement/euphoria
Increased morbidity[45]	**Behaviour[16,36]**
■ Increased risk of motor vehicle accidents ■ Higher risk of falls (elderly) ■ Delirium (elderly) ■ ?Dementia ■ ?Cancer ■ ?Infections	■ Insomnia ■ Avoidance/agoraphobia ■ Appetite/weight (anorexia, weight gain) ■ Impulsivity/disinhibition ■ Suicidality ■ Aggression

*Some of these impairments can persist after discontinuation.

incoordination, drowsiness and ataxia.[16] Impairment in many of these domains can persist even after discontinuation.[17] Many patients on long-term benzodiazepines can be largely unaware of their own deficits and may only become aware of their prior impairment after withdrawing, with consequent improvement of their concentration and increased sensory appreciation.[18] In older people, benzodiazepines can cause psychomotor impairment and delirium in addition to the effects mentioned.[19]

Significant morbidity has been attributed to the use of benzodiazepines. For example, it has been found that there is a 60–80% increase in the risk of motor vehicle accidents in benzodiazepine users,[19] and a 2.3-fold increase in accidents that are fatal,[20] compared to non-users. Z-drugs increase the risk of motor vehicle collisions 2-fold.[21] The use of benzodiazepines and z-drugs has been associated with at least a 50% increase in risk of falls in the elderly.[5] In a study of 43,000 people zolpidem increased the risk of hip fracture by 2.55 times in those older than 65 years.[22] Deleterious effects on sleep are also evident. Despite the short-term effects of benzodiazepines and z-drugs on improving insomnia, in the long term they have been found to worsen sleep quality by disturbing a number of sleep parameters.[16,23] These changes seem to resolve on cessation.[16] In a number of meta-analyses long-term use of benzodiazepines has also been associated with an increased risk of developing dementia, although there is also conflicting data.[19]

Mortality risk

There is general agreement that benzodiazepine and z-drug use increase mortality risk, though some disagreement regarding the size of the effect.[24–27] A systematic review and meta-analysis of all eligible observational studies found that people using benzodiazepines or z-drugs had a 43% (95% CI 12% to 84%) increased risk of mortality compared to non-users.[25] As these are observational studies, there remains the possibility that such findings are influenced by residual confounding.

Other morbidity

There is also some evidence that benzodiazepines increase the risk of cancer, particularly brain cancer, although there are possibilities that these associations are confounded by indication or unmeasured confounders.[19] Observational studies have also found associations between benzodiazepine use and pneumonia, suicide and pancreatitis.[19] After opioids, benzodiazepines are the drug class most frequently involved in drug-related suicide attempts.[28] Benzodiazepine-related overdose mortality has risen dramatically in the USA, from 0.6 per 100,000 adults in 1999 to 4.4 per 100,000 in 2016.[29]

The adverse effects of benzodiazepines are amplified by concurrent use of opioids, other benzodiazepines or z-drugs, and gabapentinoids.[30] An FDA boxed warning highlights the risk of respiratory sedation and death when benzodiazepines are combined with opioids and other CNS depressants.[31] Benzodiazepines were detected in half of unintentional deaths associated with prescription opioids in the USA in 2018,[32] a 4-fold increase from two decades before.[30]

Psychiatric adverse effects

Benzodiazepines may also worsen a number of psychiatric symptoms. Studies have reported increased levels of depression in chronic benzodiazepine users,[16,33,34] with one study finding that non-depressed patients who were administered benzodiazepines had

CHAPTER 3

a 4-fold increased chance of developing clinically significant depressive symptoms,[35] although it can be difficult to distinguish this from the development of a co-morbid condition. Benzodiazepines have also been observed to cause worsening of anxiety in long-term use,[36] sometimes called benzodiazepine-induced hyperanxiogenesis.[30] Indeed, in one case series, 20% of patients on benzodiazepines developed agoraphobia only after taking benzodiazepines (which resolved on cessation).[36] Speculation on the cause of this increase in anxiety ranges from the induction of tolerance and withdrawal symptoms to psychological theories centring on the promotion of avoidance and prevention of fear extinction, to the overall cognitive impairment attributed to these medications.[16,36] These effects have been compared to the long-term, seemingly paradoxical, effects of opioids (opioid-induced hyperalgesia) and nicotine (worsened anxiety, which resolves after cessation).[16,30]

In support of these observations, studies have observed improved anxiety and depression scores in those patients who discontinued benzodiazepines.[37] A case series of 50 patients noted that patients' mental state seemed to improve after tapering off long-term benzodiazepines (after the period of withdrawal effects).[36] Cases of agoraphobia and suicidality, as well as gastroenterological and neurological complaints, which developed only after benzodiazepines were started (and had been unamenable to treatment during benzodiazepine use) largely resolved after cessation.[36] Benzodiazepines can also diminish the effectiveness of psychotherapeutic interventions such as exposure therapy.[38]

Z-drug adverse effects

The perception that z-drugs are safer than benzodiazepines is largely erroneous – apart from their quicker onset and shorter duration of action they produce similar adverse (side) effects.[39] Short-term adverse effects are well recognised: next-day grogginess, daytime memory impairment, disturbances of psychomotor performance (potentially affecting driving) and partial amnesia of the night's events.[40] Z-drugs, especially zolpidem, are associated with sleepwalking, sleep-driving and hallucinations in some people.[40]

As for benzodiazepines, there is general consensus that z-drugs increase the risk of mortality compared to non-users, though some debate about the size of the effect.[24,41] There was a greater than 3-fold increase found in the risk of mortality for users of hypnotics compared to non-users, after controlling for confounders in a large US cohort,[41] whereas a UK cohort analysis found a 2-fold increased risk for z-drugs, which showed a dose–response relationship.[42] A meta-analysis found an increased relative risk of mortality of 73% that did not reach statistical significance (95% CI: –5% to 216%).[43] As these are observational studies they remain susceptible to residual confounding. In people using hypnotics more than 130 times a year there was also an increased risk of cancer, which was not attributable to pre-existing disease.[41] Hypnotics have been associated with an increased risk of infection (perhaps due to disrupted healing at night), depression, falls and other accidents.[42] In a survey of people taking z-drugs, 40% reported at least one side effect and almost half had attempted to stop treatment at some point.[43]

Beneficial effects

Anxiolytic effects

Although benzodiazepines and z-drugs have positive effects on anxiety and insomnia in the short term, because of tolerance to these drugs (which can develop after 2–4 weeks) their effectiveness wanes over the long term, and physical dependence is likely to develop, meaning that treatment is often only continued to prevent withdrawal symptoms.[46] A meta-analysis comparing the mean difference in anxiety scores between placebo and benzodiazepines in people with generalised anxiety disorder found that at week 1 the difference between the treatment groups was 8 points on the Hamilton Anxiety Rating Scale (HAM-A) in favour of benzodiazepines, but by 8 weeks this had decreased to a difference of 4 points, and by 3 months there was almost no difference detected between placebo and benzodiazepines (Figure 3.1).[45] Indeed, as outlined earlier, there is a possibility that long-term use of benzodiazepines could actually make symptoms of anxiety worse.[16,36]

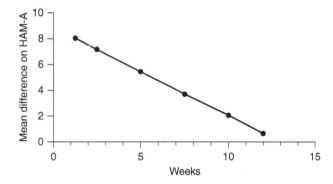

Figure 3.1 The difference between the placebo arm and the benzodiazepine arm of placebo-controlled trials in generalised anxiety disorder. This shows the difference in HAM-A scores at study end-point for the placebo and benzodiazepine treatment groups. HAM-A = Hamilton Anxiety Scale. Adapted from Gale et al. (2019).[45]

Interestingly, both tolerance and negative effects of long-term benzodiazepines have even been observed in epilepsy. In a clonazepam discontinuation study, 75% of participants showed no worsening of their epilepsy when the medication was slowly withdrawn, and 15% showed a decrease in seizure frequency.[46] Only 7.5% of participants showed a worsening in seizure activity after discontinuation.

Hypnotic effects

Sleep induced by z-drugs shows reduced slow wave sleep compared with normal sleep[47] – these stages being important for memory consolidation, physical healing and growth. Z-drugs improve time to sleep onset by 22 minutes in short-term (mostly 2 to 4 week) trials compared with placebo.[47] However, because of tolerance, these effects diminish over time, and when zolpidem, for example, is examined in studies with a duration of over 3 months, there is no difference from placebo in effect on sleep quality.[48] In short-term studies there was no difference between z-drugs and placebo for number of awakenings, total sleep time, sleep efficiency or sleep quality.[47] A systematic review found that there was no significant difference in problems with sleeping in people who continued or stopped benzodiazepine receptor agonists at 12-month follow up.[49]

There are a number of non-pharmacological interventions for insomnia that are effective. In the short-term cognitive-behavioural therapies showed a greater reduction in sleep latency than sleep medication and similar results in other measures of sleep; these effects tend to persist.[50] The American College of Physicians recommends cognitive behavioural therapy for insomnia (CBT-I) as the initial treatment for chronic insomnia.[51] Other techniques such as keeping a stable sleep–wake schedule, exposure to light in the morning, light restriction at night, exercise, a relaxation routine and limiting naps and caffeine in the afternoon can all be helpful for reducing insomnia.[52]

References

1. Roth T, Walsh JK, Krystal A, Wessel T, Roehrs TA. An evaluation of the efficacy and safety of eszopiclone over 12 months in patients with chronic primary insomnia. *Sleep Med* 2005; 6: 487–95.
2. Krystal AD, Walsh JK, Laska E, et al. Sustained efficacy of eszopiclone over 6 months of nightly treatment: results of a randomized, double-blind, placebo-controlled study in adults with chronic insomnia. *Sleep* 2003; 26: 793–9.
3. Olfson M, King M, Schoenbaum M. Benzodiazepine use in the United States. *JAMA Psychiatry* 2015; 72: 136–42.
4. Lister RG. The amnesic action of benzodiazepines in man. *Neurosci Biobehav Rev* 1985; 9: 87–94.
5. Donnelly K, Bracchi R, Hewitt J, Routledge PA, Carter B. Benzodiazepines, Z-drugs and the risk of hip fracture: a systematic review and meta-analysis. *PLoS One* 2017; 12. doi:10.1371/journal.pone.0174730.
6. De Gage SB, Moride Y, Ducruet T, et al. Benzodiazepine use and risk of Alzheimer's disease: case-control study. *BMJ* 2014; 349: 1–10.
7. Gray SL, Dublin S, Yu O, et al. Benzodiazepine use and risk of incident dementia or cognitive decline: prospective population-based study. *BMJ* 2016; 352: i90.
8. Ng BJ, Le Couteur DG, Hilmer SN. Deprescribing benzodiazepines in older patients: impact of interventions targeting physicians, pharmacists, and patients. *Drugs and Aging* 2018; 35: 493–521.
9. FDA Drug Safety Communication. FDA requiring boxed warning updated to improve safe use of benzodiazepine drug class. 2020. https://www.fda.gov/drugs/drug-safety-and-availability/fda-requiring-boxed-warning-updated-improve-safe-use-benzodiazepine-drug-class#:~:text=FDA is requiring the Boxed,and life-threatening side effects (accessed 3 July 2023).
10. Kaiser Permanente. Benzodiazepine and Z-drug safety guideline expectations for Kaiser Foundation health plan of Washington providers. 2019. https://wa.kaiserpermanente.org/static/pdf/public/guidelines/benzo-zdrug.pdf.
11. Conn DK, Hogan DB, Amdam L, et al. Canadian guidelines on benzodiazepine receptor agonist use disorder among older adults. *Can Geriatr J* 2020; 23: 116–22.
12. National Institute for Health and Care Excellence (NICE). Generalised anxiety disorder and panic disorder in adults: management. NICE clinical guideline CG113, 2011. https://www.nice.org.uk/guidance/cg113/chapter/2-Research-recommendations#the-effectiveness-of-physical-activity-compared-with-waiting-list-control-for-the-treatment-of-gad.
13. National Institute for Health and Care Excellence (NICE). Benzodiazepine and z-drug withdrawal. 2018. https://cks.nice.org.uk/benzodiazepine-and-z-drug-withdrawal#!topicsummary (accessed 8 August 2021).
14. Davies J, Rae TC, Montagu L. Long-term benzodiazepine and z-drugs use in the UK: a survey of general practice. *Br J Gen Pract* 2017; bjgp17X691865.
15. Maust DT, Lin LA, Blow FC. Benzodiazepine use and misuse among adults in the United States. *Psychiatr Serv* 2019; 70: 97–106.
16. Guina J, Merrill B. Benzodiazepines I: upping the care on downers: the evidence of risks, benefits and alternatives. *J Clin Med Res* 2018; 7: 17.
17. Crowe SF, Stranks EK. The residual medium and long-term cognitive effects of benzodiazepine use: an updated meta-analysis. *Arch Clin Neuropsychol* 2018; 33: 901–11.
18. Golombok S, Moodley P, Lader M. Cognitive impairment in long-term benzodiazepine users. *Psychol Med* 1988; 18: 365–74.
19. Brandt J, Leong C. Benzodiazepines and z-drugs: an updated review of major adverse outcomes reported on in epidemiologic research. *Drugs R D* 2017; 17: 493–507.
20. Elvik R. Risk of road accident associated with the use of drugs: a systematic review and meta-analysis of evidence from epidemiological studies. *Accid Anal Prev* 2013; 60: 254–67.
21. Gustavsen I, Bramness JG, Skurtveit S, Engeland A, Neutel I, Mørland J. Road traffic accident risk related to prescriptions of the hypnotics zopiclone, zolpidem, flunitrazepam and nitrazepam. *Sleep Med* 2008; 9: 818–22.
22. Finkle WD, Der JS, Greenland S, et al. Risk of fractures requiring hospitalization after an initial prescription for zolpidem, alprazolam, lorazepam, or diazepam in older adults. *J Am Geriatr Soc* 2011; 59: 1883–90.

23. Arbon EL, Knurowska M, Dijk D-J. Randomised clinical trial of the effects of prolonged-release melatonin, temazepam and zolpidem on slow-wave activity during sleep in healthy people. *J Psychopharmacol* 2015; 29: 764–76.

24. Weich S, Pearce HL, Croft P, et al. Effect of anxiolytic and hypnotic drug prescriptions on mortality hazards: retrospective cohort study. *BMJ* 2014; 348: g1996.

25. Parsaik AK, Mascarenhas SS, Khosh-Chashm D, et al. Mortality associated with anxiolytic and hypnotic drugs – a systematic review and meta-analysis. *Aust N Z J Psychiatry* 2016; 50: 520–33.

26. Xu KY, Hartz SM, Borodovsky JT, Bierut LJ, Grucza RA. Association between benzodiazepine use with or without opioid use and all-cause mortality in the United States, 1999–2015. *JAMA Netw Open* 2020; 3: e2028557.

27. Patorno E, Glynn RJ, Levin R, Lee MP, Huybrechts KF. Benzodiazepines and risk of all-cause mortality in adults: cohort study. *BMJ* 2017; 358: j2941.

28. Jones CM, McAninch JK. Emergency department visits and overdose deaths from combined use of opioids and benzodiazepines. *Am J Prev Med* 2015; 49: 493–501.

29. Agarwal SD, Landon BE. Patterns in outpatient benzodiazepine prescribing in the United States. *JAMA Netw Open* 2019; 2: e187399.

30. Wright SL. Benzodiazepine withdrawal: clinical aspects. In: *The Benzodiazepines* Crisis (eds. J Peppin, J Pergolizzi, R Raffa, S Wright) 2020: 117–C8.P334. Oxford: Oxford University Press. doi:10.1093/med/9780197517277.003.0008.

31. Center for Drug Evaluation, Research. FDA Drug Safety Communication: FDA warns about serious risks and death when combining opioid pain or cough medicines with benzodiazepines; requires its strongest warning. U.S. Food and Drug Administration. https://www.fda.gov/drugs/drug-safety-and-availability/fda-drug-safety-communication-fda-warns-about-serious-risks-and-death-when-combining-opioid-pain-or (accessed 2 April 2023).

32. Mattson CL, O'Donnell J, Kariisa M, Seth P, Scholl L, Gladden RM. Opportunities to prevent overdose deaths involving prescription and illicit opioids, 11 states, July 2016–June 2017. *MMWR Morb Mortal Wkly Rep* 2018; 67: 945–51.

33. Ashton H. The diagnosis and management of benzodiazepine dependence. *Curr Opin Psychiatry* 2005; 18: 249–55.

34. Michelini S, Cassano GB, Frare F, Perugi G. Long-term use of benzodiazepines: tolerance, dependence and clinical problems in anxiety and mood disorders. *Pharmacopsychiatry* 1996; 29: 127–34.

35. Patten SB, Williams JVA, Love EJ. Self-reported depressive symptoms following treatment with corticosteroids and sedative-hypnotics. *Int J Psychiatry Med* 1996; 26: 15–24.

36. Ashton H. Benzodiazepine withdrawal: outcome in 50 patients. *Br J Addict* 1987; 82: 665–71.

37. Rickels K, Case WG, Schweizer E, Garcia-Espana F, Fridman R. Long-term benzodiazepine users 3 years after participation in a discontinuation program. *Am J Psychiatry* 1991; 148: 757–61.

38. Marks IM, Swinson RP, Başoğlu M, et al. Alprazolam and exposure alone and combined in panic disorder with agoraphobia: a controlled study in London and Toronto. *Br J Psychiatry* 1993; 162: 776–87.

39. Agravat A. 'Z'-hypnotics versus benzodiazepines for the treatment of insomnia. *Prog Neurol Psychiatry* 2018; 22: 26–9.

40. Gunja N. In the zzz zone: the effects of z-drugs on human performance and driving. *J Med Toxicol* 2013; 9: 163–71.

41. Kripke DF, Langer RD, Kline LE. Hypnotics' association with mortality or cancer: a matched cohort study. *BMJ Open* 2012; 2: e000850.

42. Kripke DF. Hypnotic drug risks of mortality, infection, depression, and cancer: but lack of benefit. *F1000Res* 2016; 5: 918.

43. Siriwardena AN, Qureshi MZ, Dyas JV, Middleton H, Orner R. Magic bullets for insomnia? Patients' use and experiences of newer (z drugs) versus older (benzodiazepine) hypnotics for sleep problems in primary care. *Br J Gen Pract* 2008; 58: 417–22.

44. Gutierrez MA, Roper JM, Hahn P. Paradoxical reactions to benzodiazepines: when to expect the unexpected. *Am J Nurs* 2001; 101. https://journals.lww.com/ajnonline/Fulltext/2001/07000/Paradoxical_Reactions_to_Benzodiazepines__When_to.19.aspx.

45. Gale C, Glue P, Guaiana G, Coverdale J, McMurdo M, Wilkinson S. Influence of covariates on heterogeneity in Hamilton Anxiety Scale ratings in placebo-controlled trials of benzodiazepines in generalized anxiety disorder: systematic review and meta-analysis. *J Psychopharmacol* 2019; 33: 543–7.

46. Specht U, Boenigk HE, Wolf P. Discontinuation of clonazepam after long-term treatment. *Epilepsia* 1989; 30: 458–63.

47. Huedo-Medina TB, Kirsch I, Middlemass J, Klonizakis M, Siriwardena AN. Effectiveness of non-benzodiazepine hypnotics in treatment of adult insomnia: meta-analysis of data submitted to the Food and Drug Administration. *BMJ* 2012; 345: e8343.

48. De Crescenzo F, D'Alò GL, Ostinelli EG, et al. Comparative effects of pharmacological interventions for the acute and long-term management of insomnia disorder in adults: a systematic review and network meta-analysis. *Lancet* 2022; 400: 170–84.

49. Pottie K, Thompson W, Davies S, et al. Deprescribing benzodiazepine receptor agonists: evidence-based clinical practice guideline. *Can Fam Physician* 2018; 64: 339–51.

50. Smith MT, Perlis ML, Park A, et al. Comparative meta-analysis of pharmacotherapy and behavior therapy for persistent insomnia. *Am J Psychiatry* 2002; 159: 5–11.

51. Qaseem A, Kansagara D, Forciea MA, Cooke M, Denberg TD. Clinical Guidelines Committee of the American College of Physicians. Management of Chronic insomnia disorder in adults: a clinical practice guideline from the American College of Physicians. *Ann Intern Med* 2016; 165: 125–33.

52. Your Guide to Healthy Sleep. NHLBI, NIH. 2011; published online 8 January. https://www.nhlbi.nih.gov/resources/your-guide-healthy-sleep (accessed 8 April 2023).

Discussing deprescribing benzodiazepines and z-drugs

It is recommended that the possibility of stopping benzodiazepines or z-drugs should be brought up and discussed with each patient on long-term treatment.[1]

The main reasons for stopping these drugs are:

- adverse effects from the medication, outlined previously (some patients may not attribute these symptoms to the benzodiazepines);[2]
- the patient has been prescribed the drug for more than 4 weeks;[3,4]
- loss of efficacy (not always obvious to patients and prescribers);[2,5]
- the condition for which the drug was initially prescribed has resolved or alternative approaches have been developed;
- the person wants to stop taking the medication; and
- family, friends or clinical staff think the drug is adversely affecting the person (of course, informed consent is required from the patient to do so).

The group at highest risk for adverse effects from continuing benzodiazepines include those with the following characteristics:[4]

- age >65,
- more than 1 benzodiazepine or z-drug,
- combination with opioids or gabapentinoids,
- falls risk,
- Chronic Obstructive Pulmonary Disease (COPD), severe or uncontrolled respiratory disease or risk of respiratory depression,
- substance use disorder,
- history of overdose, and
- pregnant women or women planning for pregnancy.

Initiating the offer of deprescribing via a tailored letter from a general practitioner (GP) is effective in 25% of patients.[6] Providing patients with information about the harms and benefits of long-term use of these drugs is an important component of a deprescribing intervention. In the Eliminating Medications through Patient Ownership of End Results (EMPOWER) trial, an intervention providing education to older adults along with step-wise tapering increased the number of people who were able to stop benzodiazepine compared with care as usual by 5-fold (27% vs 5%).[7]

Patients should be informed of the adverse effects of long-term use. In a trial where GPs provided an education intervention (with or without structured follow-ups) 45% of patients were able to stop their benzodiazepines within 12 months.[8] The intervention included: information on benzodiazepine dependence, and withdrawal symptoms; the risks of long-term use, including memory and cognitive impairment, accidents and falls; reassurance about reducing medication; and a self-help leaflet to improve sleep quality if patients were taking benzodiazepines for insomnia.[8]

It is important to determine the best time to stop taking these drugs. The chances of success are improved when a person's physical and psychological health and personal circumstances are stable.[1] In some circumstances, it may be more appropriate to wait until other problems are resolved or improved before starting drug withdrawal.[1] When patients have considerable levels of anxiety, depression or insomnia, withdrawal can be especially difficult. On the one hand the presence of these symptoms will make the process of withdrawal more challenging, but on the other, being off these medications may improve these symptoms (which can be induced or worsened by these medications).[1,9] Sometimes mood symptoms are due to inter-dose withdrawal, which can be improved by more frequent dosing. Alternatively, tolerance may be the cause, which may be first alleviated by an increase in dose so that subsequent tapering is made from a position of stability.[2,5]

If these symptoms are thought to be unrelated to medication then this territory may be navigated by trying to manage these conditions with non-benzodiazepine approaches, attempting a very gradual taper or deferring tapering until a more stable period.[1] Sometimes enhancing coping skills will be required before a patient feels ready to embark on a taper. Techniques such as cognitive behavioural approaches are supported for benzodiazepine discontinuation as evidenced in meta-analyses,[10] and other approaches such as mindfulness, exercise or other forms of intentional relaxation can be useful.[11,12] If medical problems are causing significant distress then these should ideally be managed first before commencement of a taper.[1] For some people – for example, the frail and elderly – it may be prohibitively difficult to attempt a taper.

Patients may have a number of fears regarding stopping these medications (Table 3.2). These include a fear of withdrawal symptoms and a fear of a relapse of their underlying condition. There should be a discussion about the probable lack (or diminution) of long-term efficacy for these drug classes for insomnia or anxiety, due to the phenomenon of tolerance.[1] A discussion about withdrawal effects should emphasise that they can be mistaken for a return of an underlying condition, which can convince people that they may need the drug to avoid these symptoms.[1] This is a common mis-conception – 'because I can't sleep when I stop the drug I must need the drug to sleep' or 'when I stop, I have panic attacks: I must need the drug'. These ideas can be gently explored. Patients should also be reassured that deprescribing will be performed under the principle of shared decision making so that they will have control over how fast the medication is reduced and will not be subject to an imposed taper.[13] Patients should be told that stopping in this manner, at a slow pace determined by the degree of withdrawal effects, down to low doses before stopping (in a hyperbolic manner) is likely to reduce the risk and severity of withdrawal symptoms and so may make the process more tolerable than on previous attempts – which may reduce anxieties patients have about the process.[14]

Table 3.2 Barriers and facilitators for patients to stop benzodiazepines and z-drugs. Adapted from Evrard et al. (2022),[23] Maund et al. (2019)[21] and Kaiser Permanente (2022).[4]

Domain	Barriers	Facilitators
Psychological capabilities and physiological effects	■ Difficult life circumstances ■ Aversive experience of discontinuation in past ■ Lack of effective coping strategies ■ Physical dependence on benzodiazepines/z-drugs ■ Lack of resources	■ Confidence in ability to discontinue ■ Life circumstances stable ■ Well-informed about approach to tapering/trying a taper that is more gradual and more tolerable ■ Patient's perceived self-efficacy
Perceived cause and management of anxiety/insomnia	■ Long-term (perhaps life-long) condition requiring long-term treatment ■ Predominantly biochemical/genetic cause ■ Lack of awareness of alternative treatment strategies	■ Life circumstances/seasonal/ 'rough patch' ■ Knowledge or competence in other effective strategies to address underlying issues
Fears	■ Fear of relapse ■ Fear of withdrawal effects	■ Fear of 'addiction', physical dependence ■ Fear of adverse effects ■ Fear of long-term health consequences
Personal goals/ motivations	■ Self-identity as 'disabled' ■ Stopping as threat to stability ■ Benefit of continuing to others around them ■ Cure is not possible, only management	■ Self-identity as 'healthy' ■ Desire to function without a medication ■ Feeling better ■ Dislike having to take a medication
Perception of benzodiazepines/ z-drugs	■ Positive/pleasurable effect ■ Belief in effectiveness of drugs ■ Lack of concern over adverse/side effects	■ Awareness of long-term lack of efficacy ■ Ineffectual/tolerance effects ■ Unacceptable adverse/side effects ■ Benefit from drugs is caused by relief of withdrawal effects ■ Unhappy about long-term use
Information about the discontinuation process	■ Inadequate information about the discontinuation process, and risks and benefits of this	■ Information on how to safely discontinue and what to expect
Beliefs about the consequences of deprescribing	■ No expected benefit ■ Return of primary condition ■ Withdrawal symptoms ■ Increase in care burden ■ Previous failed attempts	■ Expected improvement in well-being ■ Primary condition manageable or resolved ■ Withdrawal symptoms manageable ■ Decrease in healthcare burden
Support network (friends, family, professionals)	■ Pressure to stay on medication ■ Insufficient support from prescriber/ inability to talk openly about their drugs/ feeling stigmatised by prescriber	■ Support to come off medication ■ Patient's trust in prescriber (knowledgeable about benzodiazepines, open communication, shared decision making)

Beneficial effects of deprescribing

The benefits of stopping should be outlined:

- Perhaps counter-intuitively, an improvement in anxiety.[15] In a study of patients in a benzodiazepine withdrawal clinic, the incidence of panic attacks, depression, agoraphobia, and phobia all reduced such that patients taken off benzodiazepines (with no other intervention) showed lower incidence of these symptoms than they had experienced while on benzodiazepines.[15]
- Improved psychomotor and cognitive function.[16]
- A reduction in numerous adverse (side) effects. All the following symptoms were decreased in patients who stopped their benzodiazepines in a specialised withdrawal clinic (after the period of withdrawal effects) compared to before cessation:[15]
  - CNS: headache, pain (limbs, back, neck, teeth, jaw, limbs, face), ataxia, tinnitus, dizziness, light-headedness, insomnia, nightmares;
  - muscular/neuromuscular: stiffness, muscle tremors, fasciculations;
  - gastrointestinal symptoms such as nausea, vomiting, abdominal pain, diarrhoea, constipation, appetite disturbances, dry mouth, metallic taste, dysphagia;
  - cardiovascular symptoms such as flushing, sweating, palpitations; and
  - other: thirst, polyuria, incontinence, menorrhagia, mammary pain/swelling, rash/itching, sinusitis, influenza-like symptoms.[15]
- There is likely to be a reduction in the risk of the long-term adverse consequences of benzodiazepine use, such as probable increased all-cause mortality, increased risk of falls and fractures, motor vehicle accidents and drug interactions.
- Stopping can also prevent further cascades of prescribing where tolerance leads to increased doses or the addition of further medications, or adverse effects lead to the need for other medications.[9,17]
- Stopping can also allow better engagement in therapy or other useful non-drug modalities, as cognitive impairment and emotional blunting may make aspects of therapy more difficult to access.[18,19]
- Lastly, the fact that being on these medications for longer will make them harder to stop may be a reason to try stopping sooner rather than later so as to avoid a more severe withdrawal reaction.[1]

One important note is that people who do not wish to stop benzodiazepines or z-drugs should not be pressurised to do so.[1] It may be worthwhile to advise these people of the benefits of stopping, address any concerns they may have about stopping if possible and review the issue at a later date, if that is appropriate.[1] People's circumstances should be accounted for, and although it may be in the best interests of the patient's health in the long term to stop these medications, if their circumstances do not permit this (e.g. professional or personal responsibilities), then this course of action should not be imposed. Forced tapers often backfire.[2,5] Some patients may be unable to stop their medication but a reduction of dose may be a reasonable goal.

Many people are ambivalent about continuing or discontinuing long-term benzodiazepines and z-drugs,[20] with the default position often being to continue taking the medication ('if it ain't broke, don't fix it'). There are a variety of barriers to considering stopping benzodiazepines and z-drugs that may make people ambivalent or resistant to doing so. These are shown in Table 3.2.[20,21] Motivational interviewing skills might be helpful here to draw out the advantages and disadvantages of different courses of action.[22]

References

1. National Institute for Health and Care Excellence (NICE). Benzodiazepine and z-drug withdrawal. 2018. https://cks.nice.org.uk/benzodiazepine-and-z-drug-withdrawal#!topicsummary (accessed 8 August 2021).
2. Wright SL. Benzodiazepine withdrawal: clinical aspects. In: *The Benzodiazepines* Crisis (eds. J Peppin, J Pergolizzi, R Raffa, S Wright) 2020: 117–C8.P334. Oxford: Oxford University Press. doi:10.1093/med/9780197517277.003.0008.
3. Pottie K, Thompson W, Davies S, et al. Deprescribing benzodiazepine receptor agonists: evidence-based clinical practice guideline. *Can Fam Physician* 2018; 64: 339–51.
4. Kaiser Permanente. Benzodiazepine and z-drug safety guideline. https://wa.kaiserpermanente.org/static/pdf/public/guidelines/benzo-zdrug.pdf (accessed 29 April 2023).
5. Ashton H. Benzodiazepines: how they work and how to withdraw (The Ashton Manual). Newcastle University, 2002. http://www.benzo.org.uk/manual/bzcha01.htm (accessed 11 July 2023).
6. Darker CD, Sweeney BP, Barry JM, Farrell MF, Donnelly-Swift E. Psychosocial interventions for benzodiazepine harmful use, abuse or dependence. *Cochrane Database Syst Rev* 2015; CD009652.
7. Tannenbaum C, Martin P, Tamblyn R, Benedetti A, Ahmed S. Reduction of inappropriate benzodiazepine prescriptions among older adults through direct patient education: the EMPOWER cluster randomized trial. *JAMA Intern Med* 2014; 174: 890–8.
8. Vicens C, Bejarano F, Sempere E, et al. Comparative efficacy of two interventions to discontinue long-term benzodiazepine use: cluster randomised controlled trial in primary care. *Br J Psychiatry* 2014; 204: 471–9.
9. Ashton H. Benzodiazepine withdrawal: outcome in 50 patients. *Br J Addict* 1987; 82: 665–71.
10. Parr JM, Kavanagh DJ, Cahill L, Mitchell G, McD Young R. Effectiveness of current treatment approaches for benzodiazepine discontinuation: a meta-analysis. *Addiction* 2009; 104: 13–24.
11. Framer A. What I have learnt from helping thousands of people taper off psychotropic medications. *Ther Adv Psychopharmacol* 2021; 11: 204512532199127.
12. Guy A, Davies J, Rizq R. *Guidance for Psychological Therapists: Enabling Conversations with Clients Taking or Withdrawing from prescribed Psychiatric Drugs*. London: APPG for Prescribed Drug Dependence, 2019.
13. National Institute for Health and Care Excellence (NICE). Medicines associated with dependence or withdrawal symptoms: safe prescribing and withdrawal management for adults | Guidance | NICE. 2022. https://www.nice.org.uk/guidance/ng215/chapter/Recommendations (accessed 27 June 2022).
14. Liebrenz M, Gehring MT, Buadze A, Caflisch C. High-dose benzodiazepine dependence: a qualitative study of patients' perception on cessation and withdrawal. *BMC Psychiatry* 2015; 15: 1–12.
15. Ashton H. Benzodiazepine withdrawal: an unfinished story. *Br Med J* 1984; 288: 1135–40.
16. Lader M, Tylee A, Donoghue J. Withdrawing benzodiazepines in primary care. *CNS Drugs* 2009; 23: 19–34.
17. Guina J, Merrill B. Benzodiazepines II: Waking up on sedatives: providing optimal care when inheriting benzodiazepine prescriptions in transfer patients. *J Clin Med Res* 2018; 7. doi:10.3390/jcm7020020.
18. Wilhelm FH, Roth WT. Acute and delayed effects of alprazolam on flight phobics during exposure. *Behav Res Ther* 1997; 35: 831–41.
19. Hart G, Panayi MC, Harris JA, Westbrook RF. Benzodiazepine treatment can impair or spare extinction, depending on when it is given. *Behav Res Ther* 2014; 56: 22–9.
20. Pollmann AS, Murphy AL, Bergman JC, Gardner DM. Deprescribing benzodiazepines and z-drugs in community-dwelling adults: a scoping review. *BMC Pharmacol Toxicol* 2015; 16: 19.
21. Maund E, Dewar-Haggart R, Williams S, et al. Barriers and facilitators to discontinuing antidepressant use: a systematic review and thematic synthesis. *J Affect Disord* 2019; 245: 38–62.
22. Karter JM. Conversations with clients about antidepressant withdrawal and discontinuation. *Ther Adv Psychopharmacol* 2020; 10: 2045125320922738.
23. Evrard P, Pétein C, Beuscart J-B, Spinewine A. Barriers and enablers for deprescribing benzodiazepine receptor agonists in older adults: a systematic review of qualitative and quantitative studies using the theoretical domains framework. *Implement Sci* 2022; 17: 41.

Withdrawal Symptoms from Benzodiazepines and Z-drugs

Some people experience no withdrawal symptoms on stopping benzodiazepines and z-drugs – together called benzodiazepine receptor agonists (BzRAs). Others have only mild withdrawal symptoms upon discontinuation. For others, stopping can be difficult because of withdrawal effects, which can sometimes be severe and long-lasting.

Physical dependence and withdrawal phenomena from benzodiazepines have been acknowledged for almost six decades. Normal dose physical dependence and withdrawal effects were observed in the 1960s and 1970s and these medications were put on the FDA restricted drug list in 1975. Anecdotal reports from patients and physicians about dependence and withdrawal were confirmed by trials in the 1980s, and in 1990 the American Psychiatric Association officially recognised the risk of benzodiazepine dependence and withdrawal.[1,2]

In 2020 the FDA updated the boxed warning (previously known as black box warnings) on all marketed benzodiazepines to re-emphasise the risk of physical dependence, addiction and withdrawal effects, including the warning that withdrawal syndromes could persist for more than 12 months after stopping.[3,4] The FDA found in its investigation that mis-diagnosis of benzodiazepine withdrawal (as a return of underlying symptoms) led to increased doses of benzodiazepines being prescribed, that patients were being told they could stop their drugs abruptly and that they were often tapered off too quickly.[5]

In patients that have been taking regular benzodiazepines for more than one year 58% to 100% experience a withdrawal reaction, depending on the definition used.[6] Overall, 15% to 44% of chronic benzodiazepine users will experience moderate to severe withdrawal symptoms on stopping.[7] One study found that 32% of people who were using long-half-life benzodiazepines and 42% of people using short-half-life benzodiazepine were unable to cease their medication because of withdrawal symptoms.[8] It is estimated that up to 15% of patients who stop long-term benzodiazepines will experience a protracted withdrawal syndrome, which can last months and sometimes years.[9]

The onset of withdrawal effects often occurs a day or two after stopping for shorter-acting benzodiazepines, and several days for longer-acting drugs, although delayed onset effects are also recognised, including by the NICE guidelines.[10–12] The time to peak severity is variable and symptoms can fluctuate over time.[13] The symptoms of the withdrawal syndrome can be life-threatening with fatalities recognised.[14,15] Seizures, delirium and catatonia can occur, especially when the drug is stopped abruptly. Suicidality is also a recognised withdrawal effect (which can occur as a new-onset symptom in people who have not experienced this before withdrawal).[14,15]

Short-acting benzodiazepines are associated with more severe acute withdrawal symptoms on discontinuation than longer-acting drugs such as diazepam,[16,17] but both can cause protracted withdrawal syndromes.[18,19] As the drugs have limited effectiveness for anxiety and insomnia in the long term because of tolerance, symptoms that arise on stopping are likely to be withdrawal symptoms not relapse (though symptoms can be similar).[13] Mental state often improves on stopping, after withdrawal symptoms abate, because of a reduction in the long-term adverse effects of benzodiazepines on mood and anxiety.[20]

CHAPTER 3

Withdrawal effects are generally recognised to occur after weeks of use, but the 2020 FDA boxed warning points out that withdrawal effects from benzodiazepines can even occur when the medication is taken 'steadily for several days', although presumably symptoms are more likely to be mild and short-lived in these circumstances.[3] To avoid or reduce the severity of these problems, good practice dictates that benzodiazepines (and z-drugs) should not be prescribed as hypnotics or anxiolytics for longer than 4 weeks (as also recommended widely by their manufacturers) and the risks of longer term use should be part of informed consent.[21] Intermittent use (i.e. as infrequently as possible) at the lowest possible dose is also prudent because it is thought to produce less physical dependence over time.[3]

References

1. Guina J, Merrill B. Benzodiazepines I: upping the care on downers: the evidence of risks, benefits and alternatives. *J Clin Med Res* 2018; 7: 17.

2. Lader M. History of benzodiazepine dependence. *J Subst Abuse Treat* 1991; 8: 53–9.

3. FDA Drug Safety Communication. FDA requiring boxed warning updated to improve safe use of benzodiazepine drug class. 2020. https://www.fda.gov/drugs/drug-safety-and-availability/fda-requiring-boxed-warning-updated-improve-safe-use-benzodiazepine-drug-class#:~:text=FDA is requiring the Boxed,and life-threatening side effects (accessed 3 July 2023).

4. Parsons G. Dependence on benzodiazepines or Z-drugs: having that conversation. *Pharm J* 2012; 289: 399–402.

5. FDA. Integrated drug utilization, epidemiology and pharmacovigilance review: benzodiazepine use, misuse, abuse, dependence, withdrawal, morbidity, and mortality. 2020; www.benzoinfo.com/wp-content/uploads/2020/11/Benzodiazepine-Information-Coalition-FOIA-FDA-.pdf (accessed 3 July 2023).

6. Rickels K, Schweizer E, Case WG, Greenblatt DJ. Long-term therapeutic use of benzodiazepines. I. Effects of abrupt discontinuation. *Arch Gen Psychiatry* 1990; 47: 899–907.

7. Hood SD, Norman A, Hince DA, Melichar JK, Hulse GK. Benzodiazepine dependence and its treatment with low dose flumazenil. *Br J Clin Pharmacol* 2014; 77: 285–94.

8. Schweizer E, Rickels K, Case WG, Greenblatt DJ. Long-term therapeutic use of benzodiazepines. II. Effects of gradual taper. *Arch Gen Psychiatry* 1990; 47: 908–15.

9. Ashton H. Protracted withdrawal from benzodiazepines: the post-withdrawal syndrome. *Psychiatr Ann* 1995; 25: 174–9.

10. Repplinger D, Nelson LS. Case studies in toxicology: withdrawal: another danger of diversion. 2016; published online February 1. https://www.mdedge.com/clinicianreviews/article/106391/toxicology/case-studies-toxicology-withdrawal-another-danger (accessed 13 April 2023).

11. Ishii N, Terao T, Araki Y, Hatano K. Repeated seizures in an elderly patient with alcohol dependence and mild cognitive impairment. *BMJ Case Rep* 2013; 2013. doi:10.1136/bcr-2013-201575.

12. National Institute for Health and Care Excellence (NICE). Medicines associated with dependence or withdrawal symptoms: safe prescribing and withdrawal management for adults I Guidance I NICE. 2022. https://www.nice.org.uk/guidance/ng215/chapter/Recommendations (accessed 27 June 2022).

13. Ashton H. The diagnosis and management of benzodiazepine dependence. *Curr Opin Psychiatry* 2005; 18: 249–55.

14. Murphy SM, Tyrer P. A double-blind comparison of the effects of gradual withdrawal of lorazepam, diazepam and bromazepam in benzodiazepine dependence. *Br J Psychiatry* 1991; 158: 511–16.

15. Martin-Kleisch A, Zulfiqar A-A. [Retrospective study of the assessment and management of benzodiazepine withdrawal syndrome in hospital between 2000 and 2015]. *Ann Pharm Fr* 2017; 75: 196–208.

16. Schweizer E, Rickels K. Benzodiazepine dependence and withdrawal: a review of the syndrome and its clinical management. *Acta Psychiatr Scand* 1998; 98: 95–101.

17. Uhlenhuth EH, Balter MB, Ban TA, Yang K. International study of expert judgment on therapeutic use of benzodiazepines and other psychotherapeutic medications: IV. Therapeutic dose dependence and abuse liability of benzodiazepines in the long-term treatment of anxiety disorders. *J Clin Psychopharmacol* 1999; 19: 23S–29S.

18. Lerner A, Klein M. Dependence, withdrawal and rebound of CNS drugs: an update and regulatory considerations for new drugs development. *Brain Commun* 2019; 1: fcz025.

19. Cosci F, Chouinard G. Acute and persistent withdrawal syndromes following discontinuation of psychotropic medications. *Psychother Psychosom* 2020; 89: 283–306.

20. Ashton H. Benzodiazepine withdrawal: outcome in 50 patients. *Br J Addict* 1987; 82: 665–71.

21. Clonazepam Neuraxpharm 0.5mg tablets – Summary of Product Characteristics (SmPC) - (emc). https://www.medicines.org.uk/emc/product/13633/smpc (accessed 19 March 2023).

Physical dependence vs addiction in use of benzodiazepines and z-drugs

The term 'dependence' has come to be used interchangeably with 'addiction' (to mean uncontrolled drug-seeking behaviour).[1] Inevitably this has led to some unfortunate confusion.[1] This choice of language was made in the *Diagnostic and Statistical Manual of Mental Disorders* 3rd revised edition (DSM-III-R) because the term 'addiction' was thought to be pejorative while the word 'dependence' was thought more neutral.[1] However, the original usage of 'physical dependence' (or physiological dependence) referred to 'physiological adaptation that occurs when medications acting on the central nervous system are ingested with rebound when the medication is abruptly discontinued'.[1] The FDA clarified the definition of this term in 2019: 'Physical dependence is a state that develops as a result of physiological adaptation in response to repeated drug use, manifested by withdrawal signs and symptoms after abrupt discontinuation or a significant dose reduction of a drug'.[2] The FDA also made the distinction from addiction clear:

Physical dependence is not synonymous with addiction; a patient may be physically dependent on a drug without having an addiction to the drug. Tolerance, physical dependence, and withdrawal are all expected biological phenomena that are the consequences of chronic treatment with certain drugs. These phenomena by themselves do not indicate a state of addiction.

The National Institute on Drug Abuse (NIDA) statement on this issue is consistent with this interpretation:

Dependence means that when a person stops using a drug, their body goes through 'withdrawal': a group of physical and mental symptoms that can range from mild (if the drug is caffeine) to life-threatening . . . Many people who take a prescription medicine every day over a long period of time can become dependent; when they go off the drug, they need to do it gradually, to avoid withdrawal discomfort. But people who are dependent on a drug or medicine aren't necessarily addicted.[3]

The *Diagnostic and Statistical Manual of Mental Disorders*, 5th revised edition (DSM-V) also identifies this issue:[4]

'Dependence' has been easily confused with the term 'addiction' when, in fact, the tolerance and withdrawal that previously defined dependence are actually very normal responses to prescribed medications that affect the central nervous system and do not necessarily indicate the presence of an addiction.

With benzodiazepines, both physical dependence and addiction are possible. Misuse means taking a medication in a manner or dose other than prescribed: for example, taking the drug for a legitimate medical complaint for which the drug was not prescribed.[5,6] Abuse means taking a medication to experience euphoria or for recreational purposes.[6] Addiction (synonymous with a substance use disorder) involves compulsive use of a drug, craving the drug, impaired control over drug-taking and use despite harm or negative consequences – an isolated episode of misuse or abuse is not sufficient to entail a diagnosis of addiction.[6] The majority of people who use benzodiazepines and z-drugs are taking them as prescribed by their clinician, without addiction or abuse. Only 2% have benzodiazepine use disorders (i.e. addiction), while 17.1% have misused benzodiazepines (once or more).[7] However many people taking the medication as prescribed will be physically dependent on the drug through the expected physiological process of adaptation. This means that when they stop the drug they will experience withdrawal.

A failure to appreciate this difference (which may seem merely semantic) can lead to real-life consequences. For example, people who have difficulty stopping their medications because of withdrawal effects can be accused of addiction or abuse. Requests for re-instatement to manage withdrawal effects can be characterised as 'drug seeking behaviour', and therefore refused. As the withdrawal syndrome from benzodiazepines can include seizures and occasionally be life-threatening, this response can have catastrophic consequences. Additionally, mis-diagnosis of physical dependence as addiction can lead to inappropriate management. This includes sending people to 12-step addiction-based detoxification and rehabilitation centres that focus on psychological aspects of compulsive use rather than physiological aspects of withdrawal, leading to unnecessary harms in the form of too rapid tapering regimens and consequent social and professional consequences (if people have addiction listed on their medical record).

The FDA in its 2020 boxed warning on benzodiazepine dependence and withdrawal took pains to highlight this issue: 'Physical dependence is the body's adaptation to repeated use of a drug, resulting in withdrawal reactions when the medicine is abruptly discontinued or the dose is significantly reduced. Dependence may lead some individuals to continue using the medicine to avoid symptoms of withdrawal.'[8] Moreover, the FDA's review of cases of severe withdrawal found that 'dependence and subsequent withdrawal symptoms developed even when the benzodiazepine was prescribed for therapeutic use'.[8]

This chapter deals with patients who are using benzodiazepines and z-drugs as prescribed; those with addiction issues are beyond the scope of the current textbook. Such patients will need support for the behavioural aspects of addiction that are not relevant to people with physical dependence.

References

1. O'Brien C. Addiction and dependence in DSM-V. *Addiction* 2011; 106: 866–7.
2. Center for Drug Evaluation, Research. Drug abuse and dependence section of labeling for human prescription drug and biological products — content and format guidance for industry. U.S. Food and Drug Administration. https://www.fda.gov/regulatory-information/search-fda-guidance-documents/drug-abuse-and-dependence-section-labeling-human-prescription-drug-and-biological-products-content (accessed 3 April 2023).
3. National Institute on Drug Abuse (NIDA). Is there a difference between physical dependence and addiction? National Institute on Drug Abuse. https://nida.nih.gov/publications/principles-drug-addiction-treatment-research-based-guide-third-edition/frequently-asked-questions/there-difference-between-physical-dependence-addiction (accessed 31 May 2022).
4. American Psychiatric Association. *Diagnostic and Statistical Manual of Mental Disorders* (5th ed.). Washington, DC: American Psychiatric Association, 2013. https://psychiatryonline.org/doi/10.1176/appi.books.9780890425596.dsm05.
5. National Institute on Drug Abuse (NIDA). Summary of misuse of prescription drugs. National Institute on Drug Abuse. https://nida.nih.gov/publications/research-reports/misuse-prescription-drugs/overview (accessed 8 April 2023).
6. Smith SM, Dart RC, Katz NP, et al. Classification and definition of misuse, abuse, and related events in clinical trials: ACTTION systematic review and recommendations. *Pain* 2013; 154: 2287–96.
7. Blanco C, Han B, Jones CM, Johnson K, Compton WM. Prevalence and Correlates of benzodiazepine use, misuse, and use disorders among adults in the United States. *J Clin Psychiatry* 2018; 79. doi:10.4088/JCP.18m12174.
8. FDA Drug Safety Communication. FDA requiring boxed warning updated to improve safe use of benzodiazepine drug class. 2020. https://www.fda.gov/drugs/drug-safety-and-availability/fda-requiring-boxed-warning-updated-improve-safe-use-benzodiazepine-drug-class#:~:text=FDA is requiring the Boxed,and life-threatening side effects (accessed 3 July 2023).

Pathophysiology of benzodiazepine withdrawal syndrome

Withdrawal effects from benzodiazepines occur, as for other psychotropic medications, because neuro-adaptations to the presence of a drug taken chronically take longer to dissipate than it takes for the drug to be eliminated from the body when it is stopped (Figure 3.2).[1] These compensatory adaptations act unopposed when the drug is stopped or reduced in dose. Elucidation of the exact cellular mechanisms of adaptation in benzodiazepine use has been difficult.[2] Benzodiazepines and z-drugs are positive allosteric modulators of the gamma-aminobutyric acid type A ($GABA_A$) receptor, leading to enhancement of the effect of the inhibitory neurotransmitter GABA in the nervous system.[2,3] BzRAs attach to the benzodiazepine receptor on $GABA_A$ receptors, and thereby increase the total conduction of chloride ions across the neuronal cell membrane in the presence of GABA binding to the receptor.[2] The influx of chloride ions hyperpolarises the neuron's membrane potential, making firing less likely, thought to produce sedative, hypnotic, anxiolytic, anticonvulsant and muscle relaxant properties in the short term.[4]

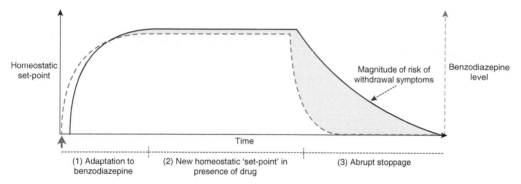

Figure 3.2 The neurobiology of benzodiazepine withdrawal. In this diagram, the homeostatic 'set-point' is shown in black and benzodiazepine drug levels are shown in purple dashed lines. (1) The system is at baseline. At the solid purple arrow, a benzodiazepine is administered; drug plasma levels increase. Physiological adaptations of the system to the presence of the drug begin. (2) At the plateau, drug plasma levels (and target receptor effects) have reached a steady state with a new homeostatic set-point of the system established. (3) The benzodiazepine is abruptly ceased and plasma drug levels drop to zero (exponentially, according to the elimination half-life of the drug). This difference between the homeostatic set-point (the 'expectations' of the system) and the level of drug in the system (dashed purple line) is experienced as withdrawal symptoms. Hence, withdrawal symptoms may worsen or peak even long after the drug has been eliminated from the system. The shaded area under the curve, representing the difference between the homeostatic set-point and the level of the drug, indicates the degree of risk of withdrawal symptoms: the larger the area the greater the risk. The time taken for adaptations to the presence of the drug to resolve after cessation will determine the duration of withdrawal symptoms.

There have been mixed findings regarding the predicted reduction in the number and sensitivity of $GABA_A$ receptors (as a homeostatic response to enhanced action of GABA) following chronic use of BzRAs.[2] However, pre-clinical models have yielded more robust findings in respect to the phenomenon of uncoupling, whereby the benzodiazepine site loses its allosteric modulatory effects over GABAergic activity after chronic benzodiazepine administration (Figure 3.3).[2] In addition, benzodiazepine administration causes down-regulation of adenosine receptors and up-regulation

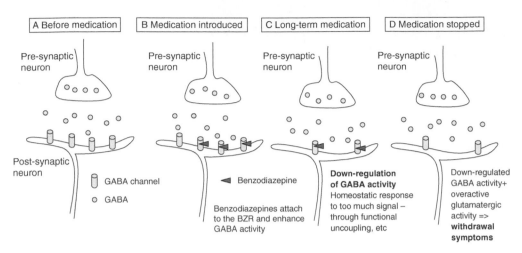

Figure 3.3 Neuro-adaptation to the presence of benzodiazepines and the effects on reduction or stopping benzo-diazepines. A – GABA is released from the pre-synaptic neuron into the synapse where it then activates the GABA$_A$ receptors on the post-synaptic neuron. B – introduction of a benzodiazepine enhances GABA effects by enhancing GABA$_A$ receptor chloride channel activity by attaching to the benzodiazepine receptor. C – Due to homeostasis, after chronic administration of BzRAs the excess GABA activity leads to down-regulation in the activity of the GABA system via mechanisms such as uncoupling of benzodiazepine receptor activation from potentiation of the GABA$_A$ chloride channel activity.[2] There is also up-regulation of the opposing glutamatergic system (not shown).[2] D – when the benzodiazepine is removed (or reduced) after long-term use the potentiation of GABA activity by benzodiaze-pines is removed (or reduced). In the context of down-regulated sensitivity or action of GABA$_A$ channels this leads to an under-activity of GABAergic action. The up-regulated glutamatergic system now acts less opposed by GABA-ergic effects. The down-regulation of GABA-ergic activity persists for some time after benzodiazepine cessation. The combination of down-regulated GABA-ergic activity and up-regulated excitatory glutamatergic activity is thought to underpin benzodiazepine withdrawal symptoms. These symptoms will persist for as long as it takes GABA-ergic receptors to be up-regulated and glutamatergic activity to be down-regulated back to their 'pre-drug' configuration.

of the ionotropic glutamate N-methyl-D-aspartate (NMDA) and α-amino-3-hydroxy-5-methyl-4-isoxazolepropionic acid (AMPA) receptors.[2,5] This up-regulation of the glutamate system is thought to represent an opponent process to compensate for enhanced GABA activation.[2,3] There are also thought to be other wide-ranging adaptations to the chronic use of benzodiazepines, involving downstream processes, including hormonal and other neural effects.[3]

Withdrawal symptoms are thought to arise as a reduction of benzodiazepine dosage causes disruption of the new homeostatic equilibrium established in the presence of benzodiazepine use (often called physical dependence).[4] In particular, underactivity of inhibitory GABA activity has been implicated in the pathogenesis of withdrawal,[4] supported by the ability of flumazenil, a short-acting selective GABA$_A$ antagonist, to induce the rapid onset of withdrawal symptoms when administered.[6] Rapid reduction in GABA transmission leads to a surge in excitatory nervous activity, as a number of neurotransmitter pathways, including glutamatergic (up-regulated to compensate for increased GABA activity) act with less opposition.[4] Blockade of glutamatergic NMDA and AMPA receptors reduces the severity of diazepam withdrawal, emphasising the role of glutamate in benzodiazepine withdrawal.[7] Increased release of dopamine, noradrenaline and serotonin is also evident in the rat brain during benzodiazepine withdrawal, consistent with the removal of inhibitory GABA activity.[8] This excess of excitatory activity is thought to be central to symptoms of benzodiazepine withdrawal.[2] It is also thought that numerous cycles on and off benzodiazepines can further enhance the potentiation of the glutamatergic system, in a process known as kindling, a form of sensitisation first identified in the case of alcohol withdrawal.[5] This may explain why withdrawal symptoms can become increasingly difficult after numerous cycles of use and cessation of benzodiazepines.[9]

The withdrawal syndrome has been thought to resolve when the neuro-adaptive changes occurring during exposure to the drug adequately reverse.[10] Although not well understood, rates at which these neuroadaptations resolve will vary between individuals, perhaps explaining the variable persistence of withdrawal symptoms.[11,12]

References

1. Reidenberg MM. Drug discontinuation effects are part of the pharmacology of a drug. *J Pharmacol Exp Ther* 2011; 339: 324–8.
2. Cheng T, Wallace DM, Ponteri B, Tuli M. Valium without dependence? Individual gabaa receptor subtype contribution toward benzodiazepine addiction, tolerance, and therapeutic effects. *Neuropsychiatr Dis Treat* 2018; 14: 1351–61.
3. Wright SL. Benzodiazepine withdrawal: clinical aspects. In: *The Benzodiazepines* Crisis (eds. J Peppin, J Pergolizzi, R Raffa, S Wright) 2020: 117–C8.P334. Oxford: Oxford University Press. doi:10.1093/med/9780197517277.003.0008.
4. Authier N, Balayssac D, Sautereau M, et al. Benzodiazepine dependence: focus on withdrawal syndrome. *Ann Pharm Fr* 2009; 67: 408–13.
5. Allison C, Pratt JA. Neuroadaptive processes in GABAergic and glutamatergic systems in benzodiazepine dependence. *Pharmacol Ther* 2003; 98: 171–95.
6. Mintzer MZ, Stoller KB, Griffiths RR. A controlled study of flumazenil-precipitated withdrawal in chronic low-dose benzodiazepine users. *Psychopharmacology (Berl)* 1999; 147: 200–9.
7. Das P, Lilly SM, Zerda R, Gunning WT, Alvarez FJ, Tietz EI. Increased AMPA receptor GluR1 subunit incorporation in rat hippocampal CA1 synapses during benzodiazepine withdrawal. *J Comp Neurol* 2008; 511: 832–46.
8. Ashton H. Benzodiazepine dependence. In: *Adverse Syndromes and Psychiatric Drugs* (eds P. Haddad, S Dursun, B Deakin), 2004: 239–60. Oxford: Oxford University Press.
9. Framer A. What I have learnt from helping thousands of people taper off psychotropic medications. *Ther Adv Psychopharmacol* 2021; 11: 204512532199127.
10. Ashton H. The diagnosis and management of benzodiazepine dependence. *Curr Opin Psychiatry* 2005; 18: 249–55.
11. Ashton H. Protracted withdrawal from benzodiazepines: the post-withdrawal syndrome. *Psychiatr Ann* 1995; 25: 174–9.
12. Lader MH, Morton SV. A pilot study of the effects of flumazenil on symptoms persisting after benzodiazepine withdrawal. *J Psychopharmacol* 1992; 6: 357–63.

Variety of withdrawal symptoms from benzodiazepines and z-drugs

As benzodiazepines have effects on myriad bodily systems, the withdrawal symptoms produced on stopping are wide-ranging. These can be broadly categorised into physical and psychological symptoms (Table 3.3).[1] Psychological symptoms can easily be mistaken for a return of an underlying condition given that this class of drugs is often prescribed for anxiety, panic and insomnia, which are also common withdrawal symptoms (evident in people even without these pre-existing conditions).[2,3]

People may be prone to characteristic patterns of emotional responses, which may be exacerbated by physiological withdrawal effects – sometimes called rebound symptoms – referring to symptoms present in the baseline condition presenting with greater severity in withdrawal.[1] The familiarity of these symptoms can make the distinction between withdrawal and the re-appearance of other symptoms somewhat confusing to clinicians unfamiliar with the phenomenology of benzodiazepine withdrawal.[4] Psychological symptoms (like anxiety or panic attacks) that emerge after stopping the medication that were not present before taking medication (or are much greater in severity) are likely to be withdrawal symptoms, but ascertaining this requires careful history taking.[4]

Physical symptoms of withdrawal are more distinctive. Benzodiazepines have muscle relaxant effects in the short term; conversely on cessation stiffness, muscle spasm, fasciculations, rigidity and trembling can be experienced.[1] Other neuromuscular effects may be related – such as akathisia (see later), dystonia, diplopia, tics, tremor, tardive dyskinesia (more often associated with long-term antipsychotic use) and myoclonus.[5,6] Failure to recognise abnormal movements as a symptom of benzodiazepine withdrawal can lead to mis-diagnosis of these symptoms as medically unexplained symptoms, functional neurological disorder, other neurological conditions, including multiple sclerosis[5] and psychogenic non-epileptic seizures.[5–7]

Benzodiazepine withdrawal also involves a number of sensory symptoms – possibly arising as a rebound of the numbing and blunting effects experienced while being on benzodiazepines. Alterations of all special senses are quite common in people experiencing withdrawal effects, including changes to vision, sound, taste, touch and smell.[1,8,9] This can involve severe and sometimes intolerable sensory hypersensitivity, tinnitus, photophobia and dysosmia.[5,10] There are numerous changes to sensation that can be disturbing, including hot and cold sensations, numbness, paraesthesiae, pruritus and formication (the sensation of insects crawling under the skin).[5,7] Increased sensitivity can also lead to pain, with allodynia and hyperaesthesia recognised: this can include shooting, twisting, burning and searing pains.[5,7]

Effects on cognition can range from impaired memory and concentration, that can impair decision making, to delirium and profound sedation, especially in older patients,[1,3,8] showing overlap with the withdrawal syndromes of other drugs.[7] Benzodiazepines inhibit REM sleep and so cessation involves a rebound effect, which can include nightmares or night terrors.[1]

The course of benzodiazepine withdrawal symptoms can be highly varied. Although benzodiazepine withdrawal syndromes are generally understood to entail an acute phase of greater intensity that gradually wanes over time, several variations on this have been observed.[7] Some patients experience protracted withdrawal syndromes that last months or years.[1,11] Others demonstrate an early improvement in the intensity of their symptoms, followed by a resurgence over time, and some have sustained chronic

Table 3.3 Withdrawal effects from benzodiazepines and z-drugs, adapted from authoritative sources.[1,2,7,9]

PHYSICAL

General	Neuromuscular	Sleep	Cardiovascular
Sweating	Paraesthesiae	Insomnia	Tachycardia/palpitations
Flu-like symptoms	Myoclonus	Nightmares	Dizziness
Headache	Tremor	Sleep problems	Chest pain
Flushing	Coordination problems		Postural hypotension
Fatigue	Numbness	**Sensory**	Flushing
Pain	Stiffness	Electric shock sensations	Hyperventilation/ dyspnoea
Malaise	Myalgia	Tinnitus	
Itching, skin rash	Fasciculations	Blurred vision/visual changes	**Gastrointestinal**
Ataxia	Cramps	Sensory hypersensitivity – touch/sound/smell	Nausea/vomiting
Increased urinary frequency		Taste/smell disturbances, metallic taste in mouth	Anorexia/weight loss
Lethargy			Diarrhoea
		Perceptual disturbances*	Abdominal pain/cramp
Cognitive	**Neurological**	**Endocrine**	Constipation
Confusion	Seizures**	Breast engorgement	Dry mouth
Amnesia	Light-headedness/vertigo	Menstrual abnormalities	Food intolerance
Impaired concentration			
Indecision			
Depersonalisation/derealisation			

PSYCHOLOGICAL

Affective		Behavioural	Psychotic**
Agoraphobia	Hypochondriasis	Restlessness	Delirium
Anger	Irritability	Aggressive behaviour	Hallucinations
Anhedonia/blunted emotions	Manic symptoms		Paranoia
Anxiety	Obsessive thinking		
Agitation	Panic		
Depression	Terror		
	Suicidality		

*For example, the perception that the floor is undulating.
**Usually only occurs in the context of abrupt or very rapid withdrawal.

symptoms.[7,8] Some patients have symptoms that fluctuate in severity in cycles that last from hours to weeks in duration, overlying a syndrome that generally gradually improves over time.[7,12] This pattern of non-linear symptoms (often described as 'windows and waves') can be perplexing to patients and clinicians, especially as the periodicity of symptoms can vary, as well as the constellation of symptoms over time (with specific groups of symptoms predominating at different points).[7,12]

There are a number of benzodiazepine withdrawal scales that are employed to track withdrawal symptoms (e.g. the Benzodiazepine Withdrawal Symptom Questionnaire and the Clinical Institute Withdrawal Assessment). These may have some utility, however, they may under-estimate the impact of a small number of symptoms of considerable intensity with marked effects on a patient's life.[7] Ratings out of 10 for the specific symptoms that an individual experiences in withdrawal may be more useful to track progress.[7]

Withdrawal akathisia

One of the most distressing consequence of benzodiazepine withdrawal is akathisia, a neuropsychiatric condition (The International Classification of Diseases, 10th Revision, Clinical Modification [ICD-10-CM] Code G25.71), characterised by severe agitation, restlessness and a sense of terror.[13-16] Although this condition is most often recognised as a side effect of antipsychotic use, it has also been observed to occur in benzodiazepine withdrawal.[3,14,17] Patients report a distressing subjective feeling of restlessness and dysphoria.[17,18] They are often fidgeting, pacing, rocking and can be unable to sit or stand still; although sometimes the manifestations are only subjective, sometimes referred to as 'inner akathisia'.[17,18] The pathophysiology is poorly understood, with theories implicating a reduction in dopaminergic activity in the mesocortical pathway projecting from the ventral tegmental area to the limbic system and prefrontal cortex, resulting in suppression of the usual inhibitory effects on motor function, leading to unwanted involuntary movements.[17]

This pronounced state of agitation can be mis-diagnosed as a manic state,[15] an anxiety disorder, a panic disorder, a personality disorder, attention deficit hyperactivity disorder (ADHD), health anxiety, drug-seeking behaviour, restless leg disorder, functional neurological disorder, or a factitious disorder by clinicians unfamiliar with the syndrome in benzodiazepine withdrawal.[17-19] It has been associated with suicidality because of the distress and agitation it engenders.[3,17,18]

Determinants of severity of withdrawal symptoms

There has been limited research into which factors determine the incidence and severity of the benzodiazepine withdrawal syndrome. The speed of tapering is thought to be one of the main determinants.[7,8] Some (mixed) evidence suggests that being older and being female increase difficulties.[7,20-22] A longer duration of use correlates with a greater intensity of withdrawal symptoms,[8] as do higher doses.[7,8,23] Shorter-acting benzodiazepines also are associated with higher risks of withdrawal, probably because their quicker elimination produces a greater difference in the homeostatic set-point of the system, after chronic use, and levels of drug present.[8,23] It has also been thought that several cycles on and off benzodiazepines (and perhaps other psychiatric medications) can make subsequent withdrawal attempts more difficult, due to increased sensitisation (often called kindling).[4,7,24,25]

References

1. Cosci F, Chouinard G. Acute and persistent withdrawal syndromes following discontinuation of psychotropic medications. *Psychother Psychosom* 2020; 89: 283–306.
2. Sokya M. Treatment of benzodiazepine dependence. *N Engl J Med.* 2017; 376: 1147–57. doi: 10.1056/NEJM1611832.
3. Reid Finlayson AJ, Macoubrie J, Huff C, Foster DE, Martin PR. Experiences with benzodiazepine use, tapering, and discontinuation: an Internet survey. *Ther Adv Psychopharmacol* 2022; 12: 20451253221082384.
4. Framer A. What I have learnt from helping thousands of people taper off psychotropic medications. *Ther Adv Psychopharmacol* 2021; 11: 204512532199127.
5. Ashton H. Benzodiazepines: how they work and how to withdraw (The Ashton Manual). Newcastle University, 2002. http://www.benzo.org.uk/manual/bzcha01.htm (accessed 11 July 2023).
6. Busto U, Sellers EM, Naranjo CA, Cappell H, Sanchez-Craig M, Sykora K. Withdrawal reaction after long-term therapeutic use of benzodiazepines. *N Engl J Med* 1986; 315: 854–9.
7. Wright SL. Benzodiazepine withdrawal: clinical aspects. In: *The Benzodiazepines* Crisis (eds J Peppin, J Pergolizzi, R Raffa, S Wright) 2020: 117–C8.P334. Oxford: Oxford University Press. doi:10.1093/med/9780197517277.003.0008.
8. Ashton H. The diagnosis and management of benzodiazepine dependence. *Curr Opin Psychiatry* 2005; 18: 249–55.
9. Petursson H. The benzodiazepine withdrawal syndrome. *Addiction* 1994; 89: 1455–9.
10. Pelissolo A, Bisserbe JC. [Dependence on benzodiazepines. Clinical and biological aspects]. *Encephale* 1994; 20: 147–57.
11. Lerner A, Klein M. Dependence, withdrawal and rebound of CNS drugs: an update and regulatory considerations for new drugs development. *Brain Commun* 2019; 1: fcz025.
12. Ashton H. Protracted withdrawal syndromes from benzodiazepines. *J Subst Abuse Treat* 1991; 8: 19–28.
13. Hirose S. Restlessness related to SSRI withdrawal. *Psychiatry Clin Neurosci* 2001; 55: 79–80.
14. Guy A, Brown M, Lewis S, Horowitz MA. The 'patient voice' – patients who experience antidepressant withdrawal symptoms are often dismissed, or mis-diagnosed with relapse, or onset of a new medical condition. *Ther Adv Psychopharmacol* 2020; 10: 204512532096718.
15. Narayan V, Haddad PM. Antidepressant discontinuation manic states: a critical review of the literature and suggested diagnostic criteria. *J Psychopharmacol* 2010; 25: 306–13.
16. Sathananthan GL, Gershon S. Imipramine withdrawal: an akathisia-like syndrome. *Am J Psychiatry* 1973; 130: 1286–7.
17. Tachere RO, Modirrousta M. Beyond anxiety and agitation: a clinical approach to akathisia. *Aust Fam Physician* 2017; 46: 296–8.
18. Akathisia Alliance for education and research. Akathisia Alliance for education and research. https://akathisiaalliance.org/about-akathisia/ (accessed 17 September 2022).
19. Lohr JB, Eidt CA, Abdulrazzaq Alfaraj A, Soliman MA. The clinical challenges of akathisia. *CNS Spectr* 2015; 20 Suppl 1: 1–14; quiz 15–16.
20. Schweizer E, Rickels K, Case WG, Greenblatt DJ. Long-term therapeutic use of benzodiazepines. II. Effects of gradual taper. *Arch Gen Psychiatry* 1990; 47: 908–15.
21. Schweizer E, Case WG, Rickels K. Benzodiazepine dependence and withdrawal in elderly patients. *Am J Psychiatry* 1989; 146: 529–31.
22. Gorgels WJMJ, Oude Voshaar RC, Mol AJJ, et al. Predictors of discontinuation of benzodiazepine prescription after sending a letter to long-term benzodiazepine users in family practice. *Fam Pract* 2006; 23: 65–72.
23. Rickels K, Schweizer E, Case WG, Greenblatt DJ. Long-term therapeutic use of benzodiazepines. I. Effects of abrupt discontinuation. *Arch Gen Psychiatry* 1990; 47: 899–907.
24. Stephens DN. A glutamatergic hypothesis of drug dependence: extrapolations from benzodiazepine receptor ligands. *Behav Pharmacol* 1995; 6: 425–46.
25. Allison C, Pratt JA. Neuroadaptive processes in GABAergic and glutamatergic systems in benzodiazepine dependence. *Pharmacol Ther* 2003; 98: 171–95.

CHAPTER 3

Protracted benzodiazepine withdrawal syndrome

While acute withdrawal symptoms from benzodiazepines are quite well recognised, there is less appreciation for the existence of protracted withdrawal symptoms from benzodiazepines, although these have been recognised since at least the 1980s.[1-3] The FDA issued a boxed warning (its highest level of warning) in 2020 in part to draw attention to the issue of a protracted withdrawal syndrome. The FDA warns that 'Protracted withdrawal syndrome persists beyond 4 to 6 weeks after initial benzodiazepine withdrawal. Symptoms may last weeks to as long as 12 months.'[4] The FDA also highlighted that the duration in some patients could be 'years',[4] supported by recent studies.[5,6] This represents an update to previous notions that benzodiazepine withdrawal symptoms normally resolve within 28 days[7,8] and are mostly mild and self-limiting.[9] Withdrawal symptoms persisting beyond 6–8 weeks are variously called protracted, prolonged or persistent or termed the 'post-acute withdrawal syndrome' (PAWS).[3,10,11]

The FDA highlighted the following symptoms of protracted withdrawal:

- anxiety,
- cognitive impairment,
- depression,
- insomnia,
- formication,
- motor symptoms (e.g. weakness, tremor, muscle twitches),
- paraesthesia, and
- tinnitus.

There has been limited formal study into the average duration of withdrawal symptoms – there are reports of weeks-long duration, but symptoms can last longer than a year, especially in the case of long-term use.[12,13] Although there is some uncertainty, people experienced in the treatment of withdrawal estimate that a sizeable minority, perhaps 10–25% of people who stop long-term benzodiazepines will experience a protracted course of withdrawal consisting of mental and physical symptoms that often fluctuate unpredictably in a pattern known as 'waves and windows'.[3,14] 'Waves' refers to periods of relatively severe symptoms, whilst 'windows' refers to periods of relative freedom from symptoms. The most common symptoms of the protracted withdrawal syndrome are shown in Table 3.4, with much overlap with acute withdrawal symptoms. Notably, anxiety and insomnia are prominent symptoms in protracted withdrawal. These were found in 50% of people with the syndrome in one survey who were originally prescribed benzodiazepines for indications other than anxiety or insomnia (for example muscle spasms, or pain).[6] Many people who experience this syndrome, finding little recognition or assistance from medical providers, seek online peer support, with the largest of these forums having 90,000 members.[15]

Sometimes clinicians are mystified on hearing about withdrawal syndromes that persist for months or years, given that it takes only days or at most weeks for benzodiazepines and z-drugs to be eliminated from the body. However, withdrawal syndromes are caused by adaptations to the presence of the drug that persist for longer than it takes the drug to be eliminated from the system.[16] There has been little study of the long-lasting changes to the brain following benzodiazepine cessation but adaptations such as down-regulation of adenosine receptors, uncoupling between allosteric linkage of GABA and the benzodiazepine site, or persistence of up-regulated glutamatergic pathways, amongst other downstream and related effects, may explain the long-lasting persistence of withdrawal effects in some patients after benzodiazepine cessation.[17] Protracted withdrawal syndromes are thought to persist for as long as it takes these adaptations to the drug to resolve after cessation, and not simply how long it takes the drug to be eliminated.[11,18]

In a large, self-selected sample of 1,200 patients who were seeking peer support for stopping benzodiazepines and the withdrawal symptoms they experienced after stopping, the vast majority reported profound consequences to their lives.[5] Most of these patients had been prescribed benzodiazepines for anxiety or insomnia. The main symptoms these people experienced after stopping were anxiety, fear, sleep disturbances, lack of energy, difficulty concentrating and memory loss, along with a variety of physical symptoms (Table 3.4).[6] In more than half of these cases the protracted withdrawal symptoms affected their marriage, almost half had lost their job or became unable to work, and half had either attempted or contemplated suicide.[5] Many patients reported that their symptoms were not recognised by doctors or were dismissed ('I was told I was making up symptoms by reading medical information').[5] Although presumably this self-selected group represents a more severe syndrome than the average patient, it demonstrates how debilitating the syndrome can be in a proportion of patients.

Table 3.4 Most commonly reported symptoms of 1,200 people with protracted withdrawal symptoms from benzodiazepines, adapted from Finlayson et al. (2022).[5]

Emotional	Neurological	Cognitive
Nervousness, anxiety, fear	Sensory sensitivity (light, noise, smell)	Concentration difficulties
Crying spells	Seizure activity	Memory loss
Anger	Trembling	
Lack of emotions (blunting)	Akathisia	
Hallucinations (rare)		

General	Gastrointestinal	Sensory
Low energy	Nausea	Balance problems
Sleep disturbance	Diarrhoea and other digestive issues	Stabbing pain
Muscle weakness	Anorexia	Joint pain
Sensitivity to alcohol, caffeine, or specific foods		Tingling sensation in skin
Difficulty breathing		Burning pains
Difficulty with swallowing		Aching sensations
Cardiac irregularities		
Hypertension		
Functional impairment (e.g. driving or walking)		
Headache		

Some researchers suggest these long-lasting neurological, cognitive, affective and somatic problems, which persist for years after stopping benzodiazepines in some people, are best conceptualised as benzodiazepine-induced neurological dysfunction (BIND), which generally shows gradual improvement over time.[6,19] There is a lack of understanding of the underlying mechanisms of this condition, but it has been postulated to relate to persistent neuro-adaptation or cumulative direct neurotoxic effects,[2,6] as seen in animal models.[20]

References

1. Ashton H. Benzodiazepine withdrawal: an unfinished story. *Br Med J* 1984; 288: 1135–40.
2. Ashton H. Protracted withdrawal syndromes from benzodiazepines. *J Subst Abuse Treat* 1991; 8: 19–28.
3. Ashton H. Protracted Withdrawal from benzodiazepines: the post-withdrawal syndrome. *Psychiatr Ann* 1995; 25: 174–9.
4. FDA Drug Safety Communication. FDA requiring boxed warning updated to improve safe use of benzodiazepine drug class. 2020. https://www.fda.gov/drugs/drug-safety-and-availability/fda-requiring-boxed-warning-updated-improve-safe-use-benzodiazepine-drug-class#:~:text=FDA is requiring the Boxed,and life-threatening side effects (accessed 3 July 2023).
5. Reid Finlayson AJ, Macoubrie J, Huff C, Foster DE, Martin PR. Experiences with benzodiazepine use, tapering, and discontinuation: an internet survey. *Ther Adv Psychopharmacol* 2022; 12: 20451253221082384.
6. Huff C, Finlayson AJR, Foster DE, Martin PR. Enduring neurological sequelae of benzodiazepine use: an internet survey. *Ther Adv Psychopharmacol* 2023; 13: 20451253221145560.
7. Petursson H. The benzodiazepine withdrawal syndrome. *Addiction* 1994; 89: 1455–9.
8. Owen RT, Tyrer P. Benzodiazepine dependence. A review of the evidence. *Drugs* 1983; 25: 385–98.
9. Busto U, Sellers EM, Naranjo CA, Cappell H, Sanchez-Craig M, Sykora K. Withdrawal reaction after long-term therapeutic use of benzodiazepines. *N Engl J Med* 1986; 315: 854–9.
10. Cosci F, Chouinard G. Acute and persistent withdrawal syndromes following discontinuation of psychotropic medications. *Psychother Psychosom* 2020; 89: 283–306.
11. Wright SL. Benzodiazepine withdrawal: clinical aspects. In: *The Benzodiazepines* Crisis (eds. J Peppin, J Pergolizzi, R Raffa, S Wright) 2020: 117–C8.P334. Oxford: Oxford University Press. doi:10.1093/med/9780197517277.003.0008.
12. Ashton H. Benzodiazepine withdrawal: outcome in 50 patients. *Br J Addict* 1987; 82: 665–71.
13. Schweizer E, Rickels K. Benzodiazepine dependence and withdrawal: a review of the syndrome and its clinical management. *Acta Psychiatr Scand* 1998; 98: 95–101.
14. Hood SD, Norman A, Hince DA, Melichar JK, Hulse GK. Benzodiazepine dependence and its treatment with low dose flumazenil. *Br J Clin Pharmacol* 2014; 77: 285–94.
15. BenzoBuddies Community Forum. http://www.benzobuddies.org/forum/index.php (accessed 18 March 2023).
16. Reidenberg MM. Drug discontinuation effects are part of the pharmacology of a drug. *J Pharmacol Exp Ther* 2011; 339: 324–8.
17. Cheng T, Wallace DM, Ponteri B, Tuli M. Valium without dependence? Individual GABA$_a$ receptor subtype contribution toward benzodiazepine addiction, tolerance, and therapeutic effects. *Neuropsychiatr Dis Treat* 2018; 14: 1351–61.
18. Ashton H. Benzodiazepines: how they work and how to withdraw (The Ashton Manual). Newcastle University. 2002. http://www.benzo.org.uk/manual/bzcha01.htm (accessed 11 July 2023).
19. Alexis D. Ritvo AD, Foster DE, et al. Long-term consequences of benzodiazepine-induced neurological dysfunction: a survey. *PLoS One* 2023; 18: e0285584.
20. Shi Y, Cui M, Ochs K, et al. Long-term diazepam treatment enhances microglial spine engulfment and impairs cognitive performance via the mitochondrial 18 kDa translocator protein (TSPO). *Nat Neurosci* 2022; 25: 317–29.

CHAPTER 3

Distinguishing benzodiazepine withdrawal symptoms from return of an underlying condition

The FDA highlighted in its report on benzodiazepine withdrawal that clinicians commonly mis-diagnose withdrawal symptoms from benzodiazepines as relapse or onset of other health conditions, leading to higher doses of the drug being prescribed.[1] Patients also report this commonly but this has not been studied systematically.[2,3] It is perhaps understandable why this may occur given limited familiarity with the withdrawal syndrome, especially in its protracted form. While anxiety, panic attacks and insomnia are common withdrawal symptoms from these drugs which in some cases can last for several months, or even years,[4] there is a general perception that these symptoms are generally minor or short-lived. When people present with severe and/or long-lasting symptoms there is a tendency to believe that these symptoms could not be explained by a withdrawal syndrome.[5]

There are several aspects that can allow distinction of withdrawal symptoms from a return of an underlying condition:

- The simplest method is when patients are able to communicate that the symptoms feel quite distinct to them from their underlying condition. Patients often say 'I've never felt this way before.'[2] In such cases it is often wise to heed advice attributed to Osler[6] 'Listen to your patient; he is telling you the diagnosis.'
- The timing of symptoms can be helpful: symptoms that occur soon after dose reduction or cessation are more likely to be withdrawal symptoms with such symptoms normally having onset within hours or days after dose reduction.[7] However, there are also reports of withdrawal symptoms being delayed for weeks after cessation for reasons that are not well understood (but often with quite distinctive characteristics of the benzodiazepine withdrawal syndrome).[8–10]
- The presence of physical withdrawal symptoms: there are numerous physical withdrawal symptoms shown in Table 3.5 that are not characteristic of the conditions for which benzodiazepines are normally prescribed, such as muscle cramping, distinctive sensory symptoms (such as increased sensitivity to sensations), cognitive impairments, cardiovascular and gastrointestinal symptoms.[5] The presence of these symptoms alongside psychological symptoms help to delineate these presentations as withdrawal syndromes.[5] It has been suggested that patients may be experiencing relapse and withdrawal that are co-incident, and while this is a possibility, Occam's razor suggests that it is more likely that one condition will cause many symptoms, rather than requiring multiple syndromes for explanation.[11]
- The presence of psychological withdrawal symptoms that are different in nature or intensity from the underlying condition. Withdrawal symptoms of a psychological nature present greater uncertainty in diagnosis; psychological symptoms that are distinct from those for which the medication was first prescribed (e.g. the emergence of panic and anxiety on dose cessation for a patient prescribed a drug for muscular problems) should suggest withdrawal.[7] Observation of psychological symptoms similar to the problems that prompted diagnosis, but of greater intensity, are often called rebound symptoms- a withdrawal phenomenon- whereby characteristic emotional patterns are amplified by the physiological withdrawal process.[2] This diagnostic uncertainty should also be framed by the limited evidence for the long-term effectiveness of BzRAs for insomnia or anxiety.[12]

Table 3.5 Benzodiazepine withdrawal symptoms – overlapping with anxiety disorders and more distinctive symptoms. Adapted from Ashton (2005).[14]

Symptoms that overlap with anxiety disorders*	Symptoms that are relatively specific to benzodiazepine withdrawal
Anxiety, panic attacks and agoraphobia	Depersonalisation/derealisation
Blurred or double vision	Distortion of body image
Depression, dysphoria	Formication ('skin crawling')
Dizziness, light-headedness	Hallucinations (visual or auditory)
Excitability, restlessness	Muscle twitches, jerks, fasciculations
Insomnia, nightmares	Perceptual distortions, sense of movement
Muscle pain, stiffness	Sensory hypersensitivity (to light, taste, sound, and smell)
Palpitations	Tingling, numbness, altered sensation
Poor memory, concentration	Tinnitus
Sweating, night sweats	Confusion, delirium**
Tremor	Convulsions**
Weakness ('jelly legs')	Psychotic symptoms**

*If these symptoms were not present in the underlying condition but appeared for the first time on dose reduction or cessation, or appeared with much greater intensity, there should be a high index of suspicion for a withdrawal syndrome.
**Usually only occurs on rapid or abrupt withdrawal from high-dose benzodiazepines, but can occur rarely in other cases.

- The presence of similar symptoms of withdrawal whilst patients were on maintenance benzodiazepines, is suggestive of withdrawal effects. Withdrawal effects can emerge while patients are taking medication due to the process of tolerance (sometimes called 'tolerance withdrawal', see later), most often seen with short-acting benzodiazepines (often observed as inter-dose withdrawal).[5]
- A pattern of waxing and waning symptom intensity. This has been described as a 'waves and windows' pattern of symptomatology, and is thought to be caused by non-linear processes in the body re-adapting to the absence of benzodiazepines but is inadequately understood.[5,13,14]

Mis-diagnosis of withdrawal as new onset of another mental or physical condition

Sometimes symptoms that emerge on dose cessation are mis-diagnosed as new onset of a mental health condition, such as an anxiety disorder, insomnia, bipolar disorder.[3,7] They can also be mis-diagnosed as another physical diagnosis such as medically unexplained symptoms (MUS), chronic fatigue syndrome (CFS) or functional neurological disorder (FND), somatoform disorder, multiple sclerosis because the myriad symptoms of the benzodiazepine withdrawal syndrome (e.g. psychiatric symptoms, fatigue, muscle fasciculations, cramps, tremor or other neurological symptoms) overlap with the diagnostic criteria of these syndromes.[3,7]

References

1. FDA. Integrated drug utilization, epidemiology and pharmacovigilance review: benzodiazepine use, misuse, abuse, dependence, withdrawal, morbidity, and mortality. 2020. www.benzoinfo.com/wp-content/uploads/2020/11/Benzodiazepine-Information-Coalition-FOIA-FDA-.pdf.

2. Framer A. What I have learnt from helping thousands of people taper off psychotropic medications. *Ther Adv Psychopharmacol* 2021; 11: 204512532199127.

3. Guy A, Brown M, Lewis S, Horowitz MA. The 'Patient voice' – patients who experience antidepressant withdrawal symptoms are often dismissed, or mis-diagnosed with relapse, or onset of a new medical condition. *Ther Adv Psychopharmacol* 2020; 10: 204512532096718.

4. FDA Drug Safety Communication. FDA requiring boxed warning updated to improve safe use of benzodiazepine drug class. 2020. https://www.fda.gov/drugs/drug-safety-and-availability/fda-requiring-boxed-warning-updated-improve-safe-use-benzodiazepine-drug-class#:~:text=FDA is requiring the Boxed,and life-threatening side effects (accessed 3 July 2023).

5. Wright SL. Benzodiazepine withdrawal: clinical aspects. In: *The Benzodiazepines* Crisis (eds. J Peppin, J Pergolizzi, R Raffa, S Wright) 2020: 117–C8.P334. Oxford: Oxford University Press. doi:10.1093/med/9780197517277.003.0008.

6. Aronson JK. When I use a word . . . . Listening to the patient. *BMJ* 2022; 376: o646.

7. Ashton H. Benzodiazepines: how they work and how to withdraw (The Ashton Manual). Newcastle University, 2002. http://www.benzo.org.uk/manual/bzcha01.htm (accessed 11 July 2023).

8. Repplinger D, Nelson LS. Case studies in toxicology: withdrawal: another danger of diversion. 2016; published online 1 February. https://www.mdedge.com/clinicianreviews/article/106391/toxicology/case-studies-toxicology-withdrawal-another-danger (accessed 13 April 2023).

9. Ishii N, Terao T, Araki Y, Hatano K. Repeated seizures in an elderly patient with alcohol dependence and mild cognitive impairment. *BMJ Case Rep* 2013; 2013. doi:10.1136/bcr-2013-201575.

10. National Institute for Health and Care Excellence (NICE). Medicines associated with dependence or withdrawal symptoms: safe prescribing and withdrawal management for adults | Guidance | NICE. 2022. https://www.nice.org.uk/guidance/ng215/chapter/Recommendations (accessed 27 June 2022).

11. Wildner M. In memory of William of Occam [16]. *Lancet* 1999; 354: 2172.

12. Gale C, Glue P, Guaiana G, Coverdale J, McMurdo M, Wilkinson S. Influence of covariates on heterogeneity in Hamilton Anxiety Scale ratings in placebo-controlled trials of benzodiazepines in generalized anxiety disorder: Systematic review and meta-analysis. *J Psychopharmacol* 2019; 33: 543–7.

13. Ashton H. Protracted withdrawal syndromes from benzodiazepines. *J Subst Abuse Treat* 1991; 8: 19–28.

14. Ashton H. The diagnosis and management of benzodiazepine dependence. *Curr Opin Psychiatry* 2005; 18: 249–55.

CHAPTER 3

Withdrawal symptoms during benzodiazepine maintenance treatment

Withdrawal symptoms, perhaps counter-intuitively, can occur during maintenance treatment and if not recognised can lead to the erroneous diagnosis of new conditions or the impression that the original condition has worsened, leading to escalation of doses or introduction of new treatments.[1,2] The situation is seen most clearly with inter-dose withdrawal in between doses of short-acting benzodiazepines.[1] For example, patients taking triazolam as a hypnotic can develop daytime anxiety, and even hallucinations or psychotic symptoms that are relieved by re-dosing the drug.[3,4] Patients taking alprazolam or lorazepam can develop increasing anxiety and panic between doses, relieved by taking the medication.[1,5]

Even with long-acting benzodiazepines such as diazepam there can be a history of steadily increasing anxiety, the development of new symptoms such as agoraphobia, along with perceptual distortions and depersonalisation, consistent with benzodiazepine withdrawal symptoms, which dissipate on discontinuation of the drug.[1] Withdrawal symptoms that emerge whilst on maintenance treatment due to the development of tolerance and consequent diminished effects of the drug are often called 'tolerance withdrawal'.[1] These symptoms can often be alleviated by an increase in dose, but re-emerge again with ongoing use and only disappear completely after the drug is stopped.[1,3,5] Withdrawal symptoms may be prompted by missed doses of the drug – which if not considered can lead to mis-diagnosis of a new-onset physical health condition or worsening mental health condition(s).[6]

References

1. Ashton H. Protracted withdrawal syndromes from benzodiazepines. *J Subst Abuse Treat* 1991; 8: 19–28.
2. Reid Finlayson AJ, Macoubrie J, Huff C, Foster DE, Martin PR. Experiences with benzodiazepine use, tapering, and discontinuation: an internet survey. *Ther Adv Psychopharmacol* 2022; 12: 20451253221082384.
3. Ashton H. Benzodiazepine withdrawal: outcome in 50 patients. *Br J Addict* 1987; 82: 665–71.
4. Oswald I. Triazolam syndrome 10 years on. *Lancet* 1989; 2: 451–2.
5. Ashton H. Benzodiazepine withdrawal: an unfinished story. *Br Med J* 1984; 288: 1135–40.
6. Framer A. What I have learnt from helping thousands of people taper off psychotropic medications. *Ther Adv Psychopharmacol* 2021; 11: 204512532199127.

How to Deprescribe Benzodiazepines and Z-drugs Safely

As discussed in the first section of Chapter 3 deprescribing of benzodiazepines and z-drugs should generally be offered to all patients who have been taking them for more than 4 weeks.[1-3] There are a few exceptions to this: those taking benzodiazepines for seizure prevention, those at the end of life, and those for whom the harms of stopping may outweigh the harms of continuing. These exceptions may also include those with serious mental illness for whom the deprescribing process might be too destabilising, those with stable, occasional use, or those for whom the withdrawal process has been previously unbearable. If the patient agrees to stop benzodiazepines, they should normally be gradually withdrawn. Tapering and stopping can be an unpleasant experience and should not therefore be imposed on a patient against their wishes.

The updated FDA boxed warning in 2020 warned of sometimes severe and long-lasting withdrawal effects from benzodiazepines. Although current deprescribing guidance is rather varied,[4] there is broad overall consensus that a gradual taper, adjusted according to withdrawal symptoms experienced by the patient is the best approach.[2,5-7] There is, however, a general message from patients that what is considered 'gradual' by most clinicians is not gradual enough to avoid unpleasant withdrawal effects. The FDA advises that a gradual taper can potentially mitigate the severity of withdrawal but does not provide specific guidance on tapering or give detailed protocols.[8] NICE in the UK has published some guidance for tapering benzodiazepines,[6] based on guidelines put forward by Professor Ashton,[5] although a proportion of patients report that the speed of the recommended tapers can be too rapid.[7]

The following guidelines on how to stop benzodiazepines and z-drugs is based on existing studies, guidelines and clinical experience, in addition to the pharmacological principles dictating benzodiazepine and z-drug action. Importantly, these guidelines are also informed by the experience of patient experts (including those with medical training) who have successfully completed a benzodiazepine taper and advise others in peer-led communities.

There is a dearth of clinical trials to inform every aspect of this guidance, and so it is suggested that shared decision making be used to guide action taken in the context of inevitable uncertainty. The guidelines outlined should not replace clinical judgement and the overarching principle should be to find a rate of taper that does not cause intolerable withdrawal symptoms for an individual patient.

Preparing to stop benzodiazepines

Preparation for deprescribing is an important part of the whole process. Patients may not have been informed of the dangers of long-term benzodiazepine and z-drug use,[9] and so education about the risks, benefits and alternatives to these medications is important (see the first section of this chapter). This educational intervention in itself has been shown to increase the likelihood of successful cessation.[7,10] Informing patients about the discontinuation process is important so that people know what to expect. This can involve education about withdrawal effects (see section on withdrawal effects) and the techniques that can be involved to mitigate these risks.

CHAPTER 3

Ongoing support can be required to prepare a patient for withdrawal and to sustain them through the process.[7] This can involve activating their network of family and friends, further engagement with professionals (e.g. therapists)[11] or connecting them to peer support (in person or online).[7] Peer-support communities can be a double-edged sword. These groups can provide camaraderie, normalisation and support during a difficult process but may also expose patients to 'horror stories' of people who have endured a very severe withdrawal process. Expectations need to be carefully managed.

Coping skills can be useful to prepare for benzodiazepine tapering as although withdrawal symptoms can be minimised by gradual, flexible, hyperbolic tapering they are unlikely to be avoided completely. So, the bolstering of existing coping skills or development of new ones can be helpful. Briefly, these skills can include intentional relaxation (mindfulness, guided meditation, etc), breathing exercises, exercise (e.g. yoga), learning to accept symptoms, distraction techniques, sleep hygiene,[12] CBT for insomnia (and anxiety), diary keeping, de-catastrophising and stress reduction.[11,13] Sometimes lightening work or family duties may be helpful, where this is feasible.

Specific treatments for the original indications for benzodiazepines and z-drugs can be helpful for the withdrawal process, especially if anxiety and insomnia are ongoing concerns. As mentioned previously, benzodiazepines and z-drugs may themselves contribute to increased levels of anxiety and depression, and tapering these medications may actually improve these symptoms.[5,14,15]

CBT-I is the first line treatment for insomnia. This has been shown to produce a greater reduction in sleep latency than medication[16] with a favourable balance of benefit and harm compared with medication.[17] Circadian rhythm disturbances are common due to a lack of light exposure in the morning and excessive exposure to light at night leading to insomnia and grogginess in the morning.[18] Where circadian rhythms play a role in insomnia, the use of light exposure in the morning (e.g. going outside or the use of a light box) and light restriction at night (dimming screens, use of lamps rather than overhead lights, various blue light blocking techniques) and possibly timed melatonin (most useful as a circadian cue at low doses taken several hours before bed, rather than as a hypnotic) can be helpful.[18]

Anxiety disorders may be treated with a variety of effective psychotherapy and non-psychotherapy modalities, for example mindfulness approaches, CBT, a variety of self-help approaches,[19] exercise[20] and other non-pharmacological approaches.[21] Learning the necessary skills to manage anxiety and insomnia may have the dual benefit of making the withdrawal process easier,[22] as well as preparing the person for life without medication.

References

1. Benzodiazepine and z-drug withdrawal. https://cks.nice.org.uk/topics/benzodiazepine-z-drug-withdrawal/ (accessed 2 April 2023).

2. Kaiser Permanente. Benzodiazepine and z-drug safety guideline expectations for Kaiser Foundation Health Plan of Washington Providers. 2019. https://wa.kaiserpermanente.org/static/pdf/public/guidelines/benzo-zdrug.pdf (accessed 3 July 2023).

3. Pottie K, Thompson W, Davies S, et al. Deprescribing benzodiazepine receptor agonists: evidence-based clinical practice guideline. *Can Fam Physician* 2018; 64: 339–51.

4. Pollmann AS, Murphy AL, Bergman JC, Gardner DM. Deprescribing benzodiazepines and z-drugs in community-dwelling adults: a scoping review. *BMC Pharmacol Toxicol* 2015; 16: 19.

5. Ashton H. Benzodiazepines: how they work and how to withdraw (The Ashton Manual). Newcastle University, 2002. http://www.benzo.org.uk/manual/bzcha01.htm (accessed 11 July 2023).

6. Scenario: benzodiazepine and z-drug withdrawal. https://cks.nice.org.uk/topics/benzodiazepine-z-drug-withdrawal/management/benzodiazepine-z-drug-withdrawal/ (accessed 7 October 2022).

7. Wright SL. Benzodiazepine withdrawal: clinical aspects. In: *The Benzodiazepines Crisis* (eds. J Peppin, J Pergolizzi, R Raffa, S Wright) 2020: 117–C8.P334. Oxford: Oxford University Press. doi:10.1093/med/9780197517277.003.0008.

8. FDA Drug Safety Communication. FDA requiring boxed warning updated to improve safe use of benzodiazepine drug class. 2020. https://www.fda.gov/drugs/drug-safety-and-availability/fda-requiring-boxed-warning-updated-improve-safe-use-benzodiazepine-drug-class#:~:text=FDA is requiring the Boxed,and life-threatening side effects (accessed 3 July 2023).

9. Reid Finlayson AJ, Macoubrie J, Huff C, Foster DE, Martin PR. Experiences with benzodiazepine use, tapering, and discontinuation: an internet survey. *Ther Adv Psychopharmacol* 2022; 12: 20451253221082384.

10. Tannenbaum C, Martin P, Tamblyn R, Benedetti A, Ahmed S. Reduction of inappropriate benzodiazepine prescriptions among older adults through direct patient education: the EMPOWER cluster randomized trial. *JAMA Intern Med* 2014; 174: 890–8.

11. Guy A, Davies J, Rizq R. *Guidance for Psychological Therapists: Enabling Conversations with Clients Taking or Withdrawing from Prescribed Psychiatric Drugs.* London: APPG for Prescribed Drug Dependence, 2019.

12. Morgan K, Dixon S, Mathers N, Thompson J, Tomeny M. Psychological treatment for insomnia in the regulation of long-term hypnotic drug use. *Health Technol Assess* 2004; 8: iii–iv, 1–68.

13. The Withdrawal Project. https://withdrawal.theinnercompass.org/.

14. Ashton H. Benzodiazepine withdrawal: outcome in 50 patients. *Br J Addict* 1987; 82: 665–71.

15. Guina J, Merrill B. Benzodiazepines I: upping the care on downers: the evidence of risks, benefits and alternatives. *J Clin Med Res* 2018; 7: 17.

16. Smith MT, Perlis ML, Park A, et al. Comparative meta-analysis of pharmacotherapy and behavior therapy for persistent insomnia. *Am J Psychiatry* 2002; 159: 5–11.

17. Buysse DJ. Insomnia. *JAMA* 2013; 309: 706–16.

18. Lack LC, Wright HR. Treating chronobiological components of chronic insomnia. *Sleep Med* 2007; 8: 637–44.

19. Lewis C, Pearce J, Bisson JI. Efficacy, cost-effectiveness and acceptability of self-help interventions for anxiety disorders: systematic review. *Br J Psychiatry* 2012; 200: 15–21.

20. Aylett E, Small N, Bower P. Exercise in the treatment of clinical anxiety in general practice – a systematic review and meta-analysis. *BMC Health Serv Res* 2018; 18: 559.

21. Moreno-Peral P, Conejo-Cerón S, Rubio-Valera M, et al. Effectiveness of psychological and/or educational interventions in the prevention of anxiety: a systematic review, meta-analysis, and meta-regression. *JAMA Psychiatry* 2017; 74: 1021–9.

22. National Institute for Health and Care Excellence (NICE). Generalised anxiety disorder and panic disorder in adults: management. *NICE clinical guideline CG113* 2011. https://www.nice.org.uk/guidance/cg113/chapter/2-Research-recommendations#the-effectiveness-of-physical-activity-compared-with-waiting-list-control-for-the-treatment-of-gad.

CHAPTER 3

Tapering benzodiazepines and z-drugs gradually

Stopping benzodiazepines abruptly risks severe withdrawal reactions, including seizures, which can be life threatening.[1] Abrupt cessation also probably presents the greatest risk of developing protracted withdrawal symptoms.[2] All manufacturers of benzodiazepines recommend that their drugs be tapered slowly to reduce risk of withdrawal. However, the rates of tapering recommended (over weeks) are often too quick for many patients to tolerate. Professor Heather Ashton, an expert in this area, said that 'the classic six weeks withdrawal period adopted by many clinics and doctors is much too fast for many long- term users'.[2] For people taking benzodiazepines long term, it may take 12 to 18 months or more to discontinue safely.[2,3]

Gradual reduction of benzodiazepine dose reduces the intensity of withdrawal probably by giving time for neural adaptations made to the drug to resolve (Figure 3.4).[4] One meta-analysis found that gradual dose reduction ('tapering') improves drug cessation rates 6-fold compared to routine clinical care.[5] Most studies find that a gradual withdrawal over at least 10 weeks is most successful in achieving long-term cessation.[6] NICE advises that stopping diazepam safely after long-term use can take between 9 and 18 months,[7] although some patients will require longer periods.[3]

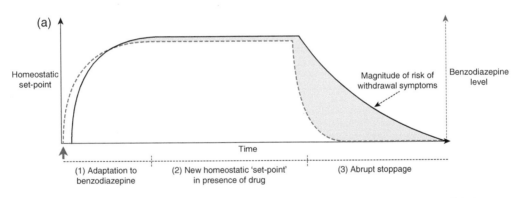

Figure 3.4 The neurobiology of tapering benzodiazepines. In this figure, the homeostatic 'set-point' of the brain is shown in black and benzodiazepine levels are shown in purple dashed lines. Adapted from Horowitz and Taylor (2021).[8] The shaded grey regions represent the degree of risk of withdrawal symptoms, the larger the area the greater the risk of withdrawal. (a) (1) A benzodiazepine is introduced (solid purple arrow). (2) The brain adapts to levels of a drug used over time. (3) The medication is abruptly ceased and plasma drug levels drop to zero (exponentially, according to the elimination half-life of the drug). This difference between the homeostatic set-point (the 'expectations' of the system) and the level of drug in the system (dashed purple line) is experienced as withdrawal symptoms.

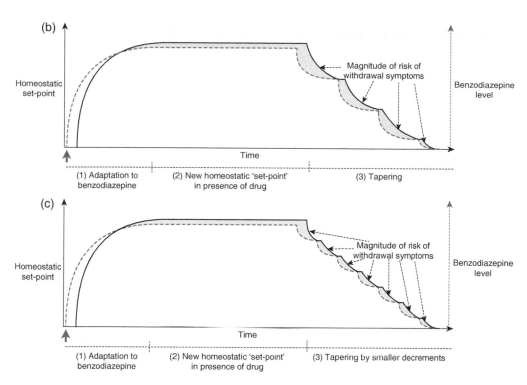

Figure 3.4 (*continued*) (b) (3) Tapering: when a drug is reduced step-wise, drug levels reduce exponentially to lower levels. At each step, there is a lag as the system adapts to a new level of drug, causing withdrawal symptoms (dashed arrows), but of lesser intensity (shaded area under the small, cupped curves) than the abrupt discontinuation shown in (a). A new (lower) homeostatic 'set-point' is established before further dose reductions are made. Drugs with longer half-lives may lessen withdrawal symptoms further by minimising the difference between the shifting homeostatic 'set-point' and plasma levels. (c) (3) An even more gradual step-wise reduction is likely to further minimise the risk of withdrawal symptoms (shaded area under the smaller, cupped curves).

References

1. FDA Drug Safety Communication. FDA requiring boxed warning updated to improve safe use of benzodiazepine drug class. 2020. https://www.fda.gov/drugs/drug-safety-and-availability/fda-requiring-boxed-warning-updated-improve-safe-use-benzodiazepine-drug-class#:~:text=FDA is requiring the Boxed,and life-threatening side effects.
2. Ashton H. Benzodiazepines: how they work and how to withdraw (The Ashton Manual). Newcastle University. 2002. http://www.benzo.org.uk/manual/bzcha01.htm (accessed 11 July 2023).
3. Wright SL. Benzodiazepine withdrawal: clinical aspects. In: *The Benzodiazepines Crisis* (eds. J Peppin, J Pergolizzi, R Raffa, S Wright). Oxford: Oxford University Press, 2020: 117–48.
4. Ashton H. The diagnosis and management of benzodiazepine dependence. *Curr Opin Psychiatry* 2005; 18: 249–55.
5. Parr JM, Kavanagh DJ, Cahill L, Mitchell G, Young RM. Effectiveness of current treatment approaches for benzodiazepine discontinuation: a meta-analysis. *Addiction* 2008; 104: 13–24.
6. Denis C, Fatseas M, Lavie E, Auriacombe M. Pharmacological interventions for benzodiazepine dependence management among benzodiazepine users in outpatient settings [Protocol]. *Cochrane Database Syst Rev* 2005. doi:10.1002/14651858.CD005194.
7. Scenario: Benzodiazepine and z-drug withdrawal. https://cks.nice.org.uk/topics/benzodiazepine-z-drug-withdrawal/management/benzodiazepine-z-drug-withdrawal/ (accessed 7 October 2022).
8. Horowitz MA, Taylor D. How to reduce and stop psychiatric medication. *Eur Neuropsychopharmacol* 2021; 55: 4–7.

Hyperbolic tapering of benzodiazepines and z-drugs

The relationship between dose of benzodiazepines and their effect on their principal target, the $GABA_A$ receptor, is hyperbolic[1] owing to the law of mass action.[2] The law of mass action dictates that when few molecules of a drug are present, most receptors are unoccupied and so even small increases in the mass of drug present at the site of action produces large effects.[2] When there is more drug in the system, receptors are increasingly saturated, leading to diminishing returns in effect on target receptors for increases in the mass of drug added.[2]

Taking diazepam as an example, this pattern of effect has the following implications:

- Reducing dose by fixed amounts (e.g. 15mg steps in Figure 3.5a) will give rise to increasingly large reductions in $GABA_A$ occupancy.
- This is consistent with clinical observations that withdrawal symptoms increase non-linearly with dose reduction. The same-sized reductions have been observed to cause greater withdrawal effects at lower doses (e.g. a 1mg reduction of diazepam is tolerable from 20mg but intolerable from 5mg).[3]
- Reducing diazepam dose by 5mg from 50mg will cause a reduction of 1.5 percentage points of $GABA_A$ occupancy, as derived from neuroimaging, but a 5mg reduction from

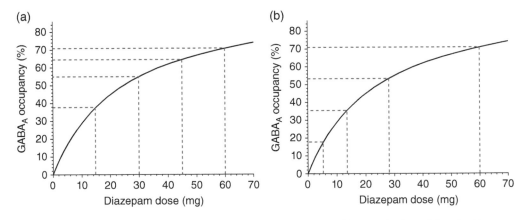

Figure 3.5 The effect of linear versus hyperbolic tapering. (a) An example of linear reductions of dose. In this case dose is reduced from 60mg in 15mg decrements to demonstrate the effect on receptor occupancy. Linear reductions of dose cause increasingly large reductions in effect on $GABA_A$ receptor occupancy. The first reduction from 60mg to 45mg will cause a reduction in receptor occupancy of 6.3 percentage points. But the final reduction from 15mg to 0mg (the same-sized reduction in terms of dose) will cause a reduction in receptor occupancy 6-fold larger (37.8 percentage points). This is likely to explain the more severe withdrawal effects patients report at lower doses when undergoing a linear regimen. (b) Hyperbolic reductions of dose. Reducing effect on $GABA_A$ receptors by even amounts, requires hyperbolically reducing doses of diazepam. In this example, the doses are reduced from 60mg (about 70 percentage points) by four equal steps in terms of receptor occupancy (about 17.5 percentage points each). The corresponding doses follow a hyperbolically reducing pattern (following the hyperbolic curve). Note how much smaller the final doses will be in such an approach (5mg) compared to the linear approach (15mg). Tapering hyperbolically is required to produce equal reductions in effect on receptor occupancy, which is likely to correspond to 'evenly spread' withdrawal symptoms. In practice, tapering will require many more intermediate steps following such a hyperbolic pattern: going down in smaller and smaller decrements and tapering down to a very small final dose so that the reduction to zero does not cause a larger reduction in receptor occupancy than previous reductions. Adapted from Brouillet et al. (1991).[1]

10mg will cause a reduction of 11.7 percentage points.[1] That is, the same-sized dose reduction will cause about an eight times larger change in effect on receptor occupancy.[1]

- To produce equal-sized reductions in receptor occupancy at each step will require making smaller and smaller dose reductions as the total dose gets lower (called hyperbolic tapering as it follows the hyperbolic curve).

There are numerous examples of a hyperbolic relationship between clinical effect and dose of benzodiazepines and z-drugs,[4] suggesting that the hyperbolic pattern of the neurobiological relationship has relevance at the level of clinical effect. For example, GABA-gated currents increase in a hyperbolic manner in response to increasing diazepam concentrations in cells.[5,6] An increasing dose of benzodiazepine produces anxiolytic effects in a hyperbolic pattern in pigeons,[7] rats[8] and non-human primates.[9] In humans there is a hyperbolic relationship between benzodiazepine dose and saccadic slowing and sedation.[10] The same is true for the effects of zolpidem on a number of sleep characteristics.[11-13] It therefore seems likely that the same hyperbolic relationship will exist between dose reductions and extent of withdrawal reactions, as observed clinically.[3]

In order to reduce benzodiazepine effects at their major target by equal amounts, hyperbolically reducing doses are required (Figure 3.4b and Table 3.6), as for other

Table 3.6 Doses of diazepam required to produce reductions in effect at the GABA$_A$ receptor of 5 percentage points. The size of the dose reductions become increasingly small to retain the same reduction in GABA$_A$ occupancy, such that a 1.3mg dose reduction at small doses produces the same change in effect as nine times the dose (11.7mg) at close to 60mg. This relationship informs the tapering regimens suggested later in this chapter.

GABA$_A$ occupancy (%)	Dose (mg)	Dose reduction from previous step (mg)
70	57.6	–
65	45.9	11.7
60	37	8.9
55	30.2	6.8
50	24.7	5.5
45	20.2	4.5
40	16.5	3.7
35	13.3	3.2
30	10.6	2.7
25	8.2	2.4
20	6.2	2.0
15	4.4	1.8
10	2.7	1.7
5	1.3	1.4
0	0	1.3

CHAPTER 3

drugs such as antidepressants.[14] Equal reductions of receptor occupancy are likely to produce an equivalent intensity of withdrawal reactions. A hyperbolic pattern of reduction means that the size of dose reductions should become smaller and smaller as the total dose reduces. Final doses before complete cessation will sometimes need to be very small (often less than 1mg of diazepam equivalent) so that this reduction is not larger (in terms of effect on reduction in receptor occupancy) than the size of the previously tolerated reductions. The suggested regimens provided in the drug-specific sections are derived from receptor occupancy relationships that follow a hyperbolic pattern of dose reduction. For example, the suggested regimens for diazepam start with reductions of 4mg when patients are taking 60mg a day, but when their daily dose is down to 2.5mg the size of the reduction suggested is just 0.5mg because these reductions produce equivalent-sized effects on $GABA_A$ receptors.

In peer-led withdrawal communities, patients have converged on a similar solution to reducing dose. Many of these communities recommend reducing by a proportion of the most recent dose every period (an exponential pattern of dose reduction). Patients often report that 10% reductions (calculated on the last dose, so that they become increasingly small) or less every 2–4 weeks are tolerable (albeit with considerable variation).[15,16]

References

1. Brouillet E, Chavoix C, Bottlaender M, et al. In vivo bidirectional modulatory effect of benzodiazepine receptor ligands on GABAergic transmission evaluated by positron emission tomography in non-human primates. *Brain Res* 1991; 557: 167–76.
2. Holford N. Pharmacodynamic principles and the time course of delayed and cumulative drug effects. *Transl Clin Pharmacol* 2018; 26: 56–59.
3. Ashton H. Benzodiazepine dependence. In: *Adverse Syndromes and Psychiatric Drugs* (eds. P Haddad, S Dursun, B Deakin). Oxford: Oxford University Press, 2004: 239–60.
4. Horowitz M, Taylor D. Withdrawing from benzodiazepines and z-drugs (in preparation).
5. Berezhnoy D, Gravielle MC, Downing S, et al. Pharmacological properties of DOV 315,090, an ocinaplon metabolite. *BMC Pharmacol* 2008; 8: 1–10.
6. Wongsamitkul N, Maldifassi MC, Simeone X, Baur R, Ernst M, Sigel E. α subunits in $GABA_A$ receptors are dispensable for GABA and diazepam action. *Sci Rep* 2017; 7: 1–11.
7. Kleven MS, Koek W. Effects of benzodiazepine agonists on punished responding in pigeons and their relationship with clinical doses in humans. *Psychopharmacology* 1999; 141: 206–12.
8. Dubinsky B, Vaidya AH, Rosenthal DI, et al. Nonbenzodiazepine anxiolytic. *Pharmacology* 2002; 303: 777–90.
9. Rowlett JK, Platt DM, Lelas S, Atack JR, Dawson GR. Different $GABA_A$ receptor subtypes mediate the anxiolytic, abuse-related, and motor effects of benzodiazepine-like drugs in primates. *Proc Natl Acad Sci USA* 2005; 102: 915–20.
10. Hommer DW, Matsuo V, Wolkowitz O, et al. Benzodiazepine sensitivity in normal human subjects. *Arch Gen Psychiatry* 1986; 43: 542–51.
11. Merlotti L, Roehrs T, Koshorek G, Zorick F, Lamphere J, Roth T. The dose effects of zolpidem on the sleep of healthy normals. *J Clin Psychopharmacol* 1989; 9: 9–14.
12. Scharf MB, Mayleben DW, Kaffeman M, Krall R, Ochs R. Dose response effects of zolpidem in normal geriatric subjects. *J Clin Psychiatry* 1991; 52: 77–83.
13. Roth T, Roehrs T, Vogel G. Zolpidem in the treatment of transient insomnia: a double-blind, randomized comparison with placebo. *Sleep* 1995; 18: 246–51.
14. Horowitz MA, Taylor D. Tapering of SSRI treatment to mitigate withdrawal symptoms. *The Lancet Psychiatry* 2019; 6: 538–46.
15. BenzoBuddies Community Forum. http://www.benzobuddies.org/forum/index.php (accessed 18 March 2023).
16. Wright SL. Benzodiazepine withdrawal: clinical aspects. In: *The Benzodiazepines Crisis* (eds. J Peppin, J Pergolizzi, R Raffa, S Wright) 2020: 117–C8.P334. Oxford: Oxford University Press. doi:10.1093/med/9780197517277.003.0008.

Switching to longer-acting benzodiazepines to taper

There are mixed views on switching to a longer-acting benzodiazepine to facilitate tapering. A Cochrane review on this topic was equivocal about switching, not finding strong evidence one way or the other.[1] Theoretically, a longer-acting drug should cause a more gradual change in plasma levels following reductions that should minimise withdrawal symptoms. This may be particularly helpful for patients who are experiencing inter-dose withdrawal from shorter-acting benzodiazepines (and sometimes z-drugs) during maintenance treatment (although more frequent dosing can also solve this issue). Other patients may find switching difficult or prefer to taper from the original, familiar drug.[2]

A conversion table for benzodiazepines is shown in Table 3.7. It should be noted that benzodiazepine equivalencies are not based on careful studies but based on expert opinion, and so can only be seen as rough estimates, and there can be significant inter-individual differences.[3–5] Consequently, switching should be performed step-wise rather than abruptly to allow a period of accommodation to the new drug and to check for withdrawal symptoms (see drug-specific chapters). Patient-reported symptoms should therefore be prioritised and adjustments should be made so as to minimise withdrawal symptoms. A period of stabilisation (e.g. 2 weeks or longer) on the new drug may be required before commencing a taper.

Diazepam is a common choice for a switch because of its long half-life (including its active metabolite) and its wide availability in small-dose tablet formulations and liquids. Extra precautions apply in patients with hepatic dysfunction as diazepam, and other longer-acting drugs, may accumulate.[6,7] As sensitised patients can be susceptible to even small perturbations in plasma levels of drugs, some patients may need to take longer-acting benzodiazepines like diazepam more than once a day (as sometimes encouraged by manufacturers).[3,4]

Z-drugs that have short half-lives and are dosed once a day may be eliminated almost completely in the 24 hours between doses. These drugs should theoretically produce less adaptation (and therefore less physical dependence) and a lower risk of withdrawal effects than drugs that affect target receptors for 24 hours a day (e.g. shorter-acting benzodiazepines dosed several times a day). Therefore, direct tapering from these medications may be more sensible than a switch to diazepam. However, an option to switch is presented as a possibility in the drug-specific sections. This is perhaps most relevant for patients who experience inter-dose withdrawal symptoms, or who have great difficulty in a direct taper from these drugs.

Table 3.7 Dose equivalencies between benzodiazepines, their half-lives and marketed indications.

Benzodiazepine or z-drug	Half-life (active metabolite)	Equivalent dose*	Marketed indication**
Diazepam	24–48 hours (up to 100 hours)[8]	10mg	a, h
Alprazolam	12–15 hours[9]	0.5mg[5]	a
Chlordiazepoxide	8–28 hours[10]	25mg[5]	a, m, w
Clonazepam	20–60 hours, mean 30 hours[1]	0.5mg[5]	e
Clorazepate	18–50 hours (1–8 days)[11]	15mg[4]	a, e, w
Estazolam	10–24 hours[12]	1mg (1–2mg)[4]	h
Eszopiclone	6 hours[13]	3mg[4]	h
Flurazepam	40–114 hours[10]	20mg (15 –30mg) [5]	h
Lorazepam	12 hours[14]	1mg[5]	a, p
Lormetazepam	10–12 hours[15]	1mg (1–2mg)[5]	h
Nitrazepam	24 hours[16]	10mg[5]	h
Oxazepam	6–20 hours[17]	20mg[5]	a
Quazepam	39 hours (73 hours)[18]	20mg[4]	h
Temazepam	7–11 hours, mean 8 hours[19]	20mg[5]	h, p
Triazolam	1.5–5 hours[20]	0.5mg[4]	h
Zaleplon	1 hour[21]	20mg[4]	h
Zolpidem tartrate	0.7–3.5 hours, mean 2.4 hours[22]	20mg[4]	h
Zopiclone	5 hours[23]	15mg[4]	h

*These equivalencies are based on clinical experience and so may not be exact and may need to be individualised, based on withdrawal symptoms.
**Marketed indications may vary between different territories.
a = anxiolytic, e = anti-epileptic, h = hypnotic, m = muscle relaxant, p = pre-medication before procedure/operation, w = alcohol withdrawal.

References

1. Denis C, Fatseas M, Lavie E, Auriacombe M. Pharmacological interventions for benzodiazepine dependence management among benzodiazepine users in outpatient settings [Protocol]. *Cochrane Database Syst Rev* 2005. doi:10.1002/14651858.CD005194.
2. benzo.org.uk : 4.1 Hypnotics and anxiolytics: British National Formulary. https://www.benzo.org.uk/BNF.htm (accessed 8 May 2023).
3. Wright SL. Benzodiazepine withdrawal: clinical aspects. In: *The Benzodiazepines Crisis* (eds. J Peppin, J Pergolizzi, R Raffa, S Wright) 2020: 117–C8.P334. Oxford: Oxford University Press. doi:10.1093/med/9780197517277.003.0008.
4. Ashton HH. Benzodiazepines: how they work and how to withdraw (The Ashton Manual). Newcastle University, 2002. http://www.benzo.org.uk/manual/bzcha01.htm (accessed 11 July 2023).
5. Hypnotics and anxiolytics. https://bnf.nice.org.uk/treatment-summaries/hypnotics-and-anxiolytics/ (accessed 19 March 2023).
6. Taylor D, Barnes T, Young A. *The Maudsley Prescribing Guidelines in Psychiatry*, 14th ed. Hoboken, NJ: Wiley-Blackwell, 2021. doi:10.1002/9781119870203.
7. Scenario: Benzodiazepine and z-drug withdrawal. https://cks.nice.org.uk/topics/benzodiazepine-z-drug-withdrawal/management/benzodiazepine-z-drug-withdrawal/ (accessed 7 October 2022).
8. FDA. Medication guide Diazepam. www.accessdata.fda.gov. https://www.accessdata.fda.gov/drugsatfda_docs/label/2021/013263s096lbl.pdf (accessed 23 March 2023).
9. FDA. Medication guide Xanax. Fda.gov. 2023; published online January. https://www.accessdata.fda.gov/drugsatfda_docs/label/2023./018276s059lbl.pdf#page=22 (accessed 27 February 2023).
10. Mylan. Summary of product characteristics. Librium 5 mg Capsules Chlordiazepoxide hydrochloride. https://www.medicines.org.uk/emc/product/1728/smpc#gref (accessed 4 July 2023).
11. Riss J, Cloyd J, Gates J, Collins S. Benzodiazepines in epilepsy: pharmacology and pharmacokinetics. *Acta Neurol Scand* 2008; 118: 69–86.
12. Estazolam Tablets, USP C-IV Rx only. https://dailymed.nlm.nih.gov/dailymed/fda/fdaDrugXsl.cfm?setid=a1e3b4bf-22e9-430a-a768-4d86ae886c9e&type=display (accessed 29 April 2023).
13. FDA. LUNESTA® (eszopiclone) tablets – Accessdata.fda.gov. FDA. https://www.accessdata.fda.gov/drugsatfda_docs/label/2014/021476s030lbl.pdf (accessed 25 March 2023).
14. Lorazepam 0.5 mg Tablets – Summary of Product Characteristics (SmPC) – (emc). https://www.medicines.org.uk/emc/product/10285/smpc (accessed 29 April 2023).
15. Dormagen 0.5 mg Tablets – Summary of Product Characteristics (SmPC) – (emc). https://www.medicines.org.uk/emc/product/5269/smpc (accessed 15 April 2023).
16. Nitrazepam 5 mg Tablets – Summary of Product Characteristics (SmPC) – (emc). https://www.medicines.org.uk/emc/product/7145/smpc (accessed 8 April 2023).
17. Oxazepam Tablets 10 mg – Summary of Product Characteristics (SmPC) – (emc). https://www.medicines.org.uk/emc/product/5338/smpc (accessed 29 April 2023).
18. DailyMed – DORAL – quazepam tablet. https://dailymed.nlm.nih.gov/dailymed/drugInfo.cfm?setid=9727e8b4-14f1-451d-9630-84eabc772e42 (accessed 29 April 2023).
19. Temazepam Tablets 20 mg – Summary of Product Characteristics (SmPC). www.hpra.ie/img/uploaded/swedocuments/Licence_PA1986-085-002_26012022100933.pdf (accessed 29 April 2023).
20. New labeling and patient insert for triazolam approved by FDA. *Clin Pharm* 1992; 11: 467.
21. FDA. Sonata (zaleplon). FDA. www.accessdata.fda.gov/drugsatfda_docs/label/2019/020859s016lbl.pdf (accessed 29 April 2023).
22. Zolpidem Tartrate 10 mg Tablets – Summary of Product Characteristics (SmPC) – (emc). https://www.medicines.org.uk/emc/product/3975/smpc (accessed 29 April 2023).
23. Zopiclone 3.75 mg Tablets – Summary of Product Characteristics (SmPC) – (emc). https://www.medicines.org.uk/emc/product/10830/smpc (accessed 29 April 2023).

CHAPTER 3

Making up smaller doses of benzodiazepines and z-drugs practically

As outlined in the following drug-specific sections, some people will need access to smaller doses of medication than are widely available as commercially produced tablets in order to taper. This is because the smallest available tablets (or even a quarter of such a tablet) produce high receptor occupancy. Reducing from the smallest tablet to zero would cause a large reduction in effect, engendering severe withdrawal symptoms for some patients (Table 3.8).[1] Various guidelines on tapering recommend using liquid versions of drugs (for which the volume of each dose is readily manipulated) in order to make gradual tapering feasible.[2,3]

Table 3.8 Tablet and liquid formulations available for commonly used benzodiazepines and z-drugs, with corresponding GABA$_A$ occupancy provided for a quarter the lowest available dose of tablet. a = UK, b = USA.

Drug	Tablets available	Liquid formulation	Quarter the dose of smallest tablet	Corresponding GABA$_A$ occupancy
Clonazepam	0.125mg, 0.25mg, 0.5mg, 1mg, 2mg	2mg/5mL[a], 0.5mg/mL[a]	0.0625mg[b] 0.125mg[a]	4.8 9.2
Diazepam	2mg, 5mg, 10mg	1mg/mL[b], 5mg/mL[b], 2mg/5mL[a]	0.5mg	2.0
Lorazepam	0.5mg, 1mg, 2mg, 2.5mg	2mg/mL[b], 1mg/mL[a]	0.125mg	4.8
Temazepam	7.5mg, 10mg	10mg/5mL[a]	1.875mg[b] 2.5mg[a]	3.7 4.8
Zopiclone	3.75mg, 7.5mg	N/A	0.94mg	2.5
Zolpidem	5mg, 10mg	N/A	1.25mg	2.5

To prepare dosages that allow steps in between or lower than doses widely available in tablet formulations, licensed and 'off-label' options are available, as outlined in the introductory chapter. Some specific remarks relevant to benzodiazepines and z-drugs are highlighted here.

Extending the dosing interval ('skipping doses')

As current tablet formulations of some benzodiazepines and z-drugs do not permit pharmacologically informed tapering regimens, it is tempting to make dose reductions by having patients miss a dose of medication once a week or more often, or to take their dose every other day (or less frequently) so that their average dose each day is reduced. However, this method is not recommended for benzodiazepines other than long-acting drugs like diazepam. Even for diazepam clinical effects sometimes require more than once-a-day dosing (perhaps because in people sensitive to benzodiazepines even small variation in plasma level can trigger withdrawal effects).[2,3] The half-lives of most benzodiazepines and z-drugs are 24 hours or less, so dosing every second day will cause plasma levels of the drug to fall to one-quarter of peak levels at their trough. It is widely recognised that skipping doses can induce withdrawal effects[4,5] from benzodiazepines, something which patients routinely report,[6] and every-other-day dosing has similar consequences. It is generally better to taper doses by giving a smaller dose each day (or as often as required to prevent inter-dose withdrawal effects) rather than a larger dose every second day.

Tablet splitting

As outlined in the introductory chapter many tablets can be easily divided into halves (or quarters if they are round) using cheaply available tablet cutters.[7] Using tablet cutters is more accurate for dividing tablets than either splitting by hand (for scored tablets), cutting with scissors (for unscored tablets) or using a kitchen knife.[8] Although in older methods of manufacturing active medication was not evenly distributed throughout a pill or tablet, this is no longer the case.[9] Tablet splitting is widely employed with almost one-quarter of all drugs administered in primary care being split.[10] Some tablets may not be suitable for splitting including those with a hard outer coat, extended-release tablets (the extended-release properties can be affected), those that are too small or have an uneven shape. Although there are concerns that the splitting process may not be completely accurate,[11] (e.g. imperfect splitting and tablet powder being formed) this can be mitigated somewhat by storing the remainder of the tablet fragment to be used over subsequent days, meaning that the correct dose will be received over 2 or 4 doses. Tablet cutters have the advantage of closing as they are used and so retain both halves of the tablet being cut.

This technique may be helpful for the first few steps of a reduction regimen. Small variation in dose from day to day whilst at higher doses of medication is unlikely to cause withdrawal issues for most people (although these differences can become more critical at lower doses). Some patients who are physically dependent on benzodiazepines can be so sensitised to benzodiazepines that even minute fluctuations in dosage can cause withdrawal effects; for these patients tablet splitting may not be appropriate and a more accurate method may be required.

Manufacturers' liquids, including dilutions

Apart from tablet splitting, the most widely available option for making up doses that are smaller than those available in tablets is the use of liquid versions of a drug. A variety of benzodiazepines are available in liquid form. Small syringes (e.g. 1mL, or sometimes 0.5mL) can be used to measure out doses. Sometimes syringes smaller than those provided by the manufacturer are required for tapering. Patients may require some education on proper syringe usage and reading. As greater errors are found when measuring less than 20% of the labelled capacity of a syringe[12] and the smallest syringe widely available is 1mL (or in some regions 0.5mL), the smallest volume that could be measured accurately with a syringe may be too large a dose to complete a taper for some benzodiazepines.

To avoid problems associated with measuring small volumes, the dilution of manufacturers' liquids may be needed. Some manufacturers recommend diluting the solution with water (or juices) before consumption.[13] For example, 0.5mL of a 5mg/mL diazepam solution could be mixed with 4.5mL of water (a 10-fold dilution) to make up a 0.5mg/mL solution.[13] The manufacturer advises that the solution will blend quickly and completely, and should be consumed 'immediately', which can be interpreted as within an hour of preparation.[13] As the stability of the dilution cannot be guaranteed, the remainder should be discarded and a new dilution prepared each day. In order to take small doses with, for example, this 0.5mg/mL dilution, 0.25mg could be taken by measuring 0.5mL of the dilution to consume.

Compounded medication

Other options, available in different territories, include having compounding pharmacies make up smaller dose tablets or capsules, or liquid suspensions or solutions. One such option is 'tapering strips', which involves small doses of benzodiazepines or z-drugs made up as tablets that successively reduce in dose over time.[14] Patients should make sure they are using a reputable compounding pharmacy.[15]

Other off-licence options for making small doses of medications

As outlined in the introductory chapter, while it may represent an unlicensed use to crush tablets or make extemporaneous suspensions, the General Medical Council (GMC) guidance on this matter states that doctors are permitted to prescribe medications off-licence when 'the dosage specified for a licensed medicine would not meet the patient's need'.[16] In the USA, such usage is also considered 'off label' or 'unapproved' use by the FDA, which, however, explains that 'healthcare providers generally may prescribe the drug for an unapproved use when they judge that it is medically appropriate for their patient'.[17]

Dispersing tablets

When liquid formulations are not available, many tablets that are not enterically coated or sustained- or extended-release can be crushed to a powdered form and dispersed in water.[18,19] The contents may sometimes taste bitter. Crushing and dispersing will not greatly alter these medications' pharmacokinetic properties according to the FDA medication guide[20] and the Royal Pharmaceutical Society (RPS) guidance on crushing, opening or splitting oral dosage forms.[7] Their time to peak plasma will be shortened because the absence of a disintegration phase allows faster gastrointestinal absorption.

Guidelines for patients who have trouble swallowing tablets (like the North East Wales NHS Trust (NEWT) guidelines in the UK[19] and similar guidance in the USA[20]) indicate that many benzodiazepine tablets will disperse in water. For example, local National Health Service (NHS) hospital guidance indicates that diazepam will disperse in water, although the process will take more than 2 minutes.[21] The process can be made faster by crushing tablets with a spoon or mortar and pestle. For other medications, such as zolpidem, guidelines for making suspensions recommend crushing instant-release preparations (e.g. Ambien) but not controlled-release preparations (e.g. Ambien CR).[20]

In order to make up a diazepam suspension, for example, water could be added to a 2mg diazepam tablet to make up a 20mL suspension, with concentration 1mg in 10mL (or 0.1mg/mL). A 0.5mg dose of diazepam could be taken by measuring out 5mL of this suspension to consume. As some benzodiazepines are poorly soluble in water, it should be noted that mixtures made by dispersing a tablet in water are suspensions (not solutions). Flakes or particles visible in a suspension are a combination of excipients (or 'fillers') and active drug. Care should be taken to vigorously shake or stir a suspension to ensure even dispersion of drug before measuring a volume to consume.[22] In the absence of stability data, a conservative approach involves consuming such suspensions immediately (within an hour). The remainder should be discarded. Although this approach presents various practical difficulties, patients who have successfully ceased benzodiazepine use reported this approach to be amongst the most useful.[2]

Benzodiazepines are more soluble in oil or fat than in water.[23] When mixed with full-fat homogenised milk, some or all of the drug will dissolve in the milk fat. This should form an evenly dispersed emulsion when shaken vigorously. This method is favoured by some patients.[24] As stability cannot be assured, the measured dose should be taken immediately after shaking and the remainder discarded.

References

1. Horowitz M, Taylor D. Withdrawing from benzodiazepines and z-drugs (in preparation).
2. Wright SL. Benzodiazepine withdrawal: clinical aspects. In: *The Benzodiazepines Crisis* (eds. J Peppin, J Pergolizzi, R Raffa, S Wright) 2020: 117–C8.P334. Oxford: Oxford University Press. doi:10.1093/med/9780197517277.003.0008.
3. Ashton H. Benzodiazepines: how they work and how to withdraw (The Ashton Manual). 2002. http://www.benzo.org.uk/manual/bzcha01.htm (accessed 11 July 2023).
4. National Institute of Health and Care Excellence (NICE). Depression in adults: treatment and management | Guidance | NICE. 2022; published online June. https://www.nice.org.uk/guidance/ng222 (accessed 16 July 2022).
5. Kaplan EM. Antidepressant noncompliance as a factor in the discontinuation syndrome. *J Clin Psychiatry* 1997; 58 Suppl 7: 31–5; discussion 36.
6. Framer A. What I have learnt from helping thousands of people taper off psychotropic medications. *Ther Adv Psychopharmacol* 2021; 11: 204512532199127.
7. Root T, Tomlin S, Erskine D, Lowey A. Pharmaceutical issues when crushing, opening or splitting oral dosage forms. *Royal Pharmaceutical Society* 2011; 1: 1–7.
8. Verrue C, Mehuys E, Boussery K, Remon J-P, Petrovic M. Tablet-splitting: a common yet not so innocent practice. *J Adv Nurs* 2011; 67: 26–32.
9. Hisada H, Okayama A, Hoshino T, et al. Determining the distribution of active pharmaceutical ingredients in combination tablets using near IR and low-frequency Raman spectroscopy imaging. *Chem Pharm Bull* 2020; 68: 155–60.
10. Chaudhri K, Kearney M, Di Tanna GL, Day RO, Rodgers A, Atkins ER. Does splitting a tablet obtain the accurate dose?: a systematic review protocol. *Medicine* 2019; 98: e17189.
11. Center for Drug Evaluation, Research. Best practices for tablet splitting. U.S. Food and Drug Administration. https://www.fda.gov/drugs/ensuring-safe-use-medicine/best-practices-tablet-splitting (accessed 22 September 2022).
12. Jordan MA, Choksi D, Lombard K, Patton LR. Development of Guidelines for Accurate Measurement of Small Volume Parenteral Products Using Syringes. *Hosp Pharm* 2021; 56: 165–71.
13. Diazepam Oral Solution, CIV, 5 mg per 5 mL and Diazepam Intensol™ Oral Solution (Concentrate), CIV, 25 mg per 5 mL (5 mg/mL). https://dailymed.nlm.nih.gov/dailymed/fda/fdaDrugXsl.cfm?setid=e435e56f-e6eb-4fe9-9a8f-e11527778fc1&type=display (accessed 23 March 2023).
14. Groot PC, van Os J. How user knowledge of psychotropic drug withdrawal resulted in the development of person-specific tapering medication. *Ther Adv Psychopharmacol* 2020; 10: 204512532093245.
15. Find A Compounder – PCCA – Professional Compounding Centers of America. https://www.pccarx.com/Resources/FindACompounder (accessed 8 May 2023).
16. General Medical Council. Prescribing unlicensed medicines. 2021.
17. Office of the Commissioner. Understanding unapproved use of approved drugs "off label." U.S. Food and Drug Administration. https://www.fda.gov/patients/learn-about-expanded-access-and-other-treatment-options/understanding-unapproved-use-approved-drugs-label (accessed 22 September 2022).
18. Brennan K. Selective serotonin reuptake inhibitor (SSRI) formulations suggested for adults with swallowing difficulties. SPS - Specialist Pharmacy Service. 2021; published online July 1. https://www.sps.nhs.uk/articles/selective-serotonin-reuptake-inhibitor-ssri-formulations-suggested-for-adults-with-swallowing-difficulties/ (accessed July 14, 2022).
19. Smyth J. The NEWT guidelines for administration of medication to patients with enteral feeding tubes or swallowing difficulties. 2011. https://www.newtguidelines.com/index.html (accessed 18 February 2023).
20. Bostwick JR, Demehri A. Pills to powder: an updated clinician's reference for crushable psychotropics. *Curr Psychiatr* 2017; 16: 46–9.
21. Colchester Medicines Information. MOC guidelines for tablet crushing in patients with swallowing difficulties. Colchester Hospital University, 2018
22. White R, Bradnam V. *Handbook of Drug Administration via Enteral Feeding Tubes*, 3rd ed. Padstow: Pharmaceutical Press, 2015.
23. Macheras PE, Koupparis MA, Antimisiaris SG. Drug binding and solubility in milk. *Pharm Res* 1990; 7: 537–41.
24. Benzodiazepine Tapering Strategies and Solutions. Benzodiazepine Information Coalition. 2020; published online September 21. https://www.benzoinfo.com/benzodiazepine-tapering-strategies/ (accessed 29 April 2023).

Other considerations in tapering benzodiazepines and z-drugs

The practical process of tapering is outlined in 'Tapering benzodiazepines and z-drugs in practice'. The key elements of a programme of tapering are:

- that it is flexible and can be adjusted so that the process is tolerable for the patient;
- that it involves close monitoring of withdrawal symptoms to facilitate timely adjustments to the rate of taper;
- that patients are provided with formulations of medication to allow the taking of doses necessary for tapering (e.g. access to liquid formulations or tablets with lower doses); and
- ensuring that patients have adequate support both psychologically and practically (knowing how to make small reductions) from friends, family and professionals.

Micro-tapering

Although the major approach outlined in the drug-specific sections involves making reductions every 1–4 weeks (sometimes called 'cut and hold')[1] an alternative approach is called micro-tapering, whereby a small change in dose is made each day. Theoretically (see Figure 3.4) making smaller reductions should produce smaller disruptions of the homeostatic equilibrium leading to less intense withdrawal symptoms.[2] This process might require further dilutions of a liquid version of the drug and the use of small-volume syringes. It also requires quite complex calculations and record keeping. Micro-tapering allows the patient great flexibility in finding a rate of reduction that is tolerable for them. It also means that doses can be evenly distributed throughout the day, which should minimise any plasma fluctuations that might provoke or exacerbate withdrawal symptoms. Where several doses of a medication are taken each day, these same small-dose reductions can be made to all doses, or sequentially to one dose at a time (e.g. morning, afternoon or night).

Micro-tapering rates can be calculated from the regimens given in the drug-specific sections by dividing the change in dose for each step by 7, 14 or 28 days, depending on the rate of desired taper. For example, if a regimen suggests that a reduction should be made from 60mg to 55mg in one step over 2 weeks, then this could be converted into a reduction of approximately 0.4mg each day for 2 weeks. The rate of tapering per day will reduce throughout the taper (hyperbolically). This rate can be slowed if withdrawal symptoms become too unpleasant. As an example, if a 0.1mg/mL suspension of diazepam is made up, as above, to a volume of 20mL, then 0.5mL less could be taken every day to reduce from 2mg (20mL) by 0.05mg each day, taking 40 days to reach 0mg (a rate that could be adjusted to withdrawal symptoms).

Adjunctive medication

Currently there are no medications approved by the FDA or other drug regulators to alleviate the symptoms of benzodiazepine withdrawal. Pharmacological adjunctive treatments for benzodiazepine withdrawal have had mixed reviews.[3,4] Many drugs that have been trialled to help people with withdrawal symptoms themselves cause physical dependence and withdrawal. These include pregabalin, paroxetine, tricyclic antidepressants, and trazodone.[4] Ultimately these agents may then in turn need to be tapered, and are, in any case, associated with their own adverse effects.[5] Clearly then, using a dependence-forming agent to assist withdrawal is ultimately likely to be self-defeating. NICE guidance on safe withdrawal of benzodiazepines states explicitly 'Do not treat withdrawal symptoms with another medicine that is associated with dependence or withdrawal symptoms.'[6] The British National Formulary (BNF) cautions: 'The addition of beta-blockers, antidepressants and antipsychotics should be avoided where possible.'[7]

When severe withdrawal symptoms occur it is generally preferable to slow the rate of taper to minimise withdrawal symptoms rather than seek to mask them with another medication. The addition of another medication also risks complicating the picture by adding in new adverse effects, and potential interactions with existing medication. In the process of withdrawal, some patients will become sensitised to a range of medications, which may include other psychiatric medications - another reason for a cautious approach to new agents.[5,8] Professor Ashton said on this issue 'Presumably the general hypersensitivity of the nervous system magnifies the reaction to any foreign substances, but no clear explanation has yet emerged.'[8]

In selected cases of severe withdrawal, the addition of an adjunctive medication may be considered.[9] The adjunct agent should be ideally one without a strong withdrawal syndrome and should have less severe adverse effects than the original benzodiazepine. In a Cochrane review, the use of valproate assisted successful benzodiazepine discontinuation,[10] as did carbamazepine.[11] Valproate and carbamazepine are less likely to produce withdrawal effects than benzodiazepines, although withdrawal is reported for both drugs.[12] These drugs also pose risk of blood dyscrasias, hepatic decompensation, and psychiatric and cognitive alterations, amongst other adverse effects, and so require careful monitoring.[13,14] Also, NICE concluded: 'Do not offer sodium valproate or buspirone to aid withdrawal from a benzodiazepine.'[6] The addition of melatonin may also be more effective[15] than tapering alone, although evidence is mixed.[16] Drugs like propranolol[17,18] and antihistamines like hydroxyzine[19] have been used in case of unpleasant withdrawal symptoms, with inconclusive findings.[11] Ideally these drugs should be used only for the short term, as some can also cause physical dependence and withdrawal with chronic use.[20]

Nutritional supplements and other products

There has been almost no formal research into the effects of supplements on withdrawal symptoms. Hypersensitivity to adverse effects may also be seen with supplements.[8] Any theories on the possible benefits of supplements in this area are mere speculation.

The use of GABA-affecting supplements (e.g. valerian, cannabinoids and phenibut)[5] seems particularly unwise as these may have similar effects to benzodiazepines. They may or may not help withdrawal but may also themselves result in dependence. Phenibut, a GABA agonist, in particular is known to cause physical dependence and withdrawal effects.[21] Carisoprodol (Soma), is metabolised into a barbiturate-like drug (meprobamate), which binds to $GABA_A$ receptors[22] and, like baclofen, a GABA analogue,[23] is associated with a withdrawal syndrome. Alcohol should be specifically avoided as it also interacts with $GABA_A$ receptors and can exacerbate withdrawal symptoms, sometimes to a surprising degree.[8]

References

1. Benzodiazepine Tapering Strategies and Solutions. Benzodiazepine Information Coalition. 2020; published online 21 September. https://www.benzoinfo.com/benzodiazepine-tapering-strategies/ (accessed 29 April 2023).

2. Horowitz MA, Taylor D. How to reduce and stop psychiatric medication. *Eur Neuropsychopharmacol* 2021; 55: 4–7.

3. Parr JM, Kavanagh DJ, Cahill L, Mitchell G, Young RM. Effectiveness of current treatment approaches for benzodiazepine discontinuation: a meta-analysis. *Addiction* 2009; 104: 13–24.

4. Baandrup L, Ebdrup BH, Rasmussen JØ, Lindschou J, Gluud C, Glenthøj BY. Pharmacological interventions for benzodiazepine discontinuation in chronic benzodiazepine users. *Cochrane Database Syst Rev* 2018; 3: CD011481.

5. Wright SL. Benzodiazepine withdrawal: clinical aspects. In: *The Benzodiazepines Crisis* (eds. J Peppin, J Pergolizzi, R Raffa, S Wright) 2020: 117–C8.P334. Oxford: Oxford University Press. doi:10.1093/med/9780197517277.003.0008.

6. National Institute for Health and Care Excellence (NICE). Medicines associated with dependence or withdrawal symptoms: safe prescribing and withdrawal management for adults | Guidance | NICE. 2022. https://www.nice.org.uk/guidance/ng215/chapter/Recommendations (accessed 27 June 2022).

7. Hypnotics and anxiolytics. https://bnf.nice.org.uk/treatment-summaries/hypnotics-and-anxiolytics/ (accessed 19 March 2023).

8. Ashton H. Benzodiazepines: how they work and how to withdraw (The Ashton Manual). Newcastle University, 2002. http://www.benzo.org.uk/manual/bzcha01.htm (accessed 11 July 2023).

9. Scenario: Benzodiazepine and z-drug withdrawal. https://cks.nice.org.uk/topics/benzodiazepine-z-drug-withdrawal/management/benzodiazepine-z-drug-withdrawal/ (accessed 7 October 2022).

10. Baandrup L, Bh E, Jø R, Lindschou J, Gluud C, By G. Pharmacological interventions for benzodiazepine discontinuation in chronic benzodiazepine users (Review) Summary of findings for the main comparison. 2018. doi:10.1002/14651858.CD011481.pub2.www.cochranelibrary.com.

11. Denis C, Fatseas M, Lavie E, Auriacombe M. Pharmacological interventions for benzodiazepine dependence management among benzodiazepine users in outpatient settings [Protocol]. *Cochrane Database Syst Rev* 2005. doi:10.1002/14651858.CD005194

12. Cosci F, Chouinard G. Acute and persistent withdrawal syndromes following discontinuation of psychotropic medications. *Psychother Psychosom* 2020; 89: 283–306.

13. Tegretol 100mg Tablets – Summary of Product Characteristics (SmPC) – (emc). https://www.medicines.org.uk/emc/product/1040/smpc (accessed 29 April 2023).

14. Sodium Valproate 500mg Gastro-Resistant Tablets – Summary of Product Characteristics (SmPC) – (emc). https://www.medicines.org.uk/emc/product/1500/smpc (accessed 29 April 2023).

15. Garfinkel D, Zisapel N, Wainstein J, Laudon M. Facilitation of benzodiazepine discontinuation by melatonin: a new clinical approach. *Arch Intern Med* 1999; 159: 2456–60.

16. Wright A, Diebold J, Otal J, et al. The effect of melatonin on benzodiazepine discontinuation and sleep quality in adults attempting to discontinue benzodiazepines: a systematic review and meta-analysis. *Drugs Aging* 2015; 32: 1009–18.

17. Cantopher T, Olivieri S, Cleave N, Edwards JG. Chronic benzodiazepine dependence: a comparative study of abrupt withdrawal under propranolol cover versus gradual withdrawal. *Br J Psychiatry* 1990; 156: 406–11.

18. Tyrer P, Rutherford D, Huggett T. Benzodiazepine withdrawal symptoms and propranolol. *Lancet* 1981; 1: 520–2.

19. Lemoine P, Touchon J, Billardon M. [Comparison of 6 different methods for lorazepam withdrawal: a controlled study, hydroxyzine versus placebo]. *Encephale* 1997; 23: 290–9.

20. Chiappini S, Schifano F, Martinotti G. Editorial: prescribing psychotropics: misuse, abuse, dependence, withdrawal and addiction. *Front Psychiatry* 2021; 12: 688434.

21. Samokhvalov AV, Paton-Gay CL, Balchand K, Rehm J. Phenibut dependence. *BMJ Case Rep* 2013; 2013. doi:10.1136/bcr-2012-008381.

22. Reeves RR, Beddingfield JJ, Mack JE. Carisoprodol withdrawal syndrome. *Pharmacotherapy* 2004; 24: 1804–6.

23. Alvis BD, Sobey CM. Oral Baclofen withdrawal resulting in progressive weakness and sedation requiring intensive care admission. *Neurohospitalist* 2017; 7: 39–40.

Psychological aspects of tapering benzodiazepines and z-drugs

The withdrawal process per se can involve intense emotions, ranging from despair, anger, anxiety, emotional lability, to hypomania and suicidal thoughts. These feelings are often unrelated (or greatly out of proportion) to events or circumstances.[1-4] Such experiences can sometimes be emotions that are familiar to the patient, at other times be quite novel (or be of much greater intensity than previously experienced emotions), and can be distressing and confusing.[2,4] Like the physical symptoms of withdrawal, psychological symptoms can often come in intense waves.[2,4,5] The emotional effects of benzodiazepine withdrawal are common to many drug-withdrawal syndromes, perhaps being most widely recognised with various recreational drugs.[1,6]

Many people cannot tolerate severe withdrawal symptoms. Severe effects can impair social and professional functioning, precipitate relapse and cause the patient to become fearful of the process of reducing their medication or of ever going off it.[4] Sometimes severe withdrawal effects will prompt people to return to a full dose of medication, or seek other medications or drugs to manage their symptoms. Occasionally severe withdrawal effects will lead people to be admitted to hospital and in some cases to attempt suicide.[7,8]

So although there are specific approaches to coping with withdrawal most people do not do well by 'white-knuckling' through the process of very severe withdrawal effects. The main tool to manage withdrawal symptoms should be to reduce the dose gradually enough to avoid severe withdrawal symptoms in the first place. Although there has been limited research in the area it seems to be the case that experiencing more severe withdrawal symptoms from rapid reductions may also increase the risk of a protracted withdrawal syndrome in the long run.[2,4]

Coping with withdrawal symptoms

There are some examples of general methods of coping with withdrawal symptoms in the introductory chapters. For benzodiazepines, there are a few interventions with supporting evidence. The addition of psychological intervention to gradual dose reduction has been found in a meta-analysis of seven studies (454 participants) to have a beneficial effect on cessation rates (Odds ratio [OR] = 1.82), with the effect maintained at follow up (OR = 1.88).[9] Note that the size of the effect is substantially smaller than the effect of gradual dose reduction (tapering), which shows an odds ratio of six compared to routine care in terms of cessation rates.[9]

Common elements in these psychological interventions included relaxation training, cognitive-behavioural treatment of insomnia, self monitoring of symptoms, goal-setting, and coping with anxiety.[9] It should be noted that CBT does not improve outcomes at longer-term follow up,[10] perhaps because the withdrawal process has a large physiological component to it that can only be accommodated by gradual tapering. Relaxation courses were shown to improve the chances of successfully stopping benzodiazepines compared to care as usual.[10]

Many patients report that it is useful to be made aware that the symptoms that are experienced during the withdrawal process are of a physiological origin and should not be given an existential weight they do not merit.[11] In peer-led withdrawal communities these symptoms are referred to as 'neuro-emotions', denoting emotions that arise because of withdrawal-associated neurological processes, as distinct from 'endogenous' emotions that relate to events in the person's life.[2] A guidebook for therapists on how to support patients undergoing psychiatric drug withdrawal suggests to therapists that they 'suspend customary assumptions about the source of distress and associated interventions (i.e. emotional processing or analysis) for the duration of withdrawal'.[11] Such symptoms, in their more extreme forms are very likely to attract mental health diagnoses from clinicians unfamiliar with this aspect of withdrawal.[2,12]

Sometimes withdrawal symptoms can be difficult to distinguish from an underlying condition, not just for the clinician but also for the patient.[2] Although timing and associated physical symptoms can be helpful in discerning this distinction, the subjective similarity of symptoms to the original condition can be confusing for some.[2] Familiar patterns of thoughts and emotions may be triggered by withdrawal symptoms. In the same way as anxiety triggered by, for example, an excess of caffeine in a given individual may have a presentation that depends on an individual's personality and habits of mind, withdrawal symptoms may interact with an individual's typical responses and then closely resemble an underlying condition. In such cases, the pattern of symptoms over time (waxing and waning and corresponding to dose reductions), and co-incident symptoms that are not typical of the patient's mental health condition are most useful to help identify these withdrawal states.[2]

Many patients go through a phase of shock when they contemplate or experience the effects of withdrawal on their lives. This sense of shock may include worries about the impact on financial, work and personal affairs and involve feelings of regret, self-blame and anger at having been prescribed these medications in the first place.[2,13] People may feel aggrieved that they were not properly informed about the difficulties in stopping medication. Another common emotional symptom in withdrawal is the opposite of intense emotion – the complete absence of emotions, sometimes referred to as 'emotional anaesthesia', or anhedonia, numbness, apathy or 'dysthymia' following drug withdrawal.[1,2,14,15] This effect, like other withdrawal effects, seems to fade over time but can take months or years to abate in some patients.[1]

Techniques such as distraction, acceptance and re-orientation can help people recognise these psychological symptoms as temporary products of the withdrawal process that resolve in time like other symptoms.[2] Peer support has been found to be helpful.[16] Some patients find that learning to manage and cope with withdrawal symptoms also translates to being able to manage the mental health conditions that first prompted medication prescriptions in a more effective way.[2]

For some people in benzodiazepine withdrawal, environmental stimuli can be overwhelming, and some patients may need to carefully manage their sensory exposure to avoid being severely disturbed.[5] Reducing stress in life, to the degree this is possible, may be helpful for the process. Activity and exercise may be useful both as distraction and to reduce tension but need to be adjusted to the degree of physiological disturbance caused by benzodiazepine withdrawal in order to avoid sensory overload, which can sometimes exacerbate symptoms.[4,5] Sleep hygiene can be helpful.[17] There has not been formal study on the role of diet during tapering benzodiazepines, but some have thought specific diets to be useful.[4]

References

1. Cosci F, Chouinard G. Acute and persistent withdrawal syndromes following discontinuation of psychotropic medications. *Psychother Psychosom* 2020; 89: 283–306.

2. Framer A. What I have learnt from helping thousands of people taper off psychotropic medications. *Ther Adv Psychopharmacol* 2021; 11: 204512532199127.

3. Reid Finlayson AJ, Macoubrie J, Huff C, Foster DE, Martin PR. Experiences with benzodiazepine use, tapering, and discontinuation: an internet survey. *Ther Adv Psychopharmacol* 2022; 12: 20451253221082384.

4. Ashton H. Benzodiazepines: how they work and how to withdraw (The Ashton Manual). Newcastle University, 2002. http://www.benzo.org. uk/manual/bzcha01.htm (accessed 11 July 2023).

5. Wright SL. Benzodiazepine withdrawal: clinical aspects. In: *The Benzodiazepines Crisis* (eds. J Peppin, J Pergolizzi, R Raffa, S Wright) 2020: 117–C8.P334. Oxford: Oxford University Press. doi:10.1093/med/9780197517277.003.0008.

6. Lerner A, Klein M. Dependence, withdrawal and rebound of CNS drugs: an update and regulatory considerations for new drugs development. *Brain Commun* 2019; 1: fcz025.

7. Guy A, Brown M, Lewis S, Horowitz M. The 'patient voice'– patients who experience antidepressant withdrawal symptoms are often dismissed, or misdiagnosed with relapse, or a new medical condition. *Ther Adv Psychopharmacol* 2020; 10: 2045125320967183.

8. Ashton H. The diagnosis and management of benzodiazepine dependence. *Curr Opin Psychiatry* 2005; 18: 249–55.

9. Parr JM, Kavanagh DJ, Cahill L, Mitchell G, Young RM. Effectiveness of current treatment approaches for benzodiazepine discontinuation: a meta-analysis. 2008; 104: 13–24.

10. Darker CD, Sweeney BP, Barry JM, Farrell MF, Donnelly-Swift E. Psychosocial interventions for benzodiazepine harmful use, abuse or dependence. *Cochrane Database Syst Rev* 2015; CD009652.

11. Guy A, Davies J, Rizq R. Guidance for psychological therapists: enabling conversations with clients taking or withdrawing from prescribed psychiatric drugs. London: APPG for Prescribed Drug Dependence, 2019. Quotation p. 95.

12. White E, Read J, Julo S. The role of Facebook groups in the management and raising of awareness of antidepressant withdrawal: is social media filling the void left by health services? *Ther Adv Psychopharmacol* 2021; 11: 2045125320981174.

13. National Institute for Health and Care Excellence (NICE). Medicines associated with dependence or withdrawal symptoms: safe prescribing and withdrawal management for adults | Guidance | NICE. 2022. https://www.nice.org.uk/guidance/ng215/chapter/Recommendations (accessed 27 June 2022).

14. El-Mallakh RS, Briscoe B. Studies of long-term use of antidepressants: how should the data from them be interpreted? *CNS Drugs* 2012; 26: 97–109.

15. Renoir T, Pang TY, Lanfumey L. Drug withdrawal-induced depression: serotonergic and plasticity changes in animal models. *Neurosci Biobehav Rev* 2012; 36: 696–726.

16. Tattersall ML, Hallstrom C. Self-help and benzodiazepine withdrawal. *J Affect Disord* 1992; 24: 193–8.

17. Morgan K, Dixon S, Mathers N, Thompson J, Tomeny M. Psychological treatment for insomnia in the regulation of long-term hypnotic drug use. *Health Technol Assess* 2004; 8: iii–iv, 1–68.

CHAPTER 3

Tapering benzodiazepines and z-drugs in practice

This chapter acts as a practical summary guide to deprescribing benzodiazepines and z-drugs.

Decision making for deprescribing

- The indications for deprescribing are:
  - adverse effects,
  - loss of efficacy (tolerance or tachyphylaxis),
  - use >1 month,[1–3]
  - patient wishes to stop, and
  - rationalising medication (e.g. reducing polypharmacy).
- Patients at higher risk from continuing benzodiazepines are those who are:[1]
  - age >65,
  - taking more than 1 benzodiazepine or z-drug,
  - also taking opioids or gabapentinoids (pregabalin or gabapentin),
  - at risk of falls,
  - diagnosed with COPD, severe or uncontrolled respiratory disease, or risk of respiratory depression,
  - have a substance use disorder or a history of overdose,
  - contemplating pregnancy[4–6] or breastfeeding.[7]
- Deprescribing decisions should be agreed between patient and prescriber. Forced tapers are not recommended (except in the case of acute severe adverse effects) and may provoke patients to seek medication from other sources.[8]
- Education about benzodiazepines and z-drugs should be provided (see first section of this chapter) – this intervention itself has been shown to increase the chances of successful cessation.[9]
  - **Benefits:** These drugs have clear short-term benefits for anxiety and insomnia. However, owing to tolerance, these benefits diminish over time and are unlikely to be effective in long-term use.[10,11] They may impair the efficacy of psychotherapeutic approaches such as exposure therapy.[12]
  - **Risks:** Adverse effects include cognitive, neurological and affective symptoms, sometimes including worsening anxiety and depression over time.[13–15] The patient may not always connect this to the use of the medication.
  - **Alternatives:** CBT for insomnia is more effective than hypnotics for sleep. Several evidence-based alternatives to benzodiazepines for the treatment of anxiety exist.[16–18]
- Initiating the offer of deprescribing with a letter can be effective and it is enhanced if there is also direct face-to-face contact with a prescriber or pharmacist.[19] Motivational interviewing might help.[19]
- Provide informed consent regarding discontinuation.
  - **Benefits.** In the long term, may lead to reduced anxiety (after the withdrawal process),[20] improve psychomotor and cognitive function,[21] possibly reduced mortality.[22,23] Lower risk of motor vehicle accidents,[24] falls[25] and drug interactions. There are numerous other neurological, cognitive, psychiatric and other symptoms that may also improve.[13,20]

- **Risks:** Withdrawal symptoms can occur – which can sometimes be severe and long-lasting – but these can generally be mitigated by tapering more slowly and adjusting the rate to one that is tolerable for the patient.[20] If tapering is performed too quickly then withdrawal effects such as suicidality, akathisia and long-term disability can occur.
- **Alternatives:** A patient may remain on their current medication if they choose.
- If deprescribing is declined (or attempted and found to be too difficult):[26]
  - patients should be advised of the benefits of stopping,
  - any concerns they have about stopping should be addressed,
  - patients should not be pressurised,
  - if appropriate, readdress discontinuation at future appointments, and
  - continue monitoring for adverse effects.
- Note that some patients may be unable to withdraw completely, and a more suitable goal may be dose reduction or maintenance of the current dose.

Before tapering

- Patients should be warned not to stop benzodiazepines abruptly if they have been used for more than 4 weeks, because in some cases this can cause severe problems (e.g. rarely, seizures)[27] and may provoke long-lasting withdrawal symptoms.[20,28]
- Reassurance may be required for those that have rapidly tapered in the past with intolerable consequences. Inform the patient that if tapering is performed gradually and adjusted to their symptoms, it can be tolerable.[8]
- Preparation for benzodiazepine tapering may be required: for example, bolstering of existing coping skills or development of new ones. These skills can include intentional relaxation (mindfulness, progressive muscle relaxation[26]), controlled breathing exercises,[29,30] physical exercise (if tolerated), sleep hygiene, acceptance, distraction techniques, CBT for insomnia, peer support and stress reduction.[31] There is a wide variety of other coping skills that people might find helpful. Sometimes lightening work or family duties may be useful.
- Specific treatments for the conditions for benzodiazepines and z-drugs were originally prescribed (i.e. anxiety and insomnia) can be helpful for the process (but may have limited effectiveness for withdrawal symptoms themselves).
  - People with insomnia may benefit from CBT for insomnia, or sleep hygiene advice. Where circadian rhythm disturbance plays a role this can be addressed.[32]
  - Anxiety disorders may be treated with psychotherapy modalities, or other non-pharmacological approaches.[20]
- Establishment of a support system. This can involve family and friends (who may require education) or more regular contact with clinical staff. Sometimes the introduction of patients to a supportive peer group in person or online can be helpful, although beware exposure to 'worst case' scenarios, and sometimes inaccurate information.[8]
- It is useful to set expectations. For people that have used benzodiazepines long term, the withdrawal process can take 6–18 months, or even longer for those sensitive to the process.[20] People who have been on short-term benzodiazepines or z-drugs may be able to stop completely in a few weeks.[33]
- Past experience of reducing can help predict symptoms that may arise again on tapering so should be noted and can be helpful for monitoring targeted symptoms, as below.

CHAPTER 3

- Familiarity of the patient and the doctor with the wide variety of withdrawal symptoms (see section on withdrawal effects) may help to mitigate unnecessary anxiety when symptoms arise. It should be impressed on patients that unpleasant withdrawal symptoms do not indicate that the drug is needed but that the taper rate should be slowed.
- If inter-dose withdrawal symptoms from benzodiazepines are present before tapering, either:
  - advise the patient to take the benzodiazepine more frequently; or
  - substitute an equivalent dose of a long-acting benzodiazepine (such as diazepam) with a step-wise cross-over (see drug-specific sections).[26]

The process of tapering

- Determine whether to perform a direct taper from the benzodiazepine or z-drug being used or to switch to a longer-acting benzodiazepine. Research evidence is equivocal about which approach is best and patient preference should be considered.[1,14,20,26] In the drug-specific tapers given in the rest of this chapter both options are provided.
  - Patients who may benefit most from a switch before tapering are those suffering from inter-dose withdrawal, or who are taking medication for which small doses are not easily available.
  - Patients who have had trouble with switching in the past or prefer to proceed with a familiar drug should be supported to do so.[34–36]
- There is consensus that a patient-directed taper, adjusted to symptoms is the most successful approach to cessation.[27] The key elements of a programme of tapering are:
  - that it is flexible and can be adjusted so that the process is tolerable for the patient,
  - that it involves close monitoring of withdrawal symptoms to facilitate timely adjustments to the rate of taper, and
  - that patients are provided with preparations of medication to make the process of creating doses that cannot be made with available tablet doses (e.g. liquid formulations or smaller dose formulations of tablets)

The process of tapering involves the following four steps (Figure 3.6).

Step one: estimation of risk of withdrawal and corresponding size of the initial dose reduction

Patients may be broadly risk stratified according to what is known about risk of withdrawal in a suggested approach below. It is better to err on the side of caution when estimating the risk category, and so the presence of any moderate- or high-risk characteristic should assign a patient to that category. Tapers can always be increased in speed if no difficulties are encountered – but the reverse can be more problematic.

Low-risk patients could start with approximately 20% (or less) dose reductions (e.g. the faster regimens given in the drug-specific sections). This group is characterised by:

- no evidence of tolerance to the medication,
- no evidence of inter-dose withdrawal,
- short-term use (weeks),
- taking longer half-life benzodiazepines,
- no or mild withdrawal symptoms in the past on stopping or skipping a dose, and
- no or limited history of benzodiazepine (or other psychiatric medication) use and cessation.[34–36]

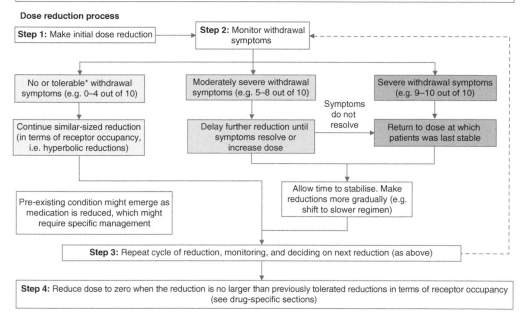

Figure 3.6 An overview of the process of tapering benzodiazepines and z-drugs.
*What constitutes tolerable withdrawal symptoms will vary from person to person.

Note that some patients who have only used benzodiazepines short term can also experience withdrawal effects,[34-36] but this is rarer than in long-term use.

- **Moderate-risk** patients could start with approximately 10% (or less) dose reduction (e.g. the moderate regimens given in the drug-specific sections). This group is characterised by:
  - some evidence of tolerance to the medication,
  - some experience of inter-dose withdrawal,
  - moderate-length use (months),
  - moderate withdrawal symptoms in the past on stopping or skipping a dose, and
  - some history of benzodiazepine (or other psychiatric medication) use and cessation.[14,20]
- **High-risk** patients could start with 5% (or less) dose reduction (e.g. the slower regimens given in the drug-specific sections). This group is characterised by:
  - evidence of significant tolerance to the medication,
  - marked experience of inter-dose withdrawal,
  - past history of severe withdrawal symptoms on dose reduction or skipping doses,
  - taking shorter half-life benzodiazepines,
  - older or otherwise physically frail, and

CHAPTER 3

- repeated cycles of benzodiazepine (or other psychiatric medication) use and cessation (which is thought to lead to sensitisation, a phenomenon sometimes called kindling).[14]
- In order to instil confidence in patients in what can be a daunting process, it may be advisable to start with an even smaller dose reduction in order to alleviate patients' fears about the process.
- None of the suggested regimens should be imposed on the patient but are a starting point to assess how the patient tolerates the process.
- If a patient prefers to try a smaller dose reduction than their risk category suggests this should be supported.
- People taking z-drugs once at night will tend to fall into the lower-risk category because z-drugs are likely to produce less physical dependence than benzodiazepines as they are probably largely eliminated in each 24 hour period.[37]

Step two: monitoring of withdrawal symptoms

- The most important information to determine the rate of reduction is how the patient experiences the process. Imposed regimens tend to backfire.[37,38] Withdrawal symptoms should be monitored for 1–4 weeks or as long as it takes for symptoms to start to ease.
- Although there are various formal scales used to measure withdrawal symptoms, these can be cumbersome because of the number of items, and potentially miss the importance of one or two significant symptoms.[39] An alternative is to rate a small number of core withdrawal symptoms such as anxiety, insomnia or other prominent symptoms out of 10 (0 = no symptoms, 10 = extreme symptoms) or to rate withdrawal symptoms out of 10 overall. This monitoring often detects a 'wave' pattern of withdrawal symptoms: where symptoms increase, reach a peak, start to resolve and return to or approach baseline (Figure 3.7).

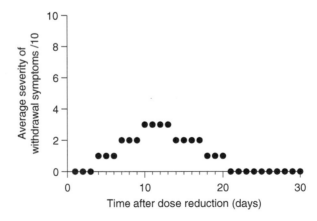

Figure 3.7 Graphical representation of withdrawal symptoms following a dose reduction of a benzodiazepine. These probably constitute mild to moderate symptoms. The y-axis shows the average patient-rated severity of withdrawal symptoms. Note the delayed onset of significant symptoms after drug reduction, probably related to drug elimination, followed by a peak and then easing of symptoms, probably related to re-adaptation of the system to a new homeostatic 'set-point' (similarly to Figures 3.4b and c).

Step three: determination of the size of the next reduction based on response to reduction

The information from monitoring can be used to determine the frequency and size of reductions (Figure 3.7). See further examples in 'Tapering antidepressants in practice' but briefly:

- if symptoms take 2 weeks to resolve and the severity is mild (e.g. less than 4 out 10) then similar-sized reductions (in terms of receptor occupancy) could be made every 1–4 weeks so that subsequent symptoms do not accumulate;
- if symptoms take longer to resolve or their severity is moderate (e.g. 5 to 8 out of 10) then further time between reductions will be required and/or smaller reductions made in future;
- if symptoms are severe (e.g. 9 or 10 out 10) then dose should be increased to the last dose at which the patient was stable, wait for stabilisation and then make reductions at half the rate, or less.

It is important that these decisions are reached jointly and that a too fast rate of taper is not imposed on patients.

Step four: repetition of cycles of reduction and monitoring until cessation

- The steps outlined above in steps 2 and 3 should be repeated. Similar-sized reductions (in terms of effect on target receptors) should produce similar withdrawal reactions, but sometimes these vary over time, so ongoing monitoring of withdrawal symptoms is warranted with adjustment of the regimen according to the experience of the patient.
  - Reductions should proceed in a hyperbolic pattern to accommodate the nature of the pharmacological effect of the drugs.[38,39] Examples of such regimens are displayed in the drug-specific sections of this chapter.
  - The taper should be flexible to accommodate periods of stress, increased responsibilities or illness.
  - The dose should be reduced to zero when the dose is low enough that the reduction to zero will not cause a larger change (in terms of effect on target receptors) than previous tolerable reductions have caused. For example, for diazepam the final dose before stopping for diazepam may be 1mg, 0.5mg 0.2mg or even lower (see diazepam section) depending on the size of the reductions tolerated throughout the taper.

Tapering techniques

Patients can taper in steps ('cut and hold', e.g. at intervals of 1–4 weeks) as outlined above or, alternatively, they can taper in smaller amounts (e.g. every day), often called micro-tapering. There are pros and cons to each approach:

- Tapering in steps is simpler and can often be performed with existing tablet formulations of some medications (e.g. halving and quartering 2mg diazepam tablets). Larger, less frequent reductions can cause greater symptoms (see Figure 3.4).

- Micro-tapering involves more complicated calculations and use of formulations other than tablets (e.g. manufacturers' liquids or suspensions of tablets). It can reduce the severity of symptoms making the process of tapering more tolerable by 'spreading' out changes to established equilibria.[40] See the drug-specific section for example regimens (e.g. by reducing by 0.05mg per day from 20mg of diazepam).

A variety of different formulations can be used for tapering:

- Commercially available tablets: small doses are preferable, with round tablets able to be divided into halves and quarters using a tablet cutter (more accurate than breaking along a score line).[41]
- Manufacturers' liquids: using a syringe for precise measurement. Further dilution in water is sometimes required for small doses.
- Compounded tablets or liquids: specialist pharmacies can prepare lower-dose tablet formulations or liquid suspensions. One example is 'tapering strips'.[42]
- Suspending tablets or capsules: tablets can be crushed and dispersed in water or milk. Capsules can be emptied to disperse in water or milk. Suspension of tablets is an off-label but widely recommended method by authoritative pharmaceutical guidance[43-45] and is commonly used by patients.[20,46]

After tapering

Some patients can have ongoing withdrawal symptoms following cessation. Sometimes this lasts just for several days or weeks but occasionally is extended for months or sometimes years, termed protracted withdrawal syndrome.[47,48] See the subsequent section 'Management of complications of benzodiazepine and z-drug discontinuation' for further details.

Other considerations

- Extending the dosing interval ('skipping doses') to taper is ill-advised as it can lead to inter-dose withdrawal symptoms, unless involving benzodiazepines with very long half-lives such as diazepam. It is preferable to give smaller doses each day using one of the techniques outlined previously.
- Withdrawal symptoms are best managed by adjustment of the taper rate, rather than 'white-knuckling' through the process. It is thought that severe withdrawal effects may make a protracted withdrawal syndrome more likely.[26]
- Adjunctive medication has mixed evidence, with authoritative guidance recommending against its use[51,52] and it should be reserved for very severe cases.[53,54]
  - Short-term use of propanolol,[20,28] and perhaps antihistamines might be warranted in severe withdrawal. Carbamazepine might be reserved for extremely difficult cases.
- People can become sensitised to various medications during the process of withdrawal for reasons that are not well understood.[20]
  - The most noteworthy of these include alcohol and antibiotics (especially fluoroquinolones which can displace benzodiazepines from the GABA receptor).[55]
  - There are reports of sensitivities to steroids, other medications, caffeine, nicotine, supplements and even specific foods.[20,28]
  - The use of some of these medications may be unavoidable, but greater caution than usual should be exercised with any supplement or medication.[20]

Potential pitfalls

- Physiological dependence can develop in a matter of days so some people will have withdrawal symptoms after just short-term use.
- Physiological dependence and the experience of withdrawal effects does not indicate addiction. Addiction centres are therefore not advised for people suffering withdrawal effects from benzodiazepines without abuse or misuse – sometimes treatment at these centres involves abrupt cessation with other medications added in to 'cover' withdrawal effects, or inappropriate 12-step approaches irrelevant to medication taken as prescribed.
- Some symptoms can seem bizarre but should not be discounted as many of these are recognised withdrawal symptoms (see section on withdrawal effects) (e.g., depersonalization/ derealization, agoraphobia, intrusive thoughts, burning nerve pain, irritable bowel).[49,56]
- Symptoms of benzodiazepine withdrawal can mimic other conditions, leading to misdiagnosis (e.g. functional neurological disorder, medically unexplained symptoms, psychosomatic conditions, chronic fatigue syndrome, anxiety disorder, depression, bipolar disorder, neurological disorders) and unnecessary testing and medical treatment.[56,57]
- The drug-specific taper protocols in the following sections are meant to be a guide only: flexibility is key. The patient's experience of withdrawal symptoms should be the main guide to the rate of taper.
- Post-withdrawal recovery may take 12–18 months, and sometimes longer.

CHAPTER 3

CHAPTER 3

References

1. Kaiser Permanente. Benzodiazepine and z-drug safety guideline. https://wa.kaiserpermanente.org/static/pdf/public/guidelines/benzo-zdrug.pdf (accessed 29 April 2023).

2. Pottie K, Thompson W, Davies S, et al. Deprescribing benzodiazepine receptor agonists: evidence-based clinical practice guideline. *Can Fam Physician* 2018; 64: 339–51.

3. Pottie K, Thompson W, Davies S, et al. Benzodiazepine & z-drug (BZRA) deprescribing algorithm. *Canadian Family Physician/ Medecin de famille canadien*. 2019; published online May. https://deprescribing.org/wp-content/uploads/2019/02/BZRA-deprescribing-algorithms-2019-English.pdf (accessed 4 July 2023).

4. Yonkers KA, Gilstad-Hayden K, Forray A, Lipkind HS. Association of panic disorder, generalized anxiety disorder, and benzodiazepine treatment during pregnancy with risk of adverse birth outcomes. *JAMA Psychiatry* 2017; 74: 1145–52.

5. Sheehy O, Zhao J-P, Bérard A. Association between incident exposure to benzodiazepines in early pregnancy and risk of spontaneous abortion. *JAMA Psychiatry* 2019; 76: 948–57.

6. Wall-Wieler E, Robakis TK, Lyell DJ, Masarwa R, Platt RW, Carmichael SL. Benzodiazepine use before conception and risk of ectopic pregnancy. *Hum Reprod* 2020; 35: 1685–92.

7. Soussan C, Gouraud A, Portolan G, et al. Drug-induced adverse reactions via breastfeeding: a descriptive study in the French Pharmacovigilance Database. *Eur J Clin Pharmacol* 2014; 70: 1361–6.

8. Colorado Consortium for Prescription Drug Abuse Prevention. Benzodiazepine Deprescribing Guidance. Colorado Consortium for Prescription Drug Abuse Prevention. 2022. https://corxconsortium.org/wp-content/uploads/Benzo-Deprescribing.pdf (accessed 16 May 2023).

9. Tannenbaum C, Martin P, Tamblyn R, Benedetti A, Ahmed S. Reduction of inappropriate benzodiazepine prescriptions among older adults through direct patient education: the EMPOWER cluster randomized trial. *JAMA Intern Med* 2014; 174: 890–8.

10. Gale C, Glue P, Guaiana G, Coverdale J, McMurdo M, Wilkinson S. Influence of covariates on heterogeneity in Hamilton Anxiety Scale ratings in placebo-controlled trials of benzodiazepines in generalized anxiety disorder: systematic review and meta-analysis. *J Psychopharmacol* 2019; 33: 543–7.

11. Curran HV, Collins R, Fletcher S, Kee SCY, Woods B, Iliffe S. Older adults and withdrawal from benzodiazepine hypnotics in general practice: effects on cognitive function, sleep, mood and quality of life. *Psychol Med* 2003; 33: 1223–37.

12. Marks IM, Swinson RP, Başoğlu M, et al. Alprazolam and exposure alone and combined in panic disorder with agoraphobia: a controlled study in London and Toronto. *Br J Psychiatry* 1993; 162: 776–87.

13. Ashton H. Benzodiazepine withdrawal: outcome in 50 patients. *Br J Addict* 1987; 82: 665–71.

14. Wright SL. Benzodiazepine withdrawal: clinical aspects. In: *The Benzodiazepines Crisis* (eds. J Peppin, J Pergolizzi, R Raffa, S Wright) 2020: 117–C8.P334. Oxford: Oxford University Press. doi:10.1093/med/9780197517277.003.0008.

15. Guina J, Merrill B. Benzodiazepines I: upping the care on downers: the evidence of risks, benefits and alternatives. *J Clin Med Res* 2018; 7: 17.

16. Moreno-Peral P, Conejo-Cerón S, Rubio-Valera M, et al. Effectiveness of psychological and/or educational interventions in the prevention of anxiety: a systematic review, meta-analysis, and meta-regression. *JAMA Psychiatry* 2017; 74: 1021–9.

17. Aylett E, Small N, Bower P. Exercise in the treatment of clinical anxiety in general practice – a systematic review and meta-analysis. *BMC Health Serv Res* 2018; 18: 559.

18. Lewis C, Pearce J, Bisson JI. Efficacy, cost-effectiveness and acceptability of self-help interventions for anxiety disorders: systematic review. *Br J Psychiatry* 2012; 200: 15–21.

19. Darker CD, Sweeney BP, Barry JM, Farrell MF, Donnelly-Swift E. Psychosocial interventions for benzodiazepine harmful use, abuse or dependence. *Cochrane Database Syst Rev* 2015: CD009652.

20. Ashton H. Benzodiazepines: how they work and how to withdraw (The Ashton Manual). Newcastle University, 2002. http://www.benzo.org.uk/manual/bzcha01.htm (accessed 11 July 20230).

21. Lader M, Tylee A, Donoghue J. Withdrawing benzodiazepines in primary care. *CNS Drugs* 2009; 23: 19–34.

22. Xu KY, Hartz SM, Borodovsky JT, Bierut LJ, Grucza RA. Association between benzodiazepine use with or without opioid use and all-cause mortality in the United States, 1999-2015. *JAMA Netw Open* 2020; 3: e2028557.

23. Belleville G. Mortality hazard associated with anxiolytic and hypnotic drug use in the National Population Health Survey. *Can J Psychiatry* 2010; 55: 558–67.

24. Brubacher JR, Chan H, Erdelyi S, Zed PJ, Staples JA, Etminan M. Medications and risk of motor vehicle collision responsibility in British Columbia, Canada: a population-based case-control study. *Lancet Public Health* 2021; 6: e374–85.

25. Pariente A, Dartigues J-F, Benichou J, Letenneur L, Moore N, Fourrier-Réglat A. Benzodiazepines and injurious falls in community dwelling elders. *Drugs Aging* 2008; 25: 61–70.

26. Scenario: Benzodiazepine and z-drug withdrawal. https://cks.nice.org.uk/topics/benzodiazepine-z-drug-withdrawal/management/benzodiazepine-z-drug-withdrawal/ (accessed 7 October 2022).

27. FDA Drug Safety Communication. FDA requiring boxed warning updated to improve safe use of benzodiazepine drug class. 2020. https://www.fda.gov/drugs/drug-safety-and-availability/fda-requiring-boxed-warning-updated-improve-safe-use-benzodiazepine-drug-class (accessed 3 July 2023).

28. Framer A. What I have learnt from helping thousands of people taper off psychotropic medications. *Ther Adv Psychopharmacol* 2021; 11: 204512532199127.

29. The Withdrawal Project. https://withdrawal.theinnercompass.org/.

30. Guy A, Davies J, Rizq R. *Guidance for Psychological Therapists: Enabling Conversations with Clients Taking or Withdrawing from Prescribed Psychiatric Drugs*. London: APPG for Prescribed Drug Dependence, 2019.

31. Lack LC, Wright HR. Treating chronobiological components of chronic insomnia. *Sleep Med* 2007; 8: 637–44.
32. National Institute for Health and Care Excellence (NICE). Generalised anxiety disorder and panic disorder in adults: management. *NICE clinical guideline CG113* 2011. https://www.nice.org.uk/guidance/cg113/chapter/2-Research-recommendations#the-effectiveness-of-physical-activity-compared-with-waiting-list-control-for-the-treatment-of-gad (accessed 3 July 2023).
33. Denis C, Fatseas M, Lavie E, Auriacombe M. Pharmacological interventions for benzodiazepine dependence management among benzodiazepine users in outpatient settings [Protocol]. *Cochrane Database Syst Rev* 2005. doi:10.1002/14651858.CD005194.
34. Rickels K, Freeman EW. Prior benzodiazepine exposure and benzodiazepine treatment outcome. *J Clin Psychiatry* 2000; 61: 409–13.
35. Stephens DN. A glutamatergic hypothesis of drug dependence: extrapolations from benzodiazepine receptor ligands. *Behav Pharmacol* 1995; 6: 425–46.
36. Rickels K, Schweizer E, Csanalosi I, Case WG, Chung H. Long-term treatment of anxiety and risk of withdrawal: prospective comparison of Clorazepate and Buspirone. *Arch Gen Psychiatry* 1988; 45: 444–50.
37. Lader MH. Managing dependence and withdrawal with newer hypnotic medications in the treatment of insomnia. The Primary Care Companion. 2002. https://www.psychiatrist.com/pcc/sleep/managing-dependence-withdrawal-newer-hypnotic-medications (accessed 20 May 2023).
38. Horowitz M, Taylor D. Withdrawing from benzodiazepines and z-drugs (in preparation).
39. Horowitz MA, Taylor D. Tapering of SSRI treatment to mitigate withdrawal symptoms. *The Lancet Psychiatry* 2019; 6: 538–46.
40. Horowitz MA, Taylor D. How to reduce and stop psychiatric medication. *Eur Neuropsychopharmacol* 2021; 55: 4–7.
41. Verrue C, Mehuys E, Boussery K, Remon J-P, Petrovic M. Tablet-splitting: a common yet not so innocent practice. *J Adv Nurs* 2011; 67: 26–32.
42. Groot PC, van Os J. How user knowledge of psychotropic drug withdrawal resulted in the development of person-specific tapering medication. *Ther Adv in Psychopharmacol* 2020; 10: 204512532093245.
43. Bostwick JR, Demehri A. Pills to powder: an updated clinician's reference for crushable psychotropics. *Curr Psychiatr* 2017; 16: 46–9.
44. Smyth J. The NEWT guidelines for administration of medication to patients with enteral feeding tubes or swallowing difficulties. 2011. https://www.newtguidelines.com/index.html (accessed 18 February 2023).
45. Stahl SM. Flurazepam. In: *Prescriber's Guide: Stahl's Essential Psychopharmacology*. Cambridge: Cambridge University Press, 2020: 321–4.
46. BenzoBuddies Community Forum. http://www.benzobuddies.org/forum/index.php (accessed 18 March 2023).
47. Cosci F, Chouinard G. Acute and persistent withdrawal syndromes following discontinuation of psychotropic medications. *Psychother Psychosom* 2020; 89: 283–306.
48. Ashton H. Protracted withdrawal from benzodiazepines: the post-withdrawal syndrome. *Psychiatr Ann* 1995; 25: 174–9.
49. Huff C, Finlayson AJR, Foster DE, Martin PR. Enduring neurological sequelae of benzodiazepine use: an internet survey. *Ther Adv Psychopharmacol* 2023; 13: 2045125322145560.
50. Allison C, Pratt JA. Neuroadaptive processes in GABAergic and glutamatergic systems in benzodiazepine dependence. *Pharmacol Ther* 2003; 98: 171–95.
51. National Institute for Health and Care Excellence (NICE). Medicines associated with dependence or withdrawal symptoms: safe prescribing and withdrawal management for adults | Guidance | NICE. 2022. https://www.nice.org.uk/guidance/ng215/chapter/Recommendations (accessed 27 June 2022).
52. Hypnotics and anxiolytics. https://bnf.nice.org.uk/treatment-summaries/hypnotics-and-anxiolytics/ (accessed 19 March 2023).
53. Parr JM, Kavanagh DJ, Cahill L, Mitchell G, Young RM. Effectiveness of current treatment approaches for benzodiazepine discontinuation: a meta-analysis. *Addiction* 2008; 104: 13–24.
54. Baandrup L, Ebdrup BH, Rasmussen JØ, Lindschou J, Gluud C, Glenthøj BY. Pharmacological interventions for benzodiazepine discontinuation in chronic benzodiazepine users. *Cochrane Database Syst Rev* 2018; 3: CD011481.
55. Unseld E, Ziegler G, Gemeinhardt A, Janssen U, Klotz U. Possible interaction of fluoroquinolones with the benzodiazepine-GABAA-receptor complex. *Br J Clin Pharmacol* 1990; 30: 63–70.
56. Reid Finlayson AJ, Macoubrie J, Huff C, Foster DE, Martin PR. Experiences with benzodiazepine use, tapering, and discontinuation: an internet survey. *Ther Adv Psychopharmacol* 2022; 12: 20451253221082384.
57. Guy A, Brown M, Lewis S, Horowitz M. The 'patient voice' – patients who experience antidepressant withdrawal symptoms are often dismissed, or misdiagnosed with relapse, or a new medical condition. *Ther Adv Psychopharmacol* 2020. https://journals.sagepub.com/doi/abs/10.1177/2045125320967183.

CHAPTER 3

Management of complications of benzodiazepine and z-drug discontinuation

Approach to withdrawal akathisia

One of the most distressing outcomes of benzodiazepine reduction or discontinuation is akathisia.[1-4] As mentioned, although akathisia has been more commonly associated with antipsychotic exposure, it can be induced by benzodiazepine withdrawal.[1-4] Gradual tapering is thought to minimise the risk of this withdrawal effect, but there have been no trials looking specifically at this topic. As people suffering from withdrawal akathisia can be agitated and quite disordered in their behaviour (pacing, restless, grimacing, etc) the condition can often mis-diagnosed as mania, psychosis or agitated depression by clinicians unfamiliar with this withdrawal effect.[5-7] For some people the condition is so unbearable it can lead to suicide.[8,9] For others it is experienced more as internal restlessness, irritability and tension without manifesting physical signs.[10] Once a patient is in such a state it is very difficult to treat and symptoms can be prolonged in some patients.[6] This risk, albeit likely small (though unknown), of too rapid discontinuation is a strong rationale for tapering gradually.

Although there has been little in the way of research on withdrawal akathisia, the most commonly successful approach in clinical practice is re-instatement of the original benzodiazepine at the dose at which the patient had been previously stable. As the response to re-introduction of a benzodiazepine can be somewhat unpredictable when patients are in this state, it is wise to cautiously re-introduce it.

The drugs most commonly recommended as useful for akathisia are beta-blockers like propranolol, and $5HT_{2A}$ receptor antagonists (e.g. mirtazapine and cyproheptadine).[6] For example, in one open label trial of patients with neuroleptic-induced akathisia most patients (15/17) treated with cyproheptadine showed marked improvement of their symptoms, which returned when cyproheptadine was ceased.[11] The degree to which this treatment effect is also relevant to benzodiazepine withdrawal-induced akathisia has not been evaluated. The evidence for beta blockers in neuroleptic-induced akathisia is limited but not encouraging, with a Cochrane review finding no evidence of improvement.[12] Anecdotally, some patients with akathisia do report an improvement in their symptoms with propranolol.

However, even medications recommended for the treatment of akathisia have been associated with worsening symptoms in some patients.[8] Patient groups advocating for wider awareness of this syndrome, report that antipsychotics, antidepressants and additional benzodiazepines, can sometimes make withdrawal akathisia worse.[8] For example, mirtazapine has been noted to cause akathisia, amongst other movement disorders, in some patients.[13] If re-instatement of the original benzodiazepine is not successful, then the treatment of withdrawal akathisia should involve the introduction of one additional medication at a time for a short period at a low dose as a test of response. Patients should be closely observed to decide whether the drug is helpful, and it should be ceased if it is not, before trialling an additional medication.[6,8]

Aside from re-instatement of the original medication, patient advocacy groups suggest that the best management may be conservative. This essentially means allowing symptoms to resolve over time with minimal intervention, although this can be difficult for some patients to tolerate, especially when symptoms are prolonged.[8] Exercise is widely found to be helpful by patients, who often report that pacing somewhat lessens unpleasant sensations. This is supported by a case study in which the distress caused by a patient's akathisia was relieved by continuously pedalling using a stationary bike.[14] However, in some cases, akathisia will be so unbearable, or the patient's consequent suicidality so acute, that the use of further medications will be unavoidable. In extremis, some clinicians have used opioids, which has some support from a case series in neuroleptic-induced akathisia,[15] although such an approach to treatment presents clear long-term risks.

Management of protracted withdrawal syndrome

The proportion of patients who experience protracted withdrawal (sometimes called post-acute withdrawal syndrome (PAWS)) after stopping benzodiazepines is uncertain,[2,3,16,17] but it has been estimated to be as high as 15%.[17] Its risk is thought to be minimised by gradual tapering, but this has not been studied formally.[18]

There is limited research on the best approach to managing protracted withdrawal syndrome. From limited data and clinical experience,[17,19] people's clinical status does improve over time without specific intervention but recovery may take long periods (e.g. months or sometimes even years).[17,18] In a (self-selected) survey of patients with protracted withdrawal syndrome (who had used benzodiazepines for on average 8 years before stopping) patients reported it taking between 1 and 60 months (average 12.2 months) after benzodiazepine discontinuation for symptoms to resolve.[4] Some authors have speculated that such long-lasting disturbance might be better conceptualised as benzodiazepine-induced neurological dysfunction (BIND).[20]

Initiation of medications other than the original drug does not appear to be particularly helpful for most patients. Although there are isolated reports of symptomatic improvement after introduction of other medications,[18] it is not clear whether this is widely applicable because of a lack of research. Equally, there are also reports of symptoms worsening following administration of new psychiatric medications, perhaps because of further perturbation to a disturbed system, especially one sensitised to drugs by the withdrawal process.[16,18] There are a wide variety of medications trialled to treat or suppress the neurological and psychological symptoms of protracted withdrawal, such as beta blockers, anti-histamines, anticonvulsants, gabapentinoids and antidepressants with little research to guide such choices.

One management option is re-instatement of the original benzodiazepine, which generally improves people's symptoms, at least partially.[18] Sometimes withdrawal symptoms take longer (i.e. weeks, and sometimes months) to resolve after re-instatement when substantial time has elapsed after cessation (or reduction) of the benzodiazepine (i.e. months or years). Re-instatement of benzodiazepines soon after cessation almost always leads to resolution of symptoms – however, there seems to be greater variation in response when re-instatement is delayed for longer periods.[18] It is not known what determines this relationship. For antidepressants, for example, a proportion of patients with protracted withdrawal syndromes improved following re-instatement months or even years after stopping.[9] It is reported that the same phenomenon is observed in clinical practice with benzodiazepines, but there have been no controlled studies.

There are also rare reports of patients who experience a paradoxical worsening in response to re-instatement of the original medication long after stopping.[18] These paradoxical responses have been linked to kindling – a sensitisation to the ceased medication.[18,21,22] This process is analogous to the kindling effect recognised in repeated cycles of exposure to and cessation of psychoactive substances, such as alcohol.[18,21,22]

One method employed to trial re-instatement whilst mitigating the possibility of a negative outcome is to re-instate a very small test dose of the original medication (generally simpler than using a novel benzodiazepine), for example 0.5 or 1 mg of diaz-epam, or equivalent.[18] If this test dose has positive effects, an increase in dose may be cautiously attempted – recognising that some patients may need titration to approximately the same dose on which they were previously stable.[18] If this test re-instatement produces a negative effect then reinstatement could be abandoned.

Patients in protracted withdrawal may need social and financial support if their ability to work and function is impaired for long periods because the above treatment options were unsuccessful or only partially successful. There is unfortunately limited recognition of protracted withdrawal syndrome by clinicians, making navigating the medical and support system difficult for these patients, adding to their suffering.[18,19,23] Such patients are often mis-diagnosed as suffering from a mental health condition, or a psychosomatic disorder.[1,4,18,19] One of the main requests from patients is that the medical system recognises the difficulties that protracted withdrawal syndromes can cause them and that sufficient support be provided (including completing disability or benefits paperwork where needed).[3]

To try to make it more explicit just how debilitating such protracted withdrawal states can be, some expert clinicians have suggested that this state may be better thought of as a neurological injury caused by use and/or cessation of a benzodiazepine.[4] Nevertheless, the vast majority of people eventually recover (albeit some taking years)[3] and one important aspect of treatment is to project optimism for a favourable outcome, as despair in response to slow improvement is common.

Increased sensitivity during withdrawal

Patients can become highly sensitive to psychoactive and neurologically active substances in the process of withdrawal.[4,19] This phenomenon is thought to be related to an increased sensitivity to stimuli secondary to the de-stabilisation produced by the drug withdrawal process,[18,24,25] though the mechanism is not fully understood. People can respond to a wide variety of substances with activation or other paradoxical effects, including alcohol, neurologically active antibiotics,[26] caffeine, St John's Wort, and sometimes even specific foods, supplements and herbs.[18,27] This is in addition to other sensitivities to light and sound, more generally recognised.[16] The fluoroquinolone class of antibiotics is particularly notorious for causing problems[28] probably because this class of antibiotic is thought to compete with benzodiazepines at the GABA receptor and so can precipitate withdrawal.[29,30]

Where these substances exacerbate withdrawal symptoms it is wise to restrict exposure to them during the withdrawal process.[18] Sensitivities often resolve or improve markedly when the patient recovers from withdrawal.[18] It may not be possible to avoid all implicated medications during the withdrawal process. Decisions will be contingent upon individual circumstances, the risks of exacerbating withdrawal, the risks of the condition to be treated and alternative treatments available.

In the process of withdrawal, or after becoming sensitised to a benzodiazepine, patients describe requiring dosing several times a day – often more frequently than manufacturers recommend in the drug labels. This may be because small reductions in plasma levels are enough to precipitate inter-dose withdrawal symptoms in people sensitised to these changes, although this phenomenon is not fully understood.[19] Some patients may require dosing twice a day with long half-life benzodiazepines (like diazepam), three to four times a day with moderately long half-life benzodiazepines (like clonazepam), four to five times a day with shorter half-life drugs (like lorazepam) and dosing five to six times a day with short-acting drugs (like alprazolam).[23] Many patients will report relief from symptoms if these regimens are instituted.

Lastly, increased sensitivity in benzodiazepine withdrawal can extend to women's menstrual cycles, with many women reporting an exacerbation of withdrawal symptoms at the time of their menses. Many sex hormones potentiate benzodiazepines including progesterone,[31] and their natural variation throughout the menstrual cycle, as well as in the menopause, post-partum or post-hysterectomy can contribute to exacerbations of benzodiazepine withdrawal symptoms.[32]

References

1. Guy A, Brown M, Lewis S, Horowitz MA. The "Patient Voice" – Patients who experience antidepressant withdrawal symptoms are often dismissed, or mis-diagnosed with relapse, or onset of a new medical condition. *Ther Adv Psychopharmacol* 2020; 10: 204512532096718.
2. Reid Finlayson AJ, Macoubrie J, Huff C, Foster DE, Martin PR. Experiences with benzodiazepine use, tapering, and discontinuation: an Internet survey. *Ther Adv Psychopharmacol* 2022; 12: 20451253221082384.
3. Huff C, Finlayson AJR, Foster DE, Martin PR. Enduring neurological sequelae of benzodiazepine use: an Internet survey. *Ther Adv Psychopharmacol* 2023; 13: 20451253221145560.
4. Wright SL. Benzodiazepine Withdrawal: Clinical Aspects. In: J Peppin, J Pergolizzi, R Raffa, S Wright, ed. The Benzodiazepines Crisis. Oxford University Press, 2020: 117–48.
5. Narayan V, Haddad PM. Antidepressant discontinuation manic states: a critical review of the literature and suggested diagnostic criteria. *J Psychopharmacol* 2010; 25: 306–13.
6. Tachere RO, Modirrousta M. Beyond anxiety and agitation: a clinical approach to akathisia. *Aust Fam Physician* 2017; 46: 296–8.
7. Lohr JB, Eidt CA, Abdulrazzaq Alfaraj A, Soliman MA. The clinical challenges of akathisia. *CNS Spectr* 2015; 20(suppl 1): 1–14; quiz 15–6.
8. Akathisia Alliance for education and research. Akathisia Alliance for education and research. https://akathisiaalliance.org/about-akathisia/ (accessed September 17, 2022).
9. Hengartner MP, Schulthess L, Sorensen A, Framer A. Protracted withdrawal syndrome after stopping antidepressants: a descriptive quantitative analysis of consumer narratives from a large internet forum. *Ther Adv Psychopharmacol* 2020; 10: 2045125320980573.
10. Duma SR, Fung VS. Drug-induced movement disorders. *Aust Prescr* 2019; 42: 56–61.
11. Weiss D, Aizenberg D, Hermesh H, et al. Cyproheptadine treatment in neuroleptic-induced akathisia. *Br J Psychiatry* 1995; 167: 483–6.
12. Lima AR, Bacaltchuk J, Barnes TRE, Soares-Weiser K. Central action beta-blockers versus placebo for neuroleptic-induced acute akathisia. *Cochrane Database Syst Rev* 2004; 2004: CD001946.
13. Rissardo JP, Caprara ALF. Mirtazapine-associated movement disorders: a literature review. *Tzu Chi Med J* 2020; 32: 318–30.
14. Taubert M, Back I. The Akathisic Cyclist - An unusual symptomatic treatment. 2007. https://orca.cardiff.ac.uk/id/eprint/117286/ (accessed September 24, 2022).
15. Walters A, Hening W, Chokroverty S, Fahn S. Opioid responsiveness in patients with neuroleptic-induced akathisia. *Mov Disord* 1986; 1: 119–27.
16. Cosci F, Chouinard G. Acute and Persistent Withdrawal Syndromes Following Discontinuation of Psychotropic Medications. *Psychother Psychosom* 2020; 89: 283–306.
17. Ashton H. Protracted Withdrawal From Benzodiazepines: The Post-Withdrawal Syndrome. *Psychiatr Ann* 1995; 25: 174–9.
18. Framer A. What I Have Learnt from Helping Thousands of People Taper Off Psychotropic Medications. *Ther Adv Psychopharmacol* 2021; 11: 204512532199127.
19. Ashton H. Benzodiazepines: How They Work & How to Withdraw (The Ashton Manual). 2002. http://www.benzo.org.uk/manual/bzcha01.htm (accessed July 11, 2023).
20. Ritvo AD, Foster DE, Huff C, Reid Finlayson AJ, Silvernail B, Martin PR. Long-term consequences of benzodiazepine-induced neurological dysfunction: A survey. *PLoS One* 2023; 18: e0285584.
21. Becker HC. Kindling in alcohol withdrawal. *Alcohol Health Res World* 1998; 22: 25–33.
22. Flemenbaum A. Postsynaptic supersensitivity and kindling: further evidence of similarities. *Am J Drug Alcohol Abuse* 1978; 5: 247–54.
23. Benzodiazepine Tapering Strategies and Solutions. Benzodiazepine Information Coalition. 2020; published online September 21. https://www.benzoinfo.com/benzodiazepine-tapering-strategies/ (accessed April 29, 2023).
24. Otis HG, King JH. Unanticipated Psychotropic Medication Reactions. *J Ment Health Couns* 2006; 28: 218–40.
25. Smith SW, Hauben M, Aronson JK. Paradoxical and bidirectional drug effects. *Drug Saf* 2012; 35: 173–89.
26. Bangert MK, Hasbun R. Neurological and Psychiatric Adverse Effects of Antimicrobials. *CNS Drugs* 2019; 33: 727–53.
27. Parker G. Psychotropic Drug Intolerance. *J Nerv Ment Dis* 2018; 206: 223–5.
28. McConnell JG. Benzodiazepine tolerance, dependency, and withdrawal syndromes and interactions with fluoroquinolone antimicrobials. *Br J Gen Pract* 2008; 58: 365–6.
29. Unseld E, Ziegler G, Gemeinhardt A, Janssen U, Klotz U. Possible interaction of fluoroquinolones with the benzodiazepine-GABAA-receptor complex. *Br J Clin Pharmacol* 1990; 30: 63–70.
30. Scavone C, Mascolo A, Ruggiero R, et al. Quinolones-Induced Musculoskeletal, Neurological, and Psychiatric ADRs: A Pharmacovigilance Study Based on Data From the Italian Spontaneous Reporting System. *Front Pharmacol* 2020; 11. doi:10.3389/fphar.2020.00428.
31. Babalonis S, Lile JA, Martin CA, Kelly TH. Physiological doses of progesterone potentiate the effects of triazolam in healthy, premenopausal women. *Psychopharmacology* 2011; 215: 429–39.
32. Smith SS, Gong QH, Hsu FC, Markowitz RS, ffrench-Mullen JM, Li X. GABA(A) receptor alpha4 subunit suppression prevents withdrawal properties of an endogenous steroid. *Nature* 1998; 392: 926–30.

CHAPTER 3

Tapering Guidance for Specific Benzodiazepines and Z-drugs

The following sections include guides to tapering the most commonly used benzodiazepines and z-drugs. Neuroimaging data for diazepam were used to derive a receptor occupancy curve.[1] The receptor occupancy curves for other benzodiazepines and z-drugs were derived from this relationship using equivalency tables.[2-4] Pharmacologically rational regimens were then calculated from these equations and are presented as 'faster', 'moderate' and 'slower' regimens.

Somewhat different regimens are recommended for different classes of drugs. Short-acting drugs (e.g. z-drugs), which are taken once a day will probably be cleared quickly enough from target receptors such that receptors are not exposed to the drug effect for an entire 24-hour period.[5] Adaptation and therefore physical dependence is less likely to occur, meaning such drugs are less likely to produce withdrawal effects. For these drugs we have suggested shorter tapering regimens. With drugs with longer half-lives, whether they are taken once a day (e.g. nitrazepam) or several times a day (e.g. clonazepam), and for shorter-acting drugs taken several times a day (e.g. alprazolam) the drug will interact with target receptors throughout a 24-hour period. This, it is assumed, will lead to greater adaptation and withdrawal potential. These drugs are given longer example tapering regimens.

There is little research to determine which of the three suggested example taper regimens is most suitable for a particular patient. Withdrawal is known to be more severe for people who have used benzodiazepines which are shorter acting, for longer periods, and for those who have experienced withdrawal in the past on reducing, stopping or missing a dose.[6,7] A rough guide to estimating initial reductions is shown in 'Tapering benzodiazepines and z-drugs in practice'. However, the response of the patient to initial reductions is the best guide as to the appropriate pace for a patient and the patient's experience should be prioritised over what an algorithm suggests. This patient-led aspect is a crucial part of our suggested regimens.

These guides include a summary of formulations available in selected countries around the world. Licensed and unlicensed (or 'off-label') options are presented. Overall, the guidance given here is consistent with the UK NICE guidelines on how to safely stop benzodiazepines and z-drugs,[8] but we offer considerably more detail in order to allow implementation of deprescribing in clinical practice. Our regimens are informed by contributions from patient advocacy groups who have wide experience in determining the most appropriate rate and manner of withdrawal.

Although there are many uncertainties in the field of deprescribing, the aim of this chapter is to provide some structure to the process of stopping these drugs, while acknowledging that clinical judgement will have to be used to modify the regimens to fit the particular circumstances of individual patients. The key feature of these suggested regimens is that they represent a framework around which deviation can take place according to patient experience. Our aim is not necessarily to encourage deprescribing but to assure it is undertaken in a manner that optimises patient experience and outcome.

References

1. Brouillet E, Chavoix C, Bottlaender M, et al. In vivo bidirectional modulatory effect of benzodiazepine receptor ligands on GABAergic transmission evaluated by positron emission tomography in non-human primates. *Brain Res* 1991; 557: 167–76.

2. Choosing an equivalent dose of oral benzodiazepine. SPS – Specialist Pharmacy Service. 2022; published online 25 January. https://www.sps.nhs.uk/articles/choosing-an-equivalent-dose-of-oral-benzodiazepine/ (accessed 8 April 2023).

3. Hypnotics and anxiolytics. https://bnf.nice.org.uk/treatment-summaries/hypnotics-and-anxiolytics/ (accessed 19 March 2023).

4. Ashton H. Benzodiazepines: how they work and how to withdraw (The Ashton Manual). Newcastle University, 2002. http://www.benzo.org.uk/manual/bzcha01.htm (accessed 11 July 2023).

5. Lader MH. Managing dependence and withdrawal with newer hypnotic medications in the treatment of insomnia. The Primary Care Companion. 2002. https://www.psychiatrist.com/pcc/sleep/managing-dependence-withdrawal-newer-hypnotic-medications (accessed 20 May 2023).

6. Guina J, Merrill B. Benzodiazepines II: waking up on sedatives: providing optimal care when inheriting benzodiazepine prescriptions in transfer patients. *J Clin Med Res* 2018; 7. doi:10.3390/jcm7020020.

7. Framer A. What I have learnt from helping thousands of people taper off psychotropic medications. *Ther Adv Psychopharmacol* 2021; 11: 204512532199127.

8. National Institute for Health and Care Excellence (NICE). Medicines associated with dependence or withdrawal symptoms: safe prescribing and withdrawal management for adults | Guidance | NICE. 2022. https://www.nice.org.uk/guidance/ng215/chapter/Recommendations (accessed 27 June 2022).

CHAPTER 3

Alprazolam

Trade names: Xanax, Xanax XR, Alprax, Alti-ALPRAZolam, Alzam, Alzolam, Farmapram, Frontin, Gabazolamine-05, Helex, Kalma, Ksalol, Misar, Mylan-Alprazolam, Neurol, Niravam, Onax, Restyl, Solanax, Tafil, Tranax, Trankimazin, Xanor, Xycalm, Zolam, Zopax.

Description: Alprazolam is a high-potency benzodiazepine.[1] It is a positive allosteric modulator of the gamma-aminobutyric acid (GABA) type A receptor, which it affects by binding to the benzodiazepine binding site with high affinity.[2] This leads to facilitation of the inhibitory neurotransmitter action of GABA, which mediates both pre- and post-synaptic inhibition in the CNS.[2] The manufacturer in the UK states that alprazolam should be used 'for the shortest period of time and for a maximum of 2–4 weeks' and that 'long term treatment is not recommended'.[2]

Withdrawal effects: Alprazolam, as for other benzodiazepines, carries a boxed warning from the FDA, which highlights that physical dependence and withdrawal effects can occur when the drug is taken 'for several days to weeks, even as prescribed'.[3,4] Not everyone who stops alprazolam will experience withdrawal and some of those who do will only experience mild symptoms – this probably depends on drug dose, duration of use and individual factors.[2] However, in a very few instances, stopping abruptly can cause seizures and can be life threatening. Numerous other physical, cognitive and psychological withdrawal symptoms (outlined earlier in this chapter) are possible, which can last 'for several weeks to more than 12 months' after stopping according to the FDA.[3,4] In a case series of eight patients[5] treated with high-dose alprazolam, upon discontinuation all eight patients developed worsening anxiety, sleep disturbance and nightmares, seven patients experienced irritability and hypervigilance, six patients had rage reactions and homicidal ideation, and four patients developed dissociative reactions and suicidal ideation, after a taper over an average period of 8 weeks.[2] These patients had been treated with a dose of at least 2mg per day for at least a year.

Peak plasma: Following oral administration peak concentration in the plasma occurs after 1–2 hours.[4]

Half-life: The mean half-life is 12–15 hours. The manufacturer recommends that alprazolam be dosed three times a day, or two to three times a day in the elderly or in the presence of a debilitating disease.[6] Dosing less often (including every-other-day dosing) is not recommended for tapering because the changes in plasma levels may precipitate inter-dose withdrawal symptoms.

Receptor occupancy: The relationship between dose of alprazolam and the occupancy of its major target $GABA_A$ is hyperbolic.[7] Benzodiazepines demonstrate a hyperbolic relationship between dose and clinical effects,[7] which may be relevant to withdrawal effects. Dose reductions made by linear amounts (e.g. 4 mg, 3 mg, 2 mg, 1 mg, 0 mg) will cause increasingly large reductions in effect, which may cause increasingly severe withdrawal effects (Figure 3.8a). To produce equal-sized reductions in effect on receptor occupancy will require hyperbolically reducing doses (Figure 3.8b),[8] which informs the reductions presented later. The relationship was derived by converting the receptor occupancy curve for diazepam[9] to the equivalent alprazolam dose.[10]

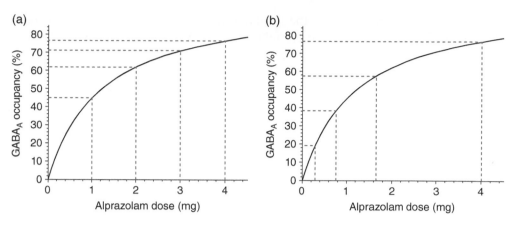

Figure 3.8 (a) Linear reductions of dose cause increasingly large reductions in effect on receptor targets, possibly associated with more withdrawal effects. (b) Even reductions of effect at target receptors requires hyperbolic dose reductions. The final dose before stopping will need to be very small so that this step down is not larger (in terms of effect on receptor occupancy) than previous reductions.

Available formulations: As tablets and liquid.

Tablets

Dosage	UK	Europe	USA	Australia	Canada
0.25mg	✓	✓	✓	✓	✓
0.5mg	✓	✓	✓*	✓	✓
1mg	–	✓	✓*	✓	✓
2mg	–	–	✓*	✓	✓
3mg	–	–	✓*	–	–

*Also available as XR (3mg only as XR)

Liquid*

Dosage	UK	Europe	USA	Australia	Canada
1mg/mL	–	–	✓	–	–

*Store at 20° to 25°C (68° to 77 °F) and protect from light.[11]

Dilutions: To make up some of the small doses outlined in the suggested regimens, dilution of the liquid available from the manufacturer will be required. Xanax liquid is dissolved in propylene glycol, succinic acid and water.[11] Dilution in water might cause precipitation of the drug and so the resulting mixture should be shaken vigorously before use to produce dispersal. As its stability cannot be assured it should be made up fresh each day.

USA dilutions	Solution required	How to prepare solution
Doses ≥ 0.2mg	1mg/mL	Original solution
Doses < 0.2 mg	0.1mg/mL	Mix 0.5mL of original solution with 4.5mL of water*

*Other dilutions are possible to produce different concentrations. The above is provided as an example.

Worked example: To illustrate how the volumes were calculated in the regimens given, a worked example is provided. To make up 0.05mg of alprazolam the 0.1mg/mL dilution can be used, prepared as above. The volume of 0.1mg/mL liquid required to give a dose of 0.05mg alprazolam is 0.05/0.1 = 0.5mL.

Off-label options: In order to follow the regimens suggested here in some cases where manufacturers' liquid versions are not available smaller doses are required than can be made using commercially available tablets and capsules. Guidelines for people who cannot swallow tablets (e.g. NEWT guidelines in the UK based on advice from the manufacturer or local hospital guidance[12]) suggest that alprazolam tablets can be dispersed in water for administration.[13] They will disperse in less than a minute. Water could be added to a 0.5mg tablet to make up a 5mL suspension (concentration 1mg in 10mL or 0.1mg/mL). The suspension should be shaken vigorously before administration. As its stability cannot be assured it should be consumed immediately, and any unused suspension discarded.

Some patients use full-fat milk to make liquid preparations. Benzodiazepines are more soluble in oil or fat than in water.[14] When mixed with milk, some or all of the drug will dissolve in the milk fat. This should form an evenly dispersed emulsion when shaken vigorously. The measured dose should be taken immediately after shaking and the remainder discarded.

Another option is to have a compounding pharmacy make up a suspension or smaller dose tablets or capsules.

Deprescribing notes: There are two main methods for tapering from alprazolam – a switch to a longer-acting benzodiazepine like diazepam or a direct taper of alprazolam itself. There are no established guides to determine the rate of taper of someone stopping benzodiazepines. Withdrawal is known to be more severe for people who have used benzodiazepines which are shorter acting, for longer periods, and who have experienced withdrawal in the past on reducing, stopping or missing a dose.[15,16] The size of the initial reduction can be estimated based on these factors (see 'Tapering benzodiazepines and z-drugs in practice'), with patient preference also taken into account. Sometimes an even smaller reduction to start with may be advisable to boost a patient's confidence that they can taper if performed carefully.

Each reduction should be made when the withdrawal symptoms from the previous reduction have largely resolved so that subsequent reductions do not lead to cumulative withdrawal symptoms. Withdrawal symptoms should not be too unpleasant: a rate of reduction should be aimed for that produces tolerable withdrawal symptoms that abate within a week or two. Allowing for a sufficient observation period, reductions can therefore be made about every 1–4 weeks, depending on how long it takes withdrawal symptoms to resolve. If withdrawal symptoms are moderately severe or take longer than a couple of weeks to resolve, dose reductions should be postponed until symptoms resolve and then made more gradually by choosing a slower tapering rate. If severe withdrawal symptoms occur then the patient should return to a higher dose, wait until symptoms resolve and thereafter taper at a slower rate.

Suggested direct taper schedules for alprazolam: Please note that none of these regimens should be seen as prescriptive – that is, patients should not be compelled to adhere strictly to them. They are given as example regimens and are not 'set and forget' but should be modified in order to ensure that withdrawal symptoms are tolerable throughout a taper. For example, intermediate steps halfway between the doses listed could be added to make a more gradual taper. Ultimately, it is the patient's experience of withdrawal that should guide the rate of taper.

A. **A faster taper** with up to 5 percentage points of GABA$_A$ occupancy between each step – with reductions made every 1–4 weeks*.

Step	RO (%)	AM (mg)	PM (mg)	Night (mg)	Total daily dose (mg)	Formulation
1	76.4	1.25	1.25	1.5	4	Use tabs
2	73.9	1.25	1	1.25	3.5	Use tabs
3	70.8	1	1	1	3	Use tabs
4	66.9	0.75	0.75	1	2.5	Use tabs
5	61.8	0.75	0.5	0.75	2	Use tabs
6	58.6	0.5	0.5	0.75	1.75	Use tabs
7	54.8	0.5	0.5	0.5	1.5	Use tabs
8	50.3	0.5	0.25	0.5	1.25	Use tabs
9	49.0	0.4375	0.25	0.5	1.1875	Use ¾ tabs**
10	47.7	0.375	0.25	0.5	1.125	Use ½ tabs**
11	46.2	0.375	0.25	0.4375	1.0625	Use ½ or ¾ tabs**
12	44.7	0.375	0.25	0.375	1	Use ½ tabs**
13	43.2	0.3125	0.25	0.375	0.9375	Use ¼ or ½ tabs**
14	41.5	0.25	0.25	0.375	0.875	Use ½ tabs**
15	39.7	0.25	0.25	0.3125	0.8125	Use ¼ tabs**
16	37.8	0.25	0.25	0.25	0.75	Use tabs
17	35.8	0.25	0.1875	0.25	0.6875	Use ¾ tabs**
18	33.6	0.1875	0.1875	0.25	0.625	Use ¾ tabs**
19	31.3	0.1875	0.1875	0.1875	0.5625	Use ¾ tabs**
20	28.8	0.1875	0.125	0.1875	0.5	Use ½ or ¾ tabs**
21	26.2	0.125	0.125	0.1875	0.4375	Use ½ or ¾ tabs**
22	23.3	0.125	0.125	0.125	0.375	Use ½ tabs**
23	20.2	0.125	0.0625	0.125	0.3125	Use ¼ or ½ tabs**
24	16.8	0.0625	0.0625	0.125	0.25	Use ¼ or ½ tabs**
25	13.2	0.0625	0.0625	0.0625	0.1875	Use ¼ tabs**
26	9.2	0.0625	0	0.0625	0.125	Use ¼ tabs**
27	4.8	0	0	0.0625	0.0625	Use ¼ tabs**
28	0	0	0	0	0	

RO = receptor occupancy, tabs = tablets

*Patients who have been on the medication for only a few weeks will probably be able to taper more quickly and might follow every second or third step of this regimen and make reductions every few days or so. Normally the duration of the taper should not be longer than the period that the patient has been on the drug for people who have only taken it for a few weeks. For example, if alprazolam is taken for 3 weeks, the taper should be less than 3 weeks. However, the FDA has issued an alert regarding dependence and withdrawal from benzodiazepines indicating that some people can experience withdrawal effects after just a few days of use,[4] therefore necessitating slower tapering in this sub-group.

**Alternatively, these doses may be made up using a liquid preparation of alprazolam, made up as above.

B. A moderate taper with up to 2.8 percentage points of GABA$_A$ occupancy between each step – with reductions made every 1–4 weeks.

Step	RO (%)	AM (mg)	PM (mg)	Night (mg)	Total daily dose (mg)	Form
1	76.4	1.25	1.25	1.5	4	Use tabs
2	75.2	1.25	1.25	1.25	3.75	Use tabs
3	73.9	1.125	1.125	1.25	3.5	Use ½ tabs*
4	72.5	1.125	1	1.125	3.25	Use ½ tabs*
5	70.8	1	1	1	3	Use tabs
6	69	0.875	0.875	1	2.75	Use ½ tabs*
7	66.9	0.875	0.75	0.875	2.5	Use ½ tabs*
8	64.6	0.75	0.75	0.75	2.25	Use tabs
9	61.8	0.625	0.625	0.75	2	Use ½ tabs*
10	60.3	0.625	0.625	0.625	1.875	Use ½ tabs*
11	58.6	0.563	0.563	0.625	1.75	Use ¼ or ½ tabs*
12	56.8	0.563	0.5	0.563	1.625	Use ¼ tabs*
13	54.8	0.5	0.5	0.5	1.5	Use tabs
14	52.7	0.438	0.438	0.5	1.375	Use ¼ tabs*
15	50.3	0.438	0.375	0.438	1.25	Use ½ and ¼ tabs*

See further steps in the right-hand column

Step	RO (%)	AM (mg)	PM (mg)	Night (mg)	Total daily dose (mg)	Form
			Switch to alprazolam **1mg/mL solution**			
16	49.3	0.4	0.35	0.4	1.15	Liquid
17	47.1	0.35	0.35	0.4	1.1	Liquid
18	44.7	0.35	0.3	0.35	1.0	Liquid
19	43.5	0.3	0.3	0.35	0.95	Liquid
20	42.2	0.3	0.3	0.3	0.9	Liquid
21	40.8	0.3	0.25	0.3	0.85	Liquid
22	39.3	0.25	0.25	0.3	0.8	Liquid
23	37.8	0.25	0.25	0.25	0.75	Liquid
24	36.2	0.25	0.2	0.25	0.7	Liquid
25	34.5	0.2	0.2	0.25	0.65	Liquid
26	32.7	0.2	0.2	0.2	0.6	Liquid
			Switch to alprazolam **0.1mg/mL dilution**			
27	30.8	0.2	0.15	0.2	0.55	Liquid
28	28.8	0.15	0.15	0.2	0.5	Liquid

(Continued)

(Continued)

Step	RO (%)	AM (mg)	PM (mg)	Night (mg)	Total daily dose (mg)	Form
29	26.7	0.15	0.15	0.15	0.45	Liquid
30	24.5	0.15	0.10	0.15	0.4	Liquid
31	22.6	0.12	0.12	0.12	0.36	Liquid
32	20.6	0.1	0.1	0.12	0.32	Liquid
33	18.5	0.09	0.09	0.1	0.28	Liquid
34	16.3	0.08	0.08	0.08	0.24	Liquid
35	13.9	0.07	0.06	0.07	0.2	Liquid
36	12.7	0.06	0.06	0.06	0.18	Liquid
37	11.5	0.05	0.05	0.06	0.16	Liquid

See further steps in the right-hand column

Step	RO (%)	AM (mg)	PM (mg)	Night (mg)	Total daily dose (mg)	Form
38	10.2	0.05	0.04	0.05	0.14	Liquid
39	8.9	0.04	0.04	0.04	0.12	Liquid
40	7.5	0.03	0.03	0.04	0.1	Liquid
41	6.1	0.03	0.02	0.03	0.08	Liquid
42	4.6	0.02	0.02	0.02	0.06	Liquid
43	3.1	0.01	0.01	0.02	0.04	Liquid
44	1.6	0.01	0	0.01	0.02	Liquid
45	0	0	0	0	0	Liquid

RO = receptor occupancy, tabs = tablets
*Alternatively, these doses may be made up using a liquid preparation of alprazolam, made up as above.

C. A slower taper with up to 1.2 percentage points of GABA$_A$ occupancy between each step – with reductions made every 1–4 weeks*

Step	RO (%)	AM (mg)	PM (mg)	Night (mg)	Daily dose (mg)	Form
1	76.4	1.25	1.25	1.5	4	Use tabs
2	75.8	1.25	1.25	1.375	3.875	Use ½ tabs*
3	75.2	1.25	1.25	1.25	3.75	Use tabs
4	74.6	1.25	1.125	1.25	3.625	Use ½ tabs*
5	73.9	1.125	1.125	1.25	3.5	Use ½ tabs*
6	73.2	1.125	1.125	1.125	3.375	Use ½ tabs*
7	72.5	1.125	1	1.125	3.25	Use ½ tabs*
8	71.7	1	1	1.125	3.125	Use ½ tabs*
9	70.8	1	1	1	3	Use tabs
10	70	1	0.875	1	2.875	Use ½ tabs*
11	69	0.875	0.875	1	2.75	Use ½ tabs*
12	68	0.875	0.875	0.875	2.625	Use ½ tabs*
13	66.9	0.875	0.75	0.875	2.5	Use ½ tabs*
14	65.8	0.75	0.75	0.875	2.375	Use ½ tabs*
15	64.6	0.75	0.75	0.75	2.25	Use tabs
16	63.2	0.75	0.625	0.75	2.125	Use ½ tabs*
17	61.8	0.625	0.625	0.75	2	Use ½ tabs*
18	61.1	0.625	0.625	0.6875	1.938	Use ½ and ¼ tabs*
19	60.3	0.625	0.625	0.625	1.875	Use ½ tabs*
20	59.5	0.625	0.563	0.625	1.813	Use ½ and ¼ tabs*
21	58.6	0.563	0.563	0.625	1.75	Use ½ and ¼ tabs*
22	57.7	0.563	0.563	0.563	1.688	Use ¼ tabs*
23	56.8	0.563	0.5	0.563	1.625	Use ¼ tabs*

See further steps in the right-hand column

Step	RO (%)	AM (mg)	PM (mg)	Night (mg)	Daily dose (mg)	Form
24	55.9	0.5	0.5	0.563	1.563	Use ¼ tabs*
25	54.8	0.5	0.5	0.5	1.5	Use tabs
26	53.8	0.5	0.438	0.5	1.438	Use ½ and ¼ tabs*
27	52.7	0.438	0.438	0.5	1.375	Use ½ and ¼ tabs*
28	51.5	0.438	0.438	0.438	1.314	Use ¼ tabs*
29	50.3	0.438	0.375	0.438	1.25	Use ½ and ¼ tabs*
			Switch to alprazolam **1mg/mL solution**			
30	49.3	0.4	0.4	0.4	1.2	Liquid
31	48.2	0.4	0.35	0.4	1.15	Liquid
32	47.1	0.35	0.35	0.4	1.1	Liquid
33	46	0.35	0.35	0.35	1.05	Liquid
34	44.7	0.35	0.3	0.35	1	Liquid
35	44.1	0.325	0.3	0.35	0.975	Liquid
36	43.5	0.325	0.3	0.325	0.95	Liquid
37	42.8	0.3	0.3	0.325	0.925	Liquid
38	42.2	0.3	0.3	0.3	0.9	Liquid
39	41.5	0.3	0.275	0.3	0.875	Liquid
40	40.8	0.275	0.275	0.3	0.85	Liquid
41	40	0.275	0.275	0.275	0.825	Liquid
42	39.3	0.275	0.25	0.275	0.8	Liquid
43	38.6	0.25	0.25	0.275	0.775	Liquid
44	37.8	0.25	0.25	0.25	0.75	Liquid
45	37	0.25	0.225	0.25	0.725	Liquid

(Continued)

(Continued)

Step	RO (%)	AM (mg)	PM (mg)	Night (mg)	Daily dose (mg)	Form
46	36.2	0.225	0.225	0.25	0.7	Liquid
47	35.3	0.225	0.225	0.225	0.675	Liquid
48	34.5	0.225	0.2	0.225	0.65	Liquid
49	33.6	0.2	0.2	0.225	0.625	Liquid
50	32.7	0.2	0.2	0.2	0.6	Liquid
Switch to alprazolam 0.1mg/mL dilution						
51	31.8	0.2	0.175	0.2	0.575	Liquid
52	30.8	0.175	0.175	0.2	0.55	Liquid
53	29.8	0.175	0.175	0.175	0.525	Liquid
54	28.8	0.175	0.15	0.175	0.5	Liquid
55	27.8	0.15	0.15	0.175	0.475	Liquid
56	26.7	0.15	0.15	0.15	0.45	Liquid
57	25.6	0.15	0.125	0.15	0.425	Liquid
58	24.5	0.125	0.125	0.15	0.4	Liquid
59	23.5	0.125	0.125	0.13	0.38	Liquid
60	22.6	0.12	0.12	0.12	0.36	Liquid
61	21.6	0.11	0.11	0.12	0.34	Liquid
62	20.6	0.10	0.10	0.12	0.32	Liquid
63	19.5	0.10	0.10	0.10	0.3	Liquid
64	18.5	0.09	0.09	0.10	0.28	Liquid
65	17.4	0.09	0.08	0.09	0.26	Liquid
66	16.3	0.08	0.08	0.08	0.24	Liquid

See further steps in the right-hand column

Step	RO (%)	AM (mg)	PM (mg)	Night (mg)	Daily dose (mg)	Form
67	15.1	0.07	0.07	0.08	0.22	Liquid
68	13.9	0.07	0.06	0.07	0.2	Liquid
69	13.3	0.06	0.06	0.07	0.19	Liquid
70	12.7	0.06	0.06	0.06	0.18	Liquid
71	12.1	0.06	0.05	0.06	0.17	Liquid
72	11.5	0.05	0.05	0.06	0.16	Liquid
73	10.8	0.05	0.05	0.05	0.15	Liquid
74	10.2	0.05	0.04	0.05	0.14	Liquid
75	9.5	0.04	0.04	0.05	0.13	Liquid
76	8.9	0.04	0.04	0.04	0.12	Liquid
77	8.2	0.04	0.03	0.04	0.11	Liquid
78	7.5	0.03	0.03	0.04	0.1	Liquid
79	6.8	0.03	0.03	0.03	0.09	Liquid
80	6.1	0.03	0.02	0.03	0.08	Liquid
81	5.4	0.02	0.02	0.03	0.07	Liquid
82	4.6	0.02	0.02	0.02	0.06	Liquid
83	3.9	0.02	0.01	0.02	0.05	Liquid
84	3.1	0.01	0.01	0.02	0.04	Liquid
85	2.4	0.01	0.01	0.01	0.03	Liquid
86	1.6	0.01	0.00	0.01	0.02	Liquid
87	0.8	0.00	0.00	0.01	0.01	Liquid
88	0	0.00	0.00	0.00	0	Liquid

RO = receptor occupancy, tabs = tablets

*Alternatively, these doses may be made up using a liquid preparation of alprazolam, made up as above.

D. **An even slower taper** Some patients will be unable to taper at the slowest rates shown here and will need to taper by even smaller decrements, thus lengthening the overall period of tapering. Such a regimen could be constructed by placing intermediate steps between those in regimen C. For example, 1mg, 0.975mg, 0.95mg, could be modified to be 1mg, 0.9875mg, 0.975mg, 0.9625mg, 0.95mg and so on. Further intermediate steps could also be added.

Micro-tapering: The tapering tables show how to make reductions at intervals of 1–4 weeks. An alternative approach is called 'micro-tapering' whereby very small dose reductions are made every day, as explained in 'Other considerations in tapering benzodiazepines and z-drugs'. Micro-tapering rates can be calculated from the above regimens by dividing the change in dose for each step by 14 or 28 days and then dividing that dose into three doses during the day. For example, for the moderate regimen, a reduction of 4mg to 3.75mg over 14 days is equivalent to a reduction of 0.018mg per day, or 0.006mg reduction per dose (when dosed three times a day). By the end of this regimen the rate of reduction would have slowed down to a reduction of 0.0014mg each day, or 0.0005mg per dose when dosed three times a day. To make these reductions a very dilute solution will be required. The rate can be adjusted if withdrawal symptoms become too unpleasant.

Switching guide from alprazolam to diazepam: An alternative to a direct taper from alprazolam is to switch to diazepam before tapering from this drug, as outlined in 'Switching to longer-acting benzodiazepines to taper'. A 1mg dose of alprazolam is equivalent to 20mg of diazepam.[17] Switching could be performed by steps of 0.5mg of alprazolam made every week (or as tolerated by the patient).

Steps	Morning	Afternoon	Evening	Daily diazepam equivalent
Start	1.25mg alprazolam	1.25mg alprazolam	1.5mg alprazolam	80mg
1	1.25mg alprazolam	1.25mg alprazolam	1mg alprazolam 10mg diazepam	80mg
2	1mg alprazolam 5mg diazepam	1mg alprazolam 5mg diazepam	1mg alprazolam 10mg diazepam	80mg
3	1mg alprazolam 5mg diazepam	0.5mg alprazolam 15mg diazepam	1 mg alprazolam 10 mg diazepam	80mg
4	0.5mg alprazolam 15mg diazepam	0.5mg alprazolam 15mg diazepam	1 mg alprazolam 10 mg diazepam	80mg
5	0.5mg alprazolam 15mg diazepam	0.5mg alprazolam 15mg diazepam	0.5 mg alprazolam 20 mg diazepam	80mg
6	0.5mg alprazolam 15mg diazepam	25mg diazepam	0.5 mg alprazolam 20 mg diazepam	80mg
7	25mg diazepam	25mg diazepam	0.5 mg alprazolam 20 mg diazepam	80mg
8	25mg diazepam	25mg diazepam	30 mg diazepam	80mg
9	40mg diazepam	Stop middle dose, divert to morning and evening dose	40 mg diazepam	80mg

(Continued)

CHAPTER 3

(Continued)

Steps	Morning	Afternoon	Evening	Daily diazepam equivalent
10	35mg diazepam	–	40 mg diazepam	75mg
11	35mg diazepam	–	35 mg diazepam	70mg
12	30mg diazepam	–	35 mg diazepam	65mg
13	30mg diazepam	–	30 mg diazepam	60mg
Continue to taper as for 60mg diazepam (see diazepam section)				

References

1. Chouinard G. Issues in the clinical use of benzodiazepines: potency, withdrawal, and rebound. *J Clin Psychiatry* 2004; 65 Suppl 5: 7–12.
2. Xanax Tablets 250 micrograms – Summary of Product Characteristics (SmPC) – (emc). https://www.medicines.org.uk/emc/product/1657/smpc (accessed 26 February 2023).
3. FDA. Medication guide Xanax. Fda.gov. 2023; published online January. https://www.accessdata.fda.gov/drugsatfda_docs/label/2023/018276s059lbl.pdf#page=22 (accessed February 27, 2023).
4. FDA Drug Safety Communication. FDA requiring boxed warning updated to improve safe use of benzodiazepine drug class. 2020. https://www.fda.gov/drugs/drug-safety-and-availability/fda-requiring-boxed-warning-updated-improve-safe-use-benzodiazepine-drug-class#:~:text=FDA is requiring the Boxed,and life-threatening side effects (accessed 3 July 2023).
5. Risse SC, Whitters A, Burke J, Chen S, Scurfield RM, Raskind MA. Severe withdrawal symptoms after discontinuation of alprazolam in eight patients with combat-induced posttraumatic stress disorder. *J Clin Psychiatry* 1990; 51: 206–9.
6. Innis RB, al-Tikriti MS, Zoghbi SS, et al. SPECT imaging of the benzodiazepine receptor: feasibility of in vivo potency measurements from stepwise displacement curves. *J Nucl Med* 1991; 32: 1754–61.
7. Horowitz M, Taylor D. Withdrawing from benzodiazepines and z-drugs (in preparation).
8. Horowitz MA, Taylor D. Tapering of SSRI treatment to mitigate withdrawal symptoms. *The Lancet Psychiatry* 2019; 6: 538–46.
9. Brouillet E, Chavoix C, Bottlaender M, et al. In vivo bidirectional modulatory effect of benzodiazepine receptor ligands on GABAergic transmission evaluated by positron emission tomography in non-human primates. *Brain Res* 1991; 557: 167–76.
10. Choosing an equivalent dose of oral benzodiazepine. SPS – Specialist Pharmacy Service. 2022; published online 25 January. https://www.sps.nhs.uk/articles/choosing-an-equivalent-dose-of-oral-benzodiazepine/ (accessed 8 April 2023).
11. DailyMed – ALPRAZOLAM solution, concentrate. https://dailymed.nlm.nih.gov/dailymed/drugInfo.cfm?setid=b945ac6f-796e-41ef-85e9-61007e4a4e9a (accessed 26 February 2023).
12. Smyth J. The NEWT Guidelines for administration of medication to patients with enteral feeding tubes or swallowing difficulties website. The NEWT Guidelines. 2011. https://www.newtguidelines.com/index.html (accessed 7 September 2022).
13. Martin TP, Hayes P, Collins DM. Tablet dispersion as an alternative to formulation of liquid dosage forms. *Australian Journal of Hospital Pharmacy* 1993; 23: 378–86.
14. Macheras PE, Koupparis MA, Antimisiaris SG. Drug binding and solubility in milk. *Pharm Res* 1990; 7: 537–41.
15. Guina J, Merrill B. Benzodiazepines II: waking up on sedatives: providing optimal care when inheriting benzodiazepine prescriptions in transfer patients. *J Clin Med Res* 2018; 7. doi:10.3390/jcm7020020.
16. Framer A. What I have learnt from helping thousands of people taper off psychotropic medications. *Ther Adv Psychopharmacol* 2021; 11: 204512532199127.
17. Hypnotics and anxiolytics. https://bnf.nice.org.uk/treatment-summaries/hypnotics-and-anxiolytics/ (accessed 19 March 2023).

Buspirone

Trade names: Buspar, Buspar Dividose, Vanspar.

Description: Buspirone is an azapirone compound licensed in the UK for short-term treatment of anxiety,[1] and in the USA for management of anxiety disorders.[2] Its mechanism of action is not fully understood; however, it has strong affinity for $5HT_{1A}$ receptors, where it is a partial agonist.[3] It also has a weak affinity for serotonin $5HT_2$ receptors and acts as a weak antagonist at dopamine D_2 autoreceptors and D_3 receptors.[4] Animal studies show that it interacts with the dopamine, serotonin, noradrenaline and acetylcholine systems. It has no or very low affinity for benzodiazepine receptors.[1,3]

Withdrawal effects: There are a limited number of studies examining the withdrawal effects from buspirone. One study found effects were less pronounced than withdrawal effects from lorazepam, although severity was not directly quantified and withdrawal effects were only monitored for 2 weeks.[5,6] Its manufacturer warns about withdrawal effects that can manifest as 'irritability, anxiety, agitation, insomnia, tremor, abdominal cramps, muscle cramps, vomiting, sweating, flu-like symptoms without fever, and occasionally, even as seizures'.[2]

Peak plasma: 60–90 minutes.[1]

Half-life: 2–11 hours.[1] The manufacturer recommends dosing two or three times per day. Every-other-day dosing is not recommended for tapering because of its short half-life. This can lead to substantial reductions in plasma levels, which might give rise to withdrawal effects.

Receptor occupancy: There appear to be no neuroimaging studies of the relationship between buspirone and $5HT_{1A}$ binding. Nonetheless, the relationship between dose of buspirone and occupancy of one of its targets, the D_3 receptor, is hyperbolic on neuroimaging.[4] Anxiolytics and antidepressants that also affect serotonergic receptors show a hyperbolic relationship between dose and clinical effects,[7,8] which may be relevant to withdrawal effects from buspirone. Dose reductions made by linear amounts (e.g. 60mg, 45mg, 30mg, 15mg, 0mg) will cause increasingly large reductions in receptor occupancy, which may in turn cause increasingly severe withdrawal effects. To produce equal-sized reductions in effect on D_3 occupancy will require hyperbolically reducing doses (Figure 3.9) which informs the reductions presented later. This hyperbolic pattern

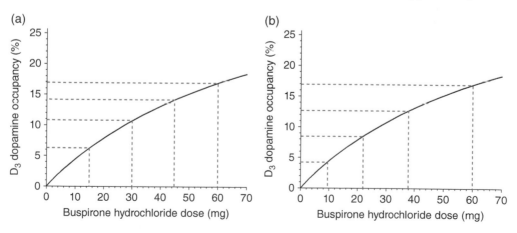

Figure 3.9 (a) Linear reductions of dose cause increasingly larger reductions in effect on receptor targets, possibly associated with more withdrawal effects. (b) Even reductions of effect at target receptors requires hyperbolic dose reductions, slightly different from linear reductions in this case. The final dose before stopping will need to be small so that this step down is not larger (in terms of effect on receptor occupancy) than previous reductions.

CHAPTER 3

also applies to its occupancy of its other target receptors, including $5HT_{1A}$, because of the law of mass action.[9] While there may be some differences in the precise dose-related activity between receptors the hyperbolic relationship remains. It is expected that the regimens given later (based on D_3 occupancy) will be broadly suitable for other receptor occupancies, such as $5\text{-}HT_{1A}$.

Available formulations: As tablets.

Tablets As buspirone hydrochloride.

Dosage	UK	Europe	USA	Australia	Canada
5mg	✓	✓	✓	✓	–
7.5mg	✓	–	✓	–	–
10mg	✓	✓	✓	✓	✓
15mg	–	–	✓	–	–
30mg	–	–	✓	–	–

Off-label options: In order to follow the regimens suggested, in some cases, where liquid versions are unavailable, smaller doses are required than can be made using commercially available tablets and capsules. According to NEWT guidance (in the UK) for people who cannot swallow tablets, buspirone can be crushed and dispersed in water.[10] Without crushing, buspirone tablets disintegrate in around 5 minutes.[10] As an example, a 5mg tablet can be made up to 5mL with water to make a 1mg/mL suspension. The tablet may be crushed with a spoon or pestle and mortar before mixing with water to speed up this process. The suspension should be shaken vigorously before administration. As its stability cannot be assured, it should be consumed immediately (within an hour of dispersal).

Another option is to have a compounding pharmacy make up a suspension or smaller dose tablets or capsules.

Worked example: To illustrate how volumes can be calculated in the regimens given below, a worked example is provided. To make up 3mg of buspirone, a 1mg/mL suspension can be used, prepared as above. The volume of 1mg/mL liquid required to give a dose of 3mg buspirone is 3/1 = 3mL.

Deprescribing notes: There are no established guides to determine the rate of taper of buspirone. In general for medications, longer duration of use, higher doses and experience of withdrawal on previous attempts to stop medication predict more severe withdrawal effects.[11] In general, reductions should be made when the withdrawal symptoms from the previous reduction have largely resolved so that subsequent reductions do not lead to cumulative withdrawal symptoms. Withdrawal symptoms should be tolerable and last at most a couple of weeks. Allowing for a sufficient observation period, reductions might therefore be made about every 2–4 weeks. If withdrawal symptoms are moderately severe or take longer than a couple of weeks to resolve, dose reductions should be postponed until symptoms resolve and then made more gradual by choosing a slower tapering rate. If severe withdrawal symptoms occur then the patient should return to a higher dose, wait until symptoms resolve and thereafter taper at a slower rate.

Suggested taper schedules for buspirone: Please note that none of these regimens should be seen as prescriptive – that is, patients should not be compelled to adhere strictly to them. They are given as example regimens and are not 'set and forget' but should be modified in order to ensure that withdrawal symptoms are tolerable throughout a taper – for example, intermediate steps halfway between the doses listed could be added to make a more gradual taper.

A. **A faster taper** with up to 5.4 percentage points of D_3 occupancy between each step – with reductions made every 2–4 weeks*.

Step	RO (%)	AM (mg)	PM (mg)	Total dose (mg)	Volume
1	16.9	30	30	60	Use tablets
2	13.1	20	20	40	Use tablets
3	9.4	10	15	25	Use tablets
4	4.4	5	5	10	Use tablets
5	0	0	0	0	–

RO = receptor occupancy
*Patients who have been on the medication for only a few weeks will probably be able to taper more quickly and might follow every second step of this regimen, and make reductions every few days or so. Normally the duration of the taper should not be longer than the period that the patient has been on the drug for people who have only taken it for a few weeks. For example, if buspirone is taken for three weeks the taper should be less than three weeks.

B. **A moderate taper** with up to 3 percentage points of D_3 occupancy between each step – with reductions made every 2–4 weeks.

Step	RO (%)	AM (mg)	PM (mg)	Total dose (mg)	Volume
1	16.9	30	30	60	Use tablets
2	14.2	20	25	45	Use tablets
3	12.6	17.5	20	37.5	Use ½ tablets*
4	10.7	15	15	30	Use tablets
5	8.6	10	12.5	22.5	Use ½ tablets*
6	6.2	7.5	7.5	15	Use ½ tablets
7	3.4	2.5	5	7.5	Use ½ tablets*
8	1.8	1.25	2.5	3.75	Use ¼ tablets*
9	0	0	0	0	–

RO = receptor occupancy
*Alternatively, these doses could be made up using a liquid preparation, made up as above.

C. **A slower taper** with up to 1.5 percentage points of D_3 occupancy between each step – with reductions made every 2–4 weeks.

Step	RO (%)	AM (mg)	PM (mg)	Total dose (mg)	Volume	Step	RO (%)	AM (mg)	PM (mg)	Total dose (mg)	Volume
1	16.9	30	30	60	Use tablets	10	7.5	8.75	10	18.75	Use ¾ tablets*
2	15.6	25	27.5	52.5	Use ½ tablets*	11	6.2	7.5	7.5	15	Use tablets
3	14.2	20	25	45	Use tablets	12	4.8	5	6.25	11.25	Use ¼ tablets*
4	13.4	20	21.25	41.25	Use ¼ tablets*	Switch to buspirone **1mg/mL** solution**					
5	12.6	17.5	20	37.5	Use ½ tablets*	13	3.6	4	4	8	4mL BD
6	11.7	15	18.75	33.75	Use ¾ tablets*	14	2.3	2.5	2.5	5	2.5mL BD***
7	10.7	15	15	30	Use tablets	15	1	1	1	2	1mL BD
8	9.7	11.25	15	26.25	Use ¼ tablets*	16	0	0	0	0	–
9	8.6	10	12.5	22.5	Use ½ tablets*						

See further steps in the right-hand column

RO = receptor occupancy
*Alternatively, these doses could be made up using a liquid preparation.
**A suspension can be made as an off-label option, as outlined above
***Alternatively, this dose could be made up using portions of a tablet.

D. **An even slower taper** Some patients will be unable to taper at the slowest rates shown here and will need to taper by even smaller decrements, thus lengthening the overall period of tapering. Such a regimen could be constructed by placing intermediate steps in regimen C. For example, 60mg, 52.5mg, 45mg could be modified to 60mg, 56.25mg, 52.5mg, 48.75mg, 45mg and so on. Further intermediate steps could also be added.

Micro-tapering: The deprescribing tables above show how to make reductions at intervals of 2–4 weeks. An alternative approach is called 'micro-tapering' whereby very small dose reductions are made every day, as explained in 'Other considerations in tapering benzodiazepines and z-drugs.' Micro-tapering rates can be calculated by dividing the change in dose for each step by 14 or 28 days. For example, for the moderate regimen a reduction of 60mg to 45mg over 14 days is equivalent to a reduction of approximately 1mg reduction per day. By the end of this regimen the rate of reduction would have slowed down to a reduction of 0.3mg each day. The rate can be adjusted if withdrawal symptoms become too unpleasant.

References

1. Buspirone hydrochloride 7.5mg tablets – Summary of Product Characteristics (SmPC) – (emc). https://www.medicines.org.uk/emc/product/10562/smpc (accessed 15 April 2023).

2. FDA. BuSPar. www.accessdata.fda.gov. https://www.accessdata.fda.gov/drugsatfda_docs/label/2010/018731s051lbl.pdf (accessed 1 May 2023).

3. Wilson TK, Tripp J. Buspirone. StatPearls Publishing, 2023. https://www.ncbi.nlm.nih.gov/books/NBK531477/ (accessed 15 April 2023).

4. Le Foll B, Payer D, Di Ciano P, et al. Occupancy of dopamine D3 and D2 receptors by buspirone: A [11C]-(+)-PHNO PET study in humans. *Neuropsychopharmacology* 2016; 4B1: 529–37.

5. Bourin M, Malinge M. Controlled comparison of the effects and abrupt discontinuation of buspirone and lorazepam. *Prog Neuropsychopharmacol Biol Psychiatry* 1995; 19: 567–75.

6. Dimitriou EC, Parashos AJ, Giouzepas JS. Buspirone vs alprazolam: a double-blind comparative study of their efficacy, adverse effects and withdrawal symptoms. *Drug Investigation* 1992; 4: 316–21.

7. Furukawa TA, Cipriani A, Cowen PJ, Leucht S, Egger M, Salanti G. Optimal dose of selective serotonin reuptake inhibitors, venlafaxine, and mirtazapine in major depression: a systematic review and dose-response meta-analysis. *The Lancet Psychiatry* 2019; 6: 601–9.

8. Horowitz M, Taylor D. Withdrawing from benzodiazepines and z-drugs (in preparation).

9. Holford N. Pharmacodynamic principles and the time course of delayed and cumulative drug effects. *Trans Clin Pharmacol* 2018; 26: 56–9.

10. Smyth J. The NEWT guidelines for administration of medication to patients with enteral feeding tubes or swallowing difficulties. 2011. https://www.newtguidelines.com/index.html (accessed 18 February 2023).

11. National Institute for Health and Care Excellence (NICE). Medicines associated with dependence or withdrawal symptoms: safe prescribing and withdrawal management for adults | Guidance | NICE. 2022. https://www.nice.org.uk/guidance/ng215/chapter/Recommendations (accessed 27 June 2022).

CHAPTER 3

Chlordiazepoxide

Trade names: Librium, Elenium, Mitran, Risolid.

Description: Chlordiazepoxide is a low-potency benzodiazepine.[1] It is a positive allosteric modulator of the gamma-aminobutyric acid (GABA) type A receptor, which it affects by binding to stereospecific benzodiazepine (BZD) binding sites with low affinity.[2] Stimulation of benzodiazepine receptors potentiates the inhibitory actions of GABA. This results in diminution of various serotonin, dopamine and noradrenergic neurotransmitter system effects.[2] The UK manufacturer states that the duration of treatment should not be longer than 4 weeks, including a tapering-off process.[2]

Withdrawal effects: Chlordiazepoxide, as for other benzodiazepines, carries a boxed warning from the FDA that highlights that physical dependence and withdrawal effects can occur when the drug is taken 'for several days to weeks, even as prescribed'.[3] Not everyone who stops chlordiazepoxide will experience withdrawal and some of those who do will only experience mild symptoms – this probably depends on drug dose, duration of use and individual factors. However, in a very few instances, stopping abruptly can cause seizures and can be life threatening. Numerous other physical, cognitive and psychological withdrawal symptoms, outlined earlier in this chapter, are possible which can last 'for several weeks to more than 12 months' after stopping according to the FDA.[3,4] A case series report of 11 hospitalised psychiatric patients (with a variety of diagnoses) abruptly switched from high-dose chlordiazepoxide to placebo reported emergence of new symptoms such as depression, worsening of psychosis, loss of appetite, nausea and agitation in 10 out of 11 patients.[5] Two patients experienced seizures on day 7 and 8 following drug cessation.[5]

Peak plasma: Following oral administration peak concentration in the plasma occurs after 1–2 hours.[2]

Half-life: The mean half-life is 8–28 hours. Chlordiazepoxide's two active metabolites, desmethyl-chlordiazepoxide and demoxepam, have half-lives of 10–18 hours and 21–78 hours, respectively. The manufacturer recommends chlordiazepoxide to be given 2 to 4 times daily in divided doses.[2] Dosing less often (including every-other-day dosing) for tapering is not recommended because the substantial changes in plasma levels may precipitate inter-dose withdrawal symptoms.

Receptor occupancy: The relationship between dose of chlordiazepoxide and the occupancy of its major target $GABA_A$ is hyperbolic, according to the law of mass action.[6,7] Benzodiazepines demonstrate a hyperbolic relationship between dose and clinical effects,[8] which may be relevant to withdrawal effects. Dose reductions made by linear amounts (e.g. 100mg, 75mg, 50mg, 25mg, 0mg) will cause increasingly large reductions in effect, which may cause increasingly severe withdrawal effects (Figure 3.10a). To produce equal-sized reductions in effect on receptor occupancy will require hyperbolically reducing doses (Figure 3.10b),[9] which informs the reductions presented later. The relationship was derived by converting the receptor occupancy curve for diazepam[6] to equivalent chlordiazepoxide dose.[10]

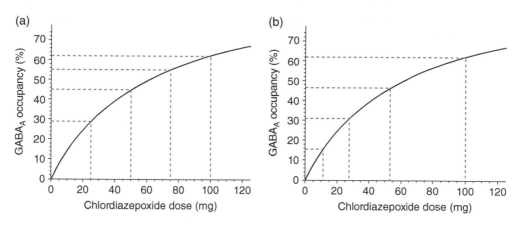

Figure 3.10 (a) Linear reductions of dose cause increasingly large reductions in effect on receptor targets, possibly associated with more withdrawal effects. (b) Even reductions of effect at target receptors requires hyperbolic dose reductions. The final dose before stopping will need to be very small so that this step down is not larger (in terms of effect on receptor occupancy) than previous reductions.

Available formulations: As tablets and capsules.

Tablets

Dosage	UK	Europe	USA	Australia	Canada
25mg	✓	✓	–	–	–

Capsules

Dosage	UK	Europe	USA	Australia	Canada
5mg	✓	–	✓	–	✓
10mg	✓	–	✓	–	✓
25mg	–	–	✓	–	✓
30mg	–	–	✓*	–	–

*Available as XR.

Off-label options: In order to follow the regimens suggested, where no liquid versions are available, in some cases smaller doses are required than can be made using commercially available tablets and capsules. Guidelines for people who cannot swallow tablets (e.g. NEWT guidelines in the UK based on advice from the manufacturer or local hospital guidance[11]) advise as a first choice to switch to an alternative medication (e.g. diazepam) if possible. Other options include the use of a custom-made suspension from a pharmacy (if available) or opening the capsule and using the contents to make a suspension. For example, the contents of a 5mg capsule could be emptied and made up to 50mL with water to make a 1mg in 10mL or 0.1mg/mL suspension.

CHAPTER 3

The suspension should be shaken vigorously before administration. As its stability cannot be assured it should be consumed immediately, and any unused suspension discarded.

Alternatively, crushing of tablets to make suspensions (e.g. 25mg tablets made up to 25mL with water to make a 1mg/mL suspension) is performed in some centres but is not recommended by the NEWT guidelines.[11] Some patients use full-fat milk to make liquid preparations. Benzodiazepines are more soluble in oil or fat than in water.[12] When mixed with milk, some or all of the drug will dissolve in the milk fat. This should form an evenly dispersed emulsion when shaken vigorously. The measured dose should be taken immediately after shaking and the remainder discarded.

Worked example: To illustrate how volumes can be calculated in the regimens suggested, a worked example is provided. To make up 0.5mg of chlordiazepoxide a 0.1mg/mL dilution can be used, prepared as above. The volume of 0.1mg/mL liquid required to give a dose of 0.5mg chlordiazepoxide is 0.5/0.1 = 5mL.

Deprescribing notes: There are two main methods for tapering from chlordiazepoxide – a switch to diazepam or a direct taper of chlordiazepoxide itself. There are no established guides to determine the rate of taper for someone stopping benzodiazepines. Withdrawal is known to be more severe for people who have used benzodiazepines with a shorter half-life, for longer periods and for those who have experienced withdrawal in the past on reducing, stopping or missing a dose.[13,14] The size of the initial reduction can be estimated based on these factors (see 'Tapering benzodiazepines and z-drugs in practice'), with patient preference also taken into account. Sometimes an even smaller reduction to start with may be advisable to boost a patient's confidence that they can taper if performed carefully.

Each reduction should be made when the withdrawal symptoms from the previous reduction have largely resolved so that subsequent reductions do not lead to cumulative withdrawal symptoms. Withdrawal symptoms should not be too unpleasant: a rate of reduction should be aimed for that produces tolerable withdrawal symptoms that abate within a week or two. Allowing for a sufficient observation period, reductions can therefore be made about every 1–4 weeks, depending on how long it takes withdrawal symptoms to resolve. If withdrawal symptoms are moderately severe or take longer than a couple of weeks to resolve, dose reductions should be postponed until symptoms resolve and then made more gradually by choosing a slower tapering rate. If severe withdrawal symptoms occur, then the patient should return to a higher dose, wait until symptoms resolve and thereafter taper at a slower rate.

Suggested direct taper schedules for chlordiazepoxide: Please note that none of these regimens should be seen as prescriptive – that is, patients should not be compelled to adhere strictly to them. They are given as example regimens and are not 'set and forget' but should be modified in order to ensure that withdrawal symptoms are tolerable throughout a taper. For example, intermediate steps halfway between the doses listed could be added to make a more gradual taper. Ultimately, it is the patient's experience of withdrawal that should guide the rate of taper.

A. **A faster taper** with up to 5 percentage points of GABA$_A$ occupancy between each step – with reductions made every 1–4 weeks*.

Step	RO (%)	AM (mg)	PM (mg)	Night (mg)	Total daily dose (mg)	Form	Step	RO (%)	AM (mg)	PM (mg)	Night (mg)	Total daily dose (mg)	Form
1	61.8	35	30	35	100	Use tabs or caps	— Switch to liquid version of chlordiazepoxide (e.g. 0.1mg/mL)***						
2	59.3	30	30	30	90	Use tabs or caps**	12	25.4	8	5	8	21	Liquid
3	56.4	25	25	30	80	Use tabs or caps**	13	21.6	6	5	6	17	Liquid
4	53.1	25	20	25	70	Use tabs or caps**	14	17.4	4	4	5	13	Liquid
5	49.3	20	20	20	60	Use tabs or caps**	15	13.3	3	3	3.5	9.5	Liquid
6	44.7	15	15	20	50	Use tabs or caps	16	10.8	2.5	2.5	2.5	7.5	Liquid
7	42.2	15	15	15	45	Use tabs or caps**	17	8.2	2	1.5	2	5.5	Liquid
8	39.3	15	10	15	40	Use tabs or caps**	18	5.4	1	1	1.5	3.5	Liquid
9	36.2	10	10	15	35	Use tabs or caps**	19	2.4	0.5	0.5	0.5	1.5	Liquid
10	32.7	10	10	10	30	Use tabs or caps**	20	0	0	0	0	0	–
11	28.8	10	5	10	25	Use tabs or caps**							

See further steps in the right-hand column

RO = receptor occupancy, caps = capsules, tabs = tablets

*Patients who have been on the medication for only a few weeks will probably be able to taper more quickly and might follow every second or third step of this regimen and make reductions every few days or so. Normally the duration of the taper should not be longer than the period that the patient has been on the drug for people who have only taken it for a few weeks. However, the FDA has issued an alert regarding benzodiazepines indicating that some people can experience withdrawal effects after just a few days of use,[3] therefore necessitating slower tapering in this sub-group.

**Where appropriate tablets or capsules are not available a liquid formulation of drug will need to be used as outlined in the off-label options.

***A liquid formulation of the drug will need to be used as outlined in the off-label options.

B. **A moderate taper** with up to 2.5 percentage points of $GABA_A$ occupancy between each step – with reductions made every 1–4 weeks.

Step	RO (%)	AM (mg)	PM (mg)	Night (mg)	Total daily dose (mg)	Form	Step	RO (%)	AM (mg)	PM (mg)	Night (mg)	Total daily dose (mg)	Form
1	61.8	35	30	35	100	Use tabs or caps*	20	30.8	10	7.5	10	27.5	Liquid
2	60.6	30	30	35	95	Use tabs or caps*	21	28.8	10	5	10	25	Liquid
3	59.3	30	30	30	90	Use tabs or caps*	22	27.1	9	5	9	23	Liquid
4	57.9	30	25	30	85	Use tabs or caps*	23	25.4	8	5	8	21	Liquid
5	56.4	25	25	30	80	Use tabs or caps*	24	23.5	6	5	8	19	Liquid
6	54.8	25	25	25	75	Use tabs or caps	25	21.6	6	5	6	17	Liquid
7	53.1	25	20	25	70	Use tabs or caps*	26	19.5	5	5	5	15	Liquid
8	51.3	20	20	25	65	Use tabs or caps*	27	17.4	4	4	5	13	Liquid
9	49.3	20	20	20	60	Use tabs or caps*	28	15.1	4	3	4	11	Liquid
10	47.1	20	15	20	55	Use tabs or caps*	29	13.3	3	3	3.5	9.5	Liquid
11	44.7	15	15	20	50	Use tabs or caps*	30	12.1	3	2.5	3	8.5	Liquid
Switch to liquid version of chlordiazepoxide (e.g. 0.1mg/mL)**							31	10.8	2.5	2.5	2.5	7.5	Liquid
12	43.5	15	15	17.5	47.5	Liquid	32	9.5	2	2	2.5	6.5	Liquid
13	42.2	15	15	15	45	Liquid	33	8.2	2	1.5	2	5.5	Liquid
14	40.8	15	12.5	15	42.5	Liquid	34	6.8	1.5	1.5	1.5	4.5	Liquid
15	39.3	15	10	15	40	Liquid	35	5.4	1	1	1.5	3.5	Liquid
16	37.8	12.5	10	15	37.5	Liquid	36	3.9	1	0.5	1	2.5	Liquid
17	36.2	10	10	15	35	Liquid	37	2.4	0.5	0.5	0.5	1.5	Liquid
18	34.5	10	10	12.5	32.5	Liquid	38	0.8	0	0	0.5	0.5	Liquid
19	32.7	10	10	10	30	Liquid	39	0	0	0	0	0	Liquid
See further steps in the right-hand column													

RO = receptor occupancy, caps = capsules, tabs = tablets
*Where appropriate tablets or capsules are not available a liquid formulation of drug will need to be used as outlined in the off-label options.
**A liquid formulation of the drug will need to be used as outlined in the off-label options. Some of these doses could be made up with capsules or half tablets and capsules where these formulations are available.

CHAPTER 3

C. **A slower taper** with up to 1.3 percentage points of GABA$_A$ occupancy between each step – with reductions made every 1–4 weeks.

Step	RO (%)	AM (mg)	PM (mg)	Night (mg)	Total daily dose (mg)	Form	Step	RO (%)	AM (mg)	PM (mg)	Night (mg)	Total daily dose (mg)	Form
1	61.8	35	30	35	100	Use tabs or caps*	30	38.6	13.75	10	15	38.75	Liquid
	Switch to liquid version of chlordiazepoxide (e.g. 0.1mg/mL)**						31	37.8	12.5	10	15	37.5	Liquid
2	61.2	32.5	30	35	97.5	Liquid	32	37	11.25	10	15	36.25	Liquid
3	60.6	30	30	35	95	Liquid	33	36.2	10	10	15	35	Liquid
4	60	30	30	32.5	92.5	Liquid	34	35.3	10	10	13.75	33.75	Liquid
5	59.3	30	30	30	90	Liquid	35	34.5	10	10	12.5	32.5	Liquid
6	58.6	30	27.5	30	87.5	Liquid	36	33.6	10	10	11.25	31.25	Liquid
7	57.9	30	25	30	85	Liquid	37	32.7	10	10	10	30	Liquid
8	57.2	27.5	25	30	82.5	Liquid	38	31.8	10	8.75	10	28.75	Liquid
9	56.4	25	25	30	80	Liquid	39	30.8	10	7.5	10	27.5	Liquid
10	55.7	25	25	27.5	77.5	Liquid	40	29.8	10	6.25	10	26.25	Liquid
11	54.8	25	25	25	75	Liquid	41	28.8	10	5	10	25	Liquid
12	54	25	22.5	25	72.5	Liquid	42	28	9	5	10	24	Liquid
13	53.1	25	20	25	70	Liquid	43	27.1	9	5	9	23	Liquid
14	52.2	22.5	20	25	67.5	Liquid	44	26.3	8	5	9	22	Liquid
15	51.3	20	20	25	65	Liquid	45	25.4	8	5	8	21	Liquid
16	50.3	20	20	22.5	62.5	Liquid	46	24.5	7	5	8	20	Liquid
17	49.3	20	20	20	60	Liquid	47	23.5	6	5	8	19	Liquid
18	48.2	20	17.5	20	57.5	Liquid	48	22.6	6	5	7	18	Liquid
19	47.1	20	15	20	55	Liquid	49	21.6	6	5	6	17	Liquid
20	46	17.5	15	20	52.5	Liquid	50	20.6	5	5	6	16	Liquid
21	44.7	15	15	20	50	Liquid	51	19.5	5	5	5	15	Liquid
22	44.1	15	15	18.75	48.75	Liquid	52	18.5	5	4	5	14	Liquid
23	43.5	15	15	17.5	47.5	Liquid	53	17.4	4	4	5	13	Liquid
24	42.8	15	15	16.25	46.25	Liquid	54	16.3	4	4	4	12	Liquid
25	42.2	15	15	15	45	Liquid	55	15.1	4	3	4	11	Liquid
26	41.5	15	13.75	15	43.75	Liquid	56	13.9	3	3	4	10	Liquid
27	40.8	15	12.5	15	42.5	Liquid	57	13.3	3	3	3.5	9.5	Liquid
28	40	15	11.25	15	41.25	Liquid	58	12.7	3	3	3	9	Liquid
29	39.3	15	10	15	40	Liquid	59	12.1	3	2.5	3	8.5	Liquid
	See further steps in the right-hand column											*(Continued)*	

(Continued)

Step	RO (%)	AM (mg)	PM (mg)	Night (mg)	Total daily dose (mg)	Form	Step	RO (%)	AM (mg)	PM (mg)	Night (mg)	Total daily dose (mg)	Form
60	11.5	2.5	2.5	3	8	Liquid	69	5.4	1	1	1.5	3.5	Liquid
61	10.8	2.5	2.5	2.5	7.5	Liquid	70	4.6	1	1	1	3	Liquid
62	10.2	2.5	2	2.5	7	Liquid	71	3.9	1	0.5	1	2.5	Liquid
63	9.5	2	2	2.5	6.5	Liquid	72	3.1	0.5	0.5	1	2	Liquid
64	8.9	2	2	2	6	Liquid	73	2.4	0.5	0.5	0.5	1.5	Liquid
65	8.2	2	1.5	2	5.5	Liquid	74	1.6	0.5	0	0.5	1	Liquid
66	7.5	1.5	1.5	2	5	Liquid	75	0.8	0	0	0.5	0.5	Liquid
67	6.8	1.5	1.5	1.5	4.5	Liquid	76	0	0	0	0	0	Liquid
68	6.1	1.5	1	1.5	4	Liquid							

See further steps in the right-hand column

RO = receptor occupancy, caps = capsules, tabs = tablets
*In Europe, a liquid formulation of drug will need to be used as outlined in the off-label options.
**A liquid formulation of the drug will need to be used as outlined in the off-label options. Some of these doses could be made up with capsules or half tablets and capsules where these formulations are available.

D. **An even slower taper** Some patients will be unable to taper at the slowest rates shown here and will need to taper by even smaller decrements, thus lengthening the overall period of tapering. Such a regimen could be constructed by placing intermediate steps in regimen C. For example, 100mg, 97.5mg, 95mg could be modified to 100mg, 98.75mg, 97.5mg, 96.25mg, 95mg and so on. Further intermediate steps could also be added.

Micro-tapering: The tables show how to make reductions at intervals of 1–4 weeks. An alternative approach is called 'micro-tapering' whereby very small dose reductions are made every day, as explained in 'Other considerations in tapering benzodiazepines and z-drugs.' Micro-tapering rates can be calculated from the above by dividing the change in dose for each step by 14 or 28 days. For example, for the moderate regimen reduction from 100mg to 95mg over 14 days is equivalent to a reduction of 0.36mg reduction per day, or a reduction of 0.12mg per dose (for three times a day dosing). By the end of this regimen the rate of reduction would have slowed down to a reduction of 0.036mg each day (or 0.012mg per dose when dosed three times a day). The rate can be adjusted if withdrawal symptoms become too unpleasant.

Switching guide from chlordiazepoxide to diazepam: An alternative to a direct taper from chlordiazepoxide is to switch to diazepam before tapering from this drug, as outlined in 'Switching to longer-acting benzodiazepines to taper'. A 25mg dose of chlordiazepoxide is equivalent to 10mg diazepam.[10] Switching could be performed by steps of 25mg of chlordiazepoxide made every week (or as tolerated by the patient).

Steps	Morning	Afternoon	Evening	Daily diazepam equivalent
1	35mg chlordiazepoxide	30mg chlordiazepoxide	35mg chlordiazepoxide	40mg
2	10mg chlordiazepoxide 10mg diazepam	30mg chlordiazepoxide	35mg chlordiazepoxide	40mg
3	10mg chlordiazepoxide 10mg diazepam	30mg chlordiazepoxide	10mg chlordiazepoxide 10mg diazepam	40mg
4	10mg chlordiazepoxide 10mg diazepam	5mg chlordiazepoxide 10mg diazepam	10mg chlordiazepoxide 10mg diazepam	40mg
5	14mg diazepam	12mg diazepam	14mg diazepam	40mg
6	20mg diazepam	divert diazepam to morning and evening	20mg diazepam	40mg

Continue to taper as for 40mg diazepam (see diazepam section)

CHAPTER 3

References

1. Chouinard G. Issues in the clinical use of benzodiazepines: potency, withdrawal, and rebound. *J Clin Psychiatry* 2004; 65 Suppl 5: 7–12.
2. Mylan. Summary of Product Characteristics. Librium 5mg Capsules Chlordiazepoxide hydrochloride. https://www.medicines.org.uk/emc/product/1728/smpc#gref.
3. FDA Drug Safety Communication. FDA requiring boxed warning updated to improve safe use of benzodiazepine drug class. 2020. https://www.fda.gov/drugs/drug-safety-and-availability/fda-requiring-boxed-warning-updated-improve-safe-use-benzodiazepine-drug-class#:~:text=FDA is requiring the Boxed,and life-threatening side effects (accessed 3 July 2023).
4. FDA. Librium – Accessdata.fda.gov. www.accessdata.fda.gov. https://www.accessdata.fda.gov/drugsatfda_docs/label/2016/012249s049lbl.pdf (accessed 8 September 2023).
5. Hollister LE, Motzenbecker FP, Degan RO. Withdrawal reactions from chlordiazepoxide ('Librium'). *Psychopharmacologia* 1961; 2: 63–8.
6. Brouillet E, Chavoix C, Bottlaender M, et al. In vivo bidirectional modulatory effect of benzodiazepine receptor ligands on GABAergic transmission evaluated by positron emission tomography in non-human primates. *Brain Res* 1991; 557: 167–76.
7. Holford N. Pharmacodynamic principles and the time course of delayed and cumulative drug effects. *Trans Clin Pharmacol* 2018; 26: 56–9.
8. Horowitz M, Taylor D. Withdrawing from benzodiazepines and z-drugs (in preparation).
9. Horowitz MA, Taylor D. Tapering of SSRI treatment to mitigate withdrawal symptoms. *The Lancet Psychiatry* 2019; 6: 538–46.
10. Hypnotics and anxiolytics. https://bnf.nice.org.uk/treatment-summaries/hypnotics-and-anxiolytics/ (accessed 19 March 2023).
11. Smyth. J. The NEWT Guidelines for administration of medication to patients with enteral feeding tubes or swallowing difficulties website. The NEWT Guidelines. 2011. http://www.newtguidelines.com (accessed 5 July 2023).
12. Macheras PE, Koupparis MA, Antimisiaris SG. Drug binding and solubility in milk. *Pharm Res* 1990; 7: 537–41.
13. Guina J, Merrill B. Benzodiazepines II: waking up on sedatives: providing optimal care when inheriting benzodiazepine prescriptions in transfer patients. *J Clin Med Res* 2018; 7. doi:10.3390/jcm7020020.
14. Framer A. What I have learnt from helping thousands of people taper off psychotropic medications. *Ther Adv Psychopharmacol* 2021; 11: 204512532199127.

Clonazepam

Trade names: Klonopin, Iktorivil, Paxam, Rivatril, Rivotril.

Description: Clonazepam is a high potency,[1] intermediate- to long-acting benzodiazepine.[2] Clonazepam is a positive allosteric modulator of the GABA$_A$ receptor, potentiating the effect of GABA on the receptor complex.[3] The manufacturer states that 'the effectiveness of Klonopin in long-term use, that is, for more than 9 weeks has not been systematically studied in controlled clinical trials'.[4]

Withdrawal effects: Clonazepam, as for other benzodiazepines, carries a boxed warning from the FDA that highlights that physical dependence and withdrawal effects can occur when the drug is taken 'for several days to weeks, even as prescribed'.[4,5] Not everyone who stops clonazepam will experience withdrawal and some of those who do will only experience mild symptoms – this probably depends on drug dose, duration of use and individual factors. However, in a very few instances, stopping abruptly can cause seizures and can be life threatening. Numerous other physical, cognitive and psychological withdrawal symptoms, outlined earlier in the chapter, are also possible, which can last 'for several weeks to more than 12 months' after stopping according to the FDA.[4,5]

Peak plasma: 1–4 hours.[1]

Half-life: 20–60 hours (mean 30 hours).[1] The manufacturer recommends that clonazepam be given in divided doses.[6] Dosing less often (including every-other-day dosing) is not recommended for tapering because the changes in plasma levels may precipitate inter-dose withdrawal symptoms.

Receptor occupancy: The relationship between dose of clonazepam and the occupancy of its major target GABA$_A$ is hyperbolic.[7,8] Benzodiazepines demonstrate a hyperbolic relationship between dose and clinical effects,[9] which may be relevant to withdrawal effects. Dose reductions made by linear amounts (e.g. 4mg, 3mg, 2mg, 1mg, 0mg) will cause increasingly large reductions in effect, which may cause increasingly severe withdrawal effects (Figure 3.11a). To produce equal-sized reductions in effect on receptor occupancy will require hyperbolically reducing doses (Figure 3.11b),[10] which informs the reductions presented later. The relationship was derived by converting the receptor occupancy curve for diazepam[7] to the equivalent clonazepam dose.[11]

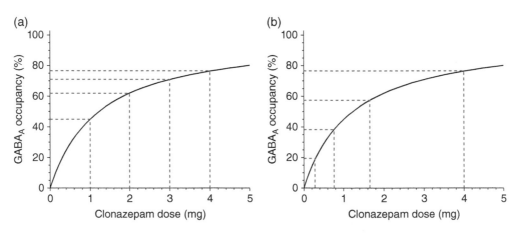

Figure 3.11 (a) Linear reductions of dose cause increasingly large reductions in effect on receptor targets, possibly associated with more withdrawal effects. (b) Even reductions of effect at target receptors requires hyperbolic dose reductions. The final dose before stopping will need to be very small so that this step down is not larger (in terms of effect on receptor occupancy) than previous reductions.

Available formulations: As tablets and liquid.

Tablets

Dosage	UK	Europe	USA	Australia	Canada
0.125mg	–	–	✓*	–	–
0.25mg	–	–	✓**	–	✓
0.5mg	✓	✓	✓*	✓	✓
1mg	✓	✓	✓*	–	✓
2mg	✓	✓	✓*	✓	✓

*Available as tablets and oral disintegrating tables (ODTs).
**Only available as ODT.

Liquids

Oral solutions	UK	Europe	USA	Australia	Canada
0.5mg/5mL (0.1mg/mL)	✓	–		–	–
2mg/5mL (0.4mg/mL)	✓	–		–	–
2.5mg/mL	–	✓	–	✓	–

Off-label options: In order to follow the regimens suggested in some cases, where no liquid versions are available, smaller doses are required than can be made using commercially available tablets and capsules. The use of tablets (or orally disintegrating tablets) to make liquid formulations is one option. Guidelines for people who cannot swallow tablets (e.g. NEWT guidelines in the UK based on advice from the manufacturer or local hospital guidance,[12] and US guidance[13]) suggest that clonazepam tablets can be dispersed in water for administration.[14] They will disintegrate in less than 2 minutes.[12] Water could be added to a 0.5mg tablet to make up a 5mL suspension (concentration of 1mg in 10mL or 0.1mg/mL). The suspension should be shaken vigorously before administration. As its stability cannot be assured it should be consumed immediately, and any unused suspension discarded. Some patients use full-fat milk to make liquid preparations. Benzodiazepines are more soluble in oil or fat than in water.[15] When mixed with milk, some or all of the drug will dissolve in the milk fat. This should form an evenly dispersed emulsion when shaken vigorously. The measured dose should be taken immediately after shaking and the remainder discarded.

Another option is to have a compounding pharmacy make up a suspension or smaller dose tablets or capsules, or to switch to diazepam to taper (see later).

Dilutions: To make up some of the small doses outlined below, dilution of the manufacturer's solutions will be required. Dilution in water might cause precipitation of the drug and so the resulting mixture should be shaken vigorously before use to produce dispersal. As its stability cannot be assured it should be made up fresh each day.

CHAPTER 3

EU/Australian dilutions	Solution required	How to prepare solution
Multiples of 0.1mg	2.5mg/mL	Drops from original solution
Doses not multiples of 0.1mg	0.1mg/mL	Add 10 drops of original solution (2.5mg/mL) to make up to 10mL of water*

*Each drop contains 0.1mg of clonazepam. Alternatively, 0.4mL of the original solution could be measured with a syringe to make up 1mg. This can be made up to 10mL of water to produce a 0.1mg/mL solution.

Worked example: To illustrate how the volumes were calculated in the regimens given, a worked example is provided. To make up 0.15mg of clonazepam a 0.1mg/mL dilution can be used, prepared as above. The volume of 0.1mg/mL liquid required to give a dose of 0.15mg clonazepam is 0.15/0.1 = 1.5mL.

Deprescribing notes: There are two main methods for tapering from clonazepam – a switch to a longer-acting benzodiazepine like diazepam (see later) or a direct taper of clonazepam itself. There are no established guides to determine the rate of taper for someone stopping benzodiazepines. Withdrawal is known to be more severe for people who have used benzodiazepines which are shorter acting, for longer periods, and for those who have experienced withdrawal in the past on reducing, stopping or missing a dose.[16,17] The size of the initial reduction can be estimated based on these factors (see 'Tapering benzodiazepines and z-drugs in practice'), with patient preference also taken into account. Sometimes an even smaller reduction to start with may be advisable to boost a patient's confidence that they can taper if performed carefully.

Each reduction should be made when the withdrawal symptoms from the previous reduction have largely resolved so that subsequent reductions do not lead to cumulative withdrawal symptoms. Withdrawal symptoms should not be too unpleasant: a rate of reduction should be aimed for that produces tolerable withdrawal symptoms that abate within a week or two. Allowing for a sufficient observation period, reductions can therefore be made about every 1–4 weeks, depending on how long it takes withdrawal symptoms to resolve. If withdrawal symptoms are moderately severe or take longer than a couple of weeks to resolve, dose reductions should be postponed until symptoms resolve and then made more gradually by choosing a slower tapering rate. If severe withdrawal symptoms occur then the patient should return to a higher dose, wait until symptoms resolve and thereafter taper at a slower rate.

Suggested direct taper schedules for clonazepam: Please note that none of these regimens should be seen as prescriptive – that is, patients should not be compelled to adhere strictly to them. They are given as example regimens and are not 'set and forget' but should be modified in order to ensure that withdrawal symptoms are tolerable throughout a taper. For example, intermediate steps halfway between the doses listed could be added to make a more gradual taper. Ultimately, it is the patient's experience of withdrawal that should guide the rate of taper.

A. **A faster taper** with up to 5.2 percentage points of $GABA_A$ occupancy between each step – with reductions made every 1–4 weeks*.

Step	RO (%)	AM (mg)	PM (mg)	Total daily dose (mg)	Form**	Step	RO (%)	AM (mg)	PM (mg)	Total daily dose (mg)	Form**
1	76.4	2	2	4	Use tablets	14	31.3	0.25	0.31	0.56	Use ¼ tablets
2	73.9	1.75	1.75	3.5	Use tablets	15	28.8	0.25	0.25	0.5	Use tablets
3	70.8	1.5	1.5	3	Use tablets	16	26.2	0.188	0.25	0.438	Use ¾ tablets
4	66.9	1.25	1.25	2.5	Use tablets	17	23.3	0.188	0.188	0.376	Use ¾ tablets
5	61.8	1	1	2	Use tablets	18	20.2	0.125	0.188	0.313	Use ¾ tablets
6	58.6	0.875	0.875	1.75	Use tablets	19	16.8	0.125	0.125	0.25	Use tablets
7	54.8	0.75	0.75	1.5	Use tablets	20	13.2	0.0625	0.125	0.1875	Use ½ tablets
8	50.3	0.625	0.625	1.25	Use tablets	21	9.2	0.0625	0.0625	0.125	Use ¼ tablets
9	47.7	0.5	0.625	1.125	Use tablets	22	7.1	0.031	0.0625	0.0938	Use ¼ and ½ tablets
10	44.7	0.5	0.5	1	Use tablets	23	4.8	0.031	0.031	0.062	Use ¼ tablets
11	41.5	0.375	0.5	0.875	Use tablets	24	2.5	0	0.031	0.031	Use ¼ tablets
12	37.8	0.375	0.375	0.75	Use tablets	25	0	0	0	0	–
13	33.6	0.25	0.375	0.625	Use tablets						

See further steps in the right-hand column

RO = receptor occupancy

*Patients who have been on the medication for only a few weeks will probably be able to taper more quickly and might follow every second or third step of this regimen and make reductions every few days or so. Normally the duration of the taper should not be longer than the period that the patient has been on the drug for people who have only taken it for a few weeks. For example, if clonazepam is taken for 3 weeks the taper should be less than 3 weeks. However, the FDA has issued an alert regarding dependence and withdrawal from benzodiazepines indicating that some people can experience withdrawal effects after just a few days of use,[5] therefore necessitating slower tapering.

**These guides are based on formulations available in the US. In other regions liquid formulations of clonazepam may be required to make up the doses suggested.

CHAPTER 3

B. **A moderate taper** with up to 2.5 percentage points of $GABA_A$ occupancy between each step – with reductions made every 1–4 weeks.

Step	RO (%)	AM (mg)	PM (mg)	Total daily dose (mg)	Form*	Step	RO (%)	AM (mg)	PM (mg)	Total daily dose (mg)	Form
1	76.4	2	2	4	Use tablets	24	36.2	0.35	0.35	0.7	Liquid
2	75.2	1.875	1.875	3.75	Use tablets	25	34.5	0.325	0.325	0.65	Liquid
3	73.9	1.75	1.75	3.5	Use tablets	26	32.7	0.30	0.30	0.6	Liquid
4	72.5	1.625	1.625	3.25	Use tablets	27	30.8	0.275	0.275	0.55	Liquid
5	70.8	1.5	1.5	3	Use tablets	28	28.8	0.25	0.25	0.5	Liquid
6	69	1.375	1.375	2.75	Use tablets	29	26.7	0.225	0.225	0.45	Liquid
7	66.9	1.25	1.25	2.5	Use tablets	30	24.5	0.20	0.20	0.4	Liquid
8	64.6	1.125	1.125	2.25	Use tablets	31	22.6	0.18	0.18	0.36	Liquid
9	61.8	1.0	1.0	2	Use tablets	32	20.6	0.16	0.16	0.32	Liquid
10	60.3	0.9375	0.9375	1.875	Use ½ tablets	33	18.5	0.14	0.14	0.28	Liquid
11	58.6	0.875	0.875	1.75	Use tablets		Switch to **0.1mg/mL** liquid formulation*				
12	56.8	0.8125	0.8125	1.625	Use ½ tablets	34	16.3	0.12	0.12	0.24	Liquid
13	54.8	0.75	0.75	1.5	Use tablets	35	13.9	0.1	0.1	0.2	Liquid
14	52.7	0.6875	0.6875	1.375	Use ½ tablets	36	12.7	0.09	0.09	0.18	Liquid
15	50.3	0.625	0.625	1.25	Use tablets	37	11.5	0.08	0.08	0.16	Liquid
	Switch to liquid formulation**					38	10.2	0.07	0.07	0.14	Liquid
16	49.3	0.55	0.6	1.15	Liquid	39	8.9	0.06	0.06	0.12	Liquid
17	47.1	0.5	0.55	1.05	Liquid	40	7.5	0.05	0.05	0.1	Liquid
18	44.7	0.5	0.5	1	Liquid	41	6.1	0.04	0.04	0.08	Liquid
19	43.5	0.475	0.475	0.95	Liquid	42	4.6	0.03	0.03	0.06	Liquid
20	42.2	0.45	0.45	0.9	Liquid	43	3.1	0.02	0.02	0.04	Liquid
21	40.8	0.425	0.425	0.85	Liquid	44	1.6	0.01	0.01	0.02	Liquid
22	39.3	0.4	0.4	0.8	Liquid	45	0	0.0	0.0	0	Liquid
23	37.8	0.375	0.375	0.75	Liquid						

See further steps in the right-hand column

RO = receptor occupancy

*These guides are based on formulations available in the US. In other regions liquid formulations of clonazepam may be required to make up the doses suggested.

**Preparation as indicated above.

C. **A slower taper** with up to 1.4 percentage points of $GABA_A$ occupancy between each step – with reductions made every 1–4 weeks.

Step	RO (%)	AM (mg)	PM (mg)	Total daily dose (mg)	Form*	Step	RO (%)	AM (mg)	PM (mg)	Total daily dose (mg)	Form
1	76.4	2	2	4	Use tabs	31	48.2	0.55	0.6	1.15	Liquid
2	75.8	1.875	2	3.875	Use tabs	32	47.1	0.55	0.55	1.1	Liquid
3	75.2	1.875	1.875	3.75	Use tabs	33	46	0.5	0.55	1.05	Liquid
4	74.6	1.75	1.875	3.625	Use tabs	34	44.7	0.5	0.5	1	Liquid
5	73.9	1.75	1.75	3.5	Use tabs	35	44.1	0.475	0.5	0.975	Liquid
6	73.2	1.625	1.75	3.375	Use tabs	36	43.5	0.475	0.475	0.95	Liquid
7	72.5	1.625	1.625	3.25	Use tabs	37	42.8	0.45	0.475	0.925	Liquid
8	71.7	1.5	1.625	3.125	Use tabs	38	42.2	0.45	0.45	0.9	Liquid
9	70.8	1.5	1.5	3	Use tabs	39	41.5	0.425	0.45	0.875	Liquid
10	70	1.375	1.5	2.875	Use tabs	40	40.8	0.425	0.425	0.85	Liquid
11	69	1.375	1.375	2.75	Use tabs	41	40	0.4	0.425	0.825	Liquid
12	68	1.25	1.375	2.625	Use tabs	42	39.3	0.4	0.4	0.8	Liquid
13	66.9	1.25	1.25	2.5	Use tabs	43	38.6	0.375	0.4	0.775	Liquid
14	65.8	1.125	1.25	2.375	Use tabs	44	37.8	0.375	0.375	0.75	Liquid
15	64.6	1.125	1.125	2.25	Use tabs	45	37	0.35	0.375	0.725	Liquid
16	63.2	1	1.125	2.125	Use tabs	46	36.2	0.35	0.35	0.7	Liquid
17	61.8	1	1	2	Use tabs	47	35.3	0.325	0.35	0.675	Liquid
18	61.1	0.9375	1	1.9375	Use ½ tabs	48	34.5	0.325	0.325	0.65	Liquid
19	60.3	0.9375	0.9375	1.875	Use ½ tabs	49	33.6	0.3	0.325	0.625	Liquid
20	59.5	0.875	0.9375	1.8125	Use ½ tabs	50	32.7	0.3	0.3	0.6	Liquid
21	58.6	0.875	0.875	1.75	Use tabs	51	31.8	0.275	0.3	0.575	Liquid
22	57.7	0.8125	0.875	1.6875	Use ½ tabs	52	30.8	0.275	0.275	0.55	Liquid
23	56.8	0.8125	0.8125	1.625	Use ½ tabs	53	29.8	0.25	0.275	0.525	Liquid
24	55.9	0.75	0.8125	1.5625	Use ½ tabs	54	28.8	0.25	0.25	0.5	Liquid
25	54.8	0.75	0.75	1.5	Use tabs	55	27.8	0.225	0.25	0.475	Liquid
26	53.8	0.6875	0.75	1.4375	Use ½ tabs	56	26.7	0.225	0.225	0.45	Liquid
27	52.7	0.6875	0.6875	1.375	Use ½ tabs						
28	51.5	0.625	0.6875	1.3125	Use ½ tabs	57	25.6	0.2	0.225	0.425	Liquid
29	50.3	0.625	0.625	1.25	Use tabs	58	24.5	0.2	0.2	0.4	Liquid
						59	23.5	0.18	0.2	0.38	Liquid
30	49.3	0.6	0.6	1.2	Liquid	60	22.6	0.18	0.18	0.36	Liquid

Left column note between steps 29 and 30: **Switch to liquid formulation****

Right column note between steps 56 and 57: Switch to **0.1mg/mL** liquid formulation*

See further steps in the right-hand column

(Continued)

(Continued)

Step	RO (%)	AM (mg)	PM (mg)	Total daily dose (mg)	Form*	Step	RO (%)	AM (mg)	PM (mg)	Total daily dose (mg)	Form
61	21.6	0.16	0.18	0.34	Liquid	75	9.5	0.06	0.07	0.13	Liquid
62	20.6	0.16	0.16	0.32	Liquid	76	8.9	0.06	0.06	0.12	Liquid
63	19.5	0.14	0.16	0.3	Liquid	77	8.2	0.05	0.06	0.11	Liquid
64	18.5	0.14	0.14	0.28	Liquid	78	7.5	0.05	0.05	0.1	Liquid
65	17.4	0.12	0.14	0.26	Liquid	79	6.8	0.04	0.05	0.09	Liquid
66	16.3	0.12	0.12	0.24	Liquid	80	6.1	0.04	0.04	0.08	Liquid
67	15.1	0.1	0.12	0.22	Liquid	81	5.4	0.03	0.04	0.07	Liquid
68	13.9	0.10	0.10	0.2	Liquid	82	4.6	0.03	0.03	0.06	Liquid
69	13.3	0.09	0.10	0.19	Liquid	83	3.9	0.02	0.03	0.05	Liquid
70	12.7	0.09	0.09	0.18	Liquid	84	3.1	0.02	0.02	0.04	Liquid
71	12.1	0.08	0.09	0.17	Liquid	85	2.4	0.01	0.02	0.03	Liquid
72	11.5	0.08	0.08	0.16	Liquid	86	1.6	0.01	0.01	0.02	Liquid
73	10.8	0.07	0.08	0.15	Liquid	87	0.8	0	0.01	0.01	Liquid
74	10.2	0.07	0.07	0.14	Liquid	88	0	0	0	0	Liquid

See further steps in the right-hand column

RO = receptor occupancy, tabs = tablets
*These guides are based on formulations available in the US. In other regions liquid formulations of clonazepam may be required to make up the doses suggested.
**Preparation as indicated above.

D. **An even slower taper** Some patients will be unable to taper at the slowest rates shown here and will need to taper by even smaller decrements, thus lengthening the overall period of tapering. Such a regimen could be constructed by placing intermediate steps in regimen C. For example, 1.2mg, 1.15mg, 1.1mg could be modified to 1.2mg, 1.175mg, 1.15mg, 1.125mg, 1.1mg and so on. Further intermediate steps could also be added.

Micro-tapering: The tables above show how to make reductions at intervals of 1–4 weeks. An alternative approach is called 'micro-tapering' whereby very small dose reductions are made every day, as explained in 'Other considerations in tapering benzodiazepines and z-drugs.' Micro-tapering rates can be calculated from the above regimens by dividing the change in dose for each step by 14 or 28 days. For example, for the moderate regime, a reduction from 4mg to 3.75mg over 14 days is equivalent to approximately 0.02mg reduction per day, or 0.01mg reduction per dose (when dosed twice daily). By the end of this regimen the rate of reduction would have slowed down to a reduction of 0.0014mg each day. The rate can be adjusted if withdrawal symptoms become too unpleasant.

Switching guide from clonazepam to diazepam: An alternative to a direct taper from clonazepam is to switch to diazepam before tapering from this drug, as outlined in 'Switching to longer-acting benzodiazepines to taper'. A 1mg dose of clonazepam is equivalent to 20mg of diazepam.[18] Switching could be performed in steps of 0.5mg of clonazepam made every week (or as tolerated by the patient).

Steps	Morning	Evening	Daily diazepam equivalent
Start	2mg clonazepam	2mg clonazepam	80mg
1	2mg clonazepam	1.5mg clonazepam+ 10mg diazepam	80mg
2	1.5mg clonazepam+ 10mg diazepam	1.5mg clonazepam+ 10mg diazepam	80mg
3	1.5mg clonazepam+ 10mg diazepam	1mg clonazepam+ 20mg diazepam	80mg
4	1mg clonazepam+ 20mg diazepam	1mg clonazepam+ 20mg diazepam	80mg
5	1mg clonazepam+ 20mg diazepam	0.5mg clonazepam+ 30mg diazepam	80mg
6	0.5mg clonazepam+ 30mg diazepam	0.5mg clonazepam+ 30mg diazepam	80mg
7	0.5mg clonazepam+ 30mg diazepam	40mg diazepam	80mg
8	40mg diazepam	40mg diazepam	80mg
10	35mg diazepam	40mg diazepam	75mg
11	35mg diazepam	35mg diazepam	70mg
12	30mg diazepam	35mg diazepam	65mg
13	30mg diazepam	30mg diazepam	60mg

Continue to taper as for 60mg diazepam (see diazepam section)

References

1. Chouinard G. Issues in the clinical use of benzodiazepines: potency, withdrawal, and rebound. *J Clin Psychiatry* 2004; 65 Suppl 5: 7–12.
2. Lexicomp: Evidence-Based Drug Referential Content. https://www.wolterskluwer.com/en/solutions/lexicomp (accessed 19 March 2023).
3. PharmGKB. PharmGKB. https://www.pharmgkb.org/literature/6754762 (accessed 19 March 2023).
4. FDA. Klonopin – Accessdata.fda.gov. www.accessdata.fda.gov. www.accessdata.fda.gov/drugsatfda_docs/label/2013/017533s053,020813s009lbl.pdf (accessed 27 March 2023).
5. FDA Drug Safety Communication. FDA requiring boxed warning updated to improve safe use of benzodiazepine drug class. 2020. https://www.fda.gov/drugs/drug-safety-and-availability/fda-requiring-boxed-warning-updated-improve-safe-use-benzodiazepine-drug-class#:~:text=FDA is requiring the Boxed,and life-threatening side effects (accessed 3 July 2023).
6. Clonazepam Neuraxpharm 0.5 mg tablets – Summary of Product Characteristics (SmPC) – (emc). https://www.medicines.org.uk/emc/product/13633/smpc (accessed 19 March 2023).
7. Brouillet E, Chavoix C, Bottlaender M, et al. In vivo bidirectional modulatory effect of benzodiazepine receptor ligands on GABAergic transmission evaluated by positron emission tomography in non-human primates. *Brain Res* 1991; 557: 167–76.
8. Innis RB, al-Tikriti MS, Zoghbi SS, et al. SPECT imaging of the benzodiazepine receptor: feasibility of in vivo potency measurements from stepwise displacement curves. *J Nucl Med* 1991; 32: 1754–61.
9. Horowitz M, Taylor D. Withdrawing from benzodiazepines and z-drugs (in preparation).
10. Horowitz MA, Taylor D. Tapering of SSRI treatment to mitigate withdrawal symptoms. *The Lancet Psychiatry* 2019; 6: 538–46.
11. Choosing an equivalent dose of oral benzodiazepine. SPS – Specialist Pharmacy Service. 2022; published online 25 January. https://www.sps.nhs.uk/articles/choosing-an-equivalent-dose-of-oral-benzodiazepine/ (accessed 8 April 2023).
12. Smyth J. The NEWT Guidelines for administration of medication to patients with enteral feeding tubes or swallowing difficulties website. The NEWT Guidelines. 2011. https://www.newtguidelines.com/index.html (accessed 7 September 2022).
13. Bostwick JR, Demehri A. Pills to powder: an updated clinician's reference for crushable psychotropics. *Curr Psychiatr* 2017; 16: 46–9.
14. Martin TP, Hayes P, Collins DM. Tablet dispersion as an alternative to formulation of liquid dosage forms. *Aust J Hosp Pharm* 1993; 23: 378–86.
15. Macheras PE, Koupparis MA, Antimisiaris SG. Drug binding and solubility in milk. *Pharm Res* 1990; 7: 537–41.
16. Guina J, Merrill B. Benzodiazepines II: waking up on sedatives: providing optimal care when inheriting benzodiazepine prescriptions in transfer patients. *J Clin Med Res* 2018; 7. doi:10.3390/jcm7020020.
17. Framer A. What I have learnt from helping thousands of people taper off psychotropic medications. *Ther Adv Psychopharmacol* 2021; 11: 204512532199127.
18. Hypnotics and anxiolytics. https://bnf.nice.org.uk/treatment-summaries/hypnotics-and-anxiolytics/ (accessed 19 March 2023).

Clorazepate

Trade names: Tranxene, Tranxilium.

Description: Clorazepate is a medium-potency benzodiazepine.[1] It is a positive allosteric modulator of the gamma-aminobutyric acid (GABA) type A receptor.

Withdrawal effects: Clorazepate, as for other benzodiazepines, carries a boxed warning from the FDA that highlights that physical dependence and withdrawal effects can occur when the drug is taken 'for several days to weeks, even as prescribed'.[2,3] Not everyone who stops clorazepate will experience withdrawal, and some of those who do will only experience mild symptoms – this probably depends on drug dose, duration of use and individual factors. However, in a very few instances, stopping abruptly can cause seizures and can be life threatening. Numerous other physical, cognitive and psychological withdrawal symptoms, outlined earlier in the chapter are also possible which can last 'for several weeks to more than 12 months' after stopping according to the FDA.[2,3] After 6 months of treatment with clorazepate 72% of patients experienced five or more withdrawal symptoms after abruptly stopping in a double blind, prospective trial.[4] Symptoms observed were anxiety, insomnia, increased sweating, loss of appetite, trembling, tiredness, difficulties sleeping, increased sensitivity to sound and smell, and muscle aches and twitching.[4]

Peak plasma: Following oral administration peak concentration in plasma occurs after 30 minutes to 2 hours.[5]

Half-life The mean half-life is 18–50 hours. The half-life of clorazepate's active metabolite ranges widely between 1 and 8 days.[5] Clorazepate can be administered in divided doses, up to three times a day. It can also be given once daily at bedtime.[5] The long half-life may enable less often than once a day dosing during tapering, but in some sensitive patients this might precipitate withdrawal effects.

Receptor occupancy: The relationship between dose of clorazepate and the occupancy of its major target GABA$_A$ receptors is hyperbolic according to the law of mass action.[6,7] Benzodiazepines demonstrate a hyperbolic relationship between dose and clinical effects,[8] which may be relevant to withdrawal effects. Dose reductions made by linear amounts (e.g. 60mg, 45mg, 30mg, 15mg, 0mg) will cause increasingly large reductions in effect, which may cause increasingly severe withdrawal effects (Figure 3.12a).

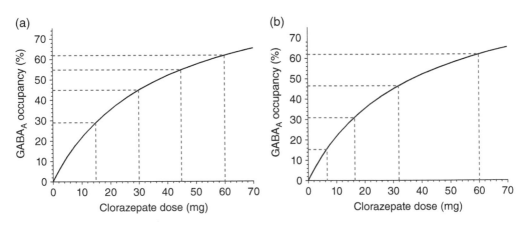

Figure 3.12 (a) Linear reductions of dose cause increasingly large reductions in effect on receptor targets, possibly associated with more withdrawal effects. (b) Even reductions of effect at target receptors requires hyperbolic dose reductions. The final dose before stopping will need to be very small so that this step down is not larger (in terms of effect on receptor occupancy) than previous reductions.

To produce equal-sized reductions in effect on receptor occupancy will require hyperbolically reducing doses (Figure 3.12b),[9] which informs the reductions presented. The relationship was derived by converting the receptor occupancy curve for diazepam[6] to equivalent clorazepate dose.[10]

Available formulations: As tablets and capsules.

Tablets

Dosage	UK	Europe	USA	Australia	Canada
3.75mg	–	–	✓	✓	–
7.5mg	–	–	✓	✓	–
15mg	–	–	✓	✓	–
20mg	–	✓	–	–	–

Capsules

Dosage	UK	Europe	USA	Australia	Canada
3.75mg	–	–	–	–	✓
5mg	–	✓	–	–	–
7.5mg	–	–	–	–	✓
15mg	–	–	–	–	✓
10mg	–	✓	–	–	–
20mg	–	✓	–	–	–

Off-label options: In order to follow the regimens suggested in some cases, where no liquid versions are available, smaller doses are required than can be made using commercially available tablets and capsules. Unusually for benzodiazepines, clorazepate is highly water soluble.[11] Water could be added to a (crushed) 3.75mg tablet to make up a 37.5mL solution with concentration 1mg in 10mL (or 0.1mg/mL). Alternatively, the contents of a 5mg capsule could be emptied into 50mL of water to make up a 0.1mg/mL solution. The mixture made will need to be shaken to facilitate dispersion. Note that the resultant liquid may be cloudy because of undissolved tablet excipients. As the stability of these solutions cannot be assured it should be consumed immediately, and any unused solution discarded.

Other options include having a compounding pharmacy make up a suspension or smaller dose tablets or capsules, or switching to diazepam (see later).

Worked example: To illustrate how the volumes could be calculated to make up doses in the regimens given, a worked example is provided. To make up 0.5mg of clorazepate a 0.1mg/mL dilution can be used, prepared as above. The volume of 0.1mg/mL liquid required to give a dose of 0.5mg clorazepate is 0.5/0.1 = 5mL.

Deprescribing notes: There are two main methods for tapering from clorazepate – a switch to diazepam or a direct taper from clorazepate. There are no established guides to determine the rate of taper of someone stopping benzodiazepines. Withdrawal is known to be more severe for people who have used benzodiazepines which are shorter acting, for longer periods, at higher doses, in the elderly and those who have experienced withdrawal in the past on reducing, stopping or missing a dose.[12,13] The size of the initial reduction can be estimated based on these factors (see 'Tapering benzodiazepines and z-drugs in practice'), with patient preference also taken into account. Sometimes an even smaller reduction to start with may be advisable to boost a patient's confidence that they can taper if performed carefully.

Each reduction should be made when the withdrawal symptoms from the previous reduction have largely resolved so that subsequent reductions do not lead to cumulative withdrawal symptoms. Withdrawal symptoms should not be too unpleasant: a rate of reduction should be aimed for that produces tolerable withdrawal symptoms that abate within a week or two. Allowing for a sufficient observation period, reductions can therefore be made about every 1–4 weeks, depending on how long it takes withdrawal symptoms to resolve. If withdrawal symptoms are moderately severe or take longer than a couple of weeks to resolve, dose reductions should be postponed until symptoms resolve and then made more gradually by choosing a slower tapering rate. If severe withdrawal symptoms occur then the patient should return to a higher dose, wait until symptoms resolve and thereafter taper at a slower rate.

Suggested direct taper schedules for clorazepate: Please note that none of these regimens should be seen as prescriptive – patients should not be compelled to adhere strictly to them. They are given as example regimens and are not 'set and forget' but should be modified in order to ensure that withdrawal symptoms are tolerable throughout a taper – for example intermediate steps halfway between the doses listed could be added to make a more gradual taper. Ultimately, it is the patient's experience of withdrawal that should guide the rate of taper.

A. **A faster taper** with up to 5 percentage points of $GABA_A$ occupancy between each step – with reductions made every 1–4 weeks*.

Step	RO (%)	Morning (mg)	Afternoon (mg)	Evening (mg)	Total daily dose (mg)	Formulation**
1	61.8	22.5	15	22.5	60	Tablets
2	58.6	15	15	22.5	52.5	Tablets
3	54.8	15	15	15	45	Tablets
4	50.3	15	7.5	15	37.5	Tablets
5	47.7	11.25	7.5	15	33.75	Tablets
6	44.7	7.5	7.5	15	30	Tablets
7	41.5	7.5	7.5	11.25	26.25	Tablets
8	37.8	7.5	7.5	7.5	22.5	Tablets
9	33.6	7.5	3.75	7.5	18.75	Tablets
10	28.8	3.75	3.75	7.5	15	Tablets
11	26.2	3.75	3.75	5.625	13.125	½ tablets
12	23.3	3.75	3.75	3.75	11.25	Tablets
13	20.2	3.75	1.875	3.75	9.375	½ tablets
14	16.8	1.875	1.875	3.75	7.5	½ tablets
15	13.2	1.875	1.875	1.875	5.625	½ tablets
16	9.2	0.9375	0.9375	1.875	3.75	¼ tablets
17	4.8	0.9375	0	0.9375	1.875	¼ tablets
18	2.5	0	0	0.9375	0.9375	¼ tablets
19	0	0	0	0	0	

RO = receptor occupancy

*Patients who have been on the medication for only a few weeks will probably be able to taper more quickly and might follow every second or third step of this regimen and make reductions every few days or so. Normally, the duration of the taper should not be longer than the period that the patient has been on the drug for people who have only taken it for a few weeks. For example, if clorazepate is taken for 3 weeks the taper should be less than 3 weeks. However the FDA has issued an alert regarding benzodiazepines indicating that some people can experience withdrawal effects after just a few days of use,[2] therefore necessitating slower tapering in this sub-group.

**Alternatively, these doses can be made up with a solution, prepared as above. In Europe, many of these doses will require a solution.

B. **A moderate taper** with up to 2.5 percentage points of $GABA_A$ occupancy between each step – with reductions made every 1–4 weeks.

Step	RO (%)	AM (mg)	PM (mg)	Night (mg)	Total daily dose (mg)	Form*	Step	RO (%)	AM (mg)	PM (mg)	Night (mg)	Total daily dose (mg)	Form*
1	61.8	18.75	18.75	22.5	60	Use tabs	19	30.8	5.25	5.25	6	16.5	Liquid
2	60.3	18.75	18.75	18.75	56.25	Use tabs	20	28.8	5	5	5	15	Liquid
3	58.6	18.75	15	18.75	52.5	Use tabs	21	26.7	4.5	4.5	4.5	13.5	Liquid
4	56.8	15	15	18.75	48.75	Use tabs	22	23.5	3.75	3.75	4.4	11.9	Liquid
5	54.8	15	15	15	45	Use tabs	23	21.6	3.3	3.3	3.7	10.3	Liquid
6	52.7	15	11.25	15	41.25	Use tabs	24	19.5	3	3	3	9	Liquid
7	50.3	11.25	11.25	15	37.5	Use tabs	25	17.4	2.7	2.4	2.7	7.8	Liquid
			Switch to clorazepate solution**				26	15.1	2.1	2.1	2.4	6.6	Liquid
8	49.3	12	11	12	35	Liquid	27	13.3	1.8	1.8	2.1	5.7	Liquid
9	47.1	10.5	10	12	32.5	Liquid	28	12.1	1.8	1.5	1.8	5.1	Liquid
10	44.7	10.5	9	10.5	30	Liquid	29	10.8	1.5	1.5	1.5	4.5	Liquid
11	43.5	9.75	9	9.75	28.5	Liquid	30	9.5	1.2	1.2	1.5	3.9	Liquid
12	42.2	9	9	9	27	Liquid	31	8.2	1.2	0.9	1.2	3.3	Liquid
13	40.8	8.25	8.25	9	25.5	Liquid	32	6.8	0.9	0.9	0.9	2.7	Liquid
14	39.3	8	8	8	24	Liquid	33	5.4	0.6	0.6	0.9	2.1	Liquid
15	37.8	7.5	7.5	7.5	22.5	Liquid	34	3.9	0.6	0.3	0.6	1.5	Liquid
16	36.2	7	7	7	21	Liquid	35	2.4	0.3	0.3	0.3	0.9	Liquid
17	34.5	6.75	6	6.75	19.5	Liquid	36	0.8	0	0	0.3	0.3	Liquid
18	32.7	6	6	6	18	Liquid	37	0	0	0	0	0	Liquid
		See further steps in the right-hand column											

RO = receptor occupancy; tabs = tablets

*Alternatively, these doses can be made up with a solution, prepared as above. In Europe, many of these doses will require a solution.

**Prepared as above.

C. **A slower taper** with up to 1.2 percentage points of $GABA_A$ occupancy between each step – with reductions made every 1–4 weeks.

Step	RO (%)	AM (mg)	PM (mg)	Night (mg)	Total daily dose (mg)	Form*	Step	RO (%)	AM (mg)	PM (mg)	Night (mg)	Total daily dose (mg)	Form*
1	61.8	22.5	15	22.5	60	Use tabs	31	35.3	7.5	5.25	7.5	20.25	Liquid
2	61.1	20.625	15	22.5	58.125	Use ½ tabs	32	34.5	7.5	4.5	7.5	19.5	Liquid
3	60.3	18.75	15	22.5	56.25	Use tabs	33	33.6	7.5	3.75	7.5	18.75	Liquid
4	59.5	16.875	15	22.5	54.375	Use ½ tabs	34	32.7	6.75	3.75	7.5	18	Liquid
5	58.6	15	15	22.5	52.5	Use tabs	35	31.8	6	3.75	7.5	17.25	Liquid
6	57.7	15	15	20.625	50.625	Use ½ tabs	36	30.8	5.25	3.75	7.5	16.5	Liquid
7	56.8	15	15	18.75	48.75	Use tabs	37	29.8	4.5	3.75	7.5	15.75	Liquid
8	55.9	15	15	16.875	46.875	Use ½ tabs	38	28.8	3.75	3.75	7.5	15	Liquid
9	54.8	15	15	15	45	Use tabs	39	27.8	3.75	3.75	6.75	14.25	Liquid
10	53.8	15	13.125	15	43.125	Use ½ tabs	40	26.7	3.75	3.75	6	13.5	Liquid
11	52.7	15	11.25	15	41.25	Use tabs	41	25.6	3.75	3.75	5.25	12.75	Liquid
12	51.5	15	9.375	15	39.375	Use ½ tabs	42	24.5	3.75	3.75	4.5	12	Liquid
13	50.3	15	7.5	15	37.5	Tablets	43	23.5	3.75	3.75	3.9	11.4	Liquid
	Switch to clorazepate solution**						44	22.6	3.75	3.15	3.9	10.8	Liquid
14	49.3	13.5	7.5	15	36	Liquid	45	21.6	3.3	3	3.9	10.2	Liquid
15	48.2	12	7.5	15	34.5	Liquid	46	20.6	3	3	3.6	9.6	Liquid
16	47.1	10.5	7.5	15	33	Liquid	47	19.5	3	3	3	9	Liquid
17	46	9	7.5	15	31.5	Liquid	48	18.5	2.7	2.7	3	8.4	Liquid
18	44.7	7.5	7.5	15	30	Liquid	49	17.4	2.7	2.4	2.7	7.8	Liquid
19	44.1	7.5	7.5	14.25	29.25	Liquid	50	16.3	2.4	2.4	2.4	7.2	Liquid
20	43.5	7.5	7.5	13.5	28.5	Liquid	51	15.1	2.1	2.1	2.4	6.6	Liquid
21	42.8	7.5	7.5	12.75	27.75	Liquid	52	13.9	2.1	1.8	2.1	6	Liquid
22	42.2	7.5	7.5	12	27	Liquid	53	13.3	1.8	1.8	2.1	5.7	Liquid
23	41.5	7.5	7.5	11.25	26.25	Liquid	54	12.7	1.8	1.8	1.8	5.4	Liquid
24	40.8	7.5	7.5	10.5	25.5	Liquid	55	12.1	1.8	1.5	1.8	5.1	Liquid
25	40	7.5	7.5	9.75	24.75	Liquid	56	11.5	1.5	1.5	1.8	4.8	Liquid
26	39.3	7.5	7.5	9	24	Liquid	57	10.8	1.5	1.5	1.5	4.5	Liquid
27	38.6	7.5	7.5	8.25	23.25	Liquid	58	10.2	1.5	1.2	1.5	4.2	Liquid
28	37.8	7.5	7.5	7.5	22.5	Liquid	59	9.5	1.2	1.2	1.5	3.9	Liquid
29	37	7.5	6.75	7.5	21.75	Liquid	60	8.9	1.2	1.2	1.2	3.6	Liquid
30	36.2	7.5	6	7.5	21	Liquid	61	8.2	1.2	0.9	1.2	3.3	Liquid
	See further steps in the right-hand column												

(Continued)

CHAPTER 3

(Continued)

Step	RO (%)	AM (mg)	PM (mg)	Night (mg)	Total daily dose (mg)	Form*	Step	RO (%)	AM (mg)	PM (mg)	Night (mg)	Total daily dose (mg)	Form*
62	7.5	0.9	0.9	1.2	3	Liquid	68	3.1	0.3	0.3	0.6	1.2	Liquid
63	6.8	0.9	0.9	0.9	2.7	Liquid	69	2.4	0.3	0.3	0.3	0.9	Liquid
64	6.1	0.9	0.6	0.9	2.4	Liquid	70	1.6	0.3	0	0.3	0.6	Liquid
65	5.4	0.6	0.6	0.9	2.1	Liquid	71	0.8	0	0	0.3	0.3	Liquid
66	4.6	0.6	0.6	0.6	1.8	Liquid	72	0	0	0	0	0	Liquid
67	3.9	0.6	0.3	0.6	1.5	Liquid							

See further steps in the right-hand column

RO = receptor occupancy; tabs = tablets
*Alternatively, these doses can be made up with a solution, prepared as above. In Europe, many of these doses will require a solution.

D. **An even slower taper** Some patients will be unable to taper at the slowest rates shown here and will need to taper by even smaller decrements, thus lengthening the overall period of tapering. Such a regimen could be constructed by placing intermediate steps in regimen C. For example, 30mg, 29.25mg, 28.5mg could be modified to 30mg, 29.625mg, 29.25mg, 28.875mg, 28.5mg and so on. Further intermediate steps could also be added.

Micro-tapering: The tables show how to make reductions at intervals of 1–4 weeks. An alternative approach is called 'micro-tapering' whereby very small dose reductions are made every day, as explained in 'Other considerations in tapering benzodiazepines and z-drugs.' Micro-tapering rates can be calculated from the table above by dividing the change in dose for each step by 14 or 28 days. For example, for the moderate regimen reduction of 60mg to 56.25mg over 14 days each day is approximately equivalent to a reduction of 0.3mg per day, or 0.1mg reduction per dose (when dosed three times a day). By the end of this regimen the rate of reduction would have slowed down to a reduction of 0.02mg each day (0.007mg reduction each dose). The rate can be adjusted if withdrawal symptoms become too unpleasant.

Switching guide from clorazepate to diazepam: An alternative to a direct taper from clorazepate is to switch to diazepam before tapering from this drug, as outlined in 'Switching to longer-acting benzodiazepines to taper'. A 15mg dose of clorazepate is equivalent to 10mg diazepam.[10] Switching could be performed by steps of 15mg of clorazepate made every week (or as tolerated by the patient).

Steps	Morning	Afternoon	Evening	Daily diazepam equivalent
Start	22.5mg clorazepate	15mg clorazepate	22.5mg clorazepate	40mg
1	7.5mg clorazepate 10mg diazepam	15mg clorazepate	22.5mg clorazepate	40mg
2	7.5mg clorazepate 10mg diazepam	stop clorazepate 10mg diazepam	22.5mg clorazepate	40mg
3	7.5mg clorazepate 10mg diazepam	stop clorazepate 10mg diazepam	7.5mg clorazepate 10mg diazepam	40mg
4	stop clorazepate 15mg diazepam	10mg diazepam	7.5mg clorazepate 10mg diazepam	40mg
5	15mg diazepam	10mg diazepam	stop clorazepate 15mg diazepam	40mg
6	20mg diazepam	switch dosing to morning and evening	20mg diazepam	40mg
	Continue to taper as for 40mg diazepam (see diazepam section).			

References

1. Chouinard G. Issues in the clinical use of benzodiazepines: potency, withdrawal, and rebound. *J Clin Psychiatry* 2004; 65 Suppl 5: 7–12.
2. FDA Drug Safety Communication. FDA requiring Boxed Warning updated to improve safe use of benzodiazepine drug class. 2020. https://www.fda.gov/drugs/drug-safety-and-availability/fda-requiring-boxed-warning-updated-improve-safe-use-benzodiazepine-drug-class#:~:text=FDA is requiring the Boxed,and life-threatening side effects.
3. National Library of Medicine NIH Daily Med. CLORAZEPATE DIPOTASSIUM tablet Boxed Warning. 2023. https://dailymed.nlm.nih.gov/dailymed/drugInfo.cfm?setid=a4b80e69-b7c7-471a-8ce8-4e992808c669.
4. Rickels K, Schweizer, E., Csanalosi I, Case WG, Chung H. Long-term treatment of anxiety and risk of withdrawal: prospective comparison of clorazepate and buspirone. *Arch Gen Psychiatry* 1988; 45: 444–50.
5. Riss J, Cloyd J, Gates J, Collins S. Benzodiazepines in epilepsy: pharmacology and pharmacokinetics. *Acta Neurol Scand* 2008; 118: 69–86.
6. Brouillet E, Chavoix C, Bottlaender M, et al. In vivo bidirectional modulatory effect of benzodiazepine receptor ligands on GABAergic transmission evaluated by positron emission tomography in non-human primates. *Brain Res* 1991; 557: 167–76.
7. Holford N. Pharmacodynamic principles and the time course of delayed and cumulative drug effects. *Transl Clin Pharmacol* 2018; 26: 56–9.
8. Horowitz M, Taylor D. Withdrawing from benzodiazepines and z-drugs (in preparation).
9. Horowitz MA, Taylor D. Tapering of SSRI treatment to mitigate withdrawal symptoms. *The Lancet Psychiatry* 2019; 6: 538–46.
10. Ashton H. Benzodiazepines: how they work and how to withdraw (The Ashton Manual). Newcastle University, 2002. http://www.benzo.org.uk/manual/bzcha01.htm (accessed 11 July 2023).
11. DRUGBANK ONLINE. Clorazepic acid. https://go.drugbank.com/drugs/DB00628 (accessed 5 July 2023).
12. Guina J, Merrill B. Benzodiazepines II: waking up on sedatives: providing optimal care when inheriting benzodiazepine prescriptions in transfer patients. *J Clin Med Res* 2018; 7. doi:10.3390/jcm7020020.
13. Framer A. What I have learnt from helping thousands of people taper off psychotropic medications. *Ther Adv Psychopharmacol* 2021; 11: 204512532199127.

CHAPTER 3

Diazepam

Trade names: Valium, Antenex, Apaurin, Apozepam, Apzepam, Diastat, Diazepam Intensol, Diazepan, Hexalid, Normabel, Pax, Stedon, Stesolid, Tranquirit, Valaxona, Valtoco, Vival.

Description: Diazepam is a medium-potency,[1] long-acting benzodiazepine. It is a positive allosteric modulator of the gamma-aminobutyric acid (GABA) type A receptor, which it affects by binding to the benzodiazepine binding site.[2]

Withdrawal effects: Diazepam, like other benzodiazepines, carries a boxed warning from the FDA that highlights that physical dependence and withdrawal effects can occur when the drug is taken 'for several days to weeks, even as prescribed'.[3,4] Not everyone who stops diazepam will experience withdrawal and some of those who do will only experience mild symptoms – this probably depends on drug dose, duration of use and individual factors. However, in a very few instances, stopping abruptly can cause seizures and can be life threatening. Numerous other physical, cognitive and psychological withdrawal symptoms, outlined earlier in the chapter are also possible, which can last 'for several weeks to more than 12 months' after stopping according to the FDA.[3,4]

Peak plasma: 1–1.5 hours.[4]

Half-life: Diazepam has a half-life of 1–2 days. Diazepam's active metabolite N-desmethyldiazepam has a half-life of up to 100 hours. The elimination half-life increases by an hour for every year over 20 years of age.[4] Diazepam accumulates upon multiple dosing and there is some evidence that the terminal elimination half-life is slightly prolonged. Diazepam is sometimes dosed as often as three times[5] a day, but because of its long elimination half-life less frequent dosing (including every-other-day) may be feasible without provoking inter-dose withdrawal. People sensitive to withdrawal effects may not tolerate the plasma level variation this produces.[6]

Receptor occupancy: The relationship between dose of diazepam and the occupancy of its major target $GABA_A$ is hyperbolic.[7] Benzodiazepines demonstrate a hyperbolic relationship between dose and clinical effects,[8] which may be relevant to withdrawal effects. Dose reductions made by linear amounts (e.g. 60mg, 45mg, 30mg, 15mg, 0mg) will cause increasingly large reductions in effect, which may cause increasingly severe withdrawal effects (Figure 3.13a). To produce equal-sized reductions in effect on receptor occupancy will require hyperbolically reducing doses (Figure 3.13b),[9] which informs the reductions presented.

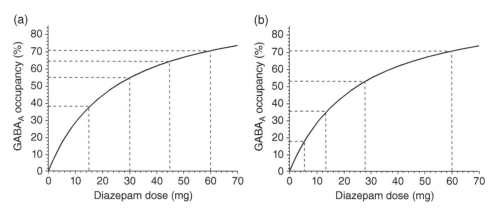

Figure 3.13 (a) Linear reductions of dose cause increasingly large reductions in effect on receptor targets, possibly associated with more withdrawal effects. (b) Even reductions of effect at target receptors requires hyperbolic dose reductions. The final dose before stopping will need to be very small so that this step down is not larger (in terms of effect on receptor occupancy) than previous reductions.

Available formulations: As tablets and liquid.

Tablets

Dosage	UK	Europe	USA	Australia	Canada
2mg	✓	✓	✓	✓	✓
5mg	✓	✓	✓	✓	✓
10mg	✓	✓	✓	✓	✓

Liquids

Oral solutions	UK	Europe	USA	Australia	Canada
5mg/mL	–	–	✓	–	–
2mg/5mL (0.4mg/mL)	✓	–	–	–	–
5mg/5mL (1mg/mL)	–	–	✓	–	–
10mg/mL	–	✓	–	–	–
10mg/10mL (1mg/mL)	–	–	–	✓	–

Dilutions: Diazepam is widely available in small dosage units so liquid dilutions may only be necessary in very slow tapering. In the USA, the manufacturer recommends that the 5mg/mL (Intensol) solution should be mixed with water or other diluents to make a less concentrated solution for use.[10] Dilution in water might cause precipitation of the drug and so the resulting mixture should be shaken vigorously before use to produce dispersal. As its stability cannot be assured it should be made up fresh each day.

USA dilutions	Solution required	How to prepare solution
Doses ≥ 1mg	5mg/mL	Original solution
Doses < 1mg	1mg/mL	Mix 0.5mL of original solution with 2mL of water*

EU dilutions	Solution required	How to prepare solution
Doses ≥ 2mg	10mg/mL	Original solution
Doses < 2mg	1mg/mL	Mix 0.5mL of original solution with 4.5mL of water*

*Other dilutions are possible to produce different concentrations. These are provided as examples.

Off-label options: In order to follow the regimens suggested in some cases, where no liquid versions are available, smaller doses are required than can be made using commercially available tablets and capsules. Guidelines for people who cannot swallow tablets[11] suggest that diazepam tablets can be dispersed in water for administration. It takes more than a couple of minutes to disintegrate.[11] The tablet may be crushed with a spoon or pestle and mortar before mixing with water to speed up this process. For example, water could be added to a 2mg tablet to make up a 20mL suspension (concentration 1mg in 10mL or 0.1mg/mL). The suspension should be shaken vigorously before use. As its stability cannot be assured it should be consumed immediately, and any unused suspension discarded. Some patients use full-fat milk to make liquid preparations. Benzodiazepines are more soluble in oil or fat than in water.[12] When mixed with milk, some or all of the drug will dissolve in the milk fat. This should form an evenly dispersed emulsion when shaken vigorously. The measured dose should be taken immediately after shaking and the remainder discarded.

Other options to make up small doses include having compounding pharmacies make up suspensions or smaller dose capsules or tablets, including the option of 'tapering strips'.[13] **Worked example:** To illustrate how to calculate volumes to make up a given dose using a liquid a worked example is provided. To make up 0.5mg of diazepam using the 2mg/5mL solution (0.4mg/mL) will require 0.5/0.4 = 1.25mL.

Deprescribing notes There are no established guides to determine the rate of taper for someone stopping benzodiazepines. Withdrawal is known to be more severe for people who have used benzodiazepines which are shorter acting for longer periods, at higher doses, and for those who have experienced withdrawal in the past on reducing, stopping or missing a dose.[14,15] The size of the initial reduction can be estimated based on these factors (see 'Tapering benzodiazepines and z-drugs in practice'), with patient preference also taken into account. Sometimes an even smaller reduction to start with may be advisable to boost a patient's confidence that they can taper if performed carefully.

Each reduction should be made when the withdrawal symptoms from the previous reduction have largely resolved so that subsequent reductions do not lead to cumulative withdrawal symptoms. Withdrawal symptoms should not be too unpleasant: a rate of reduction should be aimed at that produces tolerable withdrawal symptoms that abate within a week or two. Allowing for a sufficient observation period, reductions can therefore be made about every 1–4 weeks, depending on how long it takes withdrawal symptoms to resolve. If withdrawal symptoms are moderately severe or take longer than a couple of weeks to resolve, dose reductions should be postponed until symptoms resolve and then made more gradually by choosing a slower tapering rate. If severe withdrawal symptoms occur then the patient should return to a higher dose, wait until symptoms resolve and thereafter taper at a slower rate.

Suggested direct taper schedules for diazepam: Please note that none of these regimens should be seen as prescriptive – patients should not be compelled to adhere strictly to them. They are given as example regimens and are not 'set and forget' but should be modified in order to ensure that withdrawal symptoms are tolerable throughout a taper. For example, intermediate steps halfway between the doses listed could be added to make a more gradual taper. Ultimately, it is the patient's experience of withdrawal that should guide the rate of taper.

A. **A faster taper** with up to 5 percentage points of GABA$_A$ occupancy between each step – with reductions made every 1–4 weeks*.

Step	RO (%)	AM (mg)	PM (mg)	Total daily dose (mg)	Form	Step	RO (%)	AM (mg)	PM (mg)	Total daily dose (mg)	Form
1	70.8	30	30	60	Use tablets	13	36.2	7	7	14	Use tablets
2	69	25	30	55	Use tablets	14	32.7	6	6	12	Use tablets
3	66.9	25	25	50	Use tablets	15	28.8	5	5	10	Use tablets
4	64.6	20	25	45	Use tablets	16	24.5	4	4	8	Use tablets
5	61.8	20	20	40	Use tablets	17	22.1	3	4	7	Use ½ tablets**
6	59.3	18	18	36	Use tablets	18	19.5	3	3	6	Use ½ tablets**
7	56.4	16	16	32	Use tablets	19	16.8	2	3	5	Use ½ tablets**
8	53.1	14	14	28	Use tablets	20	13.9	2	2	4	Use tablets
9	49.3	12	12	24	Use tablets	21	10.8	1	2	3	Use ½ tablets**
10	44.7	10	10	20	Use tablets	22	7.5	1	1	2	Use ½ tablets**
11	42.2	9	9	18	Use tablets	23	3.9	0.5	0.5	1	Use ¼ tablets**
12	39.3	8	8	16	Use tablets	24	0	0	0	0	

See further steps in the right-hand column

RO = receptor occupancy

*Patients who have been on the medication for only a few weeks will probably be able to taper more quickly and might follow every second or third step of this regimen and make reductions every few days or so. Normally the duration of the taper should not be longer than the period that the patient has been on the drug for people who have only taken it for a few weeks. For example, if diazepam is taken for 3 weeks, the taper should be less than 3 weeks. However, the FDA has issued an alert regarding dependence and withdrawal from benzodiazepines indicating that some people can experience withdrawal effects after just a few days of use,[3] therefore necessitating slower tapering.

**Alternatively, a liquid formulation of the drug could be used for these doses.

CHAPTER 3

B. **A moderate taper** with up to 2.5 percentage points of $GABA_A$ occupancy between each step – with reductions made every 1–4 weeks.

Step	RO (%)	AM (mg)	PM (mg)	Total daily dose (mg)	Form*	Step	RO (%)	AM (mg)	PM (mg)	Total daily dose (mg)	Form
1	70.8	30	30	60	Use tablets	23	34.5	6.5	6.5	13	Use ¼ tablets*
2	69.4	28	28	56	Use tablets	24	32.7	6	6	12	Use tablets
3	67.8	26	26	52	Use tablets	25	30.8	5.5	5.5	11	Use ¼ tablets*
4	66	24	24	48	Use tablets	26	28.8	5	5	10	Use tablets
5	64	22	22	44	Use tablets	27	26.7	4.5	4.5	9	Use ¼ tablets*
6	61.8	20	20	40	Use tablets	28	24.5	4	4	8	Use tablets
7	60.6	19	19	38	Use tablets	29	23.3	3.5	4	7.5	Use ¼ tablets*
8	59.3	18	18	36	Use tablets	30	22.1	3.5	3.5	7	Use ¼ tablets*
9	57.9	17	17	34	Use tablets	31	20.8	3	3.5	6.5	Use ¼ tablets*
10	56.4	16	16	32	Use tablets	32	19.5	3	3	6	Use ½ tablets*
11	54.8	15	15	30	Use tablets	33	18.2	2.5	3	5.5	Use ¼ tablets*
12	53.1	14	14	28	Use tablets	34	16.8	2.5	2.5	5	Use ¼ tablets*
13	51.3	13	13	26	Use tablets	35	15.4	2	2.5	4.5	Use ¼ tablets*
14	49.3	12	12	24	Use tablets	36	13.9	2	2	4	Use tablets
15	47.1	11	11	22	Use tablets	37	12.4	1.5	2	3.5	Use ¼ tablets*
16	44.7	10	10	20	Use tablets	38	10.8	1.5	1.5	3	Use ¼ tablets*
17	43.5	9.5	9.5	19	Use ¼ tablets*	39	9.2	1	1.5	2.5	Use ¼ tablets*
18	42.2	9	9	18	Use tablets	40	7.5	1	1	2	Use ½ tablets*
19	40.8	8.5	8.5	17	Use ¼ tablets*	41	5.7	0.5	1	1.5	Use ¼ tablets*
20	39.3	8	8	16	Use tablets	42	3.9	0.5	0.5	1	Use ¼ tablets*
21	37.8	7.5	7.5	15	Use ¼ tablets*	43	2	0	0.5	0.5	Use ¼ tablets*
22	36.2	7	7	14	Use tablets	44	0	0	0	0	
See further steps in the right-hand column											

RO = receptor occupancy
*Alternatively, a liquid formulation of the drug could be used for these doses. Or, a slightly higher dose could be taken at night using half tablets. E.g. 8mg morning and 9mg night to make up 17mg total, using half tablets.

C. **A slower taper** with up to 1.3 percentage points of $GABA_A$ occupancy between each step – with reductions made every 1–4 weeks.

Step	RO (%)	AM (mg)	PM (mg)	Total daily dose (mg)	Form	Step	RO (%)	AM (mg)	PM (mg)	Total daily dose (mg)	Form
1	70.8	30	30	60	Use tablets	31	44.7	10	10	20	Use tablets
2	70.1	28	30	58	Use tablets	32	44.1	9.5	10	19.5	Use ¼ tablets*
3	69.4	28	28	56	Use tablets	33	43.5	9.5	9.5	19	Use ¼ tablets*
4	68.6	26	28	54	Use tablets	34	42.8	9	9.5	18.5	Use ¼ tablets*
5	67.8	26	26	52	Use tablets	35	42.2	9	9	18	Use tablets
6	66.9	24	26	50	Use tablets	36	41.5	8.5	9	17.5	Use ¼ tablets*
7	66	24	24	48	Use tablets	37	40.8	8.5	8.5	17	Use ¼ tablets*
8	65.1	22	24	46	Use tablets	38	40	8	8.5	16.5	Use ¼ tablets*
9	64	22	22	44	Use tablets	39	39.3	8	8	16	Use tablets
10	63	20	22	42	Use tablets	40	38.6	7.5	8	15.5	Use ¼ tablets*
11	61.8	20	20	40	Use tablets	41	37.8	7.5	7.5	15	Use ¼ tablets*
12	61.2	19	20	39	Use tablets	42	37	7	7.5	14.5	Use ¼ tablets*
13	60.6	19	19	38	Use tablets	43	36.2	7	7	14	Use tablets
14	60	18	19	37	Use tablets	44	35.3	6.5	7	13.5	Use ¼ tablets*
15	59.3	18	18	36	Use tablets	45	34.5	6.5	6.5	13	Use ¼ tablets*
16	58.6	17	18	35	Use tablets	46	33.6	6	6.5	12.5	Use ¼ tablets*
17	57.9	17	17	34	Use tablets	47	32.7	6	6	12	Use tablets
18	57.2	16	17	33	Use tablets	48	31.8	5.5	6	11.5	Use ¼ tablets*
19	56.4	16	16	32	Use tablets	49	30.8	5.5	5.5	11	Use ¼ tablets*
20	55.7	15	16	31	Use tablets	50	29.8	5	5.5	10.5	Use ¼ tablets*
21	54.8	15	15	30	Use tablets	51	28.8	5	5	10	Use tablets
22	54	14	15	29	Use tablets	Switch to liquid formulation of diazepam **					
23	53.1	14	14	28	Use tablets	52	28	4.8	4.8	9.6	Liquid
24	52.2	13	14	27	Use tablets	53	27.1	4.6	4.6	9.2	Liquid
25	51.3	13	13	26	Use tablets	54	26.3	4.4	4.4	8.8	Liquid
26	50.3	12	13	25	Use tablets	55	25.4	4.2	4.2	8.4	Liquid
27	49.3	12	12	24	Use tablets	56	24.5	4	4	8	Liquid
28	48.2	11	12	23	Use tablets	57	23.5	3.8	3.8	7.6	Liquid
29	47.1	11	11	22	Use tablets	58	22.6	3.6	3.6	7.2	Liquid
30	46	10	11	21	Use tablets	59	21.6	3.4	3.4	6.8	Liquid
See further steps in the right-hand column											*(Continued)*

CHAPTER 3

(Continued)

Step	RO (%)	AM (mg)	PM (mg)	Total daily dose (mg)	Form	Step	RO (%)	AM (mg)	PM (mg)	Total daily dose (mg)	Form
60	20.6	3.2	3.2	6.4	Liquid	74	8.9	1.2	1.2	2.4	Liquid
61	19.5	3	3	6	Liquid	75	8.2	1.1	1.1	2.2	Liquid
62	18.5	2.8	2.8	5.6	Liquid	76	7.5	1	1	2	Liquid
63	17.4	2.6	2.6	5.2	Liquid	77	6.8	0.9	0.9	1.8	Liquid
64	16.3	2.4	2.4	4.8	Liquid	78	6.1	0.8	0.8	1.6	Liquid
65	15.1	2.2	2.2	4.4	Liquid	79	5.4	0.7	0.7	1.4	Liquid
66	13.9	2	2	4	Liquid	80	4.6	0.6	0.6	1.2	Liquid
67	13.3	1.9	1.9	3.8	Liquid	81	3.9	0.5	0.5	1	Liquid
68	12.7	1.8	1.8	3.6	Liquid	82	3.1	0.4	0.4	0.8	Liquid
69	12.1	1.7	1.7	3.4	Liquid	83	2.4	0.3	0.3	0.6	Liquid
70	11.5	1.6	1.6	3.2	Liquid	84	1.6	0.2	0.2	0.4	Liquid
71	10.8	1.5	1.5	3	Liquid	85	0.8	0.1	0.1	0.2	Liquid
72	10.2	1.4	1.4	2.8	Liquid	86	0	0	0	0	
73	9.5	1.3	1.3	2.6	Liquid						

See further steps in the right-hand column

RO = receptor occupancy
*Alternatively, a liquid formulation of the drug could be used for these doses. Or, a slightly higher dose could be taken at night using half tablets where this is possible. E.g. 8mg morning and 9mg night to make up 17mg total, using half tablets.
**See above for manufacturer's liquid or off-label options.

D. **An even slower taper** Some patients will be unable to taper at the slowest rates shown here and will need to taper by even smaller decrements, thus lengthening the overall period of tapering. Such a regimen could be constructed by placing intermediate steps in regimen C. For example, 60mg, 58mg, 56mg could be modified to 60mg, 59mg, 58mg, 57mg, 56mg and so on. Further intermediate steps could also be added.

Micro-tapering: The tables above show how to make reductions at intervals of 1–4 weeks. An alternative approach is called 'micro-tapering' whereby very small dose reductions are made every day, as explained in 'Other considerations in tapering benzodiazepines and z-drugs.' Micro-tapering rates can be calculated from the above by dividing the change in dose for each step by 14 or 28 days. For example, for the moderate regimen reduction of 60mg to 56mg over 14 days is equivalent to a reduction of 0.3mg per day, or 0.15mg reduction per dose (when dosed twice a day). By the end of the taper this rate will reduce to reductions of 0.04mg a day (a rate many patients report to be tolerable).[16] This rate can be adjusted if withdrawal symptoms become too unpleasant.

References

1. Chouinard G. Issues in the clinical use of benzodiazepines: potency, withdrawal, and rebound. *J Clin Psychiatry* 2004; 65 Suppl 5: 7–12.

2. PharmGKB. PharmGKB. https://www.pharmgkb.org/literature/6754762 (accessed 19 March 2023).

3. FDA Drug Safety Communication. FDA requiring boxed warning updated to improve safe use of benzodiazepine drug class. 2020. https://www.fda.gov/drugs/drug-safety-and-availability/fda-requiring-boxed-warning-updated-improve-safe-use-benzodiazepine-drug-class#:~:text=FDA is requiring the Boxed,and life-threatening side effects (accessed 3 July 2023).

4. FDA. Medication guide Diazepam. www.accessdata.fda.gov. https://www.accessdata.fda.gov/drugsatfda_docs/label/2021/013263s096lbl.pdf (accessed 23 March 2023).

5. Diazepam 2mg/5mL Oral Suspension – Summary of Product Characteristics (SmPC) – (emc). https://www.medicines.org.uk/emc/product/7212/smpc (accessed 23 March 2023).

6. Ashton H. Benzodiazepines: how they work and how to withdraw (The Ashton Manual). Newcastle University, 2002. http://www.benzo.org.uk/manual/bzcha01.htm (accessed 11 July 2023).

7. Brouillet E, Chavoix C, Bottlaender M, et al. In vivo bidirectional modulatory effect of benzodiazepine receptor ligands on GABAergic transmission evaluated by positron emission tomography in non-human primates. *Brain Res* 1991; 557: 167–76.

8. Horowitz M, Taylor D. Withdrawing from benzodiazepines and z-drugs (in preparation).

9. Horowitz MA, Taylor D. Tapering of SSRI treatment to mitigate withdrawal symptoms. *The Lancet Psychiatry* 2019; 6: 538–46.

10. Diazepam Oral Solution, CIV, 5mg per 5mL and Diazepam Intensol™ Oral Solution (Concentrate), CIV, 25mg per 5mL (5mg/mL). https://dailymed.nlm.nih.gov/dailymed/fda/fdaDrugXsl.cfm?setid=e435e56f-e6eb-4fe9-9a8f-e11527778fc1&type=display (accessed 23 March 2023).

11. Colchester Medicines Information. MOC guidelines for tablet crushing in patients with swallowing difficulties. Colchester Hospital University, 2018.

12. Macheras PE, Koupparis MA, Antimisiaris SG. Drug binding and solubility in milk. *Pharm Res* 1990; 7: 537–41.

13. Groot PC, van Os J. Successful use of tapering strips for hyperbolic reduction of antidepressant dose: a cohort study. *Ther Adv Psychopharmacol* 2021; 11: 20451253211039330.

14. Guina J, Merrill B. Benzodiazepines II: Waking up on sedatives. providing optimal care when inheriting benzodiazepine prescriptions in transfer patients. *J Clin Med Res* 2018; 7. doi:10.3390/jcm7020020.

15. Framer A. What I have learnt from helping thousands of people taper off psychotropic medications. *Ther Adv Psychopharmacol* 2021; 11: 204512532199127.

16. BenzoBuddies Community Forum. http://www.benzobuddies.org/forum/index.php (accessed 18 March 2023).

Estazolam

Trade name: ProSom, Nuctalon.

Description: Estazolam is an intermediate-acting benzodiazepine.[1] It is a positive allosteric modulator of the gamma-aminobutyric acid (GABA) type A receptor, which it affects by binding to the benzodiazepine binding site.[2]

Withdrawal effects: The FDA warns that '[T]he continued use of estazolam may lead to clinically significant physical dependence and that abrupt discontinuation or rapid dosage reduction of estazolam may precipitate acute withdrawal reactions, which can be life threatening. Inform patients that in some cases, patients taking benzodiazepines have developed a protracted withdrawal syndrome with withdrawal symptoms lasting weeks to more than 12 months.'[1] The manufacturer of estazolam warns that the following symptoms may occur upon discontinuation: 'abnormal involuntary movements, anxiety, blurred vision, depersonalization, depression, derealization, dizziness, fatigue, gastrointestinal adverse reactions (e.g., nausea, vomiting, diarrhoea, weight loss, decreased appetite), headache, hyperacusis, hypertension, irritability, insomnia, memory impairment, muscle pain and stiffness, panic attacks, photophobia, restlessness, tachycardia, and tremor. More severe acute withdrawal signs and symptoms, including life-threatening reactions, have included catatonia, convulsions, delirium tremens, depression, hallucinations, mania, psychosis, seizures, and suicidality'.[1]

Peak plasma: 2 hours.[1]

Half-life and dosing: 10–24 hours.[1] The manufacturer recommends giving the dose once at night.[1] Dosing less often (including every-other-day dosing) is not recommended for the tapering process because the changes in plasma levels produced may precipitate withdrawal symptoms.

Receptor occupancy: The relationship between dose of estazolam and the occupancy of its major target GABA$_A$ is hyperbolic (as a consequence of the law of mass action).[3,4] Benzodiazepines demonstrate a hyperbolic relationship between dose and clinical effects,[5] which may be relevant to withdrawal effects. Dose reductions made by linear amounts (e.g. 2mg, 1.5mg, 1mg, 0.5mg, 0mg) will cause increasingly large reductions in effect, which may cause increasingly severe withdrawal effects (Figure 3.14a). To produce equal-sized reductions in effect on receptor occupancy will require hyperbolically

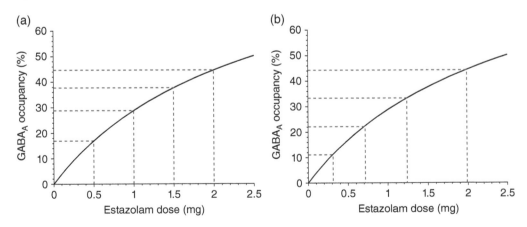

Figure 3.14 (a) Linear reductions of dose cause increasingly large reductions in effect on receptor targets, possibly associated with more withdrawal effects. (b) Even reductions of effect at target receptors requires hyperbolic dose reductions, slightly different from linear reductions in this case. The final dose before stopping will need to be small so that this step down is not larger (in terms of effect on receptor occupancy) than previous reductions.

CHAPTER 3

reducing doses (Figure 3.14b),[6] which informs the reductions presented later. This relationship was derived by converting the receptor occupancy curve for diazepam[4] to the equivalent estazolam dose.[6]

Available formulations: As tablets.

Tablets

Dosage	UK	Europe*	USA	Australia	Canada
1mg	–	–	✓	–	–
2mg	–	✓	✓	–	–

*Some formulations are available in France, Denmark, Italy, Poland and Portugal.

Off-label options: In order to follow the regimens suggested smaller doses are sometimes required than can be made using commercially available tablets and capsules (where no liquid versions of the medication are available). A suspension can be made by adding water to tablets.[7] The disintegration process can be hastened by crushing the tablet with a spoon or pestle and mortar. For example, water could be added to a crushed 1mg tablet to make up a 10mL suspension (concentration 1mg in 10mL, or 0.1mg/mL). The suspension should be shaken vigorously or stirred before use to aid dispersal so that the drug is evenly distributed within the mixture. The measured dose should be taken before settling occurs. As stability cannot be assured, the dose should be consumed immediately, and any unused suspension discarded. Benzodiazepines are more soluble in oil or fat than in water.[8] When mixed with full-fat milk, some or all of the drug will dissolve in the milk fat. This should form an evenly dispersed emulsion when shaken vigorously. The measured dose should be taken immediately after shaking and the remainder discarded.

Another option is to switch to diazepam (see later) or to have a suspension or smaller doses of tablets or capsules made up by a compounding pharmacy.

Worked example: To illustrate how the volumes can be calculated in the regimens given, a worked example is provided. To make up 0.6mg of estazolam a 0.1mg/mL suspension can be used. The volume of 0.1mg/mL liquid required to give a dose of 0.6mg of estazolam is 0.6/0.1 = 6mL.

Deprescribing notes: There are two main methods for tapering from estazolam – a switch to a longer-acting benzodiazepine like diazepam, or a direct taper of estazolam itself. There are no established guides to determine the rate of taper for someone stopping benzodiazepines. Withdrawal is known to be more severe for people who have used benzodiazepines, which are shorter acting for longer periods, at higher doses, for those who have experienced withdrawal in the past on reducing, stopping or missing a dose, as well as those with evidence of tolerance or inter-dose withdrawal effects.[9,10] The size of the initial reduction can be estimated based on these factors (see 'Tapering benzodiazepines and z-drugs in practice'), with patient preference also taken into account. Sometimes an even smaller reduction to start with may be advisable to boost a patient's confidence that they can taper if performed carefully.

Each reduction should be made when the withdrawal symptoms from the previous reduction have largely resolved so that subsequent reductions do not lead to cumulative withdrawal symptoms. Withdrawal symptoms should not be too unpleasant: a rate of reduction should be aimed for that produces tolerable withdrawal symptoms that abate within a week or two. Allowing for a sufficient observation period, reductions can therefore be made about every 1–4 weeks, depending on how long it takes withdrawal symptoms to resolve. If withdrawal symptoms are moderately severe or take longer than a couple of weeks to resolve, dose reductions should be postponed until symptoms resolve and then made more gradually by choosing a slower tapering rate. If severe withdrawal symptoms occur then the patient should return to a higher dose, wait until symptoms resolve and thereafter taper at a slower rate.

Suggested direct taper schedules for estazolam: Please note that none of these regimens should be seen as prescriptive – patients should not be compelled to adhere strictly to them. They are given as example regimens and are not 'set and forget' but should be modified in order to ensure that withdrawal symptoms are tolerable throughout a taper. For example, intermediate steps halfway between the doses listed could be added to make a more gradual taper. Ultimately, it is the patient's experience of withdrawal that should guide the rate of taper.

A. **A faster taper** with up to 5 percentage points of $GABA_A$ occupancy between each step – with reductions made every 1–4 weeks*.

Step	RO (%)	Dose (mg)	Formulation	Step	RO (%)	Dose (mg)	Formulation
1	44.7	2	Use tablets	8	22.1	0.7	7mL
Switch to liquid formulation **(0.1mg/mL)****				9	19.5	0.6	6mL
2	42.2	1.8	18mL	10	16.8	0.5	5mL***
3	39.3	1.6	16mL	11	13.9	0.4	4mL
4	36.2	1.4	14mL	12	10.8	0.3	3mL
5	32.7	1.2	12mL	13	7.5	0.2	2mL
6	28.8	1	10mL***	14	3.9	0.1	1mL
7	24.5	0.8	8mL	15	0	0	–
See further steps in the right-hand column							

RO = receptor occupancy

*Patients who have been on the medication for only a few weeks will probably be able to taper more quickly and might follow every second or third step of this regimen and make reductions every few days or so. Normally the duration of the taper should not be longer than the period that the patient has been on the drug for people who have only taken it for a few weeks. For example, if estazolam is taken for 3 weeks the taper should be less than 3 weeks. However, the FDA has issued an alert regarding dependence and withdrawal from benzodiazepines indicating that some people can experience withdrawal effects after just a few days of use,[4] therefore necessitating slower tapering in these people.

**Liquid preparation (0.1mg/mL), prepared as above.

***Alternatively, a tablet or half a tablet could be used to make up these doses.

B. **A moderate taper** with up to 2.5 percentage points of $GABA_A$ occupancy between each step – with reductions made every 1–4 weeks.

Step	RO (%)	Dose (mg)	Formulation	Step	RO (%)	Dose (mg)	Formulation
1	44.7	2	Use tablets	15	22.1	0.7	7mL
Switch to liquid formulation **(0.1mg/mL)***				16	20.8	0.65	6.5mL
2	43.5	1.9	19mL	17	19.5	0.6	6mL
3	42.2	1.8	18mL	18	18.2	0.55	5.5mL
4	40.8	1.7	17mL	19	16.8	0.5	5mL**
5	39.3	1.6	16mL	20	15.4	0.45	4.5mL
6	37.8	1.5	15mL	21	13.9	0.4	4mL
7	36.2	1.4	14mL	22	12.4	0.35	3.5mL
8	34.5	1.3	13mL	23	10.8	0.3	3mL
9	32.7	1.2	12mL	24	9.2	0.25	2.5mL
10	30.8	1.1	11mL	25	7.5	0.2	2mL
11	28.8	1	10mL**	26	5.7	0.15	1.5mL
12	26.7	0.9	9mL	27	3.9	0.1	1mL
13	24.5	0.8	8mL	28	2	0.05	0.5mL
14	23.3	0.75	7.5mL	29	0	0	–
See further steps in the right-hand column							

RO = receptor occupancy
*Liquid, prepared as above.
**Alternatively, a tablet or half a tablet could be used to make up these doses.

CHAPTER 3

C. **A slower taper** with up to 1.3 percentage points of GABA$_A$ occupancy between each step – with reductions made every 1–4 weeks.

Step	RO (%)	Dose (mg)	Formulation	Step	RO (%)	Dose (mg)	Formulation
1	44.7	2	Use tablets	29	21.6	0.68	6.8mL
Switch to liquid formulation **(0.1mg/mL)***				30	20.6	0.64	6.4mL
2	44.1	1.95	19.5mL	31	19.5	0.6	6mL
3	43.5	1.9	19mL	32	18.5	0.56	5.6mL
4	42.8	1.85	18.5mL	33	17.4	0.52	5.2mL
5	42.2	1.8	18mL	34	16.3	0.48	4.8mL
6	41.5	1.75	17.5mL	35	15.1	0.44	4.4mL
7	40.8	1.7	17mL	36	13.9	0.4	4mL
8	40	1.65	16.5mL	37	13.3	0.38	3.8mL
9	39.3	1.6	16mL	38	12.7	0.36	3.6mL
10	38.6	1.55	15.5mL	39	12.1	0.34	3.4mL
11	37.8	1.5	15mL**	40	11.5	0.32	3.2mL
12	37	1.45	14.5mL	41	10.8	0.3	3mL
13	36.2	1.4	14mL	42	10.2	0.28	2.8mL
14	35.3	1.35	13.5mL	43	9.5	0.26	2.6mL
15	34.5	1.3	13mL	44	8.9	0.24	2.4mL
16	33.6	1.25	12.5mL	45	8.2	0.22	2.2mL
17	32.7	1.2	12mL	46	7.5	0.2	2mL
18	31.8	1.15	11.5mL	47	6.8	0.18	1.8mL
19	30.8	1.1	11mL	48	6.1	0.16	1.6mL
20	29.8	1.05	10.5mL	49	5.4	0.14	1.4mL
21	28.8	1	10mL**	50	4.6	0.12	1.2mL
22	28	0.96	9.6mL	51	3.9	0.1	1mL
23	27.1	0.92	9.2mL	52	3.1	0.08	0.8mL
24	26.3	0.88	8.8mL	53	2.4	0.06	0.6mL
25	25.4	0.84	8.4mL	54	1.6	0.04	0.4mL
26	24.5	0.8	8mL	55	0.8	0.02	0.2mL
27	23.5	0.76	7.6mL	56	0	0	–
28	22.6	0.72	7.2mL				
See further steps in the right-hand column							

RO = receptor occupancy
*Liquid, prepared as above.
**Alternatively, a tablet or half a tablet could be used to make up these doses.

D. **An even slower taper** Some patients will be unable to taper at the slowest rates shown here and will need to taper by even smaller decrements, thus lengthening the overall period of tapering. Such a regimen could be constructed by placing intermediate steps in regimen C. For example, 2mg, 1.95mg, 1.9mg, could be modified to be 2mg, 1.975mg, 1.95mg, 1.925mg, 1.9mg and so on. Further intermediate steps could also be added.

Micro-tapering: The tables above show how to make reductions at intervals of 1–4 weeks. An alternative approach is called 'micro-tapering' whereby very small dose reductions are made every day, as explained in 'Other considerations in tapering benzodiazepines and z-drugs.' Micro-tapering rates can be calculated from the above by dividing the change in dose for each step by 14 or 28 days and then dividing that dose in three doses during the day. For example, for the moderate regimen a reduction of 2mg to 1.9mg over 14 days is equivalent to a reduction of 0.007mg per day. By the end of the moderate regimen the rate of reduction would have slowed down to a reduction of 0.004mg each day. The rate can be adjusted if withdrawal symptoms become too unpleasant.

Switching guide from estazolam to diazepam: An alternative to a direct taper from estazolam is to switch to diazepam before tapering from this drug, as outlined in 'Switching to longer-acting benzodiazepines to taper' 2mg of estazolam is equivalent to 20mg diazepam.[6] Conversions of 1mg of estazolam can be made every week (or as tolerated by the patient).

Steps	Evening	Daily diazepam equivalent
1	2mg estazolam	20mg
2	1mg estazolam 10mg diazepam	20mg
3	Stop estazolam 20mg diazepam	20mg
Continue to taper as for 20mg diazepam (see diazepam section).		

References

1. Estazolam Tablets, USP C-IV Rx only. https://dailymed.nlm.nih.gov/dailymed/fda/fdaDrugXsl.cfm?setid=a1e3b4bf-22e9-430a-a768-4d86ae886c9e&type=display (accessed 29 April 2023).
2. Estazolam. https://www.guidetopharmacology.org/GRAC/LigandDisplayForward?tab=clinical&ligandId=7550 (accessed 6 May 2023).
3. Holford N. Pharmacodynamic principles and the time course of delayed and cumulative drug effects. *Transl Clin Pharmacol* 2018; 26: 56–59.
4. Brouillet E, Chavoix C, Bottlaender M, et al. In vivo bidirectional modulatory effect of benzodiazepine receptor ligands on GABAergic transmission evaluated by positron emission tomography in non-human primates. *Brain Res* 1991; 557: 167–76.
5. Horowitz M, Taylor D. Withdrawing from benzodiazepines and z-drugs (in preparation).
6. Ashton H. Benzodiazepines: how they work and how to withdraw (The Ashton Manual). Newcastle University, 2002. http://www.benzo.org.uk/manual/bzcha01.htm (accessed 11 July 2023).
7. Stahl SM. Estazolam. In: *Prescriber's Guide: Stahl's Essential Psychopharmacology*. Cambridge: Cambridge University Press, 2020: 281–4.
8. Macheras PE, Koupparis MA, Antimisiaris SG. Drug binding and solubility in milk. *Pharm Res* 1990; 7: 537–41.
9. Guina J, Merrill B. Benzodiazepines II: waking up on sedatives: providing optimal care when inheriting benzodiazepine prescriptions in transfer patients. *J Clin Med Res* 2018; 7. doi:10.3390/jcm7020020.
10. Framer A. What I have learnt from helping thousands of people taper off psychotropic medications. *Ther Adv Psychopharmacol* 2021; 11: 204512532199127.

CHAPTER 3

Eszopiclone

Trade name: Lunesta.

Description: Eszopiclone is a z-drug, or non-benzodiazepine hypnotic, which acts in a similar manner to benzodiazepines as a positive allosteric modulator of the $GABA_A$ receptor by binding to domains close to or allosterically coupled to benzodiazepine receptors.[1,2]

Withdrawal effects: Stopping z-drugs even when taken as prescribed can lead to withdrawal effects in as many as 30–45% of people.[1,3,4] The longer these drugs are used and the higher the dose taken the greater the risk of withdrawal.[5] Withdrawal symptoms are usually limited to insomnia and increased dreaming, but can include fatigue, nausea, flushing, light-headedness, uncontrolled crying, emesis, stomach cramps, panic attacks, nervousness, abdominal discomfort, hyperventilation, shallow breathing, angry feelings, cramping muscles and restlessness.[3] Seizures on withdrawal have mainly been reported after higher than usual doses.[3] The existence of protracted withdrawal syndromes in z-drugs has not been investigated, but it has been suggested that there should be little difference from benzodiazepine on this issue, given similar pharmacological effects.[6] An important mitigating factor may be that eszopiclone is nearly completely cleared each day (if taken once at night) thus avoiding prolonged receptor site activity.[7]

Peak plasma: Approximately 1 hour.[5]

Half-life and dosing: The elimination half-life is approximately 6 hours.[5] The manufacturer recommends taking the drug once at night.[5] Taking the drug less frequently (including every-other-day) is not recommended in tapering because of the risk of provoking withdrawal symptoms.

Receptor occupancy: The relationship between dose of eszopiclone and the occupancy of its major target $GABA_A$ is hyperbolic as a consequence of the law of mass action.[8] Z-drugs demonstrate a hyperbolic relationship between dose and clinical effects,[9] which may be relevant to withdrawal effects. Dose reductions made by linear amounts (e.g. 3mg, 2.25mg, 1.5mg, 0.75mg, 0mg) will cause slightly larger reductions in effect in each step, which may cause increasingly severe withdrawal effects (Figure 3.15a), although because of the nature of the occupancy curve hyperbolic tapering is not

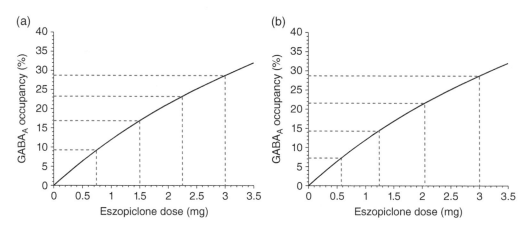

Figure 3.15 (a) Linear reductions of eszopiclone. (b) Hyperbolic reductions are fairly similar to linear reductions for eszopiclone because of the nature of the dose–occupancy relationship.

substantially different from linear tapering (Figure 3.15b),[10] which informs the reductions presented. The relationship was derived by converting the receptor occupancy curve for diazepam[11] to the equivalent eszopiclone dose.[12]

Available formulations: As tablets.

Tablets

Dosage	UK	Europe	USA	Australia	Canada
1mg	–	✓	✓	✓	✓
2mg	–	✓	✓	✓	✓
3mg	–	✓	✓	✓	✓

Off-label options: Smaller doses of eszopiclone than are commercially available as tablets may be required to assist tapering. Guidelines for people who cannot swallow tablets[13] recommend that eszopiclone tablets can be dispersed in water for administration. The tablet may be crushed with a spoon or pestle and mortar before mixing with water. For example, water could be added to a 1mg tablet to make up a 10mL suspension (concentration 1mg in 10mL or 0.1mg/mL). The suspension should be shaken vigorously before use. As its stability cannot be assured it should be consumed immediately, and any unused suspension discarded. Some patients use full-fat milk to make liquid preparations. Z-drugs are more soluble in oil or fat than in water.[14] When mixed with milk, some or all of the drug will dissolve in the milk fat. This should form an evenly dispersed emulsion when shaken vigorously. The measured dose should be taken immediately after shaking and the remainder discarded.

Other options include having a compounding pharmacy make up a suspension or smaller dose tablets or capsules, or switching to diazepam (see later).

Worked example: To illustrate how to calculate volumes to make up a given dose using a liquid, a worked example is provided. To make up 0.25mg of eszopiclone using a 0.1mg/mL suspension as outlined above will require a volume of 0.25/0.1 = 2.5mL.

Deprescribing notes: There are no established guides for determining the rate of taper for someone stopping benzodiazepines or z-drugs. The longer z-drugs are used and the higher the dose taken the greater the risk of withdrawal, according to their manufacturer.[4] The size of the initial reduction can be estimated based on these factors (see 'Tapering benzodiazepines and z-drugs in practice'), with patient preference also taken into account. Sometimes an even smaller reduction to start with may be advisable to boost a patient's confidence that they can taper if performed carefully.

Each reduction should be made when the withdrawal symptoms from the previous reduction have largely resolved so that subsequent reductions do not lead to cumulative withdrawal symptoms. Withdrawal symptoms should not be too unpleasant: a rate of reduction should be aimed for that produces tolerable withdrawal symptoms that abate within a week or two. Allowing for a sufficient observation period, reductions can therefore be made about every 1–2 weeks, depending on how long it takes withdrawal symptoms to resolve. If withdrawal symptoms are moderately severe or take longer than a couple of weeks to resolve, dose reductions should be postponed until symptoms resolve and then made more gradually by choosing a slower tapering rate. If severe withdrawal symptoms occur, then the patient should return to a higher dose, wait until symptoms resolve and thereafter taper at a slower rate.

Suggested direct taper schedules for eszopiclone: Please note that none of these regimens should be seen as prescriptive – patients should not be compelled to adhere to them strictly. They are given as example regimens and are not 'set and forget' but should be modified in order to ensure that withdrawal symptoms are tolerable throughout a taper. For example, intermediate steps halfway between the doses listed could be added to make a more gradual taper. Ultimately, it is the patient's experience of withdrawal that should guide the rate of taper.

A. **A faster taper** with up to 6.5 percentage points of $GABA_A$ occupancy between each step – with reductions made every 1–2 weeks*.

Step	RO (%)	Total daily dose (mg)	Formulation
1	28.8	3	Use tablets
2	25.2	2.5	Use ½ tablets**
3	21.2	2	Use tablets
4	16.8	1.5	Use ½ tablets**
5	11.9	1	Use tablets
6	6.3	0.5	Use ½ tablets**
7	0	0	

RO = receptor occupancy

*Patients who have been on the medication for only a few weeks will probably be able to taper more quickly and might follow every second or third step of this regimen and make reductions every few days or so. Normally the duration of the taper should not be longer than the period that the patient has been on the drug for people who have only taken it for a few weeks. For example, if eszopiclone is taken for 3 weeks the taper should be less than 3 weeks.

**Alternatively, a liquid formulation of the drug could be used for these doses, made up as above.

B. **A moderate taper** with up to 4 percentage points of $GABA_A$ occupancy between each step – with reductions made every 1–2 weeks.

Step	RO (%)	Total daily dose (mg)	Formulation	Step	RO (%)	Total daily dose (mg)	Formulation
1	28.8	3	Use tablets	7	11.9	1	Use ¼ tablets
2	25.2	2.5	Use ½ tablets*	8	9.2	0.75	Use ¾ tablets*
3	21.2	2	Use tablets	9	6.3	0.5	Use ½ tablets
4	19.1	1.75	Use ¾ tablets*	10	3.3	0.25	Use ¼ tablets*
5	16.8	1.5	Use ½ tablets*	11	0	0	
6	14.4	1.25	Use ¼ tablets*				
See further steps in the right-hand column							

RO = receptor occupancy

*Alternatively, a liquid formulation of the drug could be used for these doses.

C. **A slower taper** with up to 2.1 percentage points of $GABA_A$ occupancy between each step – with reductions made every 1–2 weeks.

Step	RO (%)	Total daily dose (mg)	Formulation	Step	RO (%)	Total daily dose (mg)	Formulation
1	28.8	3	Use tablets	11	10.8	0.9	9mL
2	27	2.75	Use ¾ tablets*	12	9.7	0.8	8mL
3	25.2	2.5	Use ½ tablets*	13	8.6	0.7	7mL
4	23.3	2.25	Use ¼ tablets*	14	7.5	0.6	6mL
5	21.2	2	Use tablets	15	6.3	0.5	5mL
Switch to **0.1mg/mL suspension****				16	5.1	0.4	4mL
6	19.5	1.8	18mL	17	3.9	0.3	3mL
7	17.7	1.6	16mL	18	2.6	0.2	2mL
8	15.9	1.4	14mL	19	1.3	0.1	1mL
9	13.9	1.2	12mL	20	0	0	
10	11.9	1	10mL***				
See further steps in the right-hand column							

RO = receptor occupancy
*Alternatively, a liquid formulation of the drug could be used for these doses.
**Prepared as above.
***Alternatively, this dose could be made with a tablet.

D. **An even slower taper** Some patients will be unable to taper at the slowest rates shown here and will need to taper by even smaller decrements, thus lengthening the overall period of tapering. Such a regimen could be constructed by placing intermediate steps in regimen C. For example, 2.5mg, 2.25mg, 2mg could be modified to 2.5mg, 2.375mg, 2.25mg, 2.125mg, 2mg and so on. Further intermediate steps could also be added.

Micro-tapering: The tables above show how to make reductions at intervals of 1–4 weeks. An alternative approach is called 'micro-tapering' whereby very small dose reductions are made every day, as explained in 'Other considerations in tapering benzodiazepines and z-drugs.' Micro-tapering rates can be calculated from the above by dividing the change in dose for each step by 14 or 28 days. For example, for the moderate regimen a reduction of 3mg to 2.5mg over 14 days is equivalent to approximately 0.04mg reduction per day. By the end of the taper this rate will be reduced to approximately 0.02mg per day. This rate can be slowed if withdrawal symptoms become too unpleasant.

Switch to diazepam: An alternative to a direct taper from eszopiclone is to switch to diazepam before tapering from this drug, as outlined in 'Switching to longer-acting benzodiazepines to taper'. However, as eszopiclone has a short half-life and is dosed once a day, it might be that less physical dependence will be produced in response to this drug than diazepam (present for the entire day).[7] Therefore, it may be easier to directly taper from eszopiclone than switching to diazepam. However, some people report inter-dose withdrawal symptoms from z-drugs – in which case a switch to a longer-acting benzodiazepine might be wise. A 3mg dose of eszopiclone is equivalent to 10mg of diazepam[12] and so a direct switch could be made to 10mg daily (or 5mg twice a day) from this dose, and then tapered according to the diazepam regimens.

References

1. What's wrong with prescribing hypnotics? *Drug Ther Bull* 2004; 42: 89–93.
2. Brielmaier BD. Eszopiclone (Lunesta): a new nonbenzodiazepine hypnotic agent. *Proc* 2006; 19: 54–9.
3. Lerner A, Klein M. Dependence, withdrawal and rebound of CNS drugs: an update and regulatory considerations for new drugs development. *Brain Commun* 2019; 1: fcz025.
4. Schifano F, Chiappini S, Corkery JM, Guirguis A. An insight into z-drug abuse and dependence: an examination of reports to the European Medicines Agency Database of suspected adverse drug reactions. *Int J Neuropsychopharmacol* 2019; 22: 270–7.
5. FDA. LUNESTA® (eszopiclone) tablets – Accessdata.fda.gov. FDA. https://www.accessdata.fda.gov/drugsatfda_docs/label/2014/021476s030lbl.pdf (accessed 25 March 2023).
6. Cosci F, Chouinard G. Acute and persistent withdrawal syndromes following discontinuation of psychotropic medications. *Psychother Psychosom* 2020; 89: 283–306.
7. Lader MH. Managing dependence and withdrawal with newer hypnotic medications in the treatment of insomnia. *The Primary Care Companion*. 2002. https://www.psychiatrist.com/pcc/sleep/managing-dependence-withdrawal-newer-hypnotic-medications (accessed 20 May 2023).
8. Holford N. Pharmacodynamic principles and the time course of delayed and cumulative drug effects. *Transl Clin Pharmacol* 2018; 26: 56–9.
9. Horowitz M, Taylor D. Withdrawing from benzodiazepines and z-drugs (in preparation).
10. Horowitz MA, Taylor D. Tapering of SSRI treatment to mitigate withdrawal symptoms. *The Lancet Psychiatry* 2019; 6: 538–46.
11. Brouillet E, Chavoix C, Bottlaender M, et al. In vivo bidirectional modulatory effect of benzodiazepine receptor ligands on GABAergic transmission evaluated by positron emission tomography in non-human primates. *Brain Res* 1991; 557: 167–76.
12. Ashton H. *Benzodiazepines: How They Work and How to Withdraw* (The Ashton Manual). Newcastle on Tyne, UK: Newcastle University, 2002. http://www.benzo.org.uk/manual/bzcha01.htm.
13. Bostwick JR, Demehri A. Pills to powder: an updated clinician's reference for crushable psychotropics. *Curr Psychiatr* 2017; 16: 46–9.
14. Macheras PE, Koupparis MA, Antimisiaris SG. Drug binding and solubility in milk. *Pharm Res* 1990; 7: 537–41.

Flurazepam

Trade names: Dalmadorm, Dalmane, Fluzepam.

Description: Flurazepam is a medium-potency benzodiazepine.[1] It is a positive allosteric modulator of the gamma-aminobutyric acid (GABA) type A receptor. It binds to the stereospecific benzodiazepine site on the receptor and enhances the inhibitory effect of GABA in the nervous system.[2] The UK manufacturer recommends that 'treatment should be as short as possible' and that generally treatment varies from a 'few days to two weeks with a maximum of four weeks, including the tapering off process'.[2]

Withdrawal effects: Flurazepam, as for other benzodiazepines, carries a boxed warning from the FDA, which highlights that physical dependence and withdrawal effects can occur when the drug is taken 'for several days to weeks, even as prescribed'.[3] Not everyone who stops flurazepam will experience withdrawal and some of those who do will only experience mild symptoms – this probably depends on drug dose, duration of use and individual factors. However, in a very few instances, stopping abruptly can cause seizures and can be life threatening. Numerous physical, cognitive and psychological withdrawal symptoms (outlined in 'Withdrawal effects from benzodiazepines and z-drugs') are possible, which can last 'for several weeks to more than 12 months' after stopping according to the FDA.[3]

Peak plasma: Following oral administration flurazepam is rapidly absorbed with peak maximum concentration after 1 to 3 hours.

Half-life and dosing: The half-life ranges from 40 to 114 hours. The manufacturer recommends taking the drug once a day at night.[2] The long half-life may enable less often than once a day dosing during tapering, but in some sensitive patients this might precipitate withdrawal effects.

Receptor occupancy: The relationship between dose of flurazepam and the occupancy of its major target GABA$_A$ is hyperbolic according to the law of mass action.[4,5] Benzodiazepines demonstrate a hyperbolic relationship between dose and clinical effects,[6] which may be relevant to withdrawal effects. Dose reductions made by linear amounts (e.g. 30mg, 22.5mg, 15mg, 7.5mg, 0mg) will cause increasingly large reductions in effect, which may cause increasingly severe withdrawal effects (Figure 3.16a). To produce equal-sized reductions in effect on receptor occupancy will require hyperbolically reducing doses (Figure 3.16b),[7]

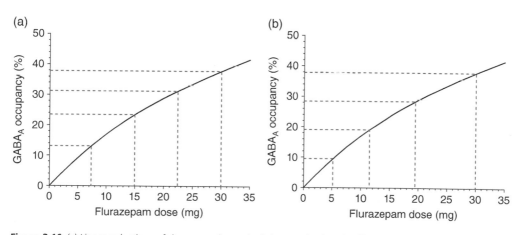

Figure 3.16 (a) Linear reductions of dose cause increasingly large reductions in effect on receptor targets, possibly associated with more withdrawal effects. (b) Even reductions of effect at target receptors requires hyperbolic dose reductions, slightly different from linear reductions in this case. The final dose before stopping will need to be small so that this step down is not larger (in terms of effect on receptor occupancy) than previous reductions.

CHAPTER 3

which informs the reductions presented. The relationship was derived by converting the receptor occupancy curve for diazepam[4] to the equivalent flurazepam dose.[8]

Available formulations: As tablets and capsules

Tablets

Dosage	UK	Europe	USA	Australia	Canada
27.42mg	–	✓	–	–	–
30mg	–	✓	–	–	–

Capsules

Dosage	UK	Europe	USA	Australia	Canada
15mg	✓	–	✓	–	✓
30mg	✓	–	✓	–	✓

Off-label options: In order to follow the regimens suggested, in some cases smaller doses are required than can be made using commercially available tablets and capsules, where no liquid versions are available. Guidelines for people who cannot swallow tablets do not cover flurazepam;[9,10] however, some authors recommend tapering by crushing a tablet and suspending or dissolving it in a liquid.[11] For example, a 30mg tablet could be made up to 30mL using water to make a 1mg/mL suspension. The speed of this process can be increased by crushing the tablet with a spoon or pestle and mortar. The suspension should be shaken vigorously before administration. As its stability cannot be assured it should be consumed immediately, and any unused suspension discarded. Some patients use full-fat milk to make liquid preparations. Benzodiazepines are more soluble in oil or fat than in water.[12] When mixed with milk, some or all of the drug will dissolve in the milk fat. This should form an evenly dispersed emulsion when shaken vigorously. The measured dose should be taken immediately after shaking and the remainder discarded. Alternatively, a capsule can be opened and the contents can be used to make up a suspension. For example, the contents of a 15mg capsule could be made up to 15mL with water to make a 1mg/mL suspension. The suspension should be shaken vigorously before administration. As its stability cannot be assured it should be consumed immediately, and any unused suspension discarded.

Another option is to switch to an alternative medication (e.g. diazepam, as below). Other options include having a compounding pharmacy make up a suspension or smaller dose tablets or capsules.

Worked example: To illustrate how volumes can be calculated in the regimens given below a worked example is provided. To make up 3.8mg of flurazepam a 1mg/mL suspension can be used, prepared as above. The volume of 1mg/mL liquid required to give a dose of 3.8mg flurazepam is 3.8/1 = 3.8mL.

Deprescribing notes: There are two main methods for tapering from flurazepam – a switch to diazepam or a direct taper from flurazepam. There are no established guides to determine the rate of taper of someone stopping benzodiazepines. Withdrawal is known to be more severe for people who have used benzodiazepines which are shorter acting for longer periods, at higher doses, in the elderly and who have experienced withdrawal in the past on reducing, stopping or missing a dose.[13,14] The size of the initial reduction can be estimated based on these factors (see 'Tapering benzodiazepines and z-drugs in practice'), with patient preference also taken into account. Sometimes an even smaller reduction to start with may be advisable to boost a patient's confidence that they can taper if performed carefully.

Each reduction should be made when the withdrawal symptoms from the previous reduction have largely resolved so that subsequent reductions do not lead to cumulative withdrawal symptoms. Withdrawal symptoms should not be too unpleasant: a rate of reduction should be aimed for that produces tolerable withdrawal symptoms that abate within a week or two. Allowing for a sufficient observation period, reductions can therefore be made about every 1–4 weeks, depending on how long it takes withdrawal symptoms to resolve. If withdrawal symptoms are moderately severe or take longer than a couple of weeks to resolve, dose reductions should be postponed until symptoms resolve and then made more gradually by choosing a slower tapering rate. If severe withdrawal symptoms occur then the patient should return to a higher dose, wait until symptoms resolve and thereafter taper at a slower rate.

Suggested direct taper schedules for flurazepam: Please note that none of these regimens should be seen as prescriptive – patients should not be compelled to adhere strictly to them. They are given as example regimens and are not 'set and forget' but should be modified in order to ensure that withdrawal symptoms are tolerable throughout a taper – for example, intermediate steps halfway between the doses listed could be added to make a more gradual taper. Ultimately, it is the patient's experience of withdrawal that should guide the rate of taper.

A. **A faster taper** with up to 8 percentage points of $GABA_A$ occupancy between each step – with reductions made every 1–4 weeks.*

Step	RO (%)	Evening dose (mg)	Formulation
1	37.8	30	Use caps or tabs
2	31.3	22.5	Use ¾ tablets**
3	23.3	15	Use ½ tablets**
Switch to flurazepam suspension **(1mg/mL)***			
4	16.8	10	10mL
5	9.2	5	5mL
6	4.8	2.5	2.5mL
7	0	0	

RO = receptor occupancy, caps = capsules, tabs = tablets

*Patients who have been on the medication for only a few weeks will probably be able to taper more quickly and might follow every second or third step of this regimen and make reductions every few days or so. Normally the duration of the taper should not be longer than the period that the patient has been on the drug for people who have only taken it for a few weeks. For example, if flurazepam is taken for 3 weeks the taper should be less than 3 weeks. However the FDA has issued an alert regarding dependence and withdrawal from benzodiazepines indicating that some people can experience withdrawal effects after just a few days of use,[15] therefore necessitating slower tapering in these people.

**Alternatively, a liquid version of the drug could be used to make up these doses.

***Prepared as above.

B. **A moderate taper:** with up to 2.6 percentage points of $GABA_A$ occupancy between each step – with reductions made every 1–4 weeks.

Step	RO (%)	Evening dose (mg)	Formulation	Step	RO (%)	Evening dose (mg)	Formulation
1	37.8	30	Use caps or tabs	12	16.3	9.6	9.6mL
Switch to flurazepam suspension **(1mg/mL)***				13	13.9	8	8mL
2	36.2	28	28mL	14	12.7	7.2	7.2mL
3	34.5	26	26mL	15	11.5	6.4	6.4mL
4	32.7	24	24mL	16	10.2	5.6	5.6mL
5	30.8	22	22mL	17	8.9	4.8	4.8mL
6	28.8	20	20mL	18	7.5	4	4mL
7	26.7	18	18mL	19	6.1	3.2	3.2mL
8	24.5	16	16mL	20	4.6	2.4	2.4mL
9	22.6	14.4	14.4mL	21	3.1	1.6	1.6mL
10	20.6	12.8	12.8mL	22	1.6	0.8	0.8mL
11	18.5	11.2	11.2mL	23	0	0	
See further steps in the right-hand column							

RO = receptor occupancy, caps = capsules, tabs = tablets
*Prepared as above.

C. **A slower taper** with up to 1.2 percentage points of $GABA_A$ occupancy between each step – with reductions made every 1–4 weeks.

Step	RO (%)	Evening dose (mg)	Form	Step	RO (%)	Evening dose (mg)	Form	Step	RO (%)	Evening dose (mg)	Form
1	37.8	30	Use caps or tabs	16	23.5	15.2	15.2mL	32	9.5	5.2	5.2mL
Switch to flurazepam suspension **(1mg/mL)***				17	22.6	14.4	14.4mL	33	8.9	4.8	4.8mL
2	37	29	29mL	18	21.6	13.6	13.6mL	34	8.2	4.4	4.4mL
3	36.2	28	28mL	19	20.6	12.8	12.8mL	35	7.5	4	4mL
4	35.3	27	27mL	20	19.5	12	12mL	36	6.8	3.6	3.6mL
5	34.5	26	26mL	21	18.5	11.2	11.2mL	37	6.1	3.2	3.2mL
6	33.6	25	25mL	22	17.4	10.4	10.4mL	38	5.4	2.8	2.8mL
7	32.7	24	24mL	23	16.3	9.6	9.6mL	39	4.6	2.4	2.4mL
8	31.8	23	23mL	24	15.1	8.8	8.8mL	40	3.9	2	2mL
9	30.8	22	22mL	25	13.9	8	8mL	41	3.1	1.6	1.6mL
10	29.8	21	21mL	26	13.3	7.6	7.6mL	42	2.4	1.2	1.2mL
11	28.8	20	20mL	27	12.7	7.2	7.2mL	43	1.6	0.8	0.8mL
12	27.8	19	19mL	28	12.1	6.8	6.8mL	44	0.8	0.4	0.4mL
13	26.7	18	18mL	29	11.5	6.4	6.4mL	45	0	0	
14	25.6	17	17mL	30	10.8	6	6mL				
15	24.5	16	16mL	31	10.2	5.6	5.6mL				
	See further steps in the middle column				**See further steps in the right-hand column**						

RO = receptor occupancy, caps = capsules, tabs = tablets
*Prepared as above.

D. **An even slower taper** Some patients will be unable to taper at the slowest rates shown here and will need to taper by even smaller decrements, thus lengthening the overall period of tapering. Such a regimen could be constructed by placing intermediate steps in regimen C. For example, 30mg, 29mg, 28mg could be modified to be 30mg, 29.5mg, 29mg, 28.5mg, 28mg and so on. Further intermediate steps could also be added.

Micro-tapering: The tables above show how to make reductions at intervals of 1–4 weeks. An alternative approach is called 'micro-tapering' whereby very small dose reductions are made every day, as explained in 'Other considerations in tapering benzodiazepines and z-drugs.' Micro-tapering rates can be calculated from the above by dividing the change in dose for each step by 14 or 28 days. For example, for the moderate regimen, a reduction of 30mg to 28mg over 14 days is equivalent to a reduction of 0.14mg per day. By the end of this regimen the rate of reduction would have slowed down to a reduction of 0.06mg each day. The rate can be adjusted if withdrawal symptoms become too unpleasant.

Switching guide from flurazepam to diazepam An alternative to a direct taper from flurazepam is to switch to diazepam before tapering from this drug, as outlined in 'Switching to longer-acting benzodiazepines to taper'. A 10mg dose of flurazepam is approximately equivalent to 5mg diazepam.[16] Switching could be performed by steps of 10mg of flurazepam made every week (or as tolerated by the patient).

Steps	Evening	Daily diazepam equivalent
Starting	30mg flurazepam	15mg
2	20mg flurazepam 5mg diazepam	15mg
3	10mg flurazepam 10mg diazepam	15mg
4	Stop flurazepam 15mg diazepam	15mg
Continue to taper as for 15mg diazepam (see diazepam section)		

References

1. Chouinard G. Issues in the clinical use of benzodiazepines: potency, withdrawal, and rebound. *J Clin Psychiatry* 2004; 65 Suppl 5: 7–12.
2. Mylan. Summary of Product Characteristics. Dalmane 30mg Capsules. Flurazepam hydrochloride. 2020. https://www.medicines.org.uk/emc/product/1726/smpc#gref (accessed 5 July 2023).
3. FDA Drug Safety Communication. FDA requiring boxed warning updated to improve safe use of benzodiazepine drug class. 2020. https://www.fda.gov/drugs/drug-safety-and-availability/fda-requiring-boxed-warning-updated-improve-safe-use-benzodiazepine-drug-class#:~:text=FDA is requiring the Boxed,and life-threatening side effects (accessed 3 July 2023).
4. Brouillet E, Chavoix C, Bottlaender M, et al. In vivo bidirectional modulatory effect of benzodiazepine receptor ligands on GABAergic transmission evaluated by positron emission tomography in non-human primates. *Brain Res* 1991; 557: 167–76.
5. Holford N. Pharmacodynamic principles and the time course of delayed and cumulative drug effects. *Transl Clin Pharmacol* 2018; 26: 56–9.
6. Horowitz M, Taylor D. Withdrawing from benzodiazepines and z-drugs (in preparation).
7. Horowitz MA, Taylor D. Tapering of SSRI treatment to mitigate withdrawal symptoms. *The Lancet Psychiatry* 2019; 6: 538–46.
8. Ashton H. Benzodiazepines: how they work and how to withdraw (The Ashton Manual). Newcastle University, 2002. http://www.benzo.org.uk/manual/bzcha01.htm (accessed 11 July 2023).
9. Smyth. J. The NEWT Guidelines for administration of medication to patients with enteral feeding tubes or swallowing difficulties website. The NEWT Guidelines. 2011. http://www.newtguidelines.com (accessed 5 July 2023).
10. Bostwick JR, Demehri A. Pills to powder: an updated clinician's reference for crushable psychotropics. *Curr Psychiatr* 2017; 16: 46–9.
11. Stahl SM. Flurazepam. In: *Prescriber's Guide: Stahl's Essential Psychopharmacology*. Cambridge: Cambridge University Press, 2020: 321–4.
12. Macheras PE, Koupparis MA, Antimisiaris SG. Drug binding and solubility in milk. *Pharm Res* 1990; 7: 537–41.
13. Guina J, Merrill B. Benzodiazepines II: waking up on sedatives: providing optimal care when inheriting benzodiazepine prescriptions in transfer patients. *J Clin Med Res* 2018; 7. doi:10.3390/jcm7020020.
14. Framer A. What I have learnt from helping thousands of people taper off antidepressants and other psychotropic medications. *Ther Adv Psychopharmacol* 2021; 11: 2045125321991274.
15. US Food & Drug Administration. FDA requiring Boxed Warning updated to improve safe use of benzodiazepine drug class. 2020. https://www.fda.gov/drugs/drug-safety-and-availability/fda-requiring-boxed-warning-updated-improve-safe-use-benzodiazepine-drug-class (accessed 5 July 2023).
16. Hypnotics and anxiolytics. https://bnf.nice.org.uk/treatment-summaries/hypnotics-and-anxiolytics/ (accessed 19 March 2023).

CHAPTER 3

Lorazepam

Trade names: Ativan, Lorabenz, Lorazepam Intensol, Loreev XR, Lorenin, Lorsilan, Orfidal, Tavor, Temesta.

Description: Lorazepam is a high-potency benzodiazepine.[1] It is a positive allosteric modulator of the gamma-aminobutyric acid (GABA) type A receptor, which it affects by binding to stereospecific benzodiazepine (BZD) binding sites. Stimulation of benzodiazepine receptors enhances the inhibitory effects of GABA.[2] The manufacturer in the UK states that the duration of treatment should not be longer than 4 weeks, and in the USA the manufacturer recommends that duration of treatment should be limited to the 'minimum required'.[2,3]

Withdrawal effects: Lorazepam, as for other benzodiazepines, carries a boxed warning from the FDA that highlights that physical dependence and withdrawal effects can occur when the drug is taken 'for several days to weeks, even as prescribed'.[2,4] Not everyone who stops lorazepam will experience withdrawal and some of those who do will only experience mild symptoms – this probably depends on drug dose, duration of use and individual factors. However, in a very few instances, stopping abruptly can cause seizures and can be life threatening. Numerous other physical, cognitive and psychological withdrawal symptoms (outlined in 'Withdrawal effects from benzodiazepines and z-drugs') are possible, which can last 'for several weeks to more than 12 months' after stopping according to the FDA.[2,4]

Peak plasma: Following oral administration peak concentration in the plasma occurs after 2 hours.[3]

Half-life: The mean half-life is 12 hours and there are no major active metabolites.[3] The manufacturer recommends lorazepam to be given 2–3 times a day in divided doses.[3] Dosing less often (including every-other-day dosing) is not recommended for tapering because the changes in plasma levels may precipitate inter-dose withdrawal symptoms.

Receptor occupancy: The relationship between dose of lorazepam and the occupancy of its major target $GABA_A$ is hyperbolic according to the law of mass action.[5,6] Benzodiazepines demonstrate a hyperbolic relationship between dose and clinical effects,[7] which may be relevant to withdrawal effects. Dose reductions made by linear amounts (e.g. 10mg, 7.5mg, 5mg, 2.5mg, 0mg) will cause increasingly large reductions in effect, which may cause increasingly severe withdrawal effects (Figure 3.17a). To produce equal-sized reductions in effect on receptor occupancy will require hyperbolically reducing doses

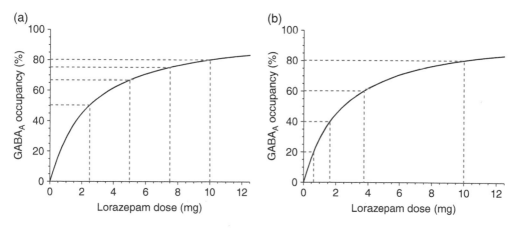

Figure 3.17 (a) Linear reductions of dose cause increasingly large reductions in effect on receptor targets, possibly associated with more withdrawal effects. (b) Even reductions of effect at target receptors requires hyperbolic dose reductions. The final dose before stopping will need to be very small so that this step down is not larger (in terms of effect on receptor occupancy) than previous reductions.

CHAPTER 3

(Figure 3.17b),[8] which informs the reductions presented. The relationship was derived by converting the receptor occupancy curve for diazepam[5] to equivalent lorazepam dose.[9]

Available formulations: As tablets, capsules and oral solution.

Tablets

Dosage	UK	Europe	USA	Australia	Canada
0.5mg	✓	✓	✓	–	✓
1mg	✓	✓	✓	✓*	✓
2mg	–	✓	✓	✓	✓
2.5mg	✓	✓	–	✓	–

* Sublingual tablet

Extended-release capsule

Dosage	UK	Europe	USA	Australia	Canada
1mg	–	–	✓	–	
1.5mg	–	–	✓	–	
2mg	–	–	✓	–	
3mg	–	–	✓	–	

Oral solution

Dosage	UK	Europe	USA	Australia	Canada
1mg/mL	✓	–	–	–	–
2mg/mL	–	–	✓	–	–

Dilution: To make up some of the small doses outlined below, dilution of the liquid available from the manufacturer will be required. Lorazepam oral concentrate is recommended by its manufacturer to be mixed with liquid or juice before being taken.[10] They recommend stirring the mixture gently for a few seconds and state that the concentrate will blend quickly and completely. They recommend that the mixture should be consumed immediately and the remainder discarded.[10] Dilution in water might cause precipitation of the drug and so the resulting mixture should be shaken vigorously before use to produce dispersal. As its stability cannot be assured it should be made up fresh each day.

UK dilutions	Solution required	How to prepare solution
Doses ≥ 0.2mg	1mg/mL	Original solution
Doses < 0.2mg	0.1mg/mL	Mix 0.5mL of original solution with 4.5mL of water*

USA dilutions	Solution required	How to prepare solution
Doses ≥ 0.4mg	2mg/mL	Original solution
Doses < 0.4mg	0.2mg/mL	Mix 0.5mL of original solution with 4.5mL of water*

* Other dilutions are possible to produce different concentrations. The above is provided as an example.

Off-label options: In order to follow the regimens suggested, in some cases smaller doses are required than can be made using commercially available tablets and capsules where no liquid versions are available. Guidelines for people who cannot swallow tablets (e.g. NEWT guidelines in the UK based on advice from the manufacturer or local hospital guidance[11], and similar guidance in the USA)[12] recommend the use of a custom-made suspension from a compounding pharmacy (if available) or making a suspension by crushing a tablet and mixing with water.[11] Crushed tablets will disintegrate in 1–5 minutes.[11] For example, a 1mg tablet could be made up to 10mL with water to make a 1mg in 10mL or 0.1mg/mL suspension. This process can be assisted by crushing the tablet with a spoon or pestle and mortar. The suspension should be shaken vigorously before administration. As its stability cannot be assured, it should be consumed immediately, and any unused suspension discarded. Some patients use full-fat milk to make liquid preparations. Benzodiazepines are more soluble in oil or fat than in water.[13] When mixed with milk, some or all of the drug will dissolve in the milk fat. This should form an evenly dispersed emulsion when shaken vigorously. The measured dose should be taken immediately after shaking and the remainder discarded.

Other options to make up small doses include having a compounding pharmacy make up smaller dose tablets, including the option of 'tapering strips'.[14]

Worked example: To illustrate how volumes can be calculated in the regimens given, a worked example is provided. To make up 0.2mg of lorazepam a 0.1mg/mL dilution can be used, prepared as above. The volume of 0.1mg/mL liquid required to give a dose of 0.1mg lorazepam is 0.2/0.1 = 2mL.

Deprescribing notes: There are two main methods for tapering from lorazepam – a switch to diazepam or a direct taper of lorazepam itself. There are no established guides to determine the rate of taper of someone stopping benzodiazepines. Withdrawal is known to be more severe for people who have used benzodiazepines which are shorter acting for longer periods, at higher doses, and in those who have experienced withdrawal in the past on reducing, stopping or missing a dose.[15,16] The size of the initial reduction can be estimated based on these factors (see 'Tapering benzodiazepines and z-drugs in practice'), with patient preference also taken into account. Sometimes an even smaller reduction to start with may be advisable to boost a patient's confidence that they can taper if performed carefully.

Each reduction should be made when the withdrawal symptoms from the previous reduction have largely resolved so that subsequent reductions do not lead to cumulative withdrawal symptoms. Withdrawal symptoms should not be too unpleasant: a rate of reduction should be aimed for that produces tolerable withdrawal symptoms that abate within a week or two. Allowing for a sufficient observation period, reductions can therefore be made about every 1–4 weeks, depending on how long it takes withdrawal symptoms to resolve. If withdrawal symptoms are moderately severe or take longer than a couple of weeks to resolve, dose reductions should be postponed until symptoms resolve and then made more gradually by choosing a slower tapering rate. If severe withdrawal symptoms occur, then the patient should return to a higher dose, wait until symptoms resolve and thereafter taper at a slower rate.

Suggested direct taper schedules for lorazepam: Please note that none of these regimens should be seen as prescriptive – patients should not be compelled to strictly adhere to them. They are given as example regimens and are not 'set and forget' but should be modified in order to ensure that withdrawal symptoms are tolerable throughout a taper. For example, intermediate steps halfway between the doses listed could be added to make a more gradual taper. Ultimately, it is the patient's experience of withdrawal that should guide the rate of taper.

A. **Fast taper** with up to 5.1 percentage points of $GABA_A$ occupancy between each step – with reductions made every 1–4 weeks*.

Step	RO (%)	Morning (mg)	Afternoon (mg)	Evening (mg)	Total daily dose (mg)	Formulation
1	80.2	3.5	3	3.5	10	Use tablets
2	76.4	2.5	2.5	3	8	Use tablets
3	73.9	2.5	2	2.5	7	Use tablets
4	70.8	2	2	2	6	Use tablets
5	66.9	1.5	1.5	2	5	Use tablets
6	61.8	1.5	1	1.5	4	Use tablets
7	58.6	1	1	1.5	3.5	Use tablets
8	54.8	1	1	1	3	Use tablets
9	50.3	1	0.5	1	2.5	Use tablets
10	47.7	0.75	0.5	1	2.25	Use ½ tablets**
11	44.7	0.5	0.5	1	2	Use tablets
12	41.5	0.5	0.5	0.75	1.75	Use ½ tablets**
13	37.8	0.5	0.5	0.5	1.5	Use tablets
14	33.6	0.5	0.25	0.5	1.25	Use ½ tablets**
15	28.8	0.25	0.25	0.5	1	Use ½ tablets**
16	26.2	0.25	0.25	0.375	0.875	Use ½ and ¾ tablets**
17	23.3	0.25	0.25	0.25	0.75	Use ½ tablets**
18	20.2	0.25	0.125	0.25	0.625	Use ¼ and ½ tablets**
19	16.8	0.125	0.125	0.25	0.5	Use ¼ and ½ tablets**
20	13.2	0.125	0.125	0.125	0.375	Use ¼ tablets**
21	9.2	0.125	0	0.125	0.25	Use ¼ tablets**
22	4.8	0	0	0.125	0.125	Use ¼ tablets**
23	0	0	0	0	0	

RO = receptor occupancy

*Patients who have been on the medication for only a few weeks will probably be able to taper more quickly and might follow every second or third step of this regimen and make reductions every few days or so. Normally the duration of the taper should not be longer than the period that the patient has been on the drug for people who have only taken it for a few weeks. However the FDA has issued an alert regarding benzodiazepines indicating that some people can experience withdrawal effects after just a few days of use,[4] therefore necessitating slower tapering in this sub-group.

**Alternatively, these doses could be made up using liquids if small-dose tablets are not available or division with a pill cutter is challenging.

B. A moderate taper with up to 2.8 percentage points of GABA$_A$ occupancy between each step - with reductions made every 1–4 weeks.

Step	RO (%)	AM (mg)	PM (mg)	Night (mg)	Total daily dose (mg)	Form
1	80.2	3.5	3	3.5	10	Use tablets
2	78.5	3	3	3	9	Use tablets
3	76.4	2.5	2.5	3	8	Use tablets
4	75.2	2.5	2.5	2.5	7.5	Use tablets
5	73.9	2.5	2	2.5	7	Use tablets
6	72.5	2	2	2.5	6.5	Use tablets
7	70.8	2	2	2	6	Use tablets
8	69	2	1.5	2	5.5	Use tablets
9	66.9	1.5	1.5	2	5	Use tablets
10	64.6	1.5	1.5	1.5	4.5	Use tablets
11	61.8	1.5	1	1.5	4	Use tablets
12	60.3	1.25	1	1.5	3.75	Use ½ tablets*
13	58.6	1	1	1.5	3.5	Use tablets
14	56.8	1	1	1.25	3.25	Use ½ tablets*
15	54.8	1	1	1	3	Use tablets
16	52.7	0.875	0.875	1	2.75	Use ¾ tablets*
17	50.3	0.875	0.75	0.875	2.5	Use ¾ tablets*

See further steps in the right-hand column

Step	RO (%)	AM (mg)	PM (mg)	Night (mg)	Total daily dose (mg)	Form
	Switch to liquid version of lorazepam (e.g. 0.1mg/mL or 1mg/mL)**					
18	48.2	0.8	0.7	0.8	2.3	Use liquid
19	46	0.7	0.7	0.7	2.1	Use liquid
20	44.7	0.7	0.6	0.7	2.0	Use liquid
21	43.5	0.6	0.6	0.7	1.9	Use liquid
22	42.2	0.6	0.6	0.6	1.8	Use liquid
23	40.8	0.6	0.5	0.6	1.7	Use liquid
24	39.3	0.5	0.5	0.6	1.6	Use liquid
25	37.8	0.5	0.5	0.5	1.5	Use liquid
26	36.2	0.5	0.4	0.5	1.4	Use liquid
27	34.5	0.4	0.4	0.5	1.3	Use liquid
28	32.7	0.4	0.4	0.4	1.2	Use liquid
29	30.8	0.4	0.3	0.4	1.1	Use liquid
30	28.8	0.3	0.3	0.4	1.0	Use liquid
31	26.7	0.3	0.3	0.3	0.9	Use liquid
32	24.5	0.3	0.2	0.3	0.8	Use liquid
33	22.1	0.2	0.2	0.3	0.7	Use liquid

(Continued)

(*Continued*)

Step	RO (%)	AM (mg)	PM (mg)	Night (mg)	Total daily dose (mg)	Form
34	19.5	0.2	0.2	0.2	0.6	Use liquid
35	18.2	0.2	0.15	0.2	0.55	Use liquid
36	16.8	0.15	0.15	0.2	0.5	Use liquid
37	15.4	0.15	0.15	0.15	0.45	Use liquid
38	13.9	0.15	0.1	0.15	0.4	Use liquid
39	12.4	0.1	0.1	0.15	0.35	Use liquid
40	10.8	0.1	0.1	0.1	0.3	Use liquid

See further steps in the right-hand column

Step	RO (%)	AM (mg)	PM (mg)	Night (mg)	Total daily dose (mg)	Form
41	9.2	0.1	0.05	0.1	0.25	Use liquid
42	8.2	0.05	0.05	0.1	0.2	Use liquid
43	5.7	0.05	0.05	0.05	0.15	Use liquid
44	3.9	0.05	0	0.05	0.1	Use liquid
45	2	0.02	0	0.03	0.05	Use liquid
46	0	0	0	0	0	

RO = receptor occupancy

*Alternatively, these doses could be made up using liquids if no small-dose tablets are available or division with a pill cutter is challenging.

**Outside the UK and US a liquid formulation of drug might be used as outlined in the off-label options.

C. A slower taper with up to 1.4 percentage points of GABA$_A$ occupancy between each step – with reductions made every 1–4 weeks.

Step	RO (%)	AM (mg)	PM (mg)	Night (mg)	Total daily dose (mg)	Form	Step	RO (%)	AM (mg)	PM (mg)	Night (mg)	Total daily dose (mg)	Form
1	80.2	3.5	3	3.5	10	Use tablets	20	63.2	1.5	1.25	1.5	4.25	Use ½ tablets*
2	79.4	3	3	3.5	9.5	Use tablets	21	61.8	1.25	1.25	1.5	4	Use ½ tablets*
3	78.5	3	3	3	9	Use tablets	22	61.1	1.25	1.25	1.375	3.875	Use ½ or ¼ tablets*
4	77.5	3	2.5	3	8.5	Use tablets	23	60.3	1.25	1.25	1.25	3.75	Use ½ tablets*
5	76.4	2.5	2.5	3	8	Use tablets	24	59.5	1.25	1.125	1.25	3.625	Use ½ or ¼ tablets*
6	75.8	2.5	2.5	2.75	7.75	Use ½ tablets*	25	58.6	1.125	1.125	1.25	3.5	Use ½ or ¼ tablets*
7	75.2	2.5	2.5	2.5	7.5	Use tablets	26	57.7	1.125	1.125	1.125	3.375	Use ¼ tablets*
8	74.6	2.5	2.25	2.5	7.25	Use ½ tablets*	27	56.8	1.125	1	1.125	3.25	Use ¼ tablets*
9	73.9	2.25	2.25	2.5	7	Use ½ tablets*	28	55.9	1	1	1.125	3.125	Use ¼ tablets*
10	73.2	2.25	2.25	2.25	6.75	Use ½ tablets*	29	54.8	1	1	1	3	Use tablets
11	72.5	2.25	2	2.25	6.5	Use ½ tablets*	30	53.8	1	0.875	1	2.875	Use ¾ tablets*
12	71.7	2	2	2.25	6.25	Use ½ tablets*	31	52.7	0.875	0.875	1	2.75	Use ¾ tablets*
13	70.8	2	2	2	6	Use tablets	32	51.5	0.875	0.875	0.875	2.625	Use ¾ tablets*
14	70	2	1.75	2	5.75	Use ½ tablets*	33	50.3	0.875	0.75	0.875	2.5	Use ½ or ¾ tablets*
15	69	1.75	1.75	2	5.5	Use ½ tablets*		Switch to liquid version of lorazepam (e.g. 0.1mg/mL or 1mg/mL)**					
16	68	1.75	1.75	1.75	5.25	Use ½ tablets*	34	49.3	0.8	0.8	0.8	2.4	Use liquid
17	66.9	1.75	1.5	1.75	5	Use ½ tablets*	35	48.2	0.8	0.7	0.8	2.3	Use liquid
18	65.8	1.5	1.5	1.75	4.75	Use ½ tablets*	36	47.1	0.7	0.7	0.8	2.2	Use liquid
19	64.6	1.5	1.5	1.5	4.5	Use tablets	37	46	0.7	0.7	0.7	2.1	Use liquid

See further steps in the right-hand column

(Continued)

(Continued)

Step	RO (%)	AM (mg)	PM (mg)	Night (mg)	Total daily dose (mg)	Form
38	44.7	0.7	0.6	0.7	2	Use liquid
39	44.1	0.65	0.6	0.7	1.95	Use liquid
40	43.5	0.65	0.6	0.65	1.9	Use liquid
41	42.8	0.6	0.6	0.65	1.85	Use liquid
42	42.2	0.6	0.6	0.6	1.8	Use liquid
43	41.5	0.6	0.55	0.6	1.75	Use liquid
44	40.8	0.55	0.55	0.6	1.7	Use liquid
45	40	0.55	0.55	0.55	1.65	Use liquid
46	39.3	0.55	0.5	0.55	1.6	Use liquid
47	38.6	0.5	0.5	0.55	1.55	Use liquid
48	37.8	0.5	0.5	0.5	1.5	Use liquid
49	37	0.5	0.45	0.5	1.45	Use liquid
50	36.2	0.45	0.45	0.5	1.4	Use liquid
51	35.3	0.45	0.45	0.45	1.35	Use liquid
52	34.5	0.45	0.4	0.45	1.3	Use liquid
53	33.6	0.4	0.4	0.45	1.25	Use liquid
54	32.7	0.4	0.4	0.4	1.2	Use liquid
55	31.8	0.4	0.35	0.4	1.15	Use liquid
56	30.8	0.35	0.35	0.4	1.1	Use liquid
57	29.8	0.35	0.35	0.35	1.05	Use liquid
58	28.8	0.35	0.3	0.35	1	Use liquid
59	27.8	0.3	0.3	0.35	0.95	Use liquid
60	26.7	0.3	0.3	0.3	0.9	Use liquid
61	25.6	0.3	0.25	0.3	0.85	Use liquid
62	24.5	0.25	0.25	0.3	0.8	Use liquid
63	23.5	0.25	0.25	0.26	0.76	Use liquid
64	22.6	0.24	0.24	0.24	0.72	Use liquid
65	21.6	0.22	0.22	0.24	0.68	Use liquid
66	20.6	0.2	0.2	0.24	0.64	Use liquid
67	19.5	0.2	0.2	0.2	0.6	Use liquid
68	18.5	0.18	0.18	0.2	0.56	Use liquid
69	17.4	0.18	0.16	0.18	0.52	Use liquid
70	16.3	0.16	0.16	0.16	0.48	Use liquid
71	15.1	0.14	0.14	0.16	0.44	Use liquid
72	13.9	0.14	0.12	0.14	0.4	Use liquid
73	13.3	0.12	0.12	0.14	0.38	Use liquid
74	12.7	0.12	0.12	0.12	0.36	Use liquid
75	12.1	0.12	0.1	0.12	0.34	Use liquid
76	11.5	0.1	0.1	0.12	0.32	Use liquid
77	10.8	0.1	0.1	0.1	0.3	Use liquid

See further steps in the right-hand column

78	10.2	0.1	0.08	0.1	0.28	Use liquid
79	9.5	0.08	0.08	0.1	0.26	Use liquid
80	8.9	0.08	0.08	0.08	0.24	Use liquid
81	8.2	0.08	0.06	0.08	0.22	Use liquid
82	7.5	0.06	0.06	0.08	0.2	Use liquid
83	6.8	0.06	0.05	0.06	0.18	Use liquid
84	6.1	0.06	0.04	0.06	0.16	Use liquid
85	5.4	0.04	0.04	0.06	0.14	Use liquid
86	4.6	0.04	0.04	0.04	0.12	Use liquid
87	3.9	0.04	0.02	0.04	0.1	Use liquid
88	3.1	0.02	0.02	0.04	0.08	Use liquid
89	2.4	0.02	0.02	0.02	0.06	Use liquid
90	1.6	0.02	0	0.02	0.04	Use liquid
91	0.8	0	0	0.02	0.02	Use liquid
92	0	0	0	0	0	Use liquid

See further steps in the right-hand column

RO = receptor occupancy

*Alternatively, these doses could be made up using liquids if no small-dose tablets are available or division with a pill cutter is challenging.

**Outside the UK and US, a liquid formulation of drug might be used as outlined in the off-label options.

D. **An even slower taper** Some patients will be unable to taper at the slowest rates shown here and will need to taper by even smaller decrements, thus lengthening the overall period of tapering. Such a regimen could be constructed by placing intermediate steps between regimen C. For example, 10mg, 9.5mg, 9mg could be modified to 10mg, 9.75mg, 9.5mg, 9.25mg, 9mg and so on. Further intermediate steps could also be added.

Micro-tapering: The tables above show how to make reductions at intervals of 1–4 weeks. An alternative approach is called 'micro-tapering' whereby very small dose reductions are made every day, as explained in 'Other considerations in tapering benzodiazepines and z-drugs.' Micro-tapering rates can be calculated from the above by dividing the change in dose for each step by 14 or 28 days. For example, for the moderate regimen a reduction from 10mg to 9mg over 14 days is equivalent to a reduction of 0.07mg per day, or 0.023mg reduction per dose (when dosed three times a day). At the end of the taper this rate will have slowed to reductions of 0.004mg per day. This rate can be slowed if withdrawal symptoms become too unpleasant.

Switching guide from lorazepam to diazepam: An alternative to a direct taper from lorazepam is to switch to diazepam before tapering from this drug, as outlined in 'Switching to longer-acting benzodiazepines to taper'. A 1mg dose of lorazepam is equivalent to 10mg diazepam.[9] Switching could be performed by steps of 1mg of lorazepam made every week (or as tolerated by the patient).

Steps	Morning	Afternoon	Evening	Daily diazepam equivalent
1	3.5mg lorazepam	3mg lorazepam	3.5mg lorazepam	100mg
2	2.5mg lorazepam 10mg diazepam	3mg lorazepam	3.5mg lorazepam	100mg
3	2.5mg lorazepam 10mg diazepam	3mg lorazepam	2.5mg lorazepam 10mg diazepam	100mg
4	2.5mg lorazepam 10mg diazepam	2mg lorazepam 10mg diazepam	2.5mg lorazepam 10mg diazepam	100mg
5	1.5mg lorazepam 20mg diazepam	2mg lorazepam 10mg diazepam	2.5mg lorazepam 10mg diazepam	100mg
6	1.5mg lorazepam 20mg diazepam	2mg lorazepam 10mg diazepam	1.5mg lorazepam 20mg diazepam	100mg
7	1.5mg lorazepam 20mg diazepam	1mg lorazepam 20mg diazepam	1.5mg lorazepam 20mg diazepam	100mg
8	0.5mg lorazepam 30mg diazepam	1mg lorazepam 20mg diazepam	0.5mg lorazepam 30mg diazepam	100mg
9	0.5mg lorazepam 30mg diazepam	Stop lorazepam 30mg diazepam	0.5mg lorazepam 30mg diazepam	100mg
10	Stop lorazepam 35mg diazepam	30mg diazepam	Stop lorazepam 35mg diazepam	100mg
11	50mg diazepam	Switch to morning and night	50mg diazepam	100mg
		Reduce from 100mg diazepam		

(Continued)

CHAPTER 3

Steps	Morning	Afternoon	Evening	Daily diazepam equivalent
12	45mg diazepam	–	50mg diazepam	95mg
13	45mg diazepam	–	45mg diazepam	90mg
14	40mg diazepam	–	45mg diazepam	85mg
15	40mg diazepam	–	40mg diazepam	80mg
16	35mg diazepam	–	40mg diazepam	75mg
17	35mg diazepam	–	35mg diazepam	70mg
18	30mg diazepam	–	35mg diazepam	65mg
19	30mg diazepam	–	30mg diazepam	60mg
Reduce as for 60mg diazepam (see diazepam section)				

References

1. Chouinard G. Issues in the clinical use of benzodiazepines: potency, withdrawal, and rebound. *J Clin Psychiatry* 2004; 65 Suppl 5: 7–12.
2. FDA. Lorazepam – Highlights of Prescribing Information 2023; published online January. www.fda.gov/medwatch. (accessed 27 March 2023).
3. SmPC. Lorazepam – Summary of Product Characteristics (SmPC). 2021. https://www.medicines.org.uk/emc/product/6137/smpc#gref (accessed 27 March 2023).
4. FDA Drug Safety Communication. FDA requiring Boxed Warning updated to improve safe use of benzodiazepine drug class. 2020. https://www.fda.gov/drugs/drug-safety-and-availability/fda-requiring-boxed-warning-updated-improve-safe-use-benzodiazepine-drug-class#:~:text=FDA is requiring the Boxed,and life-threatening side effects (accessed 3 July 2023).
5. Brouillet E, Chavoix C, Bottlaender M, et al. In vivo bidirectional modulatory effect of benzodiazepine receptor ligands on GABAergic transmission evaluated by positron emission tomography in non-human primates. *Brain Res* 1991; 557: 167–76.
6. Holford N. Pharmacodynamic principles and the time course of delayed and cumulative drug effects. *Transl Clin Pharmacol* 2018; 26: 56–9.
7. Horowitz M, Taylor D. Withdrawing from benzodiazepines and z-drugs (in preparation).
8. Horowitz MA, Taylor D. Tapering of SSRI treatment to mitigate withdrawal symptoms. *The Lancet Psychiatry* 2019; 6: 538–46.
9. Hypnotics and anxiolytics. https://bnf.nice.org.uk/treatment-summaries/hypnotics-and-anxiolytics/ (accessed 19 March 2023).
10. FDA. Lorazepam Oral Concentrate, USP. FDA. www.accessdata.fda.gov/drugsatfda_docs/label/2009/079244lbl.pdf (accessed 3 April 2023).
11. Smyth J. The NEWT guidelines for administration of medication to patients with enteral feeding tubes or swallowing difficulties. 2011. https://www.newtguidelines.com/index.html (accessed 18 February 2023).
12. Bostwick JR, Demehri A. Pills to powder: an updated clinician's reference for crushable psychotropics. *Curr Psychiatr* 2017; 16: 46–9.
13. Macheras PE, Koupparis MA, Antimisiaris SG. Drug binding and solubility in milk. *Pharm Res* 1990; 7: 537–41.
14. Groot PC, van Os J. Successful use of tapering strips for hyperbolic reduction of antidepressant dose: a cohort study. *Ther Adv Psychopharmacol* 2021; 11: 20451253211039330.
15. Guina J, Merrill B. Benzodiazepines II: waking up on sedatives: providing optimal care when inheriting benzodiazepine prescriptions in transfer patients. *Journal of Clinical Medicine* 2018; 7. doi:10.3390/JCM7020020.
16 Framer A. What I have learnt from helping thousands of people taper off antidepressants and other psychotropic medications. *Ther Adv Psychopharmacol* 2021; 11: 204512532199127.

Lormetazepam

Trade names: Dormagen, Loramet, Noctamid, Pronoctan.

Description: Lormetazepam is a high-potency benzodiazepine.[1] It is a positive allosteric modulator of the gamma-aminobutyric acid (GABA) type A receptor, which it affects by binding to the central benzodiazepine receptor with high affinity.[2] It is indicated for the short-term treatment of insomnia.[3] Its manufacturer in the UK recommends the use of the lowest effective dose for the shortest time possible and treatment for no longer than 4 weeks including the tapering off process.[3]

Withdrawal effects: The FDA has issued a boxed warning for benzodiazepines, which highlights that physical dependence and withdrawal effects can occur when the drug is taken 'for several days to weeks, even as prescribed'.[4] Not everyone who stops lormetazepam will experience withdrawal and some of those who do will only experience mild symptoms – this probably depends on drug dose, duration of use and individual factors. However, in some instances, stopping abruptly can cause seizures and can be life threatening. Numerous other physical, cognitive and psychological withdrawal symptoms, outlined in 'Withdrawal effects from benzodiazepines and z-drugs', are possible, which can last 'for several weeks to more than 12 months' after stopping according to the FDA.[4] In a study of benzodiazepine dependence in 1,112 patients in a tertiary referral centre in Italy, lormetazepam was associated with the highest risk of abuse out of all the benzodiazepines examined.[5]

Peak plasma: Following oral administration lormetazepam is rapidly absorbed and reaches peak maximum concentration after 60–90 minutes.[6]

Half-life and dosing: The mean half-life is 10–12 hours. Lormetazepam does not have any active metabolites and possesses a low risk of accumulation.[3] The manufacturer recommends taking the drug once a day at night for insomnia.[3] Dosing less often (including every-other-day dosing) is not recommended for tapering because the changes in plasma levels may precipitate inter-dose withdrawal symptoms.

Receptor occupancy: The relationship between dose of lormetazepam and the occupancy of its major target $GABA_A$ is hyperbolic, according to the law of mass action.[7,8] Benzodiazepines demonstrate a hyperbolic relationship between dose and clinical effects,[9] which may be relevant to withdrawal effects from lormetazepam. Dose reductions made by linear amounts (e.g. 1.5mg, 1.125mg, 0.75mg, 0.375mg, 0mg) will cause increasingly large reductions in effect, which may cause increasingly severe withdrawal effects (Figure 3.18a). To produce equal-sized reductions in effect on receptor occupancy will require hyperbolically reducing doses (Figure 3.18b),[10] which informs the reductions presented. The relationship was derived by converting the receptor occupancy curve for diazepam[7] to lormetazepam dose.[11]

Available formulations: As tablets and liquid.

Tablets

Dosage	UK	Europe	USA	Australia	Canada
0.5mg	✓	–	–	–	–
1mg	✓	✓	–	–	–
2mg	–	✓	–	–	–

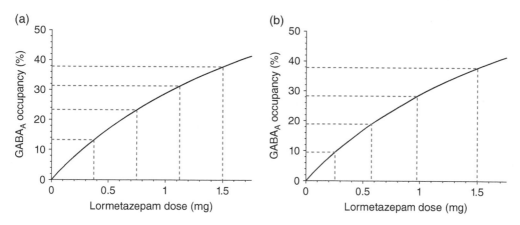

Figure 3.18 (a) Linear reductions of dose cause increasingly large reductions in effect on receptor targets, possibly associated with more withdrawal effects. (b) Even reductions of effect at target receptors requires hyperbolic dose reductions, slightly different from linear reductions in this case. The final dose before stopping will need to be small so that this step down is not larger (in terms of effect on receptor occupancy) than previous reductions.

Liquid*

Dosage	UK	Europe	USA	Australia	Canada
2mg/10mg (0.2mg/mL)	–	✓	–	–	–

*Individual dose adjustments might be required in patients taking the oral solution.[12,13] Overall pharmacokinetic examinations conclude that 1mg of oral solution is equivalent to 1mg in tablet form.[12] However, the oral solution peaks quicker and to a higher concentration than the drug in tablet form and so some patients may require 20% lower doses when transferring to liquid form.[13]

Off-label options: In order to follow the regimens suggested below in some cases smaller doses are required than can be made using commercially available tablets and capsules where no liquid versions are available. Guidelines for people who cannot swallow tablets (e.g. NEWT guidelines in the UK based on advice from the manufacturer or local hospital guidance[14]) advises crushing the tablets and dispersing them in water. For example, a 1mg tablet could be made up to 5mL with water to make a 1mg in 5mL or 0.2mg/mL suspension. This process can be hastened by crushing the tablet with a spoon or pestle and mortar. The suspension should be shaken vigorously or mixed well before administration. As its stability cannot be assured it should be consumed immediately, and any unused suspension discarded. Some patients use full-fat milk to make liquid preparations. Benzodiazepines are more soluble in oil or fat than in water.[15] When mixed with milk, some or all of the drug will dissolve in the milk fat. This should form an evenly dispersed emulsion when shaken vigorously. The measured dose should be taken immediately after shaking and the remainder discarded.

Worked example: To illustrate how volumes can be calculated in the regimens given below, a worked example is provided. To make up 0.1mg of lormetazepam a 0.2mg/mL dilution can be used, prepared as above. The volume of 0.2mg/mL liquid required to give a dose of 0.1mg lormetazepam is 0.1/0.2 = 0.5mL.

Deprescribing notes: There are two main methods for tapering from lormetazepam – a switch to diazepam or a direct taper of lormetazepam itself. There are no established guides to determine the rate of taper for someone stopping benzodiazepines. Withdrawal is known to be more severe for people who have used benzodiazepines which are shorter acting, for longer periods, at higher doses, and for those who have experienced withdrawal in the past on reducing, stopping or missing a dose.[16,17] The size of the initial reduction can be estimated based on these factors (see 'Tapering benzodiazepines and z-drugs in practice'), with patient preference also taken into account. Sometimes an even smaller reduction to start with may be advisable to boost a patient's confidence that they can taper if performed carefully.

Each reduction should be made when the withdrawal symptoms from the previous reduction have largely resolved so that subsequent reductions do not lead to cumulative withdrawal symptoms. Withdrawal symptoms should not be too unpleasant: a rate of reduction should be aimed for that produces tolerable withdrawal symptoms that abate within a week or two. Allowing for a sufficient observation period, reductions can therefore be made about every 1–4 weeks, depending on how long it takes withdrawal symptoms to resolve. If withdrawal symptoms are moderately severe or take longer than a couple of weeks to resolve, dose reductions should be postponed until symptoms resolve and then made more gradually by choosing a slower tapering rate. If severe withdrawal symptoms occur then the patient should return to a higher dose, wait until symptoms resolve and thereafter taper at a slower rate.

Suggested direct taper schedules for lormetazepam: Please note that none of these regimens should be seen as prescriptive – patients should not be compelled to adhere strictly to them. They are given as example regimens and are not 'set and forget' but should be modified in order to ensure that withdrawal symptoms are tolerable throughout a taper. For example, intermediate steps halfway between the doses listed could be added to make a more gradual taper. Ultimately, it is the patient's experience of withdrawal that should guide the rate of taper.

A. **A faster taper** with up to 8 percentage points of $GABA_A$ occupancy between each step – with reductions made every 1–4 weeks*.

Step	RO (%)	Evening dose (mg)	Formulation
1	37.8	1.5	Use tablets
2	33.6	1.25	Use ½ tablets**
3	28.8	1	Use tablets
4	23.3	0.75	Use ½ tablets**
5	16.8	0.5	Use tablets
6	9.2	0.25	Use ½ tablets**
7	4.8	0.125	Use ¼ tablets**
8	0	0	

RO = receptor occupancy

*Patients who have been on the medication for only a few weeks will probably be able to taper more quickly and might follow every second or third step of this regimen and make reductions every few days or so. Normally the duration of the taper should not be longer than the period that the patient has been on the drug for people who have only taken it for a few weeks. For example, if lormetazepam is taken for 3 weeks the taper should be less than 3 weeks. However, the FDA has issued a warning for benzodiazepines indicating that some people can experience withdrawal effects after just a few days of use,[4] therefore necessitating slower tapering in this sub-group.

**Alternatively, these doses could be made up using liquid formulations.

B. **A moderate taper** with up to 4 percentage points of $GABA_A$ occupancy between each step – with reductions made every 1–4 weeks.

Step	RO (%)	Evening dose (mg)	Formulation
1	37.8	1.5	Use tablets
2	35.8	1.375	Use ¾ tablets*
3	33.6	1.25	Use ½ tablets*
4	31.3	1.125	Use ¼ tablets*
5	28.8	1	Use tablets
6	26.2	0.875	Use ¾ tablets*
7	23.3	0.75	Use ½ tablets*
8	20.2	0.625	Use ¼ tablets*
9	16.8	0.5	Use tablets
10	13.2	0.375	Use ¾ tablets*
11	9.2	0.25	Use ½ tablets*
Switch to liquid formulation of lormetazepam **(0.2mg/mL)** *^			
12	5.6	0.15	0.75mL
13	2.0	0.05	0.25mL
14	0	0	

RO = receptor occupancy
*Alternatively, these doses could be made up using liquid formulations, prepared as above.
**Individual dose adjustments might be required in patients taking oral solution.[12,13] Overall pharmacokinetic examinations conclude that 1mg of oral solution is equivalent to 1mg in tablet form.[12] However, the oral solution peaks quicker and to a higher concentration that the drug in tablet form and so some patients may require 20% lower doses when transferring to liquid form.[13]

C. **A slower taper** with up to 2.3 percentage points of GABA$_A$ occupancy between each step – with reductions made every 1–4 weeks.

Step	RO (%)	Evening dose (mg)	Formulation	Step	RO(%)	Evening dose (mg)	Formulation
1	37.8	1.5	Use tablets	13	18.2	0.55	2.75mL
Switch to liquid formulation of lormetazepam (0.2mg/mL)*				14	16.8	0.5	2.5mL
2	36.2	1.4	7mL	15	15.4	0.45	2.25mL
3	34.5	1.3	6.5mL	16	13.9	0.4	2mL
4	32.7	1.2	6mL	17	12.4	0.35	1.75mL
5	30.8	1.1	5.5mL	18	10.8	0.3	1.5mL
6	28.8	1	5mL	19	9.2	0.25	1.25mL
7	26.7	0.9	4.5mL	20	7.5	0.2	1mL
8	24.5	0.8	4mL	21	5.7	0.15	0.75mL
9	23.3	0.75	3.75mL	22	3.9	0.1	0.5mL
10	22.1	0.7	3.5mL	23	2	0.05	0.25mL
11	20.8	0.65	3.25mL	24	0	0	
12	19.5	0.6	3mL				
See further steps in the right-hand column							

RO = receptor occupancy
*Individual dose adjustments might be required in patients taking oral solution.[12,13] Overall pharmacokinetic examinations conclude that 1mg of oral solution is equivalent to 1mg in tablet form.[12] However, the oral solution peaks quicker and to a higher concentration than the drug in tablet form and so some patients may require 20% lower doses when transferring to liquid form.[13]

D. **An even slower taper** Some patients will be unable to taper at the slowest rates shown here and will need to taper by even smaller decrements, thus lengthening the overall period of tapering. Such a regimen could be constructed by placing intermediate steps in regimen C. For example, 1.5mg, 1.4mg, 1.3mg could be modified to 1.5mg, 1.45mg, 1.4mg, 1.35mg, 1.3mg and so on. Further intermediate steps could also be added.

Micro-tapering: The tables above show how to make reductions at intervals of 1 to 4 weeks. An alternative approach is called 'micro-tapering' whereby very small dose reductions are made every day, as explained in 'Other considerations in tapering benzodiazepines and z-drugs.' Micro-tapering rates can be calculated from the above by dividing the change in dose for each step by 14 or 28 days. For example, for the moderate regimen a reduction of 1.5mg to 1.375mg over 14 days is approximately equivalent to a 0.01mg reduction per day. By the end of the taper this rate will reduce to reductions of 0.007mg a day.[18] This rate can be adjusted if withdrawal symptoms become too unpleasant.

Switching guide from lormetazepam to diazepam: An alternative to a direct taper from lormetazepam is to switch to diazepam before tapering from this drug, as outlined in 'Switching to longer-acting benzodiazepines to taper'. A 1.5mg dose of lormetazepam is equivalent to 15mg diazepam[1] with steps of 0.5mg of lormetazepam made every week (or as tolerated by the patient).

Steps	Evening	Daily diazepam equivalent
1	1.5mg lormetazepam	15mg
2	1mg lormetazepam 5mg diazepam	15mg
3	0.5mg lormetazepam 10mg diazepam	15mg
4	15mg diazepam	15mg
Continue to taper as for 15mg diazepam (see diazepam section)		

References

1. Ashton H. Benzodiazepines: how they work and how to withdraw (The Ashton Manual). Newcastle University, 2002. http://www.benzo.org.uk/manual/bzcha01.htm.

2. Dorow RG, Seidler J, Schneider HH. A radioreceptor assay to study the affinity of benzodiazepines and their receptor binding activity in human plasma including their active metabolites. *Br J Clin Pharmacol* 1982; 13: 561–5.

3. Genus Pharmaceuticals. Summary of Product Characteristics Dormagen 0.5mg Tablets. 2021. https://www.medicines.org.uk/emc/product/5269/smpc#gref (accessed 6 July 2023).

4. FDA Drug Safety Communication. FDA requiring boxed warning updated to improve safe use of benzodiazepine drug class. 2020. https://www.fda.gov/drugs/drug-safety-and-availability/fda-requiring-boxed-warning-updated-improve-safe-use-benzodiazepine-drug-class#:~:text=FDA is requiring the Boxed,and life-threatening side effects (accessed 3 July 2023).

5. Faccini M, Tamburin S, Casari R, Morbioli L, Lugoboni F. High-dose lormetazepam dependence: strange case of Dr. Jekyll and Mr. Hyde. *Intern Emerg Med* 2019; 14: 1271–8.

6. Bayer New Zealand Limited. NOCTAMID® lormetazepam 1.0mg tablet. 2019. https://www.medsafe.govt.nz/profs/datasheet/n/noctamidtab.pdf (accessed 6 July 2023).

7. Brouillet E, Chavoix C, Bottlaender M, et al. In vivo bidirectional modulatory effect of benzodiazepine receptor ligands on GABAergic transmission evaluated by positron emission tomography in non-human primates. *Brain Res* 1991; 557: 167–76.

8. Holford N. Pharmacodynamic principles and the time course of delayed and cumulative drug effects. *Transl Clin Pharmacology* 2018; 26: 56–9.

9. Horowitz M, Taylor D. Withdrawing from benzodiazepines and z-drugs (in preparation).

10. Horowitz MA, Taylor D. Tapering of SSRI treatment to mitigate withdrawal symptoms. *The Lancet Psychiatry* 2019; 6: 538–46.

11. Hypnotics and anxiolytics. https://bnf.nice.org.uk/treatment-summaries/hypnotics-and-anxiolytics/ (accessed 17 April 2023).

12. Guerra P, Soto A, Carcas AJ, Sancho A, Cassinello A, Frías-Iniesta J. Comparison of lormetazepam solution and capsules in healthy volunteers. *Clin Drug Investig* 2002; 22: 859–66.

13. Ancolio C, Tardieu S, Soubrouillard C, et al. A randomized clinical trial comparing doses and efficacy of lormetazepam tablets or oral solution for insomnia in a general practice setting. *Hum Psychopharmacol* 2004; 19: 129–34.

14. Smyth. J. The NEWT Guidelines for administration of medication to patients with enteral feeding tubes or swallowing difficulties website. The NEWT Guidelines. 2011. http://www.newtguidelines.com (accessed 6 July 2023).

15. Macheras PE, Koupparis MA, Antimisiaris SG. Drug binding and solubility in milk. *Pharm Res* 1990; 7: 537–41.

16. Guina J, Merrill B. Benzodiazepines II: waking up on sedatives: providing optimal care when inheriting benzodiazepine prescriptions in transfer patients. *J Clin Med Res* 2018; 7. doi:10.3390/jcm7020020.

17. Framer A. What I have learnt from helping thousands of people taper off psychotropic medications. *Ther Adv Psychopharmacol* 2021; 11: 204512532199127.

18. BenzoBuddies Community Forum. http://www.benzobuddies.org/forum/index.php (accessed 18 March 2023).

Nitrazepam

Trade names: Mogadon, Alodorm, Dumolid, Nitrazadon, Pacisyn.

Description: Nitrazepam is a medium-potency,[1,2] intermediate-acting benzodiazepine.[3] It is a positive allosteric modulator of the gamma-aminobutyric acid (GABA) type A receptor, which it affects by binding to the benzodiazepine binding site.[4] The manufacturer in the UK states 'Generally the duration of treatment varies from a few days to two weeks, with a maximum of four weeks; including the tapering off process' and 'long-term chronic use is not recommended'.[5]

Withdrawal effects: Benzodiazepines carry a boxed warning from the FDA that highlights that physical dependence and withdrawal effects can occur when the drugs are taken 'for several days to weeks, even as prescribed'.[6] Not everyone who stops nitrazepam will experience withdrawal and some of those who do will only experience mild symptoms – this probably depends on drug dose, duration of use and individual factors. However, in a very few instances, stopping abruptly can cause seizures and can be life threatening. Numerous other physical, cognitive and psychological withdrawal symptoms, outlined in 'Withdrawal effects from benzodiazepines and z-drugs', are possible, which can last 'for several weeks to more than 12 months' after stopping according to the FDA.[5,6]

Peak plasma: 2 hours.[5]

Half-life: 24 hours.[5] The manufacturer recommends that nitrazepam be dosed once nightly.[5] Dosing less often (including every-other-day dosing) is not recommended because the changes in plasma levels may precipitate withdrawal symptoms.

Receptor occupancy: The relationship between dose of nitrazepam and the occupancy of its major target $GABA_A$ is hyperbolic, according to the law of mass action.[7,8] Benzodiazepines demonstrate a hyperbolic relationship between dose and clinical effects,[9] which may be relevant to withdrawal effects. Dose reductions made by linear amounts (e.g. 10mg, 7.5mg, 5mg, 2.5mg, 0mg) will cause slightly larger reductions in effect each step, which may cause increasingly severe withdrawal effects (Figure 3.19a). Hyperbolic tapering is required to produce linear changes in effect on receptor occupancy,[10] although because of the nature of the occupancy curve, this pattern is not substantially different from linear tapering (Figure 3.19b),[9] which informs the

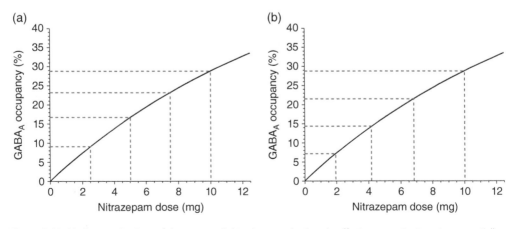

Figure 3.19 (a) Linear reductions of dose cause slighter larger reductions in effect on receptor targets sequentially, possibly associated with more withdrawal effects. (b) Even reductions of effect at target receptors requires hyperbolic dose reductions. In this case the nature of the occupancy curve is such that this pattern of dose reduction does not differ greatly from linear reductions.

reductions presented. The relationship was derived by converting the receptor occupancy curve for diazepam[11] to equivalent nitrazepam dose.[12]

Available formulations: As tablets and liquid.

Tablets

Dosage	UK	Europe	USA	Australia	Canada
5mg	✓	✓	–	✓	✓
10mg	–	✓	–	–	✓

Liquid

Oral suspension	UK	Europe	US	Australia	Canada
2.5mg/5mL (0.5mg/mL)	✓*	–	–	–	–

*Store in a refrigerator (2 °C – 8 °C). Protect from light. Do not freeze. The bottle should be shaken before use.[13]

Dilutions: To make up some of the small doses for people who need to taper slowly, dilution of the liquid available from the manufacturer may be required. In order to make a dilution a syringe will generally need to be used rather than the measuring cylinder provided by the manufacturer. Adding water to the original solution may have the effect of precipitating nitrazepam and so a suspension might be formed.[13] All dilutions need therefore to be shaken thoroughly before use.[13] As the stability of the suspension cannot be assured the dilution should be used immediately and the excess discarded.

UK dilutions	Solution required	How to prepare solution
Doses ≥ 0.1mg	0.5mg/mL	Original solution
Doses < 0.1mg	0.1mg/mL	Mix 0.5mL of original solution with 2mL of water*

*Other dilutions are possible to produce different concentrations. The above is provided as an example.

Worked example: To illustrate how the volumes can be calculated in the regimens given, a worked example is provided. The manufacturer's suspension comes with a measuring cup, but to make up small doses a syringe will have to be used instead of the measuring cup. To make up 0.4mg of nitrazepam the 2.5mg/5mL (0.5mg/mL) suspension can be used. The volume of 0.5mg/mL liquid required to give a dose of 0.4mg nitrazepam is 0.4/0.5 = 0.8mL.

Off-label options: In order to follow the regimens suggested in some cases smaller doses are required than can be made using commercially available tablets where no liquid versions are available. Guidelines for people who cannot swallow tablets[14,15] suggest that nitrazepam tablets can be dispersed in water for administration. It takes more than a couple of minutes for these to disperse.[15] The tablet may be crushed with a spoon or pestle and mortar before mixing with water to speed up this process. For example, water could be added to a 5mg tablet to make up a 10mL suspension (concentration 1mg in 2mL or 0.5mg/mL). The suspension should be shaken vigorously before use. As its stability cannot be assured, it should be

CHAPTER 3

consumed immediately, and any unused suspension discarded. Some patients use full-fat milk to make liquid preparations. Benzodiazepines are more soluble in oil or fat than in water.[16] When mixed with milk, some or all of the drug will dissolve in the milk fat. This should form an evenly dispersed emulsion when shaken vigorously. The measured dose should be taken immediately after shaking and the remainder discarded.

Another option is to switch to diazepam (see later) or to have a suspension or smaller-dose tablets or capsules made up by a compounding pharmacy.

Deprescribing notes: There are two main methods for tapering from nitrazepam – a switch to a longer-acting benzodiazepine like diazepam or a direct taper of nitrazepam itself. There are no established guides to determine the rate of taper for someone stopping benzodiazepines. Withdrawal is known to be more severe for people who have used benzodiazepines which are shorter acting, for longer periods, at higher doses, and for those who have experienced withdrawal in the past on reducing, stopping or missing a dose.[17,18] The size of the initial reduction can be estimated based on these factors (see 'Tapering benzodiazepines and z-drugs in practice'), with patient preference also taken into account. Sometimes an even smaller reduction to start with may be advisable to boost a patient's confidence that they can taper if performed carefully.

Each reduction should be made when the withdrawal symptoms from the previous reduction have largely resolved so that subsequent reductions do not lead to cumulative withdrawal symptoms. Withdrawal symptoms should not be too unpleasant: a rate of reduction should be aimed for that produces tolerable withdrawal symptoms that abate within a week or two. Allowing for a sufficient observation period, reductions can therefore be made about every 1–4 weeks, depending on how long it takes withdrawal symptoms to resolve. If withdrawal symptoms are moderately severe or take longer than a couple of weeks to resolve, dose reductions should be postponed until symptoms resolve and then made more gradually by choosing a slower tapering rate. If severe withdrawal symptoms occur then the patient should return to a higher dose, wait until symptoms resolve and thereafter taper at a slower rate.

Suggested direct taper schedules for nitrazepam Please note that none of these regimens should be seen as prescriptive – patients should not be compelled to adhere strictly to them. They are given as example regimens and are not 'set and forget' but should be modified in order to ensure that withdrawal symptoms are tolerable throughout a taper. For example, intermediate steps halfway between the doses listed could be added to make a more gradual taper. Ultimately, it is the patient's experience of withdrawal that should guide the rate of taper.

A. **A faster taper** with up to 4 percentage points of $GABA_A$ occupancy between each step – with reductions made every 1–4 weeks*.

Step	RO (%)	Dose (mg)	Formulation	Step	RO (%)	Dose (mg)	Formulation
1	28.8	10	Use tablets	7	9.2	2.5	Use ½ tablets**
2	26.2	8.75	Use ¾ tablets**	Switch to liquid suspension **(0.5mg/mL)***			
3	23.3	7.5	Use ½ tablets**	8	5.6	1.5	3mL
4	20.2	6.25	Use ¼ tablets**	9	2.0	0.5	1mL
5	16.8	5	Use tablets	10	0	0	
6	13.2	3.75	Use ¾ tablets**				
See further steps in the right-hand column							

RO = receptor occupancy

*Patients who have been on the medication for only a few weeks will probably be able to taper more quickly and might follow every second or third step of this regimen and make reductions every few days or so. Normally the duration of the taper should not be longer than the period that the patient has been on the drug for people who have only taken it for a few weeks. For example, if nitrazepam is taken for 3 weeks the taper should be less than 3 weeks. However, the FDA has issued an alert regarding dependence and withdrawal from benzodiazepines indicating that some people can experience withdrawal effects after just a few days of use,[7] therefore necessitating slower tapering in these people.

**Alternatively, these could be made up using a liquid or compounded formulation.

***Either as a licenced (UK) or off-label version (elsewhere), prepared as above.

B. **A moderate taper** with up to 2.2 percentage points of $GABA_A$ occupancy between each step – with reductions made every 1–4 weeks.

Step	RO (%)	Dose (mg)	Formulation	Step	RO (%)	Dose (mg)	Formulation
1	28.8	10	Use tablets	10	15.4	4.5	9mL
Switch to liquid suspension **(0.5mg/mL)***				11	13.9	4	8mL
2	26.7	9	18mL	12	12.4	3.5	7mL
3	24.5	8	16mL	13	10.8	3	6mL
4	23.3	7.5	15mL	14	9.2	2.5	5mL
5	22.1	7	14mL	15	7.5	2	4mL
6	20.8	6.5	13mL	16	5.7	1.5	3mL
7	19.5	6	12mL	17	3.9	1	2mL
8	18.2	5.5	11mL	18	2	0.5	1mL
9	16.8	5	10mL	19	0	0	
See further steps in the right-hand column							

RO = receptor occupancy

*Either as a licenced (UK) or off-label version (elsewhere), prepared as above. Compounded medication is another option.

C. **A slower taper** with up to 1.2 percentage points of $GABA_A$ occupancy between each step – with reductions made every 1–4 weeks.

Step	RO (%)	Dose (mg)	Formulation	Step	RO (%)	Dose (mg)	Formulation
1	28.8	10	Use tablets	19	12.1	3.4	6.8mL
Switch to liquid suspension **(0.5mg/mL)***				20	11.5	3.2	6.4mL
2	28	9.6	19.2mL	21	10.8	3	6mL
3	27.1	9.2	18.4mL	22	10.2	2.8	5.6mL
4	26.3	8.8	17.6mL	23	9.5	2.6	5.2mL
5	25.4	8.4	16.8mL	24	8.9	2.4	4.8mL
6	24.5	8	16mL	25	8.2	2.2	4.4mL
7	23.5	7.6	15.2mL	26	7.5	2	4mL
8	22.6	7.2	14.4mL	27	6.8	1.8	3.6mL
9	21.6	6.8	13.6mL	28	6.1	1.6	3.2mL
10	20.6	6.4	12.8mL	29	5.4	1.4	2.8mL
11	19.5	6	12mL	30	4.6	1.2	2.4mL
12	18.5	5.6	11.2mL	31	3.9	1	2mL
13	17.4	5.2	10.4mL	32	3.1	0.8	1.6mL
14	16.3	4.8	9.6mL	33	2.4	0.6	1.2mL
15	15.1	4.4	8.8mL	34	1.6	0.4	0.8mL
16	13.9	4	8mL	35	0.8	0.2	0.4mL
17	13.3	3.8	7.6mL	36	0	0	
18	12.7	3.6	7.2mL				
See further steps in the right-hand column							

RO = receptor occupancy
*Either as a licenced (UK) or off-label version (elsewhere), prepared as above. Compounded medication is another option.

D. **An even slower taper** Some patients will be unable to taper at the slowest rates shown here and will need to taper by even smaller decrements, thus lengthening the overall period of tapering. Such a regimen could be constructed by placing intermediate steps between those of regimen C. For example, 10mg, 9.6mg, 9.2mg could be modified to 10mg, 9.8mg, 9.6mg, 9.4mg, 9.2mg and so on. Further intermediate steps could also be added.

Micro-tapering: The tables above show how to make reductions at intervals of 1–4 weeks. An alternative approach is called 'micro-tapering' whereby very small dose reductions are made every day, as explained in 'Other considerations in tapering benzodiazepines and z-drugs.' Micro-tapering rates can be calculated from the above by dividing the change in dose for each step by 14 or 28 days. For example, for the moderate regimen a reduction of 10mg to 9mg over 14 days is equivalent to a reduction of 0.07mg per day. By the end of the moderate regimen the rate of reduction would have slowed down to a reduction of 0.036mg per day. The rate can be adjusted if withdrawal symptoms become too unpleasant.

Switching guide from nitrazepam to diazepam: An alternative to a direct taper from nitrazepam is to switch to diazepam before tapering from this drug, as outlined in 'Switching to longer-acting benzodiazepines to taper'. A 10mg dose of nitrazepam is equivalent to 10mg diazepam.[19] Conversions of 5mg of flurazepam can be made every week (or as tolerated by the patient).

Steps	Evening	Daily diazepam equivalent
1	10mg nitrazepam	10mg
2	5mg nitrazepam 5mg diazepam	10mg
3	Stop nitrazepam 10mg diazepam	10mg
Continue to taper as for 10mg diazepam (see diazepam section).		

References

1. Chouinard G. Issues in the clinical use of benzodiazepines: potency, withdrawal, and rebound. *J Clin Psychiatry* 2004; 65 Suppl 5: 7–12.

2. Choosing an equivalent dose of oral benzodiazepine. SPS — Specialist Pharmacy Service. 2022; published online 25 January. https://www.sps.nhs.uk/articles/choosing-an-equivalent-dose-of-oral-benzodiazepine/ (accessed 8 April 2023).

3. Lexicomp: Evidence-Based Drug Referential Content. https://www.wolterskluwer.com/en/solutions/lexicomp (accessed 19 March 2023).

4. PharmGKB. PharmGKB. https://www.pharmgkb.org/literature/6754762 (accessed 19 March 2023).

5. Nitrazepam 5mg Tablets – Summary of Product Characteristics (SmPC) – (emc). https://www.medicines.org.uk/emc/product/7145/smpc (accessed 8 April 2023).

6. FDA Drug Safety Communication. FDA requiring boxed warning updated to improve safe use of benzodiazepine drug class. 2020. https://www.fda.gov/drugs/drug-safety-and-availability/fda-requiring-boxed-warning-updated-improve-safe-use-benzodiazepine-drug-class#:~:text=FDA is requiring the Boxed,and life-threatening side effects (accessed 3 July 2023).

7. Innis RB, al-Tikriti MS, Zoghbi SS, et al. SPECT imaging of the benzodiazepine receptor: feasibility of in vivo potency measurements from stepwise displacement curves. *J Nucl Med* 1991; 32: 1754–61.

8. Holford N. Pharmacodynamic principles and the time course of delayed and cumulative drug effects. *Translational and Clinical Pharmacology* 2018; 26: 56–9.

9. Horowitz M, Taylor D. Withdrawing from benzodiazepines and z-drugs (in preparation).

10. Horowitz MA, Taylor D. Tapering of SSRI treatment to mitigate withdrawal symptoms. *The Lancet Psychiatry* 2019; 6: 538–46.

11. Brouillet E, Chavoix C, Bottlaender M, et al. In vivo bidirectional modulatory effect of benzodiazepine receptor ligands on GABAergic transmission evaluated by positron emission tomography in non-human primates. *Brain Res* 1991; 557: 167–76.

12. Hypnotics and anxiolytics. https://bnf.nice.org.uk/treatment-summaries/hypnotics-and-anxiolytics/ (accessed 19 March 2023).

13. Nitrazepam Mixture 2.5mg/5ml Oral Suspension BP – Summary of Product Characteristics (SmPC) – (emc). http://www.medicines.org.uk/emc/product/13277/smpc (accessed 8 April 2023).

14. AboutKidsHealth. https://www.aboutkidshealth.ca/Article?contentid=200&language=English (accessed 8 April 2023).

15. Covert medication and dysphagia - safe and cost effective administration (MHS MRG 02). https://mypsych.nhsggc.org.uk/medicines-companion/medicines-guidance-a-z/covert-medication-and-dysphagia-safe-and-cost-effective-administration-mhs-mrg-02/ (accessed 8 April 2023).

16. Macheras PE, Koupparis MA, Antimisiaris SG. Drug binding and solubility in milk. *Pharm Res* 1990; 7: 537–41.

17. Guina J, Merrill B. Benzodiazepines II: Waking up on sedatives: providing optimal care when inheriting benzodiazepine prescriptions in transfer patients. *J Clin Med Res* 2018; 7. doi:10.3390/jcm7020020.

18. Framer A. What I have learnt from helping thousands of people taper off psychotropic medications. *Ther Adv Psychopharmacol* 2021; 11: 204512532199127.

19. Ashton H. Benzodiazepines: how they work and how to withdraw (The Ashton Manual). Newcastle University, 2002. http://www.benzo.org.uk/manual/bzcha01.htm (accessed 11 July 2023).

CHAPTER 3

Oxazepam

Trade names: Serax, Alepam, Medopam, Murelax, Noripam, Opamox, Oxabenz, Oxapax, Oxascand, Ox-Pam, Purata, Serenid, Serepax, Seresta, Sobril.

Description: Oxazepam is a low-potency,[1] short-acting benzodiazepine, which binds to several sites within the CNS including the limbic system and the reticular formation.[2] It is a positive allosteric modulator of the gamma-aminobutyric acid (GABA) type A receptor.[3] The manufacturer recommends the use of the lowest effective dose for a period not exceeding 4 weeks.[2]

Withdrawal effects: Oxazepam, like other benzodiazepines, carries a boxed warning from the FDA that emphasises the risk of dependence and withdrawal with prolonged use and high doses.[4] Not everyone who stops oxazepam will experience withdrawal effects, and some might only experience mild symptoms depending on the treatment duration, dose and the patient. However, the FDA warns against abrupt discontinuation and sudden dose reduction due to its increased risk of withdrawal reactions with continued use, some of which could be life threatening.[5] Numerous other physical, cognitive and psychological withdrawal symptoms (outlined in 'Withdrawal effects from benzodiazepines and z-drugs') are also possible, which can last 'for several weeks to more than 12 months' after stopping according to the FDA.[5]

Peak plasma: Oxazepam is a pharmacologically active metabolite of diazepam. Following administration, oxazepam is rapidly absorbed and reaches peak serum levels in 1–5 hours.[2]

Half-life and dosing: The mean half-life is 5–20 hours. The manufacturer recommends dosing 3–4 times a day for anxiety or once nightly for insomnia.[2] Dosing less often (including every-other-day dosing) is not recommended for tapering because the changes in plasma levels may precipitate inter-dose withdrawal symptoms.

Receptor occupancy: The relationship between dose of oxazepam and the occupancy of its major target GABA$_A$ is hyperbolic according to the law of mass action.[6,7] Benzodiazepines demonstrate a hyperbolic relationship between dose and clinical effects,[8] which may be relevant to withdrawal effects. Dose reductions made by linear amounts (e.g. 120mg, 90mg, 60mg, 30mg, 0mg) will cause increasingly large reductions in effect, which may cause increasingly severe withdrawal effects (Figure 3.20a).

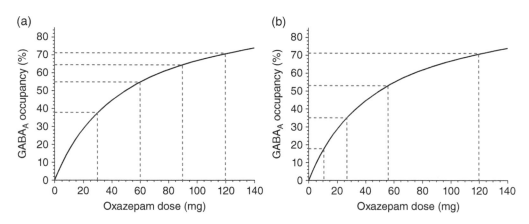

Figure 3.20 (a) Linear reductions of dose cause increasingly large reductions in effect on receptor targets, possibly associated with more withdrawal effects. (b) Even reductions of effect at target receptors requires hyperbolic dose reductions. The final dose before stopping will need to be very small so that this step down is not larger (in terms of effect on receptor occupancy) than previous reductions.

To produce equal-sized reductions in effect on receptor occupancy will require hyperbolically reducing doses (Figure 3.20b),[9] which informs the reductions presented. The relationship was derived by converting the receptor occupancy curve for diazepam[6] to equivalent oxazepam dose.[10]

Available formulations: As tablets and capsules.

Tablets

Dosage	UK	Europe	USA	Australia	Canada
10mg	✓	✓	–	–	✓
15mg	✓	✓	–	✓	✓
30mg	–	–	–	✓	✓
50mg	–	✓	–	–	–
100mg	–	✓	–	–	–

Capsules

Dosage	UK	Europe	USA	Australia	Canada
10mg	–	–	✓	–	–
15mg	–	–	✓	–	–
30mg	–	–	✓	–	–

Off- label options: In order to follow the regimens suggested in some cases, smaller doses are required than can be made using commercially available tablets and capsules where no liquid versions are available. Guidelines for people who cannot swallow tablets (e.g. NEWT guidelines in the UK based on advice from the manufacturer or local hospital guidance)[11] advise to change to the liquid formulation of diazepam. Another option would be to disperse oxazepam tablets in water. The tablets will disintegrate easily in water.[11] For example, water could be added to a 10mg tablet to make up 10mL suspension with concentration of 1mg/mL. The suspension should be shaken vigorously or mixed well before administration. As its stability cannot be assured it should be consumed immediately, and any unused suspension discarded. Some patients use full-fat milk to make liquid preparations. Benzodiazepines are more soluble in oil or fat than in water.[12] When mixed with milk, some or all of the drug will dissolve in the milk fat. This should form an evenly dispersed emulsion when shaken vigorously. The measured dose should be taken immediately after shaking and the remainder discarded.

Other options to make up small doses include having a compounding pharmacy make up a suspension or smaller dose suspensions or tablets, including the option of 'tapering strips'.[13]

Worked example: To illustrate how the volumes can be calculated for the regimens given below, a worked example is provided. To make up 0.4mg of oxazepam a 1mg/mL suspension can be used, prepared as above. The volume of 1mg/mL liquid required to give a dose of 0.4mg oxazepam is 0.4/1 = 0.4mL.

CHAPTER 3

Deprescribing notes: There are two main methods for tapering from oxazepam – a switch to diazepam or a direct taper of oxazepam itself. There are no established guides to determine the rate of taper for someone stopping benzodiazepines. Withdrawal is known to be more severe for people who have used benzodiazepines which are shorter acting, for longer periods, at higher doses, and for those who have experienced withdrawal in the past on reducing, stopping or missing a dose.[12,14] The size of the initial reduction can be estimated based on these factors (see 'Tapering benzodiazepines and z-drugs in practice'), with patient preference also taken into account. Sometimes an even smaller reduction to start with may be advisable to boost a patient's confidence that they can taper if performed carefully.

Each reduction should be made when the withdrawal symptoms from the previous reduction have largely resolved so that subsequent reductions do not lead to cumulative withdrawal symptoms. Withdrawal symptoms should not be too unpleasant: a rate of reduction should be aimed for that produces tolerable withdrawal symptoms that abate within a week or two. Allowing for a sufficient observation period, reductions can therefore be made about every 1–4 weeks, depending on how long it takes withdrawal symptoms to resolve. If withdrawal symptoms are moderately severe or take longer than a couple of weeks to resolve, dose reductions should be postponed until symptoms resolve and then made more gradually by choosing a slower tapering rate. If severe withdrawal symptoms occur then the patient should return to a higher dose, wait until symptoms resolve and thereafter taper at a slower rate.

Suggested direct taper schedules for oxazepam: Please note that none of these regimens should be seen as prescriptive – patients should not be compelled to strictly adhere to them. They are given as example regimens and are not 'set and forget' but should be modified in order to ensure that withdrawal symptoms are tolerable throughout a taper. For example, intermediate steps halfway between the doses listed could be added to make a more gradual taper. Ultimately, it is the patient's experience of withdrawal that should guide the rate of taper.

A. A faster taper with up to 5.2 percentage points of $GABA_A$ occupancy between each step – with reductions made every 1–4 weeks.*

Step	RO (%)	AM (mg)	PM (mg)	Night (mg)	Total daily dose (mg)	Form
1	70.8	40	40	40	120	Use tabs or caps
2	66.9	30	30	40	100	Use tabs or caps
3	61.8	30	20	30	80	Use tabs or caps
4	58.6	20	20	30	70	Use tabs or caps
5	54.8	20	20	20	60	Use tabs or caps
6	50.3	20	10	20	50	Use tabs or caps
7	47.7	15	10	20	45	Use tabs or caps
8	44.7	15	10	15	40	Use tabs or caps
9	41.5	10	10	15	35	Use tabs or caps
10	37.8	10	10	10	30	Use tabs or caps
Switch to liquid oxazepam (1 mg/mL)						
11	35.8	10	7.5	10	27.5	Liquid**
12	33.6	7.5	7.5	10	25	Liquid**
See further steps in the right-hand column						

Step	RO (%)	AM (mg)	PM (mg)	Night (mg)	Total daily dose (mg)	Form
13	31.3	7.5	7.5	7.5	22.5	Liquid**
14	28.8	7.5	5	7.5	20	Liquid**
15	26.2	5	5	7.5	17.5	Liquid**
16	23.3	5	5	5	15	Liquid**
17	20.2	5	2.5	5	12.5	Liquid**
18	16.8	2.5	2.5	5	10	Liquid**
19	13.2	2.5	2.5	2.5	7.5	Liquid**
20	9.2	1.25	1.25	2.5	5	Liquid
21	7.1	1.25	1.25	1.25	3.75	Liquid
22	4.8	1.25	0	1.25	2.5	Liquid
23	2.5	0	0	1.25	1.25	Liquid
24	0	0	0	0	0	

RO = receptor occupancy, caps = capsules, tabs = tablets

*Patients who have been on the medication for only a few weeks will probably be able to taper more quickly and might follow every second or third step of this regimen and make reductions every few days or so. Normally the duration of the taper should not be longer than the period that the patient has been on the drug for people who have only taken it for a few weeks. For example, if oxazepam is taken for 3 weeks, the taper should be less than 3 weeks. However the FDA has issued an warning for benzodiazepines indicating that some people can experience withdrawal effects after just a few days of use,[12] therefore necessitating slower tapering in this sub-group.

**Alternatively, these doses can be made up by half or quarter tablet portions or compounded medication.

CHAPTER 3

B. A moderate taper with up to 2.8 percentage points of GABA$_A$ occupancy between each step – with reductions made every 1–4 weeks.

Step	RO (%)	AM (mg)	PM (mg)	Night (mg)	Total daily dose (mg)	Form
1	70.8	40	40	40	120	Use tabs or caps
2	69	35	35	40	110	Use tabs or caps
3	66.9	35	30	35	100	Use tabs or caps
4	64.6	30	30	30	90	Use tabs or caps
5	61.8	25	25	30	80	Use tabs or caps
6	60.3	25	25	25	75	Use tabs or caps
7	58.6	25	20	25	70	Use tabs or caps
8	56.8	20	20	25	65	Use tabs or caps
9	54.8	20	20	20	60	Use tabs or caps
10	52.7	20	15	20	55	Use tabs or caps
11	50.3	15	15	20	50	Use tabs or caps
Switch to liquid oxazepam (1mg/mL)						
12	48.2	15	15	16	46	Liquid
13	46	14	14	14	42	Liquid
14	44.1	13	12	14	39	Liquid
15	42.8	12	12	13	37	Liquid
16	41.5	12	11	12	35	Liquid
17	40	11	11	11	33	Liquid
18	38.6	10	10	11	31	Liquid
19	37	10	9	10	29	Liquid
20	35.3	9	9	9	27	Liquid

See further steps in the right-hand column

Step	RO (%)	AM (mg)	PM (mg)	Night (mg)	Total daily dose (mg)	Form
21	33.6	8	8	9	25	Liquid
22	31.8	8	7	8	23	Liquid
23	29.8	7	7	7	21	Liquid
24	27.8	6	6	7	19	Liquid
25	25.6	6	5	6	17	Liquid
26	23.5	5	5	5.2	15.2	Liquid
27	21.6	4.4	4.4	4.8	13.6	Liquid
28	19.5	4	4	4	12	Liquid
29	17.4	3.6	3.2	3.6	10.4	Liquid
30	15.1	2.8	2.8	3.2	8.8	Liquid
31	13.3	2.4	2.4	2.8	7.6	Liquid
32	12.1	2.4	2	2.4	6.8	Liquid
33	10.8	2	2	2	6	Liquid
34	9.5	1.6	1.6	2	5.2	Liquid
35	8.2	1.6	1.2	1.6	4.4	Liquid
36	6.8	1.2	1.2	1.2	3.6	Liquid
37	5.4	0.8	0.8	1.2	2.8	Liquid
38	3.9	0.8	0.4	0.8	2	Liquid
39	2.4	0.4	0.4	0.4	1.2	Liquid
40	0.8	0.2	0	0.2	0.4	Liquid
41	0	0	0	0	0	Liquid

RO = receptor occupancy, caps = capsules, tabs = tablets

C. A slower taper with up to 1.4 percentage points of GABA$_A$ occupancy between each step – with reductions made every 1–4 weeks.

Step	RO (%)	AM (mg)	PM (mg)	Night (mg)	Total daily dose (mg)	Form
1	70.8	40	40	40	120	Use tabs or caps
2	70	40	35	40	115	Use tabs or caps
3	69	35	35	40	110	Use tabs or caps
4	68	35	35	35	105	Use tabs or caps
5	66.9	35	30	35	100	Use tabs or caps
6	65.8	30	30	35	95	Use tabs or caps
7	64.6	30	30	30	90	Use tabs or caps
8	63.2	30	25	30	85	Use tabs or caps
9	61.8	25	25	30	80	Use tabs or caps
10	61.1	25	25	27.5	77.5	Use ¼ tablets*
11	60.3	25	25	25	75	Use tabs or caps
12	59.5	25	22.5	25	72.5	Use ¼ tablets*
13	58.6	22.5	22.5	25	70	Use ¼ tablets*
14	57.7	22.5	22.5	22.5	67.5	Use ¼ tablets*
15	56.8	22.5	20	22.5	65	Use ¼ tablets*
16	55.9	20	20	22.5	62.5	Use ¼ tablets*
17	54.8	20	20	20	60	Use tabs or caps
18	53.8	20	17.5	20	57.5	Use ¼ tablets*
19	52.7	17.5	17.5	20	55	Use ¼ tablets*
20	51.5	17.5	17.5	17.5	52.5	Use ¼ tablets*
21	50.3	17.5	15	17.5	50	Use ¼ tablets*

Switch to liquid oxazepam (1mg/mL)

See further steps in the right-hand column

Step	RO (%)	AM (mg)	PM (mg)	Night (mg)	Total daily dose (mg)	Form
22	49.3	16	15	17	48	Liquid
23	48.2	15	15	16	46	Liquid
24	47.1	14	14	16	44	Liquid
25	46	14	14	14	42	Liquid
26	44.7	14	12	14	40	Liquid
27	44.1	13	12	14	39	Liquid
28	43.5	13	12	13	38	Liquid
29	42.8	12	12	13	37	Liquid
30	42.2	12	12	12	36	Liquid
31	41.5	12	11	12	35	Liquid
32	40.8	11	11	12	34	Liquid
33	40	11	11	11	33	Liquid
34	39.3	11	10	11	32	Liquid
35	38.6	10	10	11	31	Liquid
36	37.8	10	10	10	30	Liquid
37	37	10	9	10	29	Liquid
38	36.2	9	9	10	28	Liquid
39	35.3	9	9	9	27	Liquid
40	34.5	9	8	9	26	Liquid
41	33.6	8	8	9	25	Liquid
42	32.7	8	8	8	24	Liquid
43	31.8	8	7	8	23	Liquid

(Continued)

(Continued)

Step	RO (%)	AM (mg)	PM (mg)	Night (mg)	Total daily dose (mg)	Form	Step	RO (%)	AM (mg)	PM (mg)	Night (mg)	Total daily dose (mg)	Form
44	30.8	7	7	8	22	Liquid	63	12.1	2.4	2	2.4	6.8	Liquid
45	29.8	7	7	7	21	Liquid	64	11.5	2	2	2.4	6.4	Liquid
46	28.8	7	6	7	20	Liquid	65	10.8	2	2	2	6	Liquid
47	27.8	6	6	7	19	Liquid	66	10.2	2	1.6	2	5.6	Liquid
48	26.7	6	6	6	18	Liquid	67	9.5	1.6	1.6	2	5.2	Liquid
49	25.6	6	5	6	17	Liquid	68	8.9	1.6	1.6	1.6	4.8	Liquid
50	24.5	5	5	6	16	Liquid	69	8.2	1.6	1.2	1.6	4.4	Liquid
51	23.5	5	5	5.2	15.2	Liquid	70	7.5	1.2	1.2	1.6	4	Liquid
52	22.6	4.8	4.8	4.8	14.4	Liquid	71	6.8	1.2	1.2	1.2	3.6	Liquid
53	21.6	4.4	4.4	4.8	13.6	Liquid	72	6.1	1.2	0.8	1.2	3.2	Liquid
54	20.6	4	4	4.8	12.8	Liquid	73	5.4	0.8	0.8	1.2	2.8	Liquid
55	19.5	4	4	4	12	Liquid	74	4.6	0.8	0.8	0.8	2.4	Liquid
56	18.5	3.6	3.6	4	11.2	Liquid	75	3.9	0.8	0.4	0.8	2	Liquid
57	17.4	3.6	3.2	3.6	10.4	Liquid	76	3.1	0.4	0.4	0.8	1.6	Liquid
58	16.3	3.2	3.2	3.2	9.6	Liquid	77	2.4	0.4	0.4	0.4	1.2	Liquid
59	15.1	2.8	2.8	3.2	8.8	Liquid	78	1.6	0.4	0	0.4	0.8	Liquid
60	13.9	2.8	2.4	2.8	8	Liquid	79	0.8	0.2	0	0.2	0.4	Liquid
61	13.3	2.4	2.4	2.8	7.6	Liquid	80	0	0	0	0	0	
62	12.7	2.4	2.4	2.4	7.2	Liquid							

See further steps in the right-hand column

RO = receptor occupancy, caps = capsules, tabs = tablets

D. **An even slower taper** Some patients will be unable to taper at the slowest rates shown here and will need to taper by even smaller decrements, thus lengthening the overall period of tapering. Such a regimen could be constructed by placing intermediate steps in regimen C. For example, 120mg, 115mg, 110mg, 0mg could be modified to 120mg, 117.5mg, 115mg, 112.5mg, 110mg and so on. Further intermediate steps could also be added.

Micro-tapering: The tables show how to make reductions at intervals of 1–4 weeks. An alternative approach is called 'micro-tapering' whereby very small dose reductions are made every day, as explained in 'Other considerations in tapering benzodiazepines and z-drugs.' Micro-tapering rates can be calculated from the above by dividing the change in dose for each step by 14 or 28 days. For example, for the moderate regime, a reduction of 120mg to 110mg over 14 days is equivalent to a reduction of 0.7mg per day, or 0.24mg per dose (when the drug is taken three times a day). By the end of the taper this rate will reduce to reductions of 0.03mg per day.[15] This rate can be adjusted if withdrawal symptoms become too unpleasant.

Switching guide from oxazepam to diazepam: An alternative to a direct taper from oxazepam is to switch to diazepam before tapering from this drug, as outlined in 'Switching to longer-acting benzodiazepines to taper'. A 30mg dose of oxazepam is equivalent to 15mg diazepam with steps of 20mg of oxazepam[16] made every week (or as tolerated by the patient).

Steps	Morning	Afternoon	Evening	Daily diazepam equivalent
1	40mg oxazepam	40mg oxazepam	40mg oxazepam	60mg
2	40mg oxazepam	20mg oxazepam 10mg diazepam	40mg oxazepam	60mg
3	20mg oxazepam/ 10mg diazepam	20mg oxazepam 10mg diazepam	40mg oxazepam	60mg
4	20mg oxazepam/ 10mg diazepam	20mg oxazepam 10mg diazepam	20mg oxazepam 10mg diazepam	60mg
5	20mg oxazepam/ 10mg diazepam	Stop oxazepam 20mg diazepam	20mg oxazepam 10mg diazepam	60mg
6	Stop oxazepam/ 20mg diazepam	20mg diazepam	20mg oxazepam 10mg diazepam	60mg
7	20mg diazepam	20mg diazepam	Stop oxazepam 20mg diazepam	60mg
Continue to taper as for 60mg diazepam (see diazepam section).				

References

1. Chouinard G. Issues in the clinical use of benzodiazepines: potency, withdrawal, and rebound. *J Clin Psychiatry* 2004; 65 Suppl 5: 7–12.

2. Genus Pharmaceuticals. Summary of Product Characteristics Oxazepam 10mg tablets. 2018. https://www.medicines.org.uk/emc/product/5338/smpc#gref (accessed 6 July 2023).

3. PharmGKB. PharmGKB. https://www.pharmgkb.org/literature/6754762 (accessed 19 March 2023).

4. U.S Food & Drug Administration. FDA requiring boxed warning updated to improve safe use of benzodiazepine drug class. 2020. https://www.fda.gov/drugs/drug-safety-and-availability/fda-requiring-boxed-warning-updated-improve-safe-use-benzodiazepine-drug-class (accessed 3 July 2023).

5. NIH DailyMed. Drug Label Information Oxazepam 10mg capsules Boxed Warning. 2021. https://dailymed.nlm.nih.gov/dailymed/drugInfo.cfm?setid=bda8bc70-3328-46f2-89d5-7ef7a061b418#boxedwarning (accessed 6 July 2023).

6. Brouillet E, Chavoix C, Bottlaender M, et al. In vivo bidirectional modulatory effect of benzodiazepine receptor ligands on GABAergic transmission evaluated by positron emission tomography in non-human primates. *Brain Res* 1991; 557: 167–76.

7. Holford N. Pharmacodynamic principles and the time course of delayed and cumulative drug effects. *Transl Clin Pharmacol* 2018; 26: 56–9.

8. Horowitz M, Taylor D. Withdrawing from benzodiazepines and z-drugs (in preparation).

9. Horowitz MA, Taylor D. Tapering of SSRI treatment to mitigate withdrawal symptoms. *The Lancet Psychiatry* 2019; 6: 538–46.

10. Hypnotics and anxiolytics. https://bnf.nice.org.uk/treatment-summaries/hypnotics-and-anxiolytics/ (accessed 19 March 2023).

11. Smyth. J. The NEWT Guidelines for administration of medication to patients with enteral feeding tubes or swallowing difficulties website. The NEWT Guidelines. 2011. http://www.newtguidelines.com (accessed 5 July 2023).

12. Guina J, Merrill B. Benzodiazepines II: waking up on sedatives: providing optimal care when inheriting benzodiazepine prescriptions in transfer patients. *J Clin Med Res* 2018; 7. doi:10.3390/jcm7020020.

13. Groot PC, van Os J. Successful use of tapering strips for hyperbolic reduction of antidepressant dose: a cohort study. *Ther Adv Psychopharmacol* 2021; 11: 20451253211039330.

14. Framer A. What I have learnt from helping thousands of people taper off psychotropic medications. *Ther Adv Psychopharmacol* 2021; 11: 204512532199127.

15. BenzoBuddies Community Forum. http://www.benzobuddies.org/forum/index.php (accessed 6 July 2023).

16. National Institute for Health and Care Excellence (NICE). Hypnotics and anxiolytics. https://bnf.nice.org.uk/treatment-summaries/hypnotics-and-anxiolytics/ (accessed 6 July 2023).

Quazepam

Trade names: Doral, Quiedorm.

Description Quazepam is a medium-potency,[1] intermediate- to long-acting benzodiazepine.[2] Quazepam potentiates the effect of GABA by acting on the $GABA_A$ receptor.[3]

Withdrawal effects: Quazepam, as for other benzodiazepines, carries a boxed warning from the FDA that highlights that physical dependence and withdrawal effects can occur when the drug is taken 'for several days to weeks, even as prescribed'.[2,4] Not everyone who stops quazepam will experience withdrawal and some of those who do will only experience mild symptoms – this probably depends on drug dose, duration of use and individual factors. However, in a very few instances, stopping abruptly can cause seizures and can be life threatening. Numerous other physical, cognitive and psychological withdrawal symptoms, outlined in 'Withdrawal effects from benzodiazepines and z-drugs', are also possible which can last 'for several weeks to more than 12 months' after stopping according to the FDA.[2,4]

Peak plasma: 2 hours.[2]

Half-life: 39 hours and 73 hours for its metabolites.[2] The long half-life may enable less often than once-a-day dosing during tapering, but in some patients this might precipitate withdrawal effects.

Receptor occupancy: The relationship between dose of quazepam and the occupancy of its major target $GABA_A$ is hyperbolic (as a consequence of the law of mass action).[5,6] Benzodiazepines demonstrate a hyperbolic relationship between dose and clinical effects,[7] which may be relevant to withdrawal effects. Dose reductions made by linear amounts (e.g. 15mg, 11.25mg, 7.5mg, 3.75mg, 0mg) will cause slightly larger reductions in effect each step, which may cause increasingly severe withdrawal effects (Figure 3.21a). Hyperbolic tapering is required to produce linear changes in effect on receptor occupancy, although because of the nature of the occupancy curve for quazepam, this pattern is not substantially different from linear tapering (Figure 3.21b),[8] which

CHAPTER 3

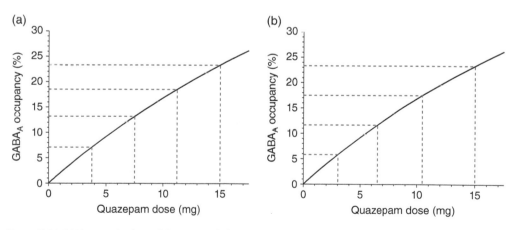

Figure 3.21 (a) Linear reductions of dose cause slighter larger reductions in effect on receptor targets sequentially, possibly associated with more withdrawal effects. (b) Even reductions of effect at target receptors requires hyperbolic dose reductions. In this case the nature of the occupancy curve is such that this pattern of dose reduction does not differ greatly from linear reductions.

informs the reductions presented. The relationship was derived by converting the receptor occupancy curve for diazepam[5] to the equivalent quazepam dose.[9]

Available formulations: As tablets.

Tablets

Dosage	UK	Europe	USA	Australia	Canada
7.5mg	–	–	✓	–	–
15mg	–	–	✓	–	–

Off-label options: In order to follow the regimens suggested, smaller doses are required than can be made using commercially available tablets and capsules (where no liquid versions of the medication are available). Quazepam tablets will disintegrate in water (or juice).[10] The disintegration process can be sped up by crushing the tablet with a spoon or pestle and mortar. For example, water could be added to a 7.5mg tablet to make up a 7.5mL suspension (concentration of 1mg/mL). The suspension should be shaken vigorously or stirred before use to aid dispersal so that the drug is distributed within the liquid. The measured dose should be taken before settling occurs. As stability cannot be assured, the dose should be consumed immediately, and any unused suspension discarded. Benzodiazepines are more soluble in oil or fat than in water.[11] When mixed with full-fat milk, some or all of the drug will dissolve in the milk fat. This should form an evenly dispersed emulsion when shaken vigorously. The measured dose should be taken immediately after shaking and the remainder discarded.

Another option is to switch to diazepam (see later) or to have a suspension, or small-dose tablets or capsules made up by a compounding pharmacy.

Worked example: To illustrate how the volumes can be calculated in the regimens given below, a worked example is provided. To make up 0.5mg of quazepam a 1mg/mL suspension can be used, prepared as above. The volume of 1mg/mL liquid required to give a dose of 0.5mg quazepam is 0.5/1 = 0.5mL.

Deprescribing notes: There are two main methods for tapering from quazepam – a switch to a longer-acting benzodiazepine like diazepam (see below) or a direct taper of quazepam itself. There are no established guides to determine the rate of taper for someone stopping benzodiazepines. Withdrawal is known to be more severe for people who have used benzodiazepines with shorter half-lives, for longer periods, at higher doses, and for those who have experienced withdrawal in the past on reducing, stopping or missing a dose.[12,13] The size of the initial reduction can be estimated based on these factors (see 'Tapering benzodiazepines and z-drugs in practice'), with patient preference also taken into account. Sometimes an even smaller reduction to start with may be advisable to boost a patient's confidence that they are able taper if performed carefully.

Each reduction should be made when the withdrawal symptoms from the previous reduction have largely resolved so that subsequent reductions do not lead to cumulative withdrawal symptoms. Withdrawal symptoms should not be too unpleasant: a rate of reduction should be aimed for that produces tolerable withdrawal symptoms that abate within a week or two. Allowing for a sufficient observation period, reductions can therefore be made about every 1–4 weeks, depending on how long it takes withdrawal symptoms to resolve. If withdrawal symptoms are moderately severe or take longer than a couple of weeks to resolve, dose reductions should be postponed until symptoms resolve and then made more gradually by choosing a slower tapering rate. If severe withdrawal symptoms occur, then the patient should return to a higher dose, wait until symptoms resolve and thereafter taper at a slower rate.

Suggested direct taper schedules for quazepam: Please note that none of these regimens should be seen as prescriptive – patients should not be compelled to adhere strictly to them. They are given as example regimens and are not 'set and forget' but should be modified in order to ensure that withdrawal symptoms are tolerable throughout a taper. For example, intermediate steps halfway between the doses listed could be added to make a more gradual taper. Ultimately, it is the patient's experience of withdrawal that should guide the rate of taper.

A. **A faster taper** with up to 3.1 percentage points of $GABA_A$ occupancy between each step – with reductions made every 1–4 weeks*.

Step	RO (%)	Total daily dose (mg)	Form
1	23.3	15	Use tablets
2	21.0	13.125	Use ¾ tablets**
3	18.5	11.25	Use ½ tablets**
4	16.0	9.375	Use ¼ tablets**
5	13.2	7.5	Use tablets
6	10.2	5.625	Use ¾ tablets**
7	7.1	3.75	Use ½ tablets**
Switch to liquid quazepam **(1mg/mL)*****			
8	5.2	2.7	2.7mL
9	2.6	1.3	1.3mL
10	0	0	

RO = receptor occupancy

*Patients who have been on the medication for only a few weeks will probably be able to taper more quickly and might follow every second or third step of this regimen and make reductions every few days or so. Normally the duration of the taper should not be longer than the period that the patient has been on the drug for people who have only taken it for a few weeks. For example, if quazepam is taken for 3 weeks, the taper should be less than 3 weeks. However, the FDA has issued an alert regarding dependence and withdrawal from benzodiazepines indicating that some people can experience withdrawal effects after just a few days of use,[13] therefore necessitating slower tapering.

**Alternatively, these doses can be made up using a liquid preparation.

***Preparation as indicated above.

B. **A moderate taper** with up to 1.5 percentage points of $GABA_A$ occupancy between each step – with reductions made every 1–4 weeks.

Step	RO (%)	Total daily dose (mg)	Form	Step	RO (%)	Total daily dose (mg)	Form
1	23.3	15	Use tablets	11	11	6.1	6.1mL
Switch to liquid quazepam **(1mg/mL)****				12	9.8	5.3	5.3mL
2	22.1	14	14mL	13	8.6	4.6	4.6mL
3	20.8	13	13mL	14	7.4	3.9	3.9mL
4	19.6	12	12mL	15	6.1	3.2	3.2mL
5	18.4	11.1	11.1mL	16	4.9	2.5	2.5mL
6	17.2	10.2	10.2mL	17	3.7	1.8	1.8mL
7	15.9	9.3	9.3mL	18	2.5	1.2	1.2mL
8	14.7	8.5	8.5mL	19	1.2	0.6	0.6mL
9	13.5	7.7	7.7mL	20	0	0	–
10	12.3	6.9	6.9mL				
See further steps in the right-hand column							

RO = receptor occupancy
*Preparation as indicated above.

C. **A slower taper** with up to 0.8 percentage points of GABA$_A$ occupancy between each step – with reductions made every 1–4 weeks.

Step	RO (%)	Total daily dose (mg)	Formulation	Step	RO(%)	Total daily dose (mg)	Formulation
1	23.3	15	Use tablets	21	11.3	6.3	6.3mL
	Switch to liquid quazepam **(1mg/mL)****			22	10.8	5.9	5.9mL
2	22.7	14.5	14.5mL	23	10.2	5.5	5.5mL
3	22.1	14	14mL	24	9.6	5.1	5.1mL
4	21.5	13.5	13.5mL	25	9	4.8	4.8mL
5	20.9	13.1	13.1mL	26	8.4	4.5	4.5mL
6	20.3	12.6	12.6mL	27	7.8	4.2	4.2mL
7	19.7	12.1	12.1mL	28	7.2	3.8	3.8mL
8	19.1	11.7	11.7mL	29	6.6	3.5	3.5mL
9	18.5	11.2	11.2mL	30	6	3.1	3.1mL
10	17.9	10.8	10.8mL	31	5.4	2.8	2.8mL
11	17.3	10.3	10.3mL	32	4.8	2.5	2.5mL
12	16.7	9.9	9.9mL	33	4.2	2.2	2.2mL
13	16.1	9.5	9.5mL	34	3.6	1.8	1.8mL
14	15.5	9.1	9.1mL	35	3	1.5	1.5mL
15	14.9	8.7	8.7mL	36	2.4	1.2	1.2mL
16	14.3	8.3	8.3mL	37	1.8	0.9	0.9mL
17	13.7	7.9	7.9mL	38	1.2	0.6	0.6mL
18	13.1	7.5	7.5mL**	39	0.6	0.3	0.3mL
19	12.5	7.1	7.1mL	40	0	0	0
20	11.9	6.7	6.7mL				
See further steps in the right-hand column							

RO = receptor occupancy
*Preparation as indicated above.
**Alternatively, this could be made up by a tablet.

D. **An even slower taper** Some patients will be unable to taper at the slowest rates shown here and will need to taper by even smaller decrements, thus lengthening the overall period of tapering. Such a regimen could be constructed by placing intermediate steps in regimen C. For example, 15mg, 14.5mg, 14mg could be modified to be 15mg, 14.75mg, 14.5mg, 14.25mg, 14mg and so on. Further intermediate steps could also be added.

Micro-tapering: The tables given show how to make reductions at intervals of 1–4 weeks. An alternative approach is called 'micro-tapering' whereby very small dose reductions are made every day, as explained in 'Other considerations in tapering benzodiazepines and z-drugs.' Micro-tapering rates can be calculated from the above by dividing the change in dose for each step by 14 or 28 days. For example, for the moderate regime, a reduction of 15mg to 14mg over 14 days is equivalent to a 0.07mg reduction per day. By the end of this regimen the rate of reduction would have slowed down to a reduction of 0.04mg each day. The rate can be adjusted if withdrawal symptoms become too unpleasant.

Switching guide from quazepam to diazepam An alternative to a direct taper from quazepam is to switch to diazepam before tapering from this drug, as outlined in 'Switching to longer-acting benzodiazepines to taper'. A 1mg dose of quazepam is equivalent to 0.5mg of diazepam.[14] Switching could be performed in steps made every week (or as tolerated by the patient).

Steps	Evening	Daily diazepam equivalent
Start	15mg quazepam	7.5mg
1	5mg quazepam 5mg diazepam	7.5mg
2	Stop quazepam 7.5mg diazepam	7.5mg
Taper from 7.5mg of diazepam (see diazepam section)		

References

1. Chouinard G. Issues in the clinical use of benzodiazepines: potency, withdrawal, and rebound. *J Clin Psychiatry* 2004; 65 Suppl 5: 7–12.
2. FDA. DORAL (Quazepam) Label. FDA. https://www.accessdata.fda.gov/drugsatfda_docs/label/2016/018708s023lbl.pdf (accessed 6 May 2023).
3. Quazepam. https://go.drugbank.com/drugs/DB01589 (accessed 6 May 2023).
4. FDA Drug Safety Communication. FDA requiring Boxed Warning updated to improve safe use of benzodiazepine drug class. 2020. https://www.fda.gov/drugs/drug-safety-and-availability/fda-requiring-boxed-warning-updated-improve-safe-use-benzodiazepine-drug-class#:~:text=FDA is requiring the Boxed,and life-threatening side effects (accessed 3 July 2023).
5. Brouillet E, Chavoix C, Bottlaender M, et al. In vivo bidirectional modulatory effect of benzodiazepine receptor ligands on GABAergic transmission evaluated by positron emission tomography in non-human primates. *Brain Res* 1991; 557: 167–76.
6. Holford N. Pharmacodynamic principles and the time course of delayed and cumulative drug effects. *Transl Clin Pharmacol* 2018; 26: 56–9.
7. Horowitz M, Taylor D. Withdrawing from benzodiazepines and z-drugs (in preparation).
8. Horowitz MA, Taylor D. Tapering of SSRI treatment to mitigate withdrawal symptoms. *The Lancet Psychiatry* 2019; 6: 538–46.
9. Ashton H. Benzodiazepines: how they work and how to withdraw (The Ashton Manual). Newcastle University, 2002. http://www.benzo.org.uk/manual/bzcha01.htm (accessed 11 July 2023).
10. Stahl SM. Quazepam. In: *Prescriber's Guide: Stahl's Essential Psychopharmacology*. Cambridge: Cambridge University Press, 2020: 663–6.
11. Macheras PE, Koupparis MA, Antimisiaris SG. Drug binding and solubility in milk. *Pharm Res* 1990; 7: 537–41.
12. Guina J, Merrill B. Benzodiazepines II: waking up on sedatives: providing optimal care when inheriting benzodiazepine prescriptions in transfer patients. *J Clin Med Res* 2018; 7. doi:10.3390/jcm7020020.
13. Framer A. What I have learnt from helping thousands of people taper off psychotropic medications. *Ther Adv in Psychopharmacol* 2021; 11: 204512532199127.
14. Hypnotics and anxiolytics. https://bnf.nice.org.uk/treatment-summaries/hypnotics-and-anxiolytics/ (accessed 19 March 2023).

Temazepam

Trade names: Restoril, Euhypnos, Normison, Temaze, Tenox.

Description: Temazepam is a low-potency benzodiazepine.[1] It increases the affinity of GABA for the GABA$_A$ receptor by binding to the central benzodiazepine receptor.[2] It is indicated for the short-term management of sleep disturbances.[3] The manufacturer in the UK recommends use for the shortest possible time and no longer than 4 weeks, including the tapering off process.[3]

Withdrawal effects: Temazepam, like other benzodiazepines, carries a boxed warning from the FDA, which highlights risk of dependence and withdrawal especially with longer duration of treatment and the use of high doses.[4] Not everyone who stops temazepam will experience withdrawal effects, and some might only experience mild symptoms depending on the treatment duration, dose and the patient. However, the FDA warns against abrupt discontinuation and sudden dose reduction due to increased risk of acute withdrawal reactions, which can occasionally be life threatening.[4] Numerous other physical, cognitive and psychological withdrawal symptoms, outlined in 'Withdrawal effects from benzodiazepines and z-drugs', are also possible which can last 'for several weeks to more than 12 months' after stopping according to the FDA.[4] The manufacturer warns that withdrawal symptoms from temazepam can include 'headaches, muscle pain, extreme anxiety, tension, restlessness, confusion and irritability. In severe cases the following symptoms may occur: derealisation, depersonalisation, hyperacusis, numbness and tingling of the extremities, hypersensitivity to light, noise and physical contact, hallucinations or epileptic seizures'.[3]

Peak plasma: Following administration, temazepam is rapidly absorbed and reaches peak plasma concentration after 1.2 to 1.6 hours.[5]

Half-life and dosing: The reported half-life for night administration is between 5.3 and 11.5 hours. A longer half-life, of up to 15 hours, has been observed in the elderly.[3] The manufacturer recommends taking the drug once at night. Dosing less often (including every-other-day dosing) is not recommended for the tapering process because the changes in plasma levels produced may precipitate withdrawal symptoms.

Receptor occupancy: The relationship between dose of temazepam and the occupancy of its major target GABA$_A$ is hyperbolic (according to the law of mass action).[6,7] Benzodiazepines demonstrate a hyperbolic relationship between dose and clinical effects,[8] which may be relevant to withdrawal effects. Dose reductions made by linear amounts (e.g. 30mg, 22.5mg, 15mg, 7.5mg, 0mg) will cause increasingly large reductions in effect that may cause increasingly severe withdrawal effects (Figure 3.22a). To produce equal-sized reductions in effect on receptor occupancy will require hyperbolically reducing doses (Figure 3.23b),[9] which informs the reductions presented. The relationship was derived by converting the receptor occupancy curve for diazepam[10] to the equivalent temazepam dose.[11]

Available formulations: As tablets, capsules and liquid

Tablets

Dosage	UK	Europe	USA	Australia	Canada
10mg	✓	–	–	✓	–
20mg	✓	–	–	–	–

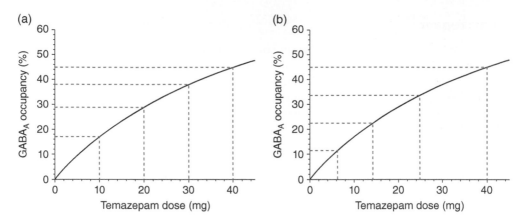

Figure 3.22 (a) Linear reductions of dose cause increasingly large reductions in effect on receptor targets, possibly associated with more withdrawal effects. (b) Even reductions of effect at target receptors requires hyperbolic dose reductions, slightly different from linear reductions in this case. The final dose before stopping will need to be small so that this step down is not larger (in terms of effect on receptor occupancy) than previous reductions.

Capsules

Dosage	UK	Europe	USA	Australia	Canada
7.5mg	–	–	✓	–	–
10mg	–	✓	–	–	–
15mg	–	–	✓	–	✓
20mg	–	✓	–	–	–
22.5mg	–	–	✓	–	✓
30mg	–	–	✓	–	–

Liquid

Dosage	UK	Europe	USA	Australia	Canada
10mg/5mL (2mg/mL)	✓	–	–	–	–

Off-label options: In order to follow the regimens suggested, sometimes smaller doses are required than can be made using commercially available tablets and capsules (where no liquid versions of the medication are available). Guidelines for people who cannot swallow tablets (e.g. the NEWT guidelines)[12] advise using the oral solution and suggest that tablets not be crushed owing to the insoluble nature of temazepam (an odd reason to give). Other individual hospital guidance advises that temazepam tablets will disintegrate in water in greater than 2 minutes.[13] For example, water could be added to a 10mg tablet to make up a 10mL suspension (concentration 1mg/mL). The suspension should be shaken vigorously or stirred before use to aid dispersal so that the drug is distributed within the liquid. The measured dose should be taken before settling occurs.

As stability cannot be assured, the dose should be consumed immediately, and any unused suspension discarded.

Benzodiazepines are more soluble in oil or fat than in water.[14] When mixed with full-fat milk, some or all of the drug will dissolve in the milk fat. This should form an evenly dispersed emulsion when shaken vigorously. The measured dose should be taken immediately after shaking and the remainder discarded. Capsules that contain powder can be opened and mixed with water, and shaken to disperse. Capsules containing a gel cannot be easily mixed with water. Another option is to switch to diazepam (see later) or to have a suspension or smaller dose capsules or tablets made up by a compounding pharmacy – one example is 'tapering strips'.[15]

Worked example: To illustrate how the volumes can be calculated in the regimens given, a worked example is provided. To make up 0.6mg of temazepam the 2mg/mL suspension can be used. The volume of 1mg/mL liquid required to give a dose of 0.6mg of temazepam is 0.6/1 = 0.6mL.

Deprescribing notes: There are two main methods for tapering from temazepam – a switch to diazepam or a direct taper of temazepam itself. There are no established guides to determine the rate of taper for someone stopping benzodiazepines. Withdrawal is known to be more severe for people who have used benzodiazepines which are shorter acting, for longer periods, at higher doses, in the elderly, and for those who have experienced withdrawal in the past on reducing, stopping or missing a dose.[16,17] The size of the initial reduction can be estimated based on these factors (see 'Tapering benzodiazepines and z-drugs in practice'), with patient preference also taken into account. Sometimes an even smaller reduction to start with may be advisable to boost a patient's confidence that they can taper if performed carefully.

Each reduction should be made when the withdrawal symptoms from the previous reduction have largely resolved so that subsequent reductions do not lead to cumulative withdrawal symptoms. Withdrawal symptoms should not be too unpleasant: a rate of reduction should be aimed for that produces tolerable withdrawal symptoms that abate within a week or two. Allowing for a sufficient observation period, reductions can therefore be made about every 1–4 weeks, depending on how long it takes withdrawal symptoms to resolve. If withdrawal symptoms are moderately severe or take longer than a couple of weeks to resolve, dose reductions should be postponed until symptoms resolve and then made more gradually by choosing a slower tapering rate. If severe withdrawal symptoms occur, then the patient should return to a higher dose, wait until symptoms resolve and thereafter taper at a slower rate.

Suggested direct taper schedules for temazepam: Please note that none of these regimens should be seen as prescriptive – patients should not be compelled to strictly adhere to them. They are given as example regimens and are not 'set and forget' but should be modified in order to ensure that withdrawal symptoms are tolerable throughout a taper. For example, intermediate steps halfway between the doses listed could be added to make a more gradual taper. Ultimately, it is the patient's experience of withdrawal that should guide the rate of taper. Note that two tapering regimens are given. This is due to different formulations availability in the UK and USA.

USA tapering regimens

A. **A faster taper** with up to 8 percentage points of GABA-A occupancy between each step – with reductions made every 1–4 weeks.[*]

Step	RO (%)	Evening dose (mg)	Formulation
1	37.8	30	Use capsules
2	31.3	22.5	Use capsules
3	23.3	15	Use capsules
Switch to temazepam liquid **(1mg/mL)**[**]			
4	18.5	11.3	11.3mL
5	13.2	7.5	7.5mL[***]
6	7.1	3.8	3.8mL
7	0	0	

RO = receptor occupancy
[*]Patients who have been on the medication for only a few weeks will probably be able to taper more quickly and might follow every second or third step of this regimen and make reductions every few days or so. Normally the duration of the taper should not be longer than the period that the patient has been on the drug for people who have only taken it for a few weeks. For example, if temazepam is taken for three weeks the taper should be less than 3 weeks. However the FDA has issued an warning for benzodiazepines indicating that some people can experience withdrawal effects after just a few days of use,[18] therefore necessitating slower tapering in this sub-group.
[**]Prepared as above. Alternatively compounded medication could be used to make up these doses.
[***]Alternatively, capsules could be used to make up these doses.

B. **A moderate taper** with up to 5 percentage points of GABA-A occupancy between each step – with reductions made every 1–4 weeks.

Step	RO (%)	Evening dose (mg)	Formulation
1	37.8	30	Use capsules
Switch to temazepam liquid **(1mg/mL)**[*]			
2	34.7	26.3	26.3mL
3	31.3	22.5	22.5mL[**]
4	27.5	18.8	18.8mL
5	23.3	15	15mL[**]
6	21	11.3	11.3mL
7	16	9.4	9.4mL
8	13.2	7.5	7.5mL[**]
9	10.2	5.6	5.6mL
10	7.1	3.8	3.8mL
11	3.7	1.9	1.9mL
12	0	0	0

RO = receptor occupancy
[*] Prepared as above. Alternatively compounded medication could be used to make up these doses.
[**]Alternatively, capsules could be used to make up these doses.

C. **A slower taper** with up to 2 percentage points of GABA-A occupancy between each step - with reductions made every 1–4 weeks.

Step	RO (%)	Evening dose (mg)	Formulation	Step	RO (%)	Evening dose (mg)	Formulation
1	37.8	30	Use tablets	13	19.5	12	12mL
Switch to temazepam liquid **(1mg/mL)***				14	18.2	11	11mL
2	36.3	28.1	28.1mL	15	16.8	10	10mL
3	34.7	26.3	26.3mL	16	15.4	9	9mL
4	33.0	24.4	24.4mL	17	13.9	8	8mL
5	31.3	22.5	22.5mL**	18	12.4	7	7mL
6	29.5	20.6	20.6mL	19	10.8	6	6mL
7	27.5	18.8	18.8mL	20	9.2	5	5mL
8	25.6	17	17mL	21	7.5	4	4mL
9	24.5	16	16mL	22	5.7	3	3mL
10	23.3	15	15mL**	23	3.9	2	2mL
11	22.1	14	14mL	24	2.0	1	1ml
12	20.8	13	13mL	25	0	0	
See further steps in the right-hand column							

RO = receptor occupancy

*Prepared as above. Alternatively compounded medication could be used to make up these doses.

**Alternatively, capsules could be used to make up these doses.

D. **An even slower taper** Some patients will be unable to taper at the slowest rates shown here and will need to taper by even smaller decrements, thus lengthening the overall period of tapering. Such a regimen could be constructed by placing intermediate steps in regimen C. For example, 5mg, 4mg, 3mg could be modified to 5mg, 4.5mg, 4mg, 3.5mg, 3mg and so on. Further intermediate steps could also be added.

UK tapering regimens

A. **A faster taper** with up to 9.2 percentage points of $GABA_A$ occupancy between each step – with reductions made every 1–4 weeks.*

Step	RO (%)	Evening dose (mg)	Formulation
1	28.8	20	Use tablets
2	23.3	15	Use ½ tablets**
3	16.8	10	Use tablets
4	9.2	5	Use ½ tablets**
5	0	0	Use tablets

RO = receptor occupancy

*Normally the duration of the taper should exceed the period that the patient has been on the drug for people who have only taken it for a few weeks. For example, if temazepam is taken for 3 weeks, the taper should be less than 3 weeks. However the FDA has issued a warning for benzodiazepines indicating that some people can experience withdrawal effects after just a few days of use,[18] therefore necessitating slower tapering in this sub-group.

**Alternatively, a liquid version of temazepam could be used instead, prepared as above.

B. **A moderate taper** with up to 5 percentage points of $GABA_A$ occupancy between each step – with reductions made every 1–4 weeks.

Step	RO (%)	Evening dose (mg)	Formulation
1	28.8	20	Use tablets
2	26.2	17.5	Use ¾ tablets*
3	23.3	15	Use ½ tablets*
4	20.2	12.5	Use ¼ tablets*
5	16.8	10	Use tablets
6	13.2	7.5	Use ¾ tablets*
7	9.2	5	Use ½ tablets*
8	4.8	2.5	Use ¼ tablets*
9	0	0	

RO = receptor occupancy
*Alternatively, a liquid version of temazepam could be used instead.

C. **A slower taper** with up to 2.5 percentage points of GABA-A occupancy between each step – with reductions made every 1–4 weeks.

Step	RO(%)	Evening dose (mg)	Formulation	Step	RO (%)	Evening dose (mg)	Formulation
1	28.8	20	Use tablets	10	13.9	8	4mL
	Switch to temazepam liquid **(2mg/mL)***			11	12.4	7	3.5mL
2	27.2	18.5	9.25mL	12	10.8	6	3mL
3	25.6	17	8.5mL	13	9.2	5	2.5mL**
4	23.9	15.5	7.75mL	14	7.5	4	2mL
5	22.1	14	7mL	15	5.7	3	1.5mL
6	20.2	12.5	6.25mL	16	3.9	2	1mL
7	18.2	11	5.5mL	17	2	1	0.5mL
8	16.8	10	5mL**	18	0	0	
9	15.4	9	4.5mL				
See further steps in the right-hand column							

RO = receptor occupancy
*Prepared as above. Alternatively compounded medication could be used to make up these doses.
**Alternatively, tablets or half tablets could be used to make these doses.

D. **An even slower taper** Some patients will be unable to taper at the slowest rates shown here and will need to taper by even smaller decrements, thus lengthening the overall period of tapering. Such a regimen could be constructed by placing intermediate steps in regimen C. For example, 5mg, 4mg, 3mg could be modified to 5mg, 4.5mg, 4mg, 3.5mg, 3mg and so on. Further intermediate steps could also be added.

Micro-tapering: The tables show how to make reductions at intervals of 1 to 4 weeks. An alternative approach is called 'micro-tapering' whereby very small dose reductions are made every day, as explained in 'Other considerations in tapering benzodiazepines and z-drugs.' Micro-tapering rates can be calculated from the above by dividing the change in dose for each step by 7 or 14 days. For example reducing from 20mg to 17.5mg in 14 days is approximately equivalent to reductions of 0.2mg per day.

Switching guide from temazepam to diazepam An alternative to a direct taper from temazepam is to switch to diazepam before tapering from this drug, as outlined in 'Switching to longer-acting benzodiazepines to taper'. A 10mg dose of temazepam is equivalent to 5mg diazepam with steps of 10mg of temazepam made every week (or as tolerated by the patient).[19]

Steps	Evening	Daily diazepam equivalent
1	40mg temazepam	20mg
2	30mg temazepam 5mg diazepam	20mg
3	20mg temazepam 10mg diazepam	20mg
4	10mg temazepam 15mg diazepam	20mg
5	Stop temazepam 20mg diazepam	20mg

Continue to taper as for 20mg diazepam (see diazepam section).

References

1. Chouinard G. Issues in the clinical use of benzodiazepines: potency, withdrawal, and rebound. *J Clin Psychiatry* 2004; 65 Suppl 5: 7–12.
2. DRUGBANK ONLINE. Temazepam. https://go.drugbank.com/drugs/DB00231 (accessed 7 July 2023).
3. Thame Laboratories. Summary of Product Characteristics. Temazepam 10mg/5mL oral solution. 2022. https://www.medicines.org.uk/emc/product/9479 (accessed 7 July 2023).
4. NIH DailyMed. Temazepam FDA drug label information boxed warning. https://dailymed.nlm.nih.gov/dailymed/drugInfo.cfm?setid=a4370eb4-b00d-4247-af8d-980e59fbbec6 (accessed 7 July 2023).
5. FDA. Restoril (temazepam) Label. FDA. https://www.accessdata.fda.gov/drugsatfda_docs/label/2016/018163s064lbl.pdf (accessed 5 May 2023).
6. Innis RB, al-Tikriti MS, Zoghbi SS, et al. SPECT imaging of the benzodiazepine receptor: feasibility of in vivo potency measurements from stepwise displacement curves. *J Nucl Med* 1991; 32: 1754–61.
7. Holford N. Pharmacodynamic principles and the time course of delayed and cumulative drug effects. *Transl Clin Pharmacol* 2018; 26: 56–9.
8. Horowitz M, Taylor D. Withdrawing from benzodiazepines and z-drugs (in preparation).
9. Horowitz MA, Taylor D. Tapering of SSRI treatment to mitigate withdrawal symptoms. *The Lancet Psychiatry* 2019; 6: 538–46.
10. Brouillet E, Chavoix C, Bottlaender M, et al. In vivo bidirectional modulatory effect of benzodiazepine receptor ligands on GABAergic transmission evaluated by positron emission tomography in non human primates. *Brain Res* 1991; 557: 167–76.
11. Choosing an equivalent dose of oral benzodiazepine. SPS – Specialist Pharmacy Service. 2022; published online January 25. https://www.sps.nhs.uk/articles/choosing-an-equivalent-dose-of-oral-benzodiazepine/ (accessed 8 April 2023).
12. Smyth. J. The NEWT Guidelines for administration of medication to patients with enteral feeding tubes or swallowing difficulties website. The NEWT Guidelines. 2011. http://www.newtguidelines.com (accessed 6 July 2023).
13. Colchester Medicines Information. MOC guidelines for tablet crushing in patients with swallowing difficulties. Colchester Hospital University, 2018.
14. Macheras PE, Koupparis MA, Antimisiaris SG. Drug binding and solubility in milk. *Pharm Res* 1990; 7: 537–41.
15. Groot PC, van Os J. How user knowledge of psychotropic drug withdrawal resulted in the development of person-specific tapering medication. *Ther Adv Psychopharmacol* 2020; 10: 204512532093245.
16. Guina J, Merrill B. Benzodiazepines II: Waking up on sedatives: providing optimal care when inheriting benzodiazepine prescriptions in transfer patients. *J Clin Med Res* 2018; 7. doi:10.3390/jcm7020020.
17. Framer A. What I have learnt from helping thousands of people taper off psychotropic medications. *Ther Adv Psychopharmacol* 2021; 11: 204512532199127.
18. US Food & Drug Administration. FDA requiring boxed warning updated to improve safe use of benzodiazepine drug class. 2020 (last accessed March 2023). https://www.fda.gov/drugs/drug-safety-and-availability/fda-requiring-boxed-warning-updated-improve-safe-use-benzodiazepine-drug-class.
19. National Institute for Health and Care Excellence (NICE). Hypnotics and anxiolytics. https://bnf.nice.org.uk/treatment-summaries/hypnotics-and-anxiolytics/ (accessed 7 July 2023).

Triazolam

Trade name: Halcion.

Description: Triazolam is a high–potency benzodiazepine.[1] It is a positive allosteric modulator of the gamma-aminobutyric acid (GABA) type A receptor, which it affects by binding to stereospecific benzodiazepine binding sites. Stimulation of benzodiazepine receptors enhances the inhibitory effects of GABA, by potentiating the conductance of chloride ions.[2] The manufacturer in the USA recommends short-term treatment (7 to 10 days) for insomnia.[2]

Withdrawal effects: Triazolam, as for other benzodiazepines, carries a boxed warning from the FDA, which highlights that physical dependence and withdrawal effects can occur when the drug is taken 'for several days to weeks, even as prescribed'.[2,3] Not everyone who stops triazolam will experience withdrawal, and some of those who do will only experience mild symptoms – this probably depends on drug dose, duration of use and individual factors. However, in a few instances, stopping abruptly can cause seizures and can be life threatening. Numerous physical, cognitive and psychological withdrawal symptoms (outlined in 'Withdrawal effects from benzodiazepines and z-drugs') are possible, which can last 'for several weeks to more than 12 months' after stopping according to the FDA.[4] The manufacturer warns that withdrawal effects can occur after discontinuing these drug following use for only a week or two, but may be more common and more severe after longer periods of continuous use.[2]

An increase in daytime anxiety can occur after as little as 10 days of use, likely a manifestation of inter-dose withdrawal.[2] Withdrawal symptoms can include 'rebound insomnia' with insomnia being worse than before triazolam was given. Other withdrawal symptoms range from mildly unpleasant feelings to a major withdrawal syndrome which may include abdominal and muscle cramps, vomiting, sweating, tremor, and convulsions.[2]

Peak plasma: Following oral administration peak concentration in the plasma occurs after 2 hours.[2]

Half-life: The half-life of triazolam is in the range of 1.5–5.5 hours and it has two primary inactive metabolites.[5] The manufacturer recommends that triazolam should be given once a day before bedtime.[2] Dosing less often to taper off the drug (including every-other-day dosing) is not recommended because the changes in plasma levels may precipitate inter-dose withdrawal symptoms.

Receptor occupancy: The relationship between dose of triazolam and the occupancy of its major target $GABA_A$ is hyperbolic.[5,6] Benzodiazepines demonstrate a hyperbolic relationship between dose and clinical effects,[7] which may be relevant to withdrawal effects from triazolam. Dose reductions made by linear amounts (e.g. 0.5mg, 0.375mg, 0.25mg, 0.125mg, 0mg) will cause increasingly large reductions in effect which may cause increasingly severe withdrawal effects (Figure 3.23a). Hyperbolic tapering is required to produce linear changes in effect on receptor occupancy, although because of the nature of the occupancy curve, this pattern is not substantially different from linear tapering (Figure 3.23b),[8] which informs the reductions presented later. The relationship was derived by converting the receptor occupancy curve for diazepam[5] to the equivalent triazolam dose.[9]

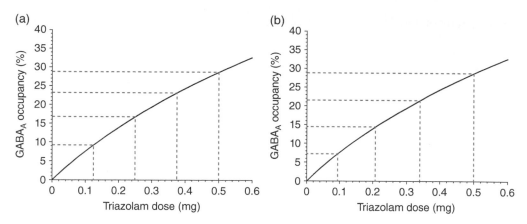

Figure 3.23 (a) Linear reductions of dose cause increasingly large reductions in effect on receptor targets, possibly associated with more withdrawal effects. (b) Even reductions of effect at target receptors requires hyperbolic dose reductions, slightly different to linear reductions in this case. The final dose before stopping will need to be small so that this step down is not larger (in terms of effect on receptor occupancy) than previous reductions.

Available formulations: As tablets

Tablets

Dosage	UK	Europe	USA	Australia	Canada
0.125mg	–	–	✓	✓	–
0.25mg	–	✓	✓	✓	✓
0.5mg	–	–	✓	–	–

Off-label options: In order to follow the regimens suggested, in some cases smaller doses are required than can be made using commercially available tablets. The use of a custom-made suspension or smaller doses in solid form from a compounding pharmacy (if available) is one option. The manufacturer states that triazolam is poorly soluble in water;[2] however, making a suspension is possible by crushing a tablet and dispersing it in water. For example, a 0.25mg tablet could be made up to 25mL with water to make a 1mg in 100mL (or 0.01mg/mL) suspension. The suspension should be shaken vigorously before administration. As its stability cannot be assured it should be consumed immediately, and any unused suspension discarded. Some patients use full-fat milk to make liquid preparations. Benzodiazepines are more soluble in oil or fat than in water.[10] When mixed with milk, some or all of the drug will dissolve in the milk fat. This should form an evenly dispersed emulsion when shaken vigorously. The measured dose should be taken immediately after shaking and the remainder discarded.

Worked example: To illustrate how volumes can be calculated for the regimens given below, a worked example is provided. To make up 0.14mg of triazolam a 0.01mg/mL suspension can be used, prepared as above. The volume of 0.01mg/mL liquid required to give a dose of 0.14mg triazolam is 0.14/0.01 = 14mL.

Deprescribing notes: There are two main methods for tapering from triazolam – a switch to diazepam or a direct taper of triazolam itself. There are no established guides to determine the rate of taper for someone stopping benzodiazepines. Withdrawal is known to be more severe for people who have used benzodiazepines which are shorter acting, for longer periods, at higher doses, and for those who have experienced withdrawal in the past on reducing, stopping or missing a dose.[11,12] The size of the initial reduction can be estimated based on these factors (see 'Tapering benzodiazepines and z-drugs in practice'), with patient preference also taken into account. Sometimes an even smaller reduction to start with may be advisable to boost a patient's confidence that they can taper if performed carefully.

Each reduction should be made when the withdrawal symptoms from the previous reduction have largely resolved so that subsequent reductions do not lead to cumulative withdrawal symptoms. Withdrawal symptoms should not be too unpleasant: a rate of reduction should be aimed for that produces tolerable withdrawal symptoms that abate within a week or two. Allowing for a sufficient observation period, reductions can therefore be made about every 1–4 weeks, depending on how long it takes withdrawal symptoms to resolve. If withdrawal symptoms are moderately severe or take longer than a couple of weeks to resolve, dose reductions should be postponed until symptoms resolve and then made more gradually by choosing a slower tapering rate. If severe withdrawal symptoms occur then the patient should return to a higher dose, wait until symptoms resolve and thereafter taper at a slower rate.

Suggested direct taper schedules for triazolam: Please note that none of these regimens should be seen as prescriptive – patients should not be compelled to adhere strictly to them. They are given as example regimens and are not 'set and forget' but should be modified in order to ensure that withdrawal symptoms are tolerable throughout a taper. For example, intermediate steps halfway between the doses listed could be added to make a more gradual taper. Ultimately, it is the patient's experience of withdrawal that should guide the rate of taper.

A. **A faster taper** with up to 9.2 percentage points of $GABA_A$ occupancy between each step – with reductions made every 1–4 weeks*.

Step	RO (%)	Total daily dose (mg)	Formulation
1	28.8	0.5	Use tablets
2	23.3	0.375	Use tablets**
3	16.8	0.25	Use tablets
4	9.2	0.125	Use tablets**
5	0	0	

RO = receptor occupancy

*Patients who have been on the medication for only a few weeks will probably be able to taper more quickly and might follow every second or third step of this regimen and make reductions every few days or so. Normally the duration of the taper should not be longer than the period that the patient has been on the drug for people who have only taken it for a few weeks. However, the FDA has issued an alert regarding benzodiazepines indicating that some people can experience withdrawal effects after just a few days of use,[13] therefore necessitating slower tapering in this sub-group.

**Alternatively, these doses could be made up using liquids, prepared as above if no small-dose tablets are available or division with a pill cutter is challenging.

B. **A moderate taper** with up to 4.8 percentage points of $GABA_A$ occupancy between each step – with reductions made every 1–4 weeks.

Step	RO (%)	Total daily dose (mg)	Formulation
1	28.8	0.5	Use tablets
2	26.2	0.4375	Use ½ tablets*
3	23.3	0.375	Use tablets
4	20.2	0.3125	Use ½ tablets*
5	16.8	0.25	Use tablets
6	13.2	0.1875	Use ½ tablets*
7	9.2	0.125	Use tablets
8	4.8	0.0625	Use ½ tablets*
9	0	0	

RO = receptor occupancy
*Alternatively, these doses could be made up using liquids, prepared as above if no small-dose tablets are available or division with a pill cutter is challenging.

C. **A slower taper** with up to 2.0 percentage points of $GABA_A$ occupancy between each step – with reductions made every 1–4 weeks.

Step	RO (%)	Dose (mg)	Formulation	Step	RO (%)	Dose (mg)	Formulation
1	28.8	0.5	Use tablets	12	11.2	0.15625	Use ¼ tablets*
2	27.5	0.46875	Use ¾ tablets*	Switch to triazolam suspension** (0.01mg/mL)			
3	26.2	0.4375	Use ½ tablets*	13	10.2	0.14	14mL
4	24.8	0.40625	Use ¼ tablets*	14	8.9	0.12	12mL
5	23.3	0.375	Use tablets	15	7.5	0.1	10mL
6	21.8	0.34375	Use ¾ tablets*	16	6.1	0.08	8mL
7	20.2	0.3125	Use ½ tablets*	17	4.6	0.06	6mL
8	18.5	0.28125	Use ¼ tablets*	18	3.1	0.04	4mL
9	16.8	0.25	Use tablets	19	1.6	0.02	2mL
10	15	0.21875	Use ¾ tablets*	20	0	0	
11	13.2	0.1875	Use ½ tablets*				
See further steps in the right-hand column							

RO = receptor occupancy
*Alternatively, these doses could be made up using liquids, prepared as above if no small-dose tablets are available or division with a pill cutter is challenging.
**A liquid formulation of drug might be used as outlined in the off-label options.

D. **An even slower taper** Some patients will be unable to taper at the slowest rates shown here and will need to taper by even smaller decrements, thus lengthening the overall period of tapering. Such a regimen could be constructed by placing intermediate steps in regimen C, for example 0.1mg, 0.08mg, 0.06mg could be modified to be 0.1mg, 0.09mg, 0.08mg, 0.07mg, 0.06mg and so on. Further intermediate steps could also be added.

Micro-tapering: The tables above show how to make reductions at intervals of 1–4 weeks. An alternative approach is called 'micro-tapering' whereby very small dose reductions are made every day, as explained in 'Other considerations in tapering benzodiazepines and z-drugs.' Micro-tapering rates can be calculated from the above by dividing the change in dose for each step by 14 or 28 days. For example, for the moderate regimen, a reduction of 0.5mg to 0.4375mg over 14 days is equivalent approximately to a 0.005mg reduction each day. This rate can be slowed if withdrawal symptoms become too unpleasant.

Switching guide from triazolam to diazepam: An alternative to a direct taper from triazolam is to switch to diazepam before tapering from this drug, as outlined in 'Switching to longer-acting benzodiazepines to taper'. However, as triazolam has a short half-life and is dosed once daily, it might be that less physical dependence will be produced in response to this drug than diazepam (present for all 24 hours). Therefore, it may be easier to directly taper from triazolam than switching to diazepam. For those patients who report inter-dose withdrawal symptoms from triazolam a switch to a longer-acting benzodiazepine might be a more reasonable option. A 0.5mg dose of triazolam is equivalent to 10mg diazepam.[9] Switching could be performed by steps of 0.25mg of triazolam made every week (or as tolerated by the patient).

Steps	Night	Daily diazepam equivalent
1	0.5mg triazolam	10mg
2	0.25mg triazolam 5mg diazepam	10mg
3	Stop triazolam 10mg diazepam	10mg
	Reduce as for 10mg diazepam (see diazepam section)	

References

1. Chouinard G. Issues in the clinical use of benzodiazepines: potency, withdrawal, and rebound. *J Clin Psychiatry* 2004; 65 Suppl 5: 7–12.

2. FDA. Triazolam – Highlights of Prescribing Information. 2019.

3. FDA Drug Safety Communication. FDA requiring boxed warning updated to improve safe use of benzodiazepine drug class. 2020. https://www.fda.gov/drugs/drug-safety-and-availability/fda-requiring-boxed-warning-updated-improve-safe-use-benzodiazepine-drug-class#:~:text=FDA is requiring the Boxed,and life-threatening side effects (accessed 5 July 2023).

4. Triazolam: Uses, Interactions, Mechanism of Action | DrugBank Online. https://go.drugbank.com/drugs/DB00897 (accessed 9 April 2023).

5. Brouillet E, Chavoix C, Bottlaender M, et al. In vivo bidirectional modulatory effect of benzodiazepine receptor ligands on GABAergic transmission evaluated by positron emission tomography in non-human primates. *Brain Res* 1991; 557: 167–76.

6. Holford N. Pharmacodynamic principles and the time course of delayed and cumulative drug effects. *Trans Clin Pharmacol* 2018; 26: 56–9.

7. Horowitz M, Taylor D. Withdrawing from benzodiazepines and z-drugs (in preparation).

8. Horowitz MA, Taylor D. Tapering of SSRI treatment to mitigate withdrawal symptoms. *The Lancet Psychiatry* 2019; 6: 538–46.

9. Ashton H. Benzodiazepines: how they work and how to withdraw (The Ashton Manual). Newcastle University, 2002. http://www.benzo.org.uk/manual/bzcha01.htm (accessed 11 July 2023).

10. Macheras PE, Koupparis MA, Antimisiaris SG. Drug binding and solubility in milk. *Pharm Res* 1990; 7: 537–41.

11. Guina J, Merrill B. Benzodiazepines II: waking up on sedatives: providing optimal care when inheriting benzodiazepine prescriptions in transfer patients. *J Clin Med Res* 2018; 7. doi:10.3390/jcm7020020.

12. Framer A. What I have learnt from helping thousands of people taper off psychotropic medications. *Ther Adv Psychopharmacol* 2021; 11: 204512532199127.

13. FDA. FDA requiring boxed warning updated to improve safe use of benzodiazepine drug class. *US Food and Drug Administration (FDA)* 2020: 1–10.

CHAPTER 3

Zaleplon

Trade names: Sonata, Starnoc.

Description: Zaleplon is z-drug, or non-benzodiazepine hypnotic, which acts in a similar manner to benzodiazepines as a positive allosteric modulator of $GABA_A$ receptors by producing conformational changes in the receptor complex.[1] Zaleplon is indicated for the short-term treatment of insomnia.[1]

Withdrawal effects: Stopping z-drugs even when taken as prescribed can lead to withdrawal effects in as many as 30–45% of people.[2,3] Zaleplon has a very short half-life.[4] This means that when taken once at night, plasma levels will fall to zero before the next dose. In theory, therefore, withdrawal reactions should be less common than with other z-drugs.[5] This seems to be true in practice although withdrawal symptoms are occasionally reported.[3] The regimens outlined are for those people who experience withdrawal symptoms in the days following the stopping of zaleplon.

Peak plasma: Approximately 1 hour after oral ingestion.[1]

Half-life and dosing: The elimination half-life is approximately 1 hour.[1] The manufacturer recommends taking the drug once at night.[1] Taking the drug less frequently (including every-other-day) is not recommended in tapering because of the risk of provoking withdrawal symptoms.

Receptor occupancy: The relationship between dose of zaleplon and the occupancy of its major target $GABA_A$ is hyperbolic as a consequence of the law of mass action.[6,7] Z-drugs demonstrate a hyperbolic relationship between dose and clinical effects,[8] which may be relevant to withdrawal effects. Dose reductions made by linear amounts (e.g. 20mg, 15mg, 10mg, 5mg, 0mg) will cause slightly larger reductions in effect each step, which may cause increasingly severe withdrawal effects (Figure 3.24a). Due to the nature of the occupancy curve hyperbolic tapering is not substantially different from linear tapering for zaleplon (Figure 3.24b),[9] which informs the reductions presented. The relationship was derived by converting the receptor occupancy curve for diazepam[10] to the equivalent zaleplon dose.[11]

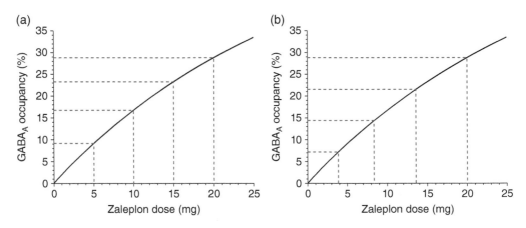

Figure 3.24 (a) Linear reductions of zaleplon. (b) Hyperbolic reductions are fairly similar to linear reductions for zaleplon because of the nature of the dose-occupancy relationship.

Available formulations: As capsules.

Capsules

Dosage	UK	Europe	USA	Australia	Canada
5mg	–	–	✓	–	–
10mg	–	–	✓	–	–

Off-label options: Smaller doses of zaleplon than those provided by commercially available capsules may be required to assist tapering. Capsules of zaleplon can be opened and emptied into water to form a suspension. For example, the contents of a 5mg capsule could be made up to 5mL with water to make up a 1mg/mL suspension. The suspension should be shaken vigorously or stirred before use. As its stability cannot be assured it should be consumed immediately, and any unused suspension discarded. Some patients use full-fat milk to make liquid preparations. Z-drugs are more soluble in oil or fat than in water.[12] When mixed with milk, some or all of the drug will dissolve in the milk fat. This should form an evenly dispersed emulsion when shaken vigorously. The measured dose should be taken immediately after shaking and the remainder discarded.

It is also possible to have a compounding pharmacy prepare a suspension or smaller-dose capsules, including the option of 'tapering strips'.[13] Another option is to switch to diazepam.

Worked example: To illustrate how to calculate volumes to make up a given dose using a liquid, a worked example is provided. To make up 2mg of zaleplon using a 1mg/mL suspension prepared as outlined above will require a volume of 2/1 = 2mL.

Deprescribing notes: There are no established guides to determine the rate of taper for someone stopping z-drugs. The longer z-drugs are used and the higher the dose taken the greater the risk of withdrawal, according to their manufacturer.[14] The size of the initial reduction can be estimated based on these factors (see 'Tapering benzodiazepines and z-drugs in practice'), with patient preference also taken into account. Sometimes an even smaller reduction to start with may be advisable to boost a patient's confidence that they can taper if performed carefully.

Each reduction should be made when the withdrawal symptoms from the previous reduction have largely resolved (most commonly insomnia with z-drugs), so that subsequent reductions do not lead to cumulative withdrawal symptoms. Withdrawal symptoms should not be too unpleasant: a rate of reduction should be aimed for that produces tolerable withdrawal symptoms that abate within a week or two. Allowing for a sufficient observation period, reductions can therefore be made about every 1–2 weeks, depending on how long it takes withdrawal symptoms to resolve. If withdrawal symptoms are moderately severe or take longer than a couple of weeks to resolve, dose reductions should be postponed until symptoms resolve, and then made more gradually by choosing a slower tapering rate. If severe withdrawal symptoms occur, the patient should return to a higher dose, wait until symptoms resolve, and thereafter taper at a slower rate.

CHAPTER 3

Suggested direct taper schedules for zaleplon: Please note that none of these regimens should be seen as prescriptive – patients should not be compelled to adhere strictly to them. They are given as example regimens and are not 'set and forget' but should be modified in order to ensure that withdrawal symptoms are tolerable throughout a taper. For example, intermediate steps halfway between the doses listed could be added to make a more gradual taper. Ultimately, it is the patient's experience of withdrawal that should guide the rate of taper.

A. **A faster taper** with up to 9.2 percentage points of $GABA_A$ occupancy between each step – with reductions made every 1–2 weeks*.

Step	RO (%)	Dose (mg)	Formulation
1	28.8	20	Use capsules
2	23.3	15	Use capsules
3	16.8	10	Use capsules
4	9.2	5	Use capsules
5	0	0	

RO = receptor occupancy
*Patients who have been on the medication for only a few weeks will probably be able to taper more quickly and might follow every second or third step of this regimen and make reductions every few days or so. Normally the duration of the taper should not be longer than the period that the patient has been on the drug for people who have only taken it for a few weeks. For example, if zaleplon is taken for 3 weeks the taper should be less than 3 weeks.

B. **A moderate taper** with up to 4 percentage points of $GABA_A$ occupancy between each step – with reductions made every 1–2 weeks.

Step	RO (%)	Dose (mg)	Formulation	Step	RO (%)	Dose (mg)	Formulation
1	28.8	20	Use tablets	6	13.2	7.5	7.5mL
Switch to liquid zaleplon (e.g. 1mg/mL)*				7	9.2	5	5mL**
2	26.2	17.5	17.5mL	8	7.1	3.75	3.75mL
3	23.3	15	15mL**	9	4.8	2.5	2.5mL
4	20.2	12.5	12.5mL	10	2.5	1.25	1.25mL
5	16.8	10	10mL**	11	0	0	
See further steps in the right-hand column							

RO = receptor occupancy
*Prepared as above
**Alternatively, these doses can be made up with capsules.

C. **A slower taper** with up to 1.9 percentage points of $GABA_A$ occupancy between each step – with reductions made every 1–2 weeks.

Step	RO (%)	Dose (mg)	Formulation	Step	RO (%)	Dose (mg)	Formulation
1	28.8	20	Capsule	11	13.9	8	8mL
Switch to liquid zaleplon (e.g. 1mg/mL)*				12	12.4	7	7mL
2	27.2	18.5	18.5mL	13	10.8	6	6mL
3	25.6	17	17mL	14	9.2	5	5mL
4	23.9	15.5	15.5mL	15	7.5	4	4mL
5	22.1	14	14mL	16	5.7	3	3mL
6	20.8	13	13mL	17	3.9	2	2mL
7	19.5	12	12mL	18	2.9	1.5	1.5mL
8	18.2	11	11mL	19	2.0	1	1mL
9	16.8	10	10mL*	20	1.0	0.5	0.5mL
10	15.4	9	9mL	21	0	0	
See further steps in the right-hand column							

RO = receptor occupancy
*Prepared as above
**Alternatively, these doses could be made up by capsules.

D. **An even slower taper** Some patients will be unable to taper at the slowest rates shown here and will need to taper by even smaller decrements, thus lengthening the overall period of tapering. Such a regimen could be constructed by placing intermediate steps in regimen C. For example, 20mg, 18.5mg, 17mg could be modified to be 20mg, 19.25mg, 18.5mg, 17.75mg, 17mg and so on. Further intermediate steps could also be added.

Micro-tapering: The tables given show how to make reductions at intervals of 1–2 weeks. An alternative approach is called 'micro-tapering' whereby very small dose reductions are made every day, as explained in 'Other considerations in tapering benzodiazepines and z-drugs.' Micro-tapering rates can be calculated from the above by dividing the change in dose for each step by 7 or 14 days and then dividing that dose into two doses during the day. For example, for the moderate regime a reduction of 20mg to 17.5mg over 14 days is approximately equivalent to a reduction of 0.2mg per day. This rate can be slowed if withdrawal symptoms become too unpleasant.
Switch to diazepam: An alternative to a direct taper from zaleplon is to switch to diazepam before tapering from this drug, as outlined in 'Switching to longer-acting benzodiazepines to taper'. However, as zaleplon has a very short half-life and is dosed once a day, it might be that less physical dependence will be produced in response to this drug than diazepam (present for the entire day). Therefore, it may be easier to directly taper

from zaleplon than switching to diazepam. A 10mg dose of zaleplon is equivalent to 5mg of diazepam,[11] with steps of 10mg of zaleplon made every week (or as tolerated by the patient).

Steps	Evening	Daily diazepam equivalent
1	20mg zaleplon	10mg
2	10mg zaleplon 5mg diazepam	10mg
3	Stop zaleplon 10mg diazepam	10mg

Continue to taper as for 10mg diazepam (see diazepam section).

References

1. FDA. Sonata FDA Label. FDA. https://www.accessdata.fda.gov/drugsatfda_docs/label/2007/020859s011lbl.pdf (accessed 20 May 2023).
2. Lerner A, Klein M. Dependence, withdrawal and rebound of CNS drugs: an update and regulatory considerations for new drugs development. *Brain Commun* 2019; 1. doi:10.1093/BRAINCOMMS/FCZ025.
3. Schifano F, Chiappini S, Corkery JM, Guirguis A. An insight into z-drug abuse and dependence: an examination of reports to the European medicines agency database of suspected adverse drug reactions. *Int J Neuropsychopharmacol* 2019; 22: 270–7.
4. FDA. Sonata (zaleplon). FDA. www.accessdata.fda.gov/drugsatfda_docs/label/2019/020859s016lbl.pdf (accessed 29 April 2023).
5. Lader MH. Managing dependence and withdrawal with newer hypnotic medications in the treatment of insomnia. The Primary Care Companion. 2002. https://www.psychiatrist.com/pcc/sleep/managing-dependence-withdrawal-newer-hypnotic-medications (accessed 20 May 2023).
6. Holford N. Pharmacodynamic principles and the time course of delayed and cumulative drug effects. *Transl Clin Pharmacol* 2018; 26: 56–9.
7. Brouillet E, Chavoix C, Bottlaender M, et al. In vivo bidirectional modulatory effect of benzodiazepine receptor ligands on GABAergic transmission evaluated by positron emission tomography in non-human primates. *Brain Res* 1991; 557: 167–76.
8. Horowitz M, Taylor D. Withdrawing from benzodiazepines and z-drugs (in preparation).
9. Horowitz MA, Taylor D. Tapering of SSRI treatment to mitigate withdrawal symptoms. *The Lancet Psychiatry* 2019; 6: 538–46.
10. Bostwick JR, Demehri A. Pills to powder: an updated clinician's reference for crushable psychotropics. *Curr Psychiatr* 2017; 16: 46–9.
11. Ashton H. Benzodiazepines: how they work and how to withdraw (The Ashton Manual). Newcastle University, 2002. http://www.benzo.org.uk/manual/bzcha01.htm (accessed 11 July 2023).
12. Macheras PE, Koupparis MA, Antimisiaris SG. Drug binding and solubility in milk. *Pharm Res* 1990; 7: 537–41.
13. Groot PC, van Os J. Successful use of tapering strips for hyperbolic reduction of antidepressant dose: a cohort study. *Ther Adv Psychopharmacol* 2021; 11: 20451253211039330.
14. FDA. LUNESTA® (eszopiclone) tablets – Accessdata.fda.gov. FDA. https://www.accessdata.fda.gov/drugsatfda_docs/label/2014/021476s030lbl.pdf (accessed 25 March 2023).

Zolpidem

Trade names: Ambien, Nytamel, Sanaval, Stilnoct, Stilnox, Sublinox, Xolnox, Zoldem, Zolnod.

Description: Zolpidem is a z-drug, or non-benzodiazepine hypnotic, which acts in a similar manner to benzodiazepines as a positive allosteric modulator of the $GABA_A$ receptor by binding to the omega-1 subtype benzodiazepine site.[1] The manufacturer recommends taking the drug for no longer than 4 weeks including the period of tapering off.[1]

Withdrawal effects: Stopping z-drugs even when taken as prescribed can lead to withdrawal effects is as many as 30–45% of people.[2-4] The longer these drugs are used and the higher the dose taken the greater the risk of withdrawal. The manufacturer states on the drug label that withdrawal effects from zolpidem include insomnia, headache or muscle pain, extreme anxiety and tension, restlessness, confusion and irritability.[1] In severe cases derealisation, depersonalisation, hyperacusis, numbness and tingling of the extremities, hypersensitivity to light, noise and touch, hallucinations or seizures may occur.[1] Inter-dose withdrawal is also possible – where withdrawal effects occur between night-time doses.[1] The existence of protracted withdrawal syndromes in z-drugs has not been investigated, but it has been suggested that there should be little difference from benzodiazepines on this issue, given their similar pharmacological effects.[5]

Peak plasma: Peak plasma concentration is reached at between 0.5 and 3 hours.

Half-life and dosing: The elimination half-life is short, with a mean of 2.4 hours (0.7–3.5) and a duration of action of up to 6 hours. Ambien-CR produces a longer period of maximal dose and a half-life of 2.8 hours.[6] Taking the drug less frequently (including every-other-day) is not recommended in tapering because of the risk of provoking withdrawal symptoms.

Receptor occupancy: The relationship between dose of zolpidem and the occupancy of its major target $GABA_A$ is hyperbolic (as a consequence of the law of mass action).[7,8] Z-drugs demonstrate a hyperbolic relationship between dose and clinical effects,[9] which may be relevant to withdrawal effects. Dose reductions made by linear amounts (e.g. 10mg, 7.5mg, 5mg, 2.5mg, 0mg) will cause slightly larger reductions in effect each step, which may cause increasingly severe withdrawal effects (Figure 3.25a). Hyperbolic tapering is required to produce linear changes in effect on receptor occupancy, although because of the nature of the occupancy curve, this pattern is not substantially different from linear tapering (Figure 3.25b),[10] which informs the reductions presented. The relationship was derived by converting the receptor occupancy curve for diazepam[8] to the equivalent zolpidem dose.[11]

Available formulations: As tablets.

Tablets*

Dosage	UK	Europe	USA	Australia	Canada
5mg	✓	✓	✓	✓	✓
10mg	✓	✓	✓	✓	✓

*As zolpidem tartrate

CHAPTER 3

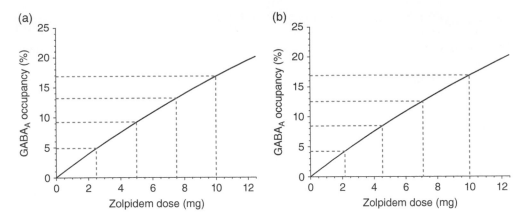

Figure 3.25 (a) Linear reductions of dose cause increasingly large reductions in effect on receptor targets, possibly associated with more withdrawal effects. (b) Even reductions of effect at target receptors requires hyperbolic dose reductions, slightly different from linear reductions in this case. The final dose before stopping will need to be small so that this step down is not larger (in terms of effect on receptor occupancy) than previous reductions.

Sublingual tablets*

Dosage	UK	Europe	USA	Australia	Canada
1.75mg	–	–	✓	–	–
3.5mg	–	–	✓	–	–
5mg	–	–	✓	–	–
10mg	–	–	✓	–	–

* As zolpidem tartrate

Extended-release tablets*

Dosage	UK	Europe	USA	Australia	Canada
6.25mg	–	–	✓	✓	–
12.5mg	–	–	✓	✓	–

*As zolpidem tartrate

Off-label options: Smaller doses of zolpidem than those provided by commercially available tablets may be required to assist tapering. Guidelines for people who cannot swallow tablets[12,13] recommend that instant-release zolpidem tablets can be mixed in water for administration. This process may be sped up by crushing the tablet with a spoon or pestle and mortar before mixing with water. For example, water could be added to a 5mg tablet to make up a 5mL suspension (concentration 1mg/mL). The suspension should be shaken vigorously before use. As its stability cannot be assured it should be consumed immediately and any unused suspension discarded. Some patients use full-fat milk to make liquid preparations. Z-drugs are more soluble in oil or fat than in water.[14] When mixed with milk, some or all of the drug will dissolve in the milk fat. This should form an evenly dispersed emulsion when shaken vigorously. The measured dose should be taken immediately after shaking and the remainder discarded.

Other options to make up small doses include compounding smaller-dose tablets or suspensions at specialist pharmacies.

Worked example: To illustrate how to calculate volumes to make up a given dose using a liquid, a worked example is provided. To make up 3.5mg of zolpidem using a 1mg/mL suspension as outlined above will require a volume of 3.5/1 = 3.5mL.

Deprescribing notes: There are no established guides to determine the rate of taper for someone stopping z-drugs. The longer z-drugs are used and the higher the dose taken the greater the risk of withdrawal, according to their manufacturer.[15] The size of the initial reduction can be estimated based on these factors (see 'Tapering benzodiazepines and z-drugs in practice'), with patient preference also taken into account. Sometimes an even smaller reduction to start with may be advisable to boost a patient's confidence that they can taper if performed carefully.

Each reduction should be made when the withdrawal symptoms from the previous reduction have largely resolved, so that subsequent reductions do not lead to cumulative withdrawal symptoms. Withdrawal symptoms should be tolerable and last at most a couple of weeks. Allowing for a sufficient observation period, reductions can therefore be made about every 1–2 weeks. If withdrawal symptoms are moderately severe or take longer than a couple of weeks to resolve, dose reductions should be postponed until symptoms resolve, and then made more gradually by choosing a slower tapering rate. If severe withdrawal symptoms occur, the patient should return to a higher dose, wait until symptoms resolve, and thereafter taper at a slower rate.

Suggested direct taper schedules for zolpidem: Please note that none of these regimens should be seen as prescriptive – patients should not be compelled to adhere strictly to them. They are given as example regimens and are not 'set and forget' but should be modified in order to ensure that withdrawal symptoms are tolerable throughout a taper. For example, intermediate steps halfway between the doses listed could be added to make a more gradual taper. Ultimately, it is the patient's experience of withdrawal that should guide the rate of taper.

A. **A faster taper** with up to 4.8 percentage points of $GABA_A$ occupancy between each step – with reductions made every 1–2 weeks*.

Step	RO (%)	Total daily dose (mg)	Formulation
1	16.8	10	Use tablets
2	13.2	7.5	Use ½ tablets**
3	9.2	5	Use tablets
4	4.8	2.5	Use ½ tablets**
5	0	0	

RO = receptor occupancy

*Patients who have been on the medication for only a few weeks will probably be able to taper more quickly and might follow every second or third step of this regimen and make reductions every few days or so. Normally the duration of the taper should not be longer than the period that the patient has been on the drug for people who have only taken it for a few weeks. For example, if zolpidem is taken for 3 weeks the taper should be less than 3 weeks.

**These should be instant-release tablets. Alternatively, a liquid formulation of the drug could be used for these doses, made up as above.

B. **A moderate taper** with up to 2.5 percentage points of $GABA_A$ occupancy between each step – with reductions made every 1–2 weeks.

Step	RO (%)	Total daily dose (mg)	Formulation	Step	RO (%)	Total daily dose (mg)	Formulation
1	16.8	10	Use tablets	6	7.1	3.75	Use ¾ tablets*
2	15	8.75	Use ¾ tablets*	7	4.8	2.5	Use ½ tablets*
3	13.2	7.5	Use ½ tablets*	8	2.5	1.25	Use ¼ tablets*
4	11.2	6.25	Use ¼ tablets*	9	0	0	0
5	9.2	5	Use tablets				
See further steps in the right-hand column							

RO = receptor occupancy
*These should be instant-release tablets. Alternatively, a liquid formulation of the drug, prepared as above, could be used for these doses.

C. **A slower taper** with up to 1.3 percentage points of $GABA_A$ occupancy between each step – with reductions made every 1–2 weeks. Liquid formulation or compounded medication will be required for this taper schedule.

Step	RO (%)	Total daily dose (mg)	Formulation	Step	RO (%)	Total daily dose (mg)	Formulation
1	16.8	10	Use tablets	9	9.2	5	5mL**
Switch to **1mg/mL** zolpidem suspension*				10	8.2	4.4	4.4mL
2	16	9.4	9.4mL	11	7.1	3.75	3.75mL**
3	15	8.75	8.75mL**	12	5.9	3.1	3.1mL
4	14.1	8.1	8.1mL	13	4.8	2.5	2.5mL**
5	13.2	7.5	7.5mL**	14	3.7	1.9	1.9mL
6	12.3	6.9	6.9mL	15	2.5	1.25	1.25mL**
7	11.2	6.25	6.25mL**	16	1.2	0.6	0.6mL
8	10.2	5.6	5.6mL	17	0	0	
See further steps in the right-hand column							

RO = receptor occupancy
*This suspension can be made up as above. Alternatively, compounded tablets or capsules of medication could be used.
**Alternatively, these doses could be made up using tablets, or fractions of tablets.

D. **An even slower taper** Some patients will be unable to taper at the slowest rates shown here and will need to taper by even smaller decrements, thus lengthening the overall period of tapering. Such a regimen could be constructed by placing intermediate steps in regimen C. For example, 10mg, 9.4mg, 8.75mg could be modified to be 10mg, 9.7mg, 9.4mg, 9.1mg, 8.75mg and so on. Further intermediate steps could also be added.

Micro-tapering The tables above show how to make reductions at intervals of 1 to 2 weeks. An alternative approach is called 'micro-tapering' whereby very small dose

CHAPTER 3

reductions are made every day, as explained in 'Other considerations in tapering benzodiazepines and z-drugs.' Micro-tapering rates can be calculated from the above by dividing the change in dose for each step by 7 or 14 days. For example, for the moderate regime, a reduction from 10mg to 8.75mg over 14 days, each day is equivalent to a reduction of approximately 0.1mg each day. This rate can be slowed if withdrawal symptoms become too unpleasant.

Switch to diazepam An alternative to a direct taper from zolpidem is to switch to diazepam before tapering from this drug, as outlined in 'Switching to longer-acting benzodiazepines to taper'. However, as zolpidem has a short half-life and is dosed once a day, it might be that less physical dependence will be produced in response to this drug than diazepam (present for the entire day). Therefore, it may be easier to directly taper from zolpidem than switching to diazepam. For those people who report inter-dose withdrawal symptoms from z-drugs a switch to a longer-acting benzodiazepine might be more reasonable. A 10mg dose of zolpidem is equivalent to 5mg of diazepam[11] and so a direct switch could be made to 5mg diazepam daily from this dose, and then tapered according to the diazepam section.

References

1. SmPC. Zolpidem – Summary of Product Characteristics. 2021. https://www.medicines.org.uk/emc/product/3975/smpc#gref (accessed 15 April 2023).

2. Anon. What's wrong with prescribing hypnotics? *Drug Ther Bull* 2004; 42: 89–93.

3. Lerner A, Klein M. Dependence, withdrawal and rebound of CNS drugs: an update and regulatory considerations for new drugs development. *Brain Communications* 2019; 1. doi:10.1093/BRAINCOMMS/FCZ025.

4. Schifano F, Chiappini S, Corkery JM, Guirguis A. An insight into z-drug abuse and dependence: an examination of reports to the European medicines agency database of suspected adverse drug reactions. *Int J Neuropsychopharmacol* 2019; 22: 270–7.

5. Cosci F, Chouinard G. Acute and persistent withdrawal syndromes following discontinuation of psychotropic medications. *Psychother Psychosom* 2020; 89: 283–306.

6. Ambien CR. RxList. https://www.rxlist.com/ambien-cr-drug.htm (accessed 4 May 2023).

7. Holford N. Pharmacodynamic principles and the time course of delayed and cumulative drug effects. *Transl Clin Pharmacol* 2018; 26: 56–9.

8. Brouillet E, Chavoix C, Bottlaender M, et al. In vivo bidirectional modulatory effect of benzodiazepine receptor ligands on GABAergic transmission evaluated by positron emission tomography in non-human primates. *Brain Res* 1991; 557: 167–76.

9. Horowitz M, Taylor D. Withdrawing from benzodiazepines and z-drugs (in preparation).

10. Horowitz MA, Taylor D. Tapering of SSRI treatment to mitigate withdrawal symptoms. *The Lancet Psychiatry* 2019; 6: 538–46.

11. Ashton H. Benzodiazepines: how they work and how to withdraw (The Ashton Manual). University of Newcastle, 2002. http://www.benzo.org.uk/manual/bzcha01.htm (accessed 11 July 2023).

12. Smyth J. The NEWT guidelines for administration of medication to patients with enteral feeding tubes or swallowing difficulties. 2011. https://www.newtguidelines.com/index.html (accessed 6 July 2023).

13. Bostwick JR, Demehri A. Pills to powder: an updated clinician's reference for crushable psychotropics. *Curr Psychiatr* 2017; 16: 46–9.

14. Macheras PE, Koupparis MA, Antimisiaris SG. Drug binding and solubility in milk. *Pharm Res* 1990; 7: 537–41.

15. FDA. Zolpidem – Highlights of Information. 2016.

CHAPTER 3

Zopiclone

Trade names: Imovane, Rhovane, Ximovan, Zileze, Zimoclone, Zimovane, Zopiklone, Zopitan, Zorclone.

Description: Zopiclone is a z-drug, or non-benzodiazepine hypnotic, which acts in a similar manner to benzodiazepines as a positive allosteric modulator of $GABA_A$ receptors by producing conformational changes in the receptor complex.[1] The manufacturer states 'long term continuous use is not recommended'.[1]

Withdrawal effects: Stopping z-drugs even when taken as prescribed can lead to withdrawal effects in as many as 30–45% of people.[1-3] The longer these drugs are used and the higher the dose taken, the greater the risk of withdrawal.[1] According to the manufacturer, withdrawal symptoms include 'insomnia, muscle pain, anxiety, tremor, sweating, agitation, confusion, headache, palpitations, tachycardia, delirium, nightmares, hallucinations, panic attacks, muscle aches/cramps, gastrointestinal disturbances and irritability. In severe cases the following symptoms may occur: derealisation, depersonalisation, hyperacusis, numbness and tingling of the extremities, hypersensitivity to light, noise and physical contact, hallucinations. In very rare cases, seizures may occur'.[1] Seizures on withdrawal have mainly been reported after higher than usual doses.[2] The existence of protracted withdrawal syndromes with z-drugs has not been investigated, but it has been suggested that there should be little difference from benzodiazepines, given the similar pharmacological effects.[4]

Peak plasma: Approximately 1.5–2 hours.[1]

Half-life and dosing: The elimination half-life is approximately 5 hours. The manufacturer recommends taking the drug once a day at night.[1] Taking the drug less frequently (including every-other-day) is not recommended in tapering because of the risk of provoking withdrawal symptoms.

Receptor occupancy: The relationship between dose of zopiclone and the occupancy of its major target $GABA_A$ is hyperbolic as a consequence of the law of mass action.[5,6] Z-drugs demonstrate a hyperbolic relationship between dose and clinical effects,[7] which may be relevant to withdrawal effects from zopiclone. Dose reductions made by linear amounts (e.g. 7.5mg, 5.6mg, 3.75mg, 1.875mg, 0mg) will cause slightly larger reductions in effect each step, which may cause increasingly severe withdrawal effects (Figure 3.26a). Due to the nature of the occupancy curve hyperbolic tapering is not substantially different from linear tapering for zopiclone (Figure 3.26b),[8] which informs the reductions presented. The relationship was derived by converting the receptor occupancy curve for diazepam[9] to the equivalent zopiclone dose.[10]

Available formulations: As tablets.

Tablets

Dosage	UK	Europe	USA	Australia	Canada
3.75mg	✓	✓	–	–	✓
5mg	–	–	–	–	✓
7.5mg	✓	✓	–	✓	✓

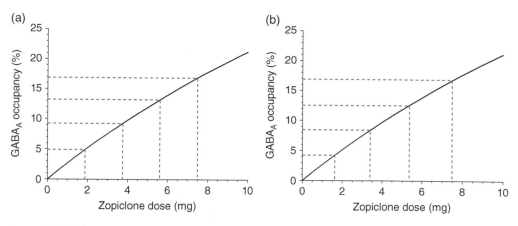

Figure 3.26 (a) Linear reductions of zopiclone. (b) Hyperbolic reductions are fairly similar to linear reductions for zopiclone because of the nature of the dose–occupancy relationship.

Off-label options: Smaller doses of zopiclone than those provided by commercially available tablets may be required to assist tapering. Guidelines for people who cannot swallow tablets[11] state that zopiclone tablets should not be crushed because zopiclone has a bitter taste, normally concealed by a film coating. However, the taste may be masked somewhat with juice and many may not find the taste too unpleasant. To make a suspension, water could be added to a 3.75mg tablet to make up a 37.5mL suspension (concentration 1mg in 10mL or 0.1mg/mL). The suspension should be shaken vigorously before use. As its stability cannot be assured it should be consumed immediately, and any unused suspension discarded. Some patients use full-fat milk to make liquid preparations. Z-drugs are more soluble in oil or fat than in water.[12] When mixed with milk, some or all of the drug will dissolve in the milk fat. This should form an evenly dispersed emulsion when shaken vigorously. The measured dose should be taken immediately after shaking and the remainder discarded.

Other options to make up small doses include compounding smaller-dose tablets, including the option of 'tapering strips'.[13] Another option is to switch to diazepam (see below).

Worked example: To illustrate how to calculate volumes to make up a given dose using a liquid, a worked example is provided. To make up 2mg of zopiclone using a 0.1mg/mL suspension prepared as outlined above will require a volume of 2/0.1 = 20mL.

Deprescribing notes: There are no established guides to determine the rate of taper for someone stopping z-drugs. The longer z-drugs are used and the higher the dose taken, the greater the risk of withdrawal, according to their manufacturer.[14] The size of the initial reduction can be estimated based on these factors (see 'Tapering benzodiazepines and z-drugs in practice'), with patient preference also taken into account. Sometimes an even smaller reduction to start with may be advisable to boost a patient's confidence that they can taper if performed carefully.

Each reduction should be made when the withdrawal symptoms from the previous reduction have largely resolved (most commonly insomnia with z-drugs), so that subsequent reductions do not lead to cumulative withdrawal symptoms. Withdrawal symptoms should not be too unpleasant: a rate of reduction should be aimed for that produces tolerable withdrawal symptoms that abate within a week or two. Allowing for a sufficient observation period, reductions can therefore be made about every 1–2 weeks, depending on how long it takes withdrawal symptoms to resolve. If withdrawal symptoms are moderately severe or take longer than a couple of weeks to resolve, dose reductions should be postponed until symptoms resolve, and then made more gradually by choosing a slower tapering rate. If severe withdrawal symptoms occur, the patient should return to a higher dose, wait until symptoms resolve, and thereafter taper at a slower rate.

Suggested direct taper schedules for zopiclone: Please note that none of these regimens should be seen as prescriptive – patients should not be compelled to adhere strictly to them. They are given as example regimens and are not 'set and forget' but should be modified in order to ensure that withdrawal symptoms are tolerable throughout a taper. For example, intermediate steps halfway between the doses listed could be added to make a more gradual taper. Ultimately, it is the patient's experience of withdrawal that should guide the rate of taper.

A. **A faster taper** with up to 4.8 percentage points of $GABA_A$ occupancy between each step – with reductions made every 1–2 weeks*.

Step	RO (%)	Dose (mg)	Formulation
1	16.8	7.5	Use tablets
2	13.2	5.625	Use ½ tablets**
3	9.2	3.75	Use tablets**
4	4.8	1.875	Use ½ tablets**
5	0	0	

RO = receptor occupancy
*Patients who have been on the medication for only a few weeks will probably be able to taper more quickly and might follow every second or third step of this regimen and make reductions every few days or so. Normally the duration of the taper should not be longer than the period that the patient has been on the drug for people who have only taken it for a few weeks. For example, if zopiclone is taken for 3 weeks the taper should be less than 3 weeks.
**Alternatively, a liquid version of zopiclone could be used to make up these doses, prepared as above.

B. **A moderate taper** with up to 2.5 percentage points of $GABA_A$ occupancy between each step – with reductions made every 1–2 weeks.

Step	RO (%)	Dose (mg)	Formulation	Step	RO (%)	Dose (mg)	Formulation
1	16.8	7.5	Use tablets	6	7.1	2.8125	Use ¾ tablets*
2	15	6.5625	Use ¾ tablets*	7	4.8	1.875	Use ½ tablets*
3	13.2	5.625	Use ½ tablets*	8	2.5	0.9375	Use ¼ tablets*
4	11.2	4.6875	Use ¼ tablets*	9	0	0	
5	9.2	3.75	Use tablets*				
See further steps in the right-hand column							

RO = receptor occupancy
*Alternatively, a liquid version of zopiclone could be used to make up these doses, prepared as above.

C. **A slower taper** with up to 1.3 percentage points of GABA$_A$ occupancy between each step – with reductions made every 1–2 weeks.

Step	RO (%)	Dose (mg)	Formulation	Step	RO (%)	Dose (mg)	Formulation
1	16.8	7.5	Use tablets	9	9.2	3.75	37.5mL**
Switch to liquid zopiclone (e.g. 0.1mg/mL)*				10	8.2	3.3	33mL
2	15.9	7	70mL	11	7.1	2.8	28mL**
3	15	6.55	65.5mL**	12	5.8	2.3	23mL
4	14.1	6.1	61mL	13	4.8	1.85	18.5mL**
5	13.2	5.65	56.5mL**	14	3.6	1.4	14mL
6	12.3	5.2	52mL	15	2.5	0.9	9mL**
7	11.2	4.7	47mL**	16	1.3	0.45	4.5mL
8	10.2	4.2	42mL	17	0	0	
See further steps in the right-hand column							

RO = receptor occupancy
*Prepared as above.
**Alternatively, these doses could be made up by tablets or fragments of tablets.

D. **An even slower taper** Some patients will be unable to taper at the slowest rates shown here and will need to taper by even smaller decrements, thus lengthening the overall period of tapering. Such a regimen could be constructed by placing intermediate steps in regimen C. For example, 7.5mg, 7mg, 6.6mg could be modified to 7.5mg, 7.25mg, 7mg, 6.8mg and so on. Further intermediate steps could also be added.

Micro-tapering The tables above show how to make reductions at intervals of 1–2 weeks. An alternative approach is called 'micro-tapering' whereby very small dose reductions are made every day, as explained in 'Other considerations in tapering benzodiazepines and z-drugs.' Micro-tapering rates can be calculated from the above by dividing the change in dose for each step by 7 or 14 days. For example, for the moderate regime a reduction from 7.5mg to 6.6mg over 14 days is equivalent to a reduction of 0.06mg per day. This rate can be slowed if withdrawal symptoms become too unpleasant.

Switch to diazepam: An alternative to a direct taper from zopiclone is to switch to diazepam before tapering from this drug, as outlined in 'Switching to longer-acting benzodiazepines to taper'. However, as zopiclone has a short half-life and is dosed once a day, it might be that less physical dependence will be produced in response to this drug than diazepam (present for the entire day). Therefore, it may be easier to directly taper from zopiclone than switching to diazepam. For people who report inter-dose withdrawal symptoms from z-drugs a switch to a longer-acting benzodiazepine might be more reasonable. A 7.5mg dose of zopiclone is equivalent to 5mg of diazepam[10] and so a direct switch could be made to 5mg daily from this dose, and then tapered according to the diazepam section.

References

1. Zopiclone 3.75mg Tablets – Summary of Product Characteristics (SmPC) – (emc). https://www.medicines.org.uk/emc/product/10830/smpc (accessed 29 April 2023).
2. Lerner A, Klein M. Dependence, withdrawal and rebound of CNS drugs: an update and regulatory considerations for new drugs development. *Brain Commun* 2019; 1. doi:10.1093/BRAINCOMMS/FCZ025.
3. Schifano F, Chiappini S, Corkery JM, Guirguis A. An insight into z-drug abuse and dependence: an examination of reports to the European medicines agency database of suspected adverse drug reactions. *Int J Neuropsychopharmacol* 2019; 22: 270–7.
4. Cosci F, Chouinard G. Acute and persistent withdrawal syndromes following discontinuation of psychotropic medications. *Psychother Psychosom* 2020; 89: 283–306.
5. Holford N. Pharmacodynamic principles and the time course of delayed and cumulative drug effects. *Transl Clin Pharmacol* 2018; 26: 56–9.
6. Brouillet E, Chavoix C, Bottlaender M, et al. In vivo bidirectional modulatory effect of benzodiazepine receptor ligands on GABAergic transmission evaluated by positron emission tomography in non-human primates. *Brain Res* 1991; 557: 167–76.
7. Horowitz M, Taylor D. Withdrawing from benzodiazepines and z-drugs (in preparation).
8. Horowitz MA, Taylor D. Tapering of SSRI treatment to mitigate withdrawal symptoms. *The Lancet Psychiatry* 2019; 6: 538–46.
9. Bostwick JR, Demehri A. Pills to powder: An updated clinician's reference for crushable psychotropics. *Curr Psychiatr* 2017; 16: 46–9.
10. Ashton H. Benzodiazepines: how they work and how to withdraw (The Ashton Manual). Newcastle University, 2002. http://www.benzo.org.uk/manual/bzcha01.htm (accessed 11 July 2023).
11. Smyth J. The NEWT guidelines for administration of medication to patients with enteral feeding tubes or swallowing difficulties. 2011. https://www.newtguidelines.com/index.html (accessed 18 February 2023).
12. Macheras PE, Koupparis MA, Antimisiaris SG. Drug binding and solubility in milk. *Pharm Res* 1990; 7: 537–41.
13. Groot PC, van Os J. Successful use of tapering strips for hyperbolic reduction of antidepressant dose: a cohort study. *Ther Adv Psychopharmacol* 2021; 11: 20451253211039330.
14. FDA. LUNESTA® (eszopiclone) tablets - Accessdata.fda.gov. FDA. https://www.accessdata.fda.gov/drugsatfda_docs/label/2014/021476s030lbl.pdf (accessed 25 March 2023).

Chapter 4

Safe Deprescribing of Gabapentinoids

When and Why to Stop Gabapentinoids

The gabapentinoids, gabapentin and pregabalin, are derivatives of the neurotransmitter gamma-aminobutyric acid (GABA). Both are licensed for the treatment of seizure disorders and neuropathic pain conditions in the UK and USA, and, additionally, in the USA for restless leg syndrome (RLS).[1,2] Pregabalin is also licensed for generalised anxiety disorder (GAD) in the UK although it is not recommended as a first-line option and reserved for use if SSRIs or SNRIs are not tolerated.[3] Pregabalin and gabapentin are also often used off-licence ('off-label') for a number of conditions for which there is a lack of evidence of efficacy[4] including migraine, low back pain, sciatica, alcohol use disorders, insomnia and bipolar disorder, and anxiety disorders (off-licence for gabapentin). Off-label use may mean that patients are exposed to harms without clear benefits (Table 4.1).[4-7] Up to 80% of gabapentin use is off-label in the USA.[8] Gabapentin, in particular, has been described as a 'catch-all' medication that has come to be used in a wide variety of disorders.[9]

The prescribing of gabapentinoids in England has increased dramatically in recent years, rising from less than 1 million prescriptions in 2008 to 16 million in 2022 with roughly equal representation of the two drugs.[15,16] In 2017–2018 1.46 million people in England received at least one prescription for a gabapentinoid.[15] In the USA the use of gabapentinoids more than trebled from 2002 to 2015, from 1.2% of adults to 3.9% of adults, with more than 80% of these prescriptions for gabapentin.[17] In 2018 gabapentin became the sixth most commonly prescribed medication in the USA.[18] It has been suggested that this rise in prescribing has been due to a desire to avoid opioid analgesics.[7] Approximately one tenth of the prescriptions for pregabalin are for anxiety.[19]

Off-label prescribing of gabapentinoids is widespread. In the UK around half (51.4%) of patients prescribed pregabalin and just over a third (36.9%) of patients prescribed gabapentin had a diagnosis for a licensed indication.[11] As with the case of OxyContin,

The Maudsley® Deprescribing Guidelines: Antidepressants, Benzodiazepines, Gabapentinoids and Z-drugs, First Edition. Mark Horowitz and David Taylor.
© 2024 John Wiley & Sons Ltd. Published 2024 by John Wiley & Sons Ltd.

Table 4.1 Licensed indications and unlicensed uses for gabapentinoids in the USA and UK.[10–14]

Drug		Licensed indications	Unlicensed uses
Pregabalin	USA[10]	■ Neuropathic pain associated with diabetic peripheral neuropathy ■ Neuropathic pain associated with spinal cord injury ■ Postherpetic neuralgia ■ Fibromyalgia ■ Adjunctive therapy for partial-onset seizures in patients 4 years of age and older	■ GAD ■ Social anxiety disorder ■ Bipolar disorder ■ Insomnia ■ Other chronic pain conditions ■ Chronic pruritus ■ Chronic cough ■ RLS ■ Insomnia ■ Alcohol use disorder
	UK[11,12]	■ Peripheral and central neuropathic pain ■ Adjunctive therapy for focal seizures with or without secondary generalisation ■ GAD	■ Chronic abdominal pain ■ Chronic back pain ■ Chronic headache ■ Fibromyalgia ■ Migraine ■ Osteoarthritis ■ RLS ■ Alcohol dependency
Gabapentin	USA[13]	■ Postherpetic neuralgia ■ Adjunctive therapy in the treatment of partial seizures with or without secondary generalisation in patients over the age of 12 with epilepsy, and 3 to 12 year olds with a partial seizure ■ Moderate to severe RLS	■ Neuropathic pain ■ Fibromyalgia ■ Bipolar disorder ■ Postmenopausal hot flushes ■ Essential tremors ■ Anxiety ■ Resistant depressant and mood disorders ■ Irritable bowel syndrome (IBS) ■ Alcohol withdrawal ■ Postoperative analgesia ■ Nausea and vomiting ■ Migraine prophylaxis ■ Headache ■ Interstitial cystitis ■ Painful diabetic neuropathy ■ Social phobia ■ Generalized tonic-clonic seizures ■ Pruritus (itching) ■ Insomnia ■ Post-traumatic stress disorder (PTSD) ■ Refractory chronic cough
	UK[11,12]	■ Epilepsy ■ Peripheral neuropathic pain ■ Menopausal symptoms, particularly hot flushes, in women with breast cancer ■ Muscular symptoms in motor neurone disease ■ Spasticity in multiple sclerosis ■ Oscillopsia in multiple sclerosis	■ Chronic abdominal pain ■ Chronic back pain ■ Chronic headache ■ Fibromyalgia ■ Migraine ■ Osteoarthritis ■ Restless leg syndrome ■ Alcohol dependency ■ Drug dependency[14]

pharmaceutical companies marketing gabapentinoids have paid large fines for misrepresentation of their safety and misuse potential, as well as for promoting prescribing for off-label indications, and so inflating demand.[20] In the USA, gabapentinoids are now prescribed during one in four post-surgical admissions, often in combination with opioids or other analgesics, presumably with an aim to reduce opioid consumption, despite a lack of evidence for peri-operative pain or for opioid-sparing effects.[21] Longer-term off-label prescribing of gabapentinoids has mostly been seen in the treatment of chronic low back pain. This use leads to wide availability among a population already vulnerable to misuse, and often in conjunctive with multiple co-prescribed sedative or analgesic medications, increasing the risk of harms.[22]

Recognition of dependence and misuse

In the UK gabapentinoids were re-classified as Class C Controlled Drugs under the Misuse of Drugs Act from 2019 and Schedule 3 controlled drugs under the Misuse of Drugs Regulation. This was in recognition of escalating misuse, diversion and addiction, as well as growing numbers of deaths associated with their use.[23,24] This scheduling places them in the same category as higher-risk benzodiazepines (e.g. midazolam and temazepam).[23,24] Under the Misuse of Drugs Act unlawful possession, production or supply of these drugs is subject to potential punishment and fines. In the USA, the FDA has issued warnings about the use of gabapentinoids in people with respiratory depression especially in those patients also using opioid medication, those with lung conditions like chronic obstructive pulmonary disease (COPD), and the elderly.[2] Pregabalin has been a Schedule V drug (indicating the lowest potential for abuse compared to other scheduled drugs) under the Controlled Substances Act since 2005,[25] and some states have classified gabapentin under the same schedule.[26]

Public Health England conducted a review of dependence-forming medicine in England in 2019 and reflected:

Recurring patterns are evident in the history of medicines that may cause dependence or withdrawal. New medicines are seen as an important part of the solution to a condition, resulting in widespread use. Their dependence or withdrawal potential are either unknown at this point, due to a lack of research, or perhaps downplayed. As evidence of harm from dependence or withdrawal emerges, efforts are made to curtail prescribing. The repetition of this pattern is striking.

Some commentators have suggested that gabapentinoid use is a clear example of this pattern.[27]

Pharmacological actions

Gabapentinoids are structurally similar to GABA, rapidly cross the blood–brain barrier and although their mechanism of action is poorly understood, seem to exert their effects through inhibition of alpha-2-delta sub-unit-containing voltage-dependent calcium channels.[28] This inhibition prevents synaptic release of glutamate and norepinephrine, and is thought to reduce neuronal excitation.[28] Although gabapentinoids are not thought to directly bind to GABA receptors they do dose-dependently increase levels of

GABA, and thus have weak GABA-mimetic effects.[28,29] They therefore have some overlap with the pharmacological effects of benzodiazepines, which also increase GABA activity.[5] This pharmacological similarity is reflected in their shared short-term anxiolytic, anticonvulsant and analgesic properties, as well as their ability to cause dissociation, relaxation, a sense of calm and, in some, euphoria.[21,30]

There are some pharmacological differences between the gabapentinoids. Pregabalin has higher potency, greater bioavailability (90%, or greater, compared with 33–60% for gabapentin) and quicker absorption than gabapentin (reaching maximum plasma concentrations within 1 hour compared with 3–4 hours for gabapentin).[28,30] It has been observed that pregabalin is more prone to abuse than gabapentin, which may be because of its ability to induce a more rapid euphoria due to its pharmacodynamic and pharmacokinetic characteristics.[28]

Efficacy in anxiety disorders

The evidence for the efficacy of pregabalin in anxiety is somewhat limited. Anxiety can be a long-term condition requiring long-term treatment that necessitates long-term trial data. However, the manufacturer's guide to pregabalin states that it has been studied in six controlled trials of 4–6 weeks duration and in one study of 8 weeks.[31] If the results of these trials are presented as response (greater than a 50% improvement in Hamilton Anxiety (HAM-A) scores), pregabalin is superior to placebo (52% response for pregabalin, 38% for placebo).[31] However, examination of the raw HAM-A data before dichotomisation can be informative. A recent meta-analysis of these short-term studies, in addition to unpublished studies by drug manufacturers, found pregabalin reduced HAM-A scores by 2.8 points compared with placebo at 4–10 weeks follow-up.[32] On the 56-point HAM-A, it is unclear whether this effect is clinically meaningful. More importantly, the short duration of treatment (average 7.3 weeks)[32] in these studies may not be informative about the treatment of anxiety, an often chronic condition commonly needing to be treated for months or years.

In a similar manner to benzodiazepines, tolerance to the effects of pregabalin develops over time.[33] It is therefore likely that, as for benzodiazepines,[34] its anxiolytic properties will lessen over time, diminishing or eliminating these short-term effects. Unfortunately, no useful study has been conducted that lasts longer than 10 weeks to evaluate this possibility.

These studies also did not examine the difficulty of withdrawing from these drugs. There is one discontinuation study evaluating relapse-prevention properties in GAD, which involved abrupt stoppage of pregabalin from a dose of 300mg after 8 weeks of treatment.[35] The authors neglected measurement of the recognised withdrawal effects that can mimic the symptoms of relapse and can inflate the detection of relapse in the discontinuation arm, rendering this study difficult to interpret.[35]

Efficacy in pain disorders

According to NHS guidance, no more than one-quarter of patients with certain long-term pain conditions (including painful diabetic neuropathy, pain following stroke and post-herpetic neuralgia) receive any benefit from gabapentinoids.[36–38] A 50% reduction in pain is experienced by even fewer.[36–38]

NHS guidance encourages review of gabapentinoids for neuropathic pain and advises that they should be gradually discontinued if ineffective.[39] This guidance suggests that even people who think they are obtaining benefit from the use of pregabalin or gabapentin should undertake a trial dose reduction periodically, to ensure they are benefiting and to see if they can derive the same benefit on a lower dose.[39] This guidance also highlights that gabapentinoids are licenced for neuropathic pain and are very unlikely to be of benefit when prescribed for non-neuropathic pain.[40]

Moderate-quality evidence supports the use of gabapentinoids to improve pain in post-herpetic neuralgia or diabetic peripheral neuropathy in short-term studies (up to 16 weeks).[36,37] At time points up to 16 weeks almost 40% of people taking pregabalin and 30% of people taking gabapentin had at least 50% pain relief.[36,37] There are no long-term studies of the effect of these drugs, but tolerance might be anticipated, as with opioids.[33]

Only 10% of patients with moderate to severe fibromyalgia experienced a 50% reduction in pain over several months of treatment according to high-quality evidence from a Cochrane review.[41] Evidence for gabapentin is inconclusive because of the small number of low-quality trials.[42] These drugs are probably not effective for pain relief in other conditions and their use is not advised.[7] Systematic reviews have found no benefit of gabapentinoids over placebo in low back pain, sciatica, spinal stenosis or episodic migraine in adults.[7] Currently, there is insufficient evidence to support the use of pregabalin in acute pain, HIV neuropathy, neuropathic cancer pain and other forms of neuropathic pain.[7]

In chronic primary pain (pain which lasts for more than 3 months and for which no underlying condition is identified as the cause), UK NICE guidelines advise against using gabapentinoids, unless as part of a research trial.[43] This guideline recommends that patients who are already on gabapentinoids for primacy pain should be informed of the lack of evidence for these medications and the risks of continuing. Those with little benefit or evidence of significant harm should be encouraged to reduce and stop.[43] For those who report benefit and few harms continuing safely is also presented as an option.[43]

Adverse effects

According to the UK manufacturer for pregabalin there are 47 adverse effects that are either common or very common (though the baseline rate for placebo was not taken into account) (Table 4.2).[31] Nearly two-thirds of patients taking these drugs for neuropathic pain experience an adverse event.[7] Very common adverse effects as reported by the manufacturer or Cochrane review include dizziness (19%), somnolence (14%) and headache (more than 10% of patients).[31,36] Other common psychiatric adverse effects include euphoric mood, confusion, irritability, decreased libido, disorientation and insomnia, all occurring in 1–10% of patients.[31] The manufacturer also reports on the patient label that increased risk of new-onset suicidal behaviour and death by suicide has been demonstrated in self-controlled studies (where periods on a drug are compared to periods off the drug in the same individual).[31] NHS guidance also highlights problems with sedation, weight gain, mood changes, hallucinations, muscle and joint pain, sexual dysfunction and impaired immune response.[39] Adverse events from gabapentinoids frequently result in discontinuation of the drug. For example, almost 30% of patients with fibromyalgia withdrew from studies because of adverse effects (compared with 11% for placebo).[41]

CHAPTER 4

There are specific risks when gabapentinoids are given with opioids. Co-prescription should usually be avoided because of an increased risk of respiratory depression, accidental overdose and death.[39] The Medicines and Healthcare Products Regulatory Agency (MHRA) warning states that in cases of existing co-prescription the patient should be evaluated for these risks and either the gabapentinoid or the opioid reduced appropriately.[44]

Table 4.2 Very common (experienced by more than 10% of participants) and common (1–10% of participants) adverse effects of pregabalin.[31] The effects of gabapentin are similar.[45]

Psychiatric	Cognitive	Neurological
Euphoric mood	Disorientation	*Dizziness*
Irritability	Memory impairment	*Somnolence*
Insomnia	Impaired attention	*Headache*
Panic attacks	Confusion	Ataxia
Restlessness		Abnormal co-ordination
Agitation		Tremor
Depressed mood		Dysarthria
Aggression		Paraesthesia
Mood swings		Sedation
Depersonalisation		Balance problems
Abnormal dreams		
Apathy		

Miscellaneous	Musculoskeletal	Gastrointestinal
Blurred vision	Muscle cramp	Vomiting
Diplopia	Arthralgia	Nausea
Vertigo	Back pain	Dry mouth
Erectile dysfunction	Pain in limb	Constipation
Nasopharyngitis	Cervical spasm	Diarrhoea
Weight gain		Flatulence
Increased appetite		Abdominal distension
Decreased libido/anorgasmia		

Very common effects are italicised.

Longitudinal studies have found that gabapentin is associated with neurocognitive and functional decline in older adults, including a more than doubling in risk of falls.[46] Gabapentinoids have also been associated with sexual dysfunction in people with epilepsy.[47] In young people, gabapentinoids have also been associated with increased risk of suicide, unintentional overdose, road traffic accidents, and head and body injuries – with stronger associations for pregabalin than for gabapentin.[30]

In 2022, the UK's MHRA issued an updated warning on pregabalin use during pregnancy, recommending effective contraception throughout treatment and to avoid pregabalin use during pregnancy unless clearly necessary.[48,49] These recommendations were updated in the context of a Nordic study of over 2,700 pregnancies, demonstrating higher crude rates of major congenital malformations in pregnancies exposed to pregabalin compared to pregnancies unexposed to pregabalin or other antiepileptic drugs (5.9% vs 4.1%, respectively), and a modestly increased risk of major congenital malformations in neonates exposed to first-trimester pregabalin compared to those exposed to lamotrigine or duloxetine.[50]

Mortality risk

According to the UK Office of National Statistics (ONS) records of coroners' reports deaths associated with pregabalin have increased more than 10-fold in the 7 years from 2014 to 2021 (perhaps partially explained by more testing).[51] In 2021 there were more deaths in England and Wales involving pregabalin (409) than diazepam (290) or fentanyl (58).[51] It should be noted that, like diazepam, pregabalin's lethality is probably attributable to combined use with opioids, possibly because of the ability of pregabalin to reverse tolerance to opioid depression of respiration:[52] indeed pregabalin is rarely the sole drug present in poisonings.[53]

When mortality is corrected to prescriptions issued per year, mortality for pregabalin has also risen approximately 10-fold in the last 7 years.[54] Its mortality per prescription is less than that for diazepam and fentanyl, although rising more steeply.[54] Gabapentinoids (along with z-drugs) have been associated with a 3-fold increase in overdose deaths in the USA from 2000 to 2018, leading to a warning to prescribers that replacing benzodiazepines and opioids with these medications did not necessarily lower the risk to the patient.[55]

Alternative treatments

Anxiety

Most analyses find little difference between psychotherapy and pharmacotherapy for anxiety disorders.[56,57] There is a non-significant benefit for psychotherapy over pharmacotherapy for anxiety disorders in general (though strongly significant ($g = 0.64$) for OCD).[57] An umbrella review of meta-analyses found that psychotherapies achieved SMDs (standard mean differences) of between 0.28 and 0.44, while pharmacotherapies achieved SMDs of 0.33 and 0.45.[58] Most guidelines recommend psychotherapeutic options, including CBT and other modalities for the treatment of generalised anxiety disorders.[3]

Pain

For chronic primary pain the NICE guidelines recommend supervised group exercise, remaining physically active, acceptance and commitment and cognitive behavioural therapies, specific acupuncture interventions and antidepressant medication.[43] (However, in a recent overview of systematic reviews, antidepressants were found to be ineffective, effective to a clinically dubious degree or analyses were found to be inconclusive,[59] leading to a re-consideration of the guidance.)[60] The provision of individualised therapy, support and social activities encouraging de-medicalisation, independence and personal development in one community pain clinic working with a charity led to a 50% reduction in prescribing, as well as improved pain and function.[61] It also reduced use of specialist outpatient services by 50%.[61] In the US, the department of Health and Human Services in its Best Practice guide for pain management, outlines four approaches to pain aside from medication including restorative therapies, interventional procedures, behavioural health approaches and complementary and integrative health.[62]

CHAPTER 4

References

1. Montastruc F, Loo SY, Renoux C. Trends in first gabapentin and pregabalin prescriptions in primary care in the United Kingdom, 1993–2017. *JAMA* 2018; 320: 2149–51.

2. Center for Drug Evaluation, Research. FDA warns about serious breathing problems with seizure and nerve pain medicines gabapentin (Neurontin, Gralise, Horizant) and pregabalin (Lyrica, Lyrica CR). U.S. Food and Drug Administration. https://www.fda.gov/drugs/drug-safety-and-availability/fda-warns-about-serious-breathing-problems-seizure-and-nerve-pain-medicines-gabapentin-neurontin (accessed 4 June 2023).

3. National Institute for Health and Care Excellence (NICE). Generalised anxiety disorder and panic disorder in adults: management. *NICE Clinical Guideline CG113* 2011. https://www.nice.org.uk/guidance/cg113/chapter/2-Research-recommendations#the-effectiveness-of-physical-activity-compared-with-waiting-list-control-for-the-treatment-of-gad (accessed 10 July 2023).

4. Goodman CW, Brett AS. A clinical overview of off-label use of gabapentinoid drugs. *JAMA Intern Med* 2019; 179: 695–701.

5. Horowitz MA, Kelleher M, Taylor D. Should gabapentinoids be prescribed long-term for anxiety and other mental health conditions? *Addict Behav* 2021; 119: 106943.

6. Peckham AM, Evoy KE, Ochs L, Covvey JR. Gabapentin for off-label use: evidence-based or cause for concern? *Subst Abuse* 2018; 12: 1178221818801311.

7. Mathieson S, Lin C-WC, Underwood M, Eldabe S. Pregabalin and gabapentin for pain. *BMJ* 2020; 369: m1315.

8. Radley DC, Finkelstein SN, Stafford RS. Off-label prescribing among office-based physicians. *Arch Intern Med* 2006; 166: 1021–6.

9. Fukada C, Kohler JC, Boon H, Austin Z, Krahn M. Prescribing gabapentin off label: perspectives from psychiatry, pain and neurology specialists. *Can Pharm J* 2012; 145: 280–4.e1.

10. Cross AL, Viswanath O, Sherman Al. Pregabalin. StatPearls Publishing, 2022 https://www.ncbi.nlm.nih.gov/books/NBK470341/ (accessed 8 June 2023).

11. Ashworth J, Bajpai R, Muller S, et al. Trends in gabapentinoid prescribing in UK primary care using the Clinical Practice Research Datalink: an observational study. *Lancet Reg Health Eur* 2023; 27: 100579.

12. Joint Formulary Committee. British National Formulary (BNF). 2021. https://bnf.nice.org.uk (accessed 10 July 2023).

13. Yasaei R, Katta S, Saadabadi A. Gabapentin. StatPearls Publishing, 2022 https://www.ncbi.nlm.nih.gov/books/NBK493228/ (accessed 8 June 2023).

14. Chiappini S, Schifano F. A decade of gabapentinoid misuse: an analysis of the European Medicines Agency's 'Suspected adverse drug reactions' database. *CNS Drugs* 2016; 30: 647–54.

15. Public Health England. Dependence and withdrawal associated with some prescribed medicines: an evidence review. 2019. https://www.gov.uk/government/publications/prescribed-medicines-review-report (accessed 25 May 2021).

16. EBM DataLab. Openprescribing.net. 2017. https://openprescribing.net/chemical/0408010AE/ (accessed 10 July 2023).

17. Johansen ME. Gabapentinoid use in the United States 2002 through 2015. *JAMA Intern Med* 2018; 178: 292–4.

18. Anderson PA, McLachlan AJ, Shaheed CA, Gnjidic D, Ivers R, Mathieson S. Deprescribing interventions for gabapentinoids in adults: a scoping review. *Br J Clin Pharmacol* 2023; published online May 23. doi:10.1111/bcp.15798.

19. Wettermark B, Brandt L, Kieler H, Bodén R. Pregabalin is increasingly prescribed for neuropathic pain, generalised anxiety disorder and epilepsy but many patients discontinue treatment. *Int J Clin Pract* 2014; 68: 104–10.

20. Landefeld CS, Steinman MA. The Neurontin legacy--marketing through misinformation and manipulation. *N Engl J Med* 2009; 360: 103–6.

21. Murnion B, Schaffer A, Cairns R, Brett J. Gabapentinoids: repeating mistakes of the past? *Addiction* 2022; 117: 2969–71.

22. Schaffer AL, Busingye D, Chidwick K, Brett J, Blogg S. Pregabalin prescribing patterns in Australian general practice, 2012–2018: a cross-sectional study. *BJGP Open* 2021; 5. doi:10.3399/bjgpopen20X101120.

23. Iacobucci G. UK government to reclassify pregabalin and gabapentin after rise in deaths. *BMJ* 2017; 358: j4441.

24. Controlled drugs: pregabalin and gabapentin. https://www.cqc.org.uk/guidance-providers/adult-social-care/controlled-drugs-pregabalin-gabapentin (accessed 4 June 2023).

25. Drug Enforcement Administration. Schedules of controlled substances: placement of pregabalin into schedule V. Federal Register. 2005; 70: 43633–5.

26. Leigh Ann Anderson P. Is gabapentin a controlled substance / narcotic? Drugs.com. https://www.drugs.com/medical-answers/gabapentin-narcotic-controlled-substance-3555993/ (accessed 8 June 2023).

27. Byng R. Should we, can we, halt the rise in prescribing for pain and distress? *Br J Gen Pract* 2020; 70: 432–3.

28. Bonnet U, Richter EL, Isbruch K, Scherbaum N. On the addictive power of gabapentinoids: a mini-review. *Psychiatr Danub* 2018; 30: 142–9.

29. Evoy KE, Morrison MD, Saklad SR. Abuse and misuse of pregabalin and gabapentin. *Drugs* 2017; 77: 403–26.

30. Molero Y, Larsson H, D'Onofrio BM, Sharp DJ, Fazel S. Associations between gabapentinoids and suicidal behaviour, unintentional overdoses, injuries, road traffic incidents, and violent crime: population based cohort study in Sweden. *BMJ* 2019; 365. DOI:10.1136/bmj.l2147.

31. Electronic Medicines Compendium. Pregabalin (SmPC). 2021. https://www.medicines.org.uk/emc/product/7132/smpc#gref.

32. Slee A, Nazareth I, Bondaronek P, Liu Y, Cheng Z, Freemantle N. Pharmacological treatments for generalised anxiety disorder: a systematic review and network meta-analysis. *Lancet* 2019; 393: 768–77.

33. Bonnet U, Scherbaum N. How addictive are gabapentin and pregabalin? A systematic review. *Eur Neuropsychopharmacol* 2017; 27: 1185–215.

34. Gale C, Glue P, Guaiana G, Coverdale J, McMurdo M, Wilkinson S. Influence of covariates on heterogeneity in Hamilton Anxiety Scale ratings in placebo-controlled trials of benzodiazepines in generalized anxiety disorder: systematic review and meta-analysis. *J Psychopharmacol* 2019; 33: 543–7.

35. Feltner D, Wittchen H-U, Kavoussi R, Brock J, Baldinetti F, Pande AC. Long-term efficacy of pregabalin in generalized anxiety disorder. *Int Clin Psychopharmacol* 2008; 23: 18–28.

36. Wiffen PJ, Derry S, Bell RF, et al. Gabapentin for chronic neuropathic pain in adults. *Cochrane Database Syst Rev* 2017; 6: CD007938.

37. Derry S, Bell RF, Straube S, Wiffen PJ, Aldington D, Moore RA. Pregabalin for neuropathic pain in adults. *Cochrane Database Syst Rev* 2019; 1: CD007076.

38. Wiffen PJ, Derry S, Moore RA, et al. Antiepileptic drugs for neuropathic pain and fibromyalgia – an overview of Cochrane reviews. *Cochrane Database Syst Rev* 2013; 2013: CD010567.

39. Somerset CCG. Gabapentinoid – suggested tapering regimes. Somerset CCG. www.somersetccg.nhs.uk/wp-content/uploads/2021/05/Tapering-gabapentinoid-1.pdf (accessed June 17, 2023).

40. Gabapentin. https://bnf.nice.org.uk/drugs/gabapentin/ (accessed June 17, 2023).

41. Derry S, Cording M, Wiffen PJ, Law S, Phillips T, Moore RA. Pregabalin for pain in fibromyalgia in adults. *Cochrane Database Syst Rev* 2016; 9: CD011790.

42. Cooper TE, Derry S, Wiffen PJ, Moore RA. Gabapentin for fibromyalgia pain in adults. *Cochrane Database Syst Rev* 2017; 1: CD012188.

43. Recommendations | Chronic pain (primary and secondary) in over 16s: assessment of all chronic pain and management of chronic primary pain | Guidance | NICE. https://www.nice.org.uk/guidance/ng193/chapter/Recommendations (accessed 4 June 2023).

44. Gabapentin (Neurontin): risk of severe respiratory depression. Gov.uk. 2017; published online 26 October https://www.gov.uk/drug-safety-update/gabapentin-neurontin-risk-of-severe-respiratory-depression (accessed 17 June 2023).

45. Gabapentin 100mg capsules – Summary of Product Characteristics (SmPC) – (emc). https://www.medicines.org.uk/emc/product/4121/smpc (accessed 5 June 2023).

46. Oh G, Moga DC, Fardo DW, Abner EL. The association of gabapentin initiation and neurocognitive changes in older adults with normal cognition. *Front Pharmacol* 2022; 13: 910719.

47. Yang Y, Wang X. Sexual dysfunction related to antiepileptic drugs in patients with epilepsy. *Expert Opin Drug Saf* 2016; 15: 31–42.

48. Wise J. Avoid prescribing pregabalin during pregnancy if possible, says UK drug regulator. *BMJ* 2022; 377: o1010.

49. Pregabalin (Lyrica): findings of safety study on risks during pregnancy. Gov.uk. 2022; published online April 19. https://www.gov.uk/drug-safety-update/pregabalin-lyrica-findings-of-safety-study-on-risks-during-pregnancy (accessed 5 June 2023).

50. Pfizer. EUPAS register non-interventional final study report: a population-based cohort study of pregabalin to characterize pregnancy outcomes. European Network of Centres for Pharmacoepidemiology and Pharmacovigilance. 2020. www.encepp.eu/encepp/openAttachment/documentsLatest.otherDocument-0/36879;jsessionid=MBGgBWcicUGrEwu0bGLQm2mFJ8x7uMvZQRb9EkDqCPMxQZS3StP2!-180077824 (accessed 5 June 2023).

51. Breen P, Butt A. Deaths related to drug poisoning by selected substances, England and Wales. 2022; published online 3 August. https://www.ons.gov.uk/peoplepopulationandcommunity/birthsdeathsandmarriages/deaths/datasets/deathsrelatedtodrugpoisoningbyselectedsubstances (accessed 4 June 2023).

52. Lyndon A, Audrey S, Wells C, et al. Risk to heroin users of polydrug use of pregabalin or gabapentin. *Addiction* 2017; 112: 1580–9.

53. Nahar LK, Murphy KG, Paterson S. Misuse and mortality related to gabapentin and pregabalin are being under-estimated: a two-year post-mortem population study. *J Anal Toxicol* 2019; 43: 564–70.

54. Office for National Statistics. Deaths related to drug poisoning by selected substances. 2020. https://www.ons.gov.uk/peoplepopulationandcommunity/birthsdeathsandmarriages/deaths/datasets/deathsrelatedtodrugpoisoningbyselectedsubstances.

55. Tardelli VS, Bianco MCM, Prakash R, et al. Overdose deaths involving non-BZD hypnotic/sedatives in the USA: trends analyses. *Lancet Reg Health Am* 2022; 10: 100190.

56. Carl E, Witcraft SM, Kauffman BY, et al. Psychological and pharmacological treatments for generalized anxiety disorder (GAD): a meta-analysis of randomized controlled trials. *Cogn Behav Ther* 2019; 00: 1–21.

57. Cuijpers P, Sijbrandij M, Koole SL, Andersson G, Beekman AT, Reynolds CF. The efficacy of psychotherapy and pharmacotherapy in treating depressive and anxiety disorders: a meta-analysis of direct comparisons. *World Psychiatry* 2013; 12: 137–48.

58. Leichsenring F, Steinert C, Rabung S, Ioannidis JPA. The efficacy of psychotherapies and pharmacotherapies for mental disorders in adults: an umbrella review and meta-analytic evaluation of recent meta-analyses. *World Psychiatry* 2022; 21: 133–45.

59. Ferreira GE, Abdel-Shaheed C, Underwood M, et al. Efficacy, safety, and tolerability of antidepressants for pain in adults: overview of systematic reviews. *BMJ* 2023; 380: e072415.

60. Stannard C, Wilkinson C. Rethinking use of medicines for chronic pain. *BMJ* 2023; 380: 170.

61. Wright E, Zarnegar R, Hermansen I, McGavin D, A clinical evaluation of a community-based rehabilitation and social intervention programme for patients with chronic pain with associated multi-morbidity. *J Pain Manag* 2017; 10: 149–59.

62. Digital Communications Division (DCD). Pain management best practices inter-agency task force report. Hhs.gov. 2018; published online 18 April. https://www.hhs.gov/opioids/prevention/pain-management-options/index.html (accessed June 2023).

CHAPTER 4

Discussing deprescribing gabapentinoids

The likelihood of considerable harms from gabapentinoid treatment in contrast to limited demonstrated benefit for various indications suggests that a substantial portion of patients may benefit from deprescribing.

NICE guidance recommends that stopping a gabapentinoid should be considered if:[1]

- it is no longer benefiting the person;
- the condition for which the medication was prescribed has resolved;
- the harms of the medicine outweigh the benefits;
- the person wants to stop taking the medication; or
- problems with dependence or addiction have developed.

NHS guidance specifically suggests that patients prescribed gabapentinoids for chronic neuropathic pain should have a trial reduction of medication considered every 6 to 12 months in order to establish whether the pain is still an issue, whether the gabapentinoid is beneficial and to determine whether it is causing adverse (side) effects.[2]

There are specific groups in whom deprescribing may be of a higher priority including:

- patients with concomitant use of opioids or benzodiazepines,
- patients with respiratory conditions (e.g. COPD, neuromuscular disorders) for whom the risk of respiratory depression is greatest,
- patients with current or previous substance use disorders, and
- women who are pregnant or are planning pregnancy, given the MHRA warning of increased risk of foetal malformations.

However, as for previous chapters on benzodiazepines and z-drugs, there are a variety of reasons why stopping gabapentinoids may be beneficial for a wider group of patients.

- Adverse effects – dizziness, headache, somnolence, difficulty with concentration or memory, weight gain, depressed mood (see more in Table 4.2).
- Lack of benefits – efficacy data suggests that a substantial portion of patients will not benefit from ongoing treatment with gabapentinoids for anxiety and some pain conditions. Tolerance may diminish the effect in a number of conditions.
- The patient's condition has improved or alternative coping strategies developed – anxiety may resolve when circumstances change, or may be managed with other approaches.
- Reducing polypharmacy – especially in the elderly, polypharmacy may have negative health consequences. As deprescribing in old age can be challenging, reducing medications while people are healthy enough to do so may be wise.
- Patient wishes to stop – there are a variety of reasons why patients may wish to stop medication that should be supported.
- Stopping before tolerance and dependence accumulate in order to minimise the degree of withdrawal produced by stopping. Longer-term use is associated with greater withdrawal effects for dependence-forming medications,[1] and, increasingly, dependence and withdrawal phenomena from gabapentinoids are a concern.[3,4]

There is no formal recommendation for a minimum period of treatment with a gabapentinoid – nor recommendations for a maximum duration of treatment. This lack of recommendations and clinical inertia can lead to patients being prescribed these medications indefinitely. Although not studied for gabapentinoids in particular, it is known from other drug classes that this uncertainty leads to a situation where both patient and prescriber is expecting the other to lead on discussing stopping.[5] There is also fear about 'rocking the boat'.[5] It has been suggested that short-term use of pregabalin in anxiety as a crisis measure only, analogous to benzodiazepines, may be warranted.[6] The NICE guidelines on safe withdrawal encourage clinicians to regularly review patients taking gabapentinoids and to consider deprescribing.[1]

There has been little work performed on the best approach to stopping gabapentinoids.[7] Those few studies have focused on educational interventions to inform patients about the possibility of deprescribing.[7] In one study highlighting opportunities for deprescribing, provision of information and tapering instructions to clinicians in an inpatient setting increased deprescribing rates for gabapentinoids in older patients from 21% to 35%.[8]

General principles from deprescribing in other drug classes may also be applicable.[9] Education of patients about the risks, benefits and alternatives to these drugs can help motivate patients to stop.[10] Many patients will be unaware of the wide variety of adverse effects of these medications and so may not have attributed these symptoms to the medication, especially after long-term use. Adverse effects of psychotropic drugs are often insidious, and patients may struggle to compare present symptoms with a pretreatment baseline. This material can be presented in a written format, with some studies in similar medication classes showing that a face-to-face discussion can enhance effectiveness.[11] Patients should have it explained to them that their anxiety or pain may not worsen if the drug is reduced in dose because of a lack of evidence for effectiveness, especially in the long-term, due to tolerance effects.

Outlining a gradual and flexible taper involving tolerable dose-reductions (see subsequent sections) may help alleviate fears patients have about the process. Patients with specific fears relating to prior unsuccessful attempts to stop medications may be reassured that reducing doses more carefully can help to avoid severe withdrawal symptoms. Patients may have falsely come to believe that their medication is helpful for pain or anxiety because when they stop it they experience worsening of these symptoms – and conversely when they take a dose they experience an improvement in anxiety or pain. Sometimes this relief may be caused by improvement of withdrawal symptoms (which can include depressed mood, anxiety and pain)[12,13] rather than direct evidence of their effectiveness for underlying conditions, analogous to the situation for benzodiazepines. If alternative means for managing pain or anxiety are available, for example, physiotherapy, psychological therapy or support, this may also give a patient greater confidence in stopping, and help to manage the issues that prompted the prescription in the first place.

CHAPTER 4

References

1. National Institute for Health and Care Excellence (NICE). Medicines associated with dependence or withdrawal symptoms: safe prescribing and withdrawal management for adults | Guidance | NICE. 2022. https://www.nice.org.uk/guidance/ng215/chapter/Recommendations (accessed June 27, 2022).

2. Fife NHS. Gabapentinoid reduction patient information leaflet. NHS Fife. https://www.nhsfife.org/media/32617/gabapentinoid-reduction-leaflet.pdf (accessed 17 June 2023).

3. Mersfelder TL, Nichols WH. Gabapentin: abuse, dependence, and withdrawal. *Ann Pharmacother* 2016; 50: 229–33.

4. Bonnet U, Scherbaum N. How addictive are gabapentin and pregabalin? A systematic review. *Eur Neuropsychopharmacol* 2017; 27: 1185–215.

5. Maund E, Dewar-Haggart R, Williams S, et al. Barriers and facilitators to discontinuing antidepressant use: a systematic review and thematic synthesis. *J Affect Disord* 2019; 245: 38–62.

6. Horowitz MA, Kelleher M, Taylor D. Should gabapentinoids be prescribed long-term for anxiety and other mental health conditions? *Addict Behav* 2021; 119: 106943.

7. Anderson PA, McLachlan AJ, Shaheed CA, Gnjidic D, Ivers R, Mathieson S. Deprescribing interventions for gabapentinoids in adults: a scoping review. *Br J Clin Pharmacol* 2023; published online 23 May. doi:10.1111/bcp.15798.

8. McDonald EG, Wu PE, Rashidi B, et al. The MedSafer Study – electronic decision support for deprescribing in hospitalized older adults: a cluster randomized clinical trial. *JAMA Intern Med* 2022; 182: 265–73.

9. Williams J, Gingras M-A, Dubé R, Lee TC, McDonald EG. Patient empowerment brochures to increase gabapentinoid deprescribing: protocol for the prospective, controlled before-and-after GABA-WHY trial. *Can Med Assoc J* 2022; 10: E652–6.

10. Tannenbaum C, Martin P, Tamblyn R, Benedetti A, Ahmed S. Reduction of inappropriate benzodiazepine prescriptions among older adults through direct patient education: the EMPOWER cluster randomized trial. *JAMA Intern Med* 2014; 174: 890–8.

11. Vicens C, Bejarano F, Sempere E, et al. Comparative efficacy of two interventions to discontinue long-term benzodiazepine use: cluster randomised controlled trial in primary care. *Br J Psychiatry* 2014; 204: 471–9.

12. Ishikawa H, Takeshima M, Ishikawa H, Ayabe N, Ohta H, Mishima K. Pregabalin withdrawal in patients without psychiatric disorders taking a regular dose of pregabalin: a case series and literature review. *Neuropsychopharmacol Rep* 2021; 41: 434–9.

13. Naveed S, Faquih AE, Chaudhary AMD. Pregabalin-associated Discontinuation symptoms: a case report. *Cureus* 2018; 10: e3425.

Overview of Gabapentinoid Withdrawal Effects

Withdrawal symptoms from gabapentinoids, along with physical dependence and, less often, addiction, are increasingly recognised.[1,2] From 2006 to 2015 the European Medicines Agency (EMA) received 7,600 reports about withdrawal effects (as well as misuse and abuse) regarding pregabalin and 4,300 similar reports for gabapentin.[2]

The gabapentinoid withdrawal syndrome resembles that for benzodiazepine withdrawal and, to a lesser extent, for SSRIs (Table 4.3).[3] A variety of withdrawal symptoms have been described after gabapentin discontinuation, typically occurring within days of treatment cessation.[4] These symptoms have been observed both after abrupt cessation and during, and after, a slow taper, including one case of a taper lasting 18 months.[4,5]

The most typical withdrawal symptoms are anxiety, insomnia, nausea, pain and diaphoresis.[6] Agitation, confusion and disorientation occur in around half of cases of abrupt discontinuation of gabapentin.[4] Sympathetic activation including tachycardia, hypertension and tremor are commonly reported.[4,5] There is one report of a discontinuation-emergent seizure in a patient taking very high dose (8,000mg) gabapentin.[4] Withdrawal symptoms in newborns whose mothers use gabapentinoids have also been documented.[7]

CHAPTER 4

Table 4.3 Typical withdrawal symptoms from gabapentinoids.[1,4,5,9]

General	Emotional
Insomnia	*Agitation*
Diaphoresis	Dysphoria
Pain	Irritability
Light-headedness	Depersonalisation
Dizziness	Anxiety
Fatigue	
Flu-like symptoms	**Gut**
Chills	*Gastrointestinal discomfort/symptoms*
Neurological	Nausea
Confusion	**Cardiovascular**
Disorientation	*Tachycardia*
Tremor	*Hypertension*
Gait instability	Palpitations
Vertigo	
Myoclonus	**Psychiatric**
Muscle spasms	Delusions*
Numbness	Hallucinations*
Asterixis	
Increased tactile sensations	
Akathisia*	
Catatonia*	
Seizures*	

*Rare symptoms. Common symptoms are italicised.

Risk factors for gabapentinoid withdrawal have not been specifically identified, but duration of treatment, dosage strength and documented history of withdrawal symptoms may correlate with the severity and duration of these symptoms, as for other dependence-forming medications.[8] Gabapentinoid withdrawal symptoms have often been observed to rapidly abate when restarting treatment.[4]

There has been little work undertaken so far to evaluate the incidence, severity and duration of withdrawal effects from gabapentinoids. Some academics have estimated, based on a review of the literature, that the risk of physical dependence (i.e. tolerance and withdrawal effects) is slightly less than for benzodiazepines or alcohol.[1] Additionally, it is not known whether a protracted withdrawal syndrome is likely following gabapentinoid cessation. Nonetheless, given the similarity of the acute withdrawal syndrome to other medications that do produce protracted withdrawal (such as benzodiazepines and SSRIs), it remains a possibility,[9] supported by reports of such long-lasting syndromes in peer support communities.[10]

Pathophysiology of gabapentinoid withdrawal syndrome

There has been little research into the mechanism by which gabapentinoids produce withdrawal effects. Presumably, as for other psychotropic medications, withdrawal symptoms occur because neuro-adaptations to the presence of gabapentinoids take longer to dissipate than it takes for the drug to be eliminated from the body when it is reduced in dose or stopped.[11] The specific changes have not been investigated but as gabapentinoids have (weak) GABA-mimetic features,[1] there may be an overlap with the pathophysiology of the benzodiazepine withdrawal syndrome. Other recognised effects of gabapentinoids on voltage-dependent calcium channels, as well as the downstream inhibitory effects on excitatory neurotransmitters like glutamate and noradrenaline may also play a role.[1] For example, chronic inhibition of glutamate and noradrenaline may lead to hypersensitivity of these receptors, possibly producing the symptoms of excitatory over-drive evident in the cardiovascular symptoms when gabapentinoids are ceased.[9]

Distinguishing withdrawal symptoms from return of underlying disorder

As pain and anxiety are recognised withdrawal symptoms from gabapentinoid dose reduction and discontinuation,[1,9] the withdrawal syndrome can be mistaken for a return of the condition for which the medication was initiated. This can lead to the erroneous conclusion that the medication is required for treatment of the condition, as opposed to the need for a more gradual, careful tapering process.[12] Although it has not been studied in detail there is also the possibility that if new-onset cardiovascular, neurological, gastrointestinal and other withdrawal symptoms from gabapentinoids are not recognised as such, physical health diagnoses can be made instead, with consequent unnecessary investigation and treatment.

Withdrawal symptoms can also occur during maintenance treatment, as for other psychotropic medications, when doses are missed.[13] If withdrawal symptoms caused by forgotten doses or erratic dosing are not recognised, they can be misinterpreted as evidence of worsening of an underlying condition or onset of a new mental or physical health disorder, given the myriad potential symptoms.[13]

References

1. Bonnet U, Richter EL, Isbruch K, Scherbaum N. On the addictive power of gabapentinoids: a mini-review. *Psychiatr Danub* 2018; 30: 142–9.
2. Chiappini S, Schifano F. A decade of gabapentinoid misuse: an analysis of the European Medicines Agency's 'suspected adverse drug reactions' database. *CNS Drugs* 2016; 30: 647–54.
3. Bonnet U, Scherbaum N. How addictive are gabapentin and pregabalin? A systematic review. *Eur Neuropsychopharmacol* 2017; 27: 1185–215.
4. Mersfelder TL, Nichols WH. Gabapentin: abuse, dependence, and withdrawal. *Ann Pharmacother* 2016; 50: 229–33.
5. Deng H, Benhamou O-M, Lembke A. Gabapentin dependence and withdrawal requiring an 18-month taper in a patient with alcohol use disorder: a case report. *J Addict Dis* 2021; 39: 575–8.
6. Fife NHS. Gabapentinoid Reduction Patient Information Leaflet. NHS Fife. https://www.nhsfife.org/media/32617/gabapentinoid-reduction-leaflet.pdf (accessed 17 June 2023).
7. Carrasco M, Rao SC, Bearer CF, Sundararajan S. Neonatal gabapentin withdrawal syndrome. *Pediatr Neurol* 2015; 53: 445–7.
8. National Institute for Social and Care Excellence (NICE). Medicines associated with dependence or withdrawal symptoms: safe prescribing and withdrawal management for adults | Guidance | NICE. 2022. https://www.nice.org.uk/guidance/ng215/chapter/Recommendations (accessed 27 June 2022).
9. Lerner A, Klein M. Dependence, withdrawal and rebound of CNS drugs: an update and regulatory considerations for new drugs development. *Brain Commun* 2019; 1: fcz025.
10. Gabapentin/Lyrica Withdrawal Support. https://www.facebook.com/groups/1438525646474773/ (accessed 17 June 2023).
11. Reidenberg MM. Drug discontinuation effects are part of the pharmacology of a drug. *J Pharmacol Exp Ther* 2011; 339: 324–8.
12. Horowitz MA, Taylor D. Distinguishing relapse from antidepressant withdrawal: clinical practice and antidepressant discontinuation studies. *BJPsych Advances* 2022; 28: 297–311.
13. Framer A. What I have learnt from helping thousands of people taper off psychotropic medications. *Ther Adv Psychopharmacol* 2021; 11: 2045125321991127.

CHAPTER 4

Physical dependence vs addiction in use of gabapentinoids

As for benzodiazepines, gabapentinoids are more commonly associated with physical dependence than addiction.[1,2] As discussed previously (see chapter on benzodiazepines), the terms 'dependence' and 'addiction' (the latter meaning uncontrolled drug-seeking behaviour) are often used interchangeably, since a conflation of the terms in DSM-III-R.[3] The FDA clarified the definition in 2019: 'Physical dependence is a state that develops as a result of physiological adaptation in response to repeated drug use, manifested by withdrawal signs and symptoms after abrupt discontinuation or a significant dose reduction of a drug.'[4]

This is distinct from addiction, which also involves compulsion, craving, impaired control over use and use despite harm or negative consequences.[5] The FDA also highlighted the distinction between physical dependence and addiction:

Physical dependence is not synonymous with addiction; a patient may be physically dependent on a drug without having an addiction to the drug. Tolerance, physical dependence, and withdrawal are all expected biological phenomena that are the consequences of chronic treatment with certain drugs. These phenomena by themselves do not indicate a state of addiction.

Public Health England defined the terms similarly in its 2019 report on prescribed drug dependence:[6]

'**Addiction** *Dependence* plus a compulsive preoccupation to seek and take a substance despite consequences

Dependence An adaptation to repeated exposure to some drugs and medicines usually characterised by *tolerance and withdrawal,* though *tolerance* may not occur with some. Dependence is an inevitable (and often acceptable) consequence of long-term use of some medicines and is distinguished here from *addiction.*'

For gabapentinoids, physical dependence (tolerance, withdrawal effects) is often associated with regular use, and addiction is less frequently reported, and generally amongst those patients with another current or previous substance use disorder.[1]

This distinction may seem merely semantic, but it has important practical ramifications: difficulty stopping gabapentinoids due to withdrawal effects does not mean the patient is misusing or abusing the drug, or that they are addicted or 'drug-seeking'.[7] Rather, it indicates physical dependence to the drug (predictable adaptation to its effects following chronic use) with the natural consequence of withdrawal effects occurring when the dose is reduced. A failure to appreciate this can lead to accusations of abuse, referral to inappropriate addiction-based treatment (e.g. 12-step programmes, rapid detoxification) and consequent social and professional consequences (if people have addiction listed on their medical records).

This chapter deals with patients who are using gabapentinoids as prescribed by their clinician. Those with addiction issues to the drugs are beyond the scope of the current book. Such patients will need support for the behavioural aspects of addiction that are not relevant to people with only physical dependence. Note, however, that an isolated episode of misuse (taking the drug for a legitimate medical complaint for which the drug was not expressly prescribed) or abuse (taking a medication to experience euphoria) is not sufficient to entail a diagnosis of addiction.[5]

References

1. Bonnet U, Richter EL, Isbruch K, Scherbaum N. On the addictive power of gabapentinoids: a mini-review. *Psychiatr Danub* 2018; 30: 142–9.
2. Lerner A, Klein M. Dependence, withdrawal and rebound of CNS drugs: an update and regulatory considerations for new drugs development. *Brain Commun* 2019; 1: fcz025.
3. O'Brien C. Addiction and dependence in DSM-V. *Addiction* 2011; 106: 866–7.
4. Center for Drug Evaluation, Research. Drug Abuse and Dependence Section of Labeling for Human Prescription Drug and Biological Products — Content and Format Guidance for Industry. U.S. Food and Drug Administration. https://www.fda.gov/regulatory-information/search-fda-guidance-documents/drug-abuse-and-dependence-section-labeling-human-prescription-drug-and-biological-products-content (accessed 3 April 2023).
5. Smith SM, Dart RC, Katz NP, et al. Classification and definition of misuse, abuse, and related events in clinical trials: ACTTION systematic review and recommendations. *Pain* 2013; 154: 2287–96.
6. Public Health England. Dependence and withdrawal associated with some prescribed medicines: an evidence review. 2019. https://www.gov.uk/government/publications/prescribed-medicines-review-report (accessed 25 May 2021).
7. Horowitz M, Taylor D. Addiction and physical dependence are not the same thing. 2023; published online 6 July. https://www.thelancet.com/pdfs/journals/lanpsy/PIIS2215-0366(23)00230-4.pdf (accessed 26 July 2023).

CHAPTER 4

How to Deprescribe Gabapentinoids Safely

Principles for tapering gabapentinoids

There has been little research performed specifically on how to taper gabapentinoids.[1] Nonetheless broad principles can be derived from existing guidance, knowledge about similar medication classes and existing clinical experience, including patient-led experience (see previous chapters on tapering antidepressants and benzodiazepines). Given the uncertainty in this area, the process of withdrawal is best managed using shared decision making so that the experience of the individual patient can be given priority.[2]

Withdrawal symptoms and a return of an underlying condition are the major concerns when deprescribing. Withdrawal symptoms are caused by disruption of existing equilibria formed during exposure to the drug.[3] The more rapidly doses are reduced the more severe withdrawal symptoms are likely to be. There is general consensus that gradual tapering, with the rate titrated to the individual's ability to tolerate the process, is likely to make the process less aversive and more likely to be successful.[2-4] As it is difficult to determine a priori what rate of tapering a particular patient might tolerate there is a certain amount of trial and error inherent to the process.[5]

In the UK, NICE guidance on tapering gabapentinoids warns against abrupt cessation, and emphasises the importance of the rate of withdrawal being acceptable to the patient rather than imposed upon them.[2] The guidance specifies that it can be useful to provide the patient with a formulation of their drug that allows them to make small decrements 'at a pace of their choosing' to give them control over the process, rather than issuing successive prescriptions for reduced daily doses.[2] NICE advises that the reduction schedule should be adjusted to avoid intolerable withdrawal symptoms by monitoring the patient's experience, including adjustments made if circumstances change (such as period of increased stress) or their preferences change and providing them with support during the process.[2]

Tapering gradually

Local hospital guidance in the UK advises gradual tapering.[4] For pregabalin, such guidance recommends reducing by 50mg of pregabalin every 1–4 weeks or 300mg of gabapentin every 1–4 weeks.[4] From maximum licensed doses (600mg for pregabalin and 3,600mg for gabapentin), tapering in this manner would take between 3 and 12 months.[4] The guidance also emphasises that the dose changes should be individualised to the person. There are case reports of patients requiring much longer to taper off these drugs in a tolerable manner, including a published report of a patient requiring an 18-month taper after 20-months use of gabapentin.[6]

A large number of patients express dissatisfaction with the manner in which these medications are tapered by clinicians, with the principal complaint being that tapers are too fast, especially at lower doses (as observed for other medication classes).[5,7] One manifestation of this dissatisfaction is the growing number of patients (more than 10,000) on peer-support websites and social-media sites who are seeking guidance from other patients, having found medical advice on this topic lacking (and often leading to intolerable withdrawal symptoms).[5,8,9] Patients in these groups report that tapering can sometimes take years because withdrawal symptoms are so unpleasant.[5,9]

Tapering hyperbolically

Existing guidance for tapering gabapentinoids, for example from NICE, advises linear dose reductions, where the same-sized reduction of dose is recommended at each interval (e.g. 50mg per month).[2,4] However, as for other medications, the relationship between the dose of gabapentinoids and its effect on target receptors is hyperbolic, as dictated by the law of mass action.[10] This hyperbolic relationship arises because when small amounts of the drug are present in the system, most receptor targets will be unsaturated so that every extra milligram of drug produces a large increase in effect.[10] When larger amounts of the drug are present (e.g. at clinically employed doses) most receptor targets will be saturated such that every extra milligram of drug has less and less incremental effect.[10]

There has been no neuroimaging conducted to determine the receptor occupancy of gabapentinoids to our knowledge. However, various clinical effects of gabapentinoids demonstrate a hyperbolic relationship with dose, which can be used to infer the relationship between dose and receptor occupancy. For example, the anticonvulsant properties of pregabalin in rats shows a hyperbolic relationship to dose.[11] The same hyperbolic relationship is also evident for anticonvulsant properties in patients.[12] As for other medications, the clinical effect presumably mirrors the hyperbolic relationship at the receptor level. It is plausible that such a relationship is also relevant to withdrawal effects and so may be informative in regard to devising withdrawal schedules.

In Figure 4.1a the relationship between the dose of gabapentin and its effect on seizure suppression (labelled 'clinical effect') can be seen. Reducing from a dose of 4,800mg in a linear manner (for example, four increments of 1,200mg) produces increasingly large reductions in clinical effect. For example, the reduction from 4,800mg to 3,600mg of gabapentin produces a 1.4% difference in clinical effect, the reduction from 3,600mg to 2,400mg produces a reduction in effect of 2.7%, from 2,400 to 1,200mg of 7.3% and from 1,200mg to 0mg a change of 84.0%. The final 1,200mg therefore produces a change in effect 60-fold that of the first 1,200mg reduction, which may plausibly also relate to withdrawal effects.

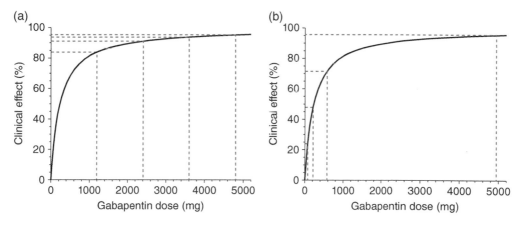

Figure 4.1 Different approaches to tapering gabapentin. (a) Linear dose reductions produced increasingly large reductions in clinical effect, plausibly related to withdrawal effects. (b) Hyperbolic dose reductions are required to produce even reductions in clinical effect and likely withdrawal effects.

CHAPTER 4

In Figure 4.1b, dose reductions are made from 4,800mg according to equal reductions in clinical effect instead of dose. This produces a hyperbolic pattern of dose reduction, following the dose–effect curve. This requires making dose reductions by smaller and smaller decrements, down to very small final doses (in this case about 70mg) so that the final reduction in dose (to zero) does not cause a larger change in effect than previous dose reductions. The drug-specific guidance, provided in later sections, follows the principles of hyperbolic dose reductions.

One case study provides some practical evidence of the utility of hyperbolic tapering. A high-functioning female patient seen in a specialist clinic taking 1,200mg/day of gabapentin for 20 months for alcohol use disorder required an 18-month taper.[6] The patient was not able to tolerate a reduction from 1,200mg to 900mg because of withdrawal effects, but was able to tolerate a reduction to 1,000mg/day. Subsequently, she was able to endure reductions of 100mg per month, until she reached 300mg/day total dose, when these reductions became unbearable. At this point she could only tolerate 20–30mg dose decrements per month. At 100mg/day total dose these decrements became intolerable, and she could only bear reductions of as little as 5mg per month. She ceased her dose at 60mg total (5% of her original dose) (Figure 4.2).[6] In order to make these small reductions the patient measured out small amounts of the contents of capsules. The observation that withdrawal symptoms become increasingly severe as the total dose of medication becomes lower is consistent with other medication classes such as benzodiazepines[13] and antidepressants.[5] This non-linear pattern of withdrawal symptoms (Figure 4.2) probably arises from the hyperbolic pattern of effect for gabapentinoids.[3,14,15]

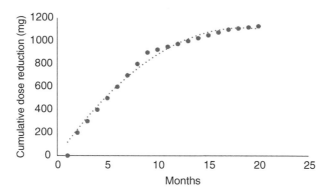

Figure 4.2 Cumulative dose reductions of gabapentin over time in a case study by Deng et al. (2021).[6] The shape of this curve is consistent with the dose effect graphs in Figure 4.1. As this graph helps to give a sense of withdrawal symptoms experienced in this case, it suggests that withdrawal effects occur according to a hyperbolic pattern as expected.

References

1. Anderson PA, McLachlan AJ, Shaheed CA, Gnjidic D, Ivers R, Mathieson S. Deprescribing interventions for gabapentinoids in adults: a scoping review. *Br J Clin Pharmacol* 2023; published online May 23. doi:10.1111/bcp.15798.
2. National Institute for Health and Care Excellence (NICE). Medicines associated with dependence or withdrawal symptoms: safe prescribing and withdrawal management for adults | Guidance | NICE. 2022. https://www.nice.org.uk/guidance/ng215/chapter/Recommendations (accessed 27 June 2022).
3. Horowitz MA, Taylor D. How to reduce and stop psychiatric medication. *Eur Neuropsychopharmacol* 2021; 55: 4–7.
4. Somerset CCG. Gabapentinoid suggested tapering regimes. Somerset CCG. www.somersetccg.nhs.uk/wp-content/uploads/2021/05/Tapering-gabapentinoid-1.pdf (accessed 17 June 2023).
5. Framer A. What I have learnt from helping thousands of people taper off psychotropic medications. *Ther Adv Psychopharmacol* 2021; 11: 204512532199127.
6. Deng H, Benhamou O-M, Lembke A. Gabapentin dependence and withdrawal requiring an 18-month taper in a patient with alcohol use disorder: a case report. *J Addict Dis* 2021; 39: 575–8.
7. Read J, Moncrieff J, Horowitz MA. Designing withdrawal support services for antidepressant users: patients' views on existing services and what they really need. *J Psychiatr Res* 2023. https://www.sciencedirect.com/science/article/pii/S0022395623001309.
8. White E, Read J, Julo S. The role of Facebook groups in the management and raising of awareness of antidepressant withdrawal: is social media filling the void left by health services? *Ther Adv Psychopharmacol* 2021; 11: 2045125320981174.
9. Gabapentin/Lyrica Withdrawal Support. https://www.facebook.com/groups/1438525646474773/ (accessed 17 June 2023).
10. Holford N. Pharmacodynamic principles and the time course of delayed and cumulative drug effects. *Transl Clin* 2018; 26: 56–9.
11. Ben-Menachem E. Pregabalin pharmacology and its relevance to clinical practice. *Epilepsia* 2004; 45 Suppl 6: 13–18.
12. Delahoy P, Thompson S, Marschner IC. Pregabalin versus gabapentin in partial epilepsy: a meta-analysis of dose-response relationships. *BMC Neurol* 2010; 10: 104.
13. Ashton H. The diagnosis and management of benzodiazepine dependence. *Curr Opin Psychiatry* 2005; 18: 249–55.
14. Horowitz MA, Taylor D. Tapering of SSRI treatment to mitigate withdrawal symptoms. *The Lancet Psychiatry* 2019; 6: 538–46.
15. Shapiro BB. Subtherapeutic doses of SSRI antidepressants demonstrate considerable serotonin transporter occupancy: implications for tapering SSRIs. *Psychopharmacology* 2018; 235: 2779–81.

CHAPTER 4

Making up smaller doses of gabapentinoids practically

In order to implement hyperbolic dose reductions many people will need to make smaller reductions in dose than are feasible with commercially available tablets. This is because the smallest available tablets (or even a quarter of such a tablet) produce high receptor occupancy such that stopping these minimum dosages would cause a large reduction in effect, engendering sometimes severe withdrawal symptoms. In the UK the NICE guidance on this topic specifically advises that it can be useful to provide the patient with a formulation of drug that allows them to make small decrements 'at a pace of their choosing' to give them control over the process,[1] mirroring advice for tapering off other psychiatric drugs.[2,3]

To prepare dosages that allow steps in between or lower than doses widely available in tablet formulations, licensed and 'off-label' options are available, as outlined in the introductory section of this chapter. Some specific remarks relevant to gabapentinoids are highlighted here.

Extending the dosing interval ('skipping doses')

As current tablet or capsule formulations of gabapentinoids in some regions do not permit pharmacologically informed tapering regimens, it is tempting to make dose reductions by having patients miss a dose of medication once a week or more often, or take their dose every other day (or less frequently) so that their average dose each day is reduced. However, this method is not recommended for gabapentinoids because both drugs have half-lives of about 6 hours so dosing every second day will cause plasma levels of the drug to fall to a tiny fraction of peak levels at their trough. It is widely recognised that skipping doses can induce withdrawal effects[4,5] and every-other-day dosing has similar consequences. It is generally better to taper doses by giving a smaller dose each day (or as often as required to prevent inter-dose withdrawal effects) rather than a larger dose every second day.

Tablet splitting

Gabapentin and pregabalin are more commonly prescribed as capsules rather than tablets in the US. Pregabalin comes as an extended-release tablet in the US that is not scored as to discourage altering the drug's pharmacokinetic profile. Instant release tablets can be easily divided into halves (or quarters if they are round) using cheaply available tablet cutters.[6] Using tablet cutters is more accurate for dividing tablets than either splitting by hand (for scored tablets), cutting with scissors (for unscored tablets) or using a kitchen knife.[7] Although in older methods of manufacturing active medication was not evenly distributed throughout a tablet, this is no longer the case.[8] Tablet splitting is widely employed, with almost a quarter of all drugs administered in primary care being split.[9] Some tablets are not suitable for splitting including those with a hard outer coat, extended-release tablets (the extended release properties can be affected) or those that are too small or have an uneven shape. Although there are concerns that the splitting process may not be completely accurate[10] (e.g. imperfect splitting, and tablet powder being formed), this can be mitigated somewhat by storing the remainder of the tablet fragment to be used over subsequent days, meaning that the correct dose will be received over 2 or 4 days. Tablet cutters have the advantage of closing as they are used and so retain both halves of the tablet being cut.

This technique may be helpful for the first few steps of a reduction regimen but may not be suitable after this stage as the doses required will be smaller than one-quarter of the smallest available tablet for some medications. Small variation in dose from day to day whilst at higher doses of medication is unlikely to cause withdrawal issues for most people (although these differences can become more critical at lower doses).

Manufacturers' liquids, including dilutions

Apart from tablet splitting, the most widely available option for making up doses that are smaller than those available in tablets is the use of liquid versions of a drug. Gabapentin and pregabalin are both widely available in liquid form. Sometimes smaller syringes (e.g. 1mL) are required for tapering than are provided by the manufacturer. Patients may require some education on proper syringe usage and reading. As greater errors are found when measuring less than 20% of the labelled capacity of a syringe[11] and the smallest syringe widely available is 1mL syringe (or in some regions a 0.5mL syringes), the smallest volume that could be measured accurately with a syringe may be too large a dose to complete a taper for some patients.

To avoid problems associated with measuring small volumes, dilution of manufacturers' liquids may be needed by some patients. Gabapentinoid manufacturers do not provide guidance on dilution of their solution with water (or juice) before consumption. Although gabapentin is freely soluble in water (pregabalin less so), the manufacturers' solutions contain non-aqueous solvents in addition to water and so there is the possibility that dilution with water will cause precipitation of the active drug.[12,13] These mixtures should therefore be shaken well before use to ensure thorough mixing. For example, 0.5mL of a 20mg/mL pregabalin solution could be mixed with 4.5mL of water (a 10-fold dilution) to make up a 2mg/mL solution. As the stability of the dilution cannot be guaranteed, the remainder should be discarded and a new dilution prepared each day.

Compounded medication

Other options, available in different territories, include having compounding pharmacies make up smaller-dose tablets or capsules, or liquid suspensions or solutions. One such option is 'tapering strips' that involves small doses of gabapentinoids made up as tablets that successively reduce in dose over time.[14] Patients should make sure they are using a reputable compounding pharmacy.[15]

Off-licence options for making small doses of medications

As outlined in the introductory section, while it may represent off-label use to crush tablets or make extemporaneous suspensions, the General Medical Council (GMC) guidance on this matter states that doctors are permitted to prescribe medications off-licence when 'the dosage specified for a licensed medicine would not meet the patient's need'.[16] In the USA, such usage is also considered 'off-label' or 'unapproved' use by the FDA, which, however, explains that 'healthcare providers generally may prescribe the drug for an unapproved use when they judge that it is medically appropriate for their patient'.[17]

CHAPTER 4

Dissolving crushed tablets

When liquid formulations are not available, tablets that are not enterically coated or sustained- or extended-release can be crushed to a powdered form and/or dispersed in water.[18,19] Crushing and dispersing will not greatly alter these medications' pharmacokinetic properties (their time to peak plasma will be shortened because the absence of a disintegration phase allows faster gastrointestinal absorption), according to the FDA medication guide,[20] and the Royal Pharmaceutical Society (RPS) guidance on crushing, opening or splitting oral dosage forms.[6] There are various guides that demonstrate to patients how to suspend tablets in water.[21]

Dissolving capsule contents

Guidelines for patients who have trouble swallowing tablets (e.g. the NEWT guidelines in the UK)[12,13,18] also indicate that the contents of gabapentin and pregabalin capsules will dissolve in water due to their high solubility.[18] These guidelines advise that these solutions can taste unpleasant and that juice might be used to mask their taste.[18] In order to make up a pregabalin solution, for example, water could be added to the contents of a 25mg capsule to make up a 25mL solution, with concentration 1mg/mL. A 5mg dose of pregabalin could be taken by measuring out 5mL of this solution to consume. The mixture should be shaken vigorously before consumption to make sure that the medication is dissolved. In the absence of stability data, a conservative approach involves consuming such liquids immediately (within an hour). The remainder should be discarded. Sometimes compounding pharmacies are able to provide suspensions of medication to make up smaller doses.

References

1. National Institute for Social and Care Excellence (NICE). Medicines associated with dependence or withdrawal symptoms: safe prescribing and withdrawal management for adults | Guidance | NICE. 2022. https://www.nice.org.uk/guidance/ng215/chapter/Recommendations (accessed 27 June 2022).

2. Wright SL. Benzodiazepine withdrawal: clinical aspects. In: *The Benzodiazepines Crisis* (ed. J Peppin, J Pergolizzi, R Raffa, S Wright). Oxford: Oxford University Press, 2020: 117–48.

3. Ashton H. Benzodiazepines: how they work and how to withdraw (The Ashton Manual). 2002. Newcastle University. http://www.benzo.org.uk/manual/bzcha01.htm (accessed 11 July 2023).

4. National Institute of Social and Care Excellence (NICE). Depression in adults: treatment and management | Guidance | NICE. 2022; published online June. https://www.nice.org.uk/guidance/ng222 (accessed 16 July 2022).

5. Kaplan EM. Antidepressant noncompliance as a factor in the discontinuation syndrome. *J Clin Psychiatry* 1997; 58 Suppl 7: 31–5; discussion 36.

6. Root T, Tomlin S, Erskine D, Lowey A. Pharmaceutical issues when crushing, opening or splitting oral dosage forms. *Royal Pharmaceutical Society* 2011; 1: 1–7.

7. Verrue C, Mehuys E, Boussery K, Remon J-P, Petrovic M. Tablet-splitting: a common yet not so innocent practice. *J Adv Nurs* 2011; 67: 26–32.

8. Hisada H, Okayama A, Hoshino T, et al. Determining the distribution of active pharmaceutical ingredients in combination tablets using near IR and low-frequency Raman spectroscopy imaging. *Chem Pharm Bull* 2020; 68: 155–60.

9. Chaudhri K, Kearney M, Di Tanna GL, Day RO, Rodgers A, Atkins ER. Does splitting a tablet obtain the accurate dose? A systematic review protocol. *Medicine* 2019; 98: e17189.

10. Center for Drug Evaluation, Research. Best practices for tablet splitting. U.S. Food and Drug Administration. https://www.fda.gov/drugs/ensuring-safe-use-medicine/best-practices-tablet-splitting (accessed 22 September 2022).

11. Jordan MA, Choksi D, Lombard K, Patton LR. Development of guidelines for accurate measurement of small volume parenteral products using syringes. *Hosp Pharm* 2021; 56: 165–71.

12. FDA. Gabapentin: Highlights of prescribing information. FDA. www.accessdata.fda.gov/drugsatfda_docs/label/2017/020235s064_020882s047_021129s046lbl.pdf (accessed 17 June 2023).

13. FDA. Lyrica CR: Highlights of prescribing information. FDA. www.accessdata.fda.gov/drugsatfda_docs/label/2017/209501s000lbl.pdf (accessed 17 June 2023).

14. Groot PC, van Os J. How user knowledge of psychotropic drug withdrawal resulted in the development of person-specific tapering medication. *Ther Adv Psychopharmacol* 2020; 10: 204512532093245.

15. Find A Compounder – PCCA – Professional Compounding Centers of America. https://www.pccarx.com/Resources/FindACompounder (accessed 8 May 2023).

16. General Medical Council. Prescribing unlicensed medicines. 2021. https://www.gmc-uk.org/ethical-guidance/ethical-guidance-for-doctors/good-practice-in-prescribing-and-managing-medicines-and-devices/prescribing-unlicensed-medicines (accessed 30 September 2023).

17. Office of the Commissioner. Understanding unapproved use of approved drugs 'off label.' U.S. Food and Drug Administration. https://www.fda.gov/patients/learn-about-expanded-access-and-other-treatment-options/understanding-unapproved-use-approved-drugs-label (accessed 22 September 2022).

18. Smyth J. The NEWT guidelines for administration of medication to patients with enteral feeding tubes or swallowing difficulties. 2011. https://www.newtguidelines.com/index.html (accessed 18 February 2023).

19. Brennan K. Selective serotonin reuptake inhibitor (SSRI) formulations suggested for adults with swallowing difficulties. SPS – Specialist Pharmacy Service. 2021; published online 1 July. https://www.sps.nhs.uk/articles/selective-serotonin-reuptake-inhibitor-ssri-formulations-suggested-for-adults-with-swallowing-difficulties/ (accessed 14 July 2022).

20. Bostwick JR, Demehri A. Pills to powder: a clinician's reference for crushable psychotropic medications. *Curr Psychiatr* 2014; 13.

21. How to give medicines: tablets. https://www.medicinesforchildren.org.uk/advice-guides/giving-medicines/how-to-give-medicines-tablets/ (accessed 27 September 2022).

Other considerations in tapering gabapentinoids

Pharmacokinetic considerations

The absorption characteristics of gabapentinoids differ markedly. Gabapentin demonstrates saturable absorption. Its bioavailability decreases from 60% to 33% as its dosage is increased from 900mg/day to 3,600mg/day. This property results in non-linear changes in plasma concentration within its clinical dosage range. In contrast, pregabalin's absorption is non-saturable and bioavailability is high (≥ 90%) throughout its dosage range.[1]

Gabapentin shows a ceiling of clinical effects at higher doses both when examined in post-herpetic neuralgia[1] and in seizure disorders,[1,2] with effects plateauing above 1,800mg/day. These data suggest that gabapentin can be tapered relatively quickly at dosages higher than 1,800mg/day but when below 1,800mg/day, gabapentin should probably be tapered more cautiously. This is reflected in the gabapentin-specific tapers presented in this chapter.

Micro-tapering

Although the major approach outlined in the drug-specific sections involves making reductions every 2–4 weeks (sometimes called 'cut and hold')[3] an alternative approach is called micro-tapering, whereby a small change in dose is made each day. Theoretically (see Figure 3.4) making smaller reductions should produce smaller disruptions of the homeostatic equilibrium leading to less intense withdrawal symptoms.[4] In practice, this process might require further dilutions of a liquid version of the drug and the use of small-volume syringes. It also requires quite complex calculations and record keeping. Micro-tapering allows the patient great flexibility in finding a rate of reduction that is tolerable for them. Where several doses of a medication are taken each day, these same small dose reductions can be made to all doses, or sequentially to one dose at a time (e.g. morning, afternoon or night).

Micro-tapering rates can be calculated from the regimens given in the drug-specific sections by dividing the change in dose for each step by 14 or 28 days, depending on the rate of desired taper. For example, if a regimen suggests that a reduction should be made from 3,600mg per day to 2,400mg per day in one step over 4 weeks then this could be converted into a reduction of 40mg each day for approximately 4 weeks. For example, 40mg per day reductions could be implemented using the manufacturer's 50mg/mL solution of gabapentin by reducing the volume taken from 72mL (3,600mg) per day by 0.8mL each day. If the drug is taken several times a day these daily reductions can be divided between the different doses. As the size of the reductions made diminishes the rate of tapering per day will also reduce – for example, a reduction from 125mg to 100mg over 4 weeks would involve a reduction of approximately 1mg per day. This rate can be slowed if withdrawal symptoms become too unpleasant.

Adjunctive medication

There is little research into adjunctive medications used in assisting gabapentinoids tapering. Currently there are no medications approved by the FDA or other drug regulators to alleviate the symptoms of withdrawal from gabapentinoids. Pharmacological adjunctive treatments for other dependence-forming medications such as benzodiazepines have had mixed reviews.[5,6] Many drugs that have been trialled to help people with withdrawal symptoms from dependence-forming medications themselves cause physical dependence and withdrawal.[6] Ultimately these agents may then in turn need to be tapered, and are associated with their own adverse effects.[7] Clearly then, using a dependence-forming agent to assist withdrawal is ultimately likely to be self-defeating. The NICE guidance on safe withdrawal of dependence-forming medication states explicitly 'Do not treat withdrawal symptoms with another medicine that is associated with dependence or withdrawal symptoms.'[8] The advice of the British National Formulary (BNF) as regards benzodiazepines may be relevant: 'The addition of beta-blockers, antidepressants and antipsychotics should be avoided where possible.'[9]

When severe withdrawal symptoms occur it is generally preferable to slow the rate of taper to minimise withdrawal symptoms rather than seek to mask them with another medication. In case studies the drug most effective at resolving withdrawal symptoms from gabapentinoids was the original gabapentinoid (successful in 18 out of 18 cases recorded).[10] In case studies of patients suffering from gabapentinoid withdrawal 7 out of 8 patients who were treated with an adjunctive benzodiazepine (including 2 cases where haloperidol was used in addition to a benzodiazepine) did not experience control of their withdrawal symptoms.[10] The addition of another medication also risks complicating the picture by adding in new adverse effects, and potential interactions with existing medication. In the process of withdrawal, some patients will become sensitised to a range of medications, which may include other psychiatric agents.[7,11] This is another reason that a cautious approach should be taken to the introduction of new agents.[7,11]

In some cases of severe withdrawal, the addition of an adjunctive medication might be considered.[12] The adjunct agent should be ideally one without a strong withdrawal syndrome and with less severe adverse effects than the original gabapentinoid. Drugs like propranolol[13,14] and antihistamines like hydroxyzine[15] have been used in case of unpleasant withdrawal symptoms for benzodiazepines, with inconclusive findings. These drugs might be considered in difficult cases of gabapentinoid withdrawal.[16] Ideally these agents should be used only for the short term, given the risk of physical dependence and withdrawal with chronic use.[17]

Nutritional supplements and other products

There has been almost no formal research into the effects of supplements on withdrawal symptoms from gabapentinoids. Any theories on the possible benefits of supplements in this area are mere speculation. Hypersensitivity to adverse effects may also be seen with supplements when used for patients in withdrawal from other dependence-forming medications, such as benzodiazepines, which may relate to gabapentinoid withdrawal as well,[18] so a cautious approach should be employed.

References

1. Bockbrader HN, Wesche D, Miller R, Chapel S, Janiczek N, Burger P. A comparison of the pharmacokinetics and pharmacodynamics of pregabalin and gabapentin. *Clin Pharmacokinet* 2010; 49: 661–9.

2. Delahoy P, Thompson S, Marschner IC. Pregabalin versus gabapentin in partial epilepsy: a meta-analysis of dose-response relationships. *BMC Neurol* 2010; 10: 104.

3. Benzodiazepine tapering strategies and solutions. Benzodiazepine Information Coalition. 2020; published online 21 September. https://www.benzoinfo.com/benzodiazepine-tapering-strategies/ (accessed 29 April 2023).

4. Horowitz MA, Taylor D. How to reduce and stop psychiatric medication. *Eur Neuropsychopharmacol* 2021; 55: 4–7.

5. Parr JM, Kavanagh DJ, Cahill L, Mitchell G, McD Young R. Effectiveness of current treatment approaches for benzodiazepine discontinuation: a meta-analysis. *Addiction* 2009; 104(1): 13–24.

6. Baandrup L, Ebdrup BH, Rasmussen JØ, Lindschou J, Gluud C, Glenthøj BY. Pharmacological interventions for benzodiazepine discontinuation in chronic benzodiazepine users. *Cochrane Database Syst Rev* 2018; 3: CD011481.

7. Wright SL. Benzodiazepine withdrawal: clinical aspects. In: *The Benzodiazepines Crisis* (eds. J Peppin, J Pergolizzi, R Raffa, S Wright) Oxford: Oxford University Press, 2020: 117–C8.P334. doi:10.1093/med/9780197517277.003.0008.

8. National Institute for Health and Care Excellence (NICE). Medicines associated with dependence or withdrawal symptoms: safe prescribing and withdrawal management for adults | Guidance | NICE. 2022. https://www.nice.org.uk/guidance/ng215/chapter/Recommendations (accessed 27 June 2022).

9. Hypnotics and anxiolytics. https://bnf.nice.org.uk/treatment-summaries/hypnotics-and-anxiolytics/ (accessed 19 March 2023).

10. Mersfelder TL, Nichols WH. Gabapentin: abuse, dependence, and withdrawal. *Ann Pharmacother* 2016; 50: 229–33.

11. Framer A. What I have learnt from helping thousands of people taper off psychotropic medications. *Ther Adv Psychopharmacol* 2021; 11: 204512532199127.

12. Scenario: benzodiazepine and z-drug withdrawal. https://cks.nice.org.uk/topics/benzodiazepine-z-drug-withdrawal/management/benzodiazepine-z-drug-withdrawal/ (accessed 7 October 2022).

13. Cantopher T, Olivieri S, Cleave N, Edwards JG. Chronic benzodiazepine dependence: a comparative study of abrupt withdrawal under propranolol cover versus gradual withdrawal. *Br J Psychiatry* 1990; 156: 406–11.

14. Tyrer P, Rutherford D, Huggett T. Benzodiazepine withdrawal symptoms and propranolol. *The Lancet* 1981; 1: 520–2.

15. Lemoine P, Touchon J, Billardon M. [Comparison of 6 different methods for lorazepam withdrawal: a controlled study, hydroxyzine versus placebo]. *Encephale* 1997; 23: 290–9.

16. Denis C, Fatseas M, Lavie E, Auriacombe M. Pharmacological interventions for benzodiazepine dependence management among benzodiazepine users in outpatient settings [Protocol]. *Cochrane Database Syst Rev* 2005. doi:10.1002/14651858.CD005194.

17. Chiappini S, Schifano F, Martinotti G. Editorial: prescribing psychotropics: misuse, abuse, dependence, withdrawal and addiction. *Front Psychiatry* 2021; 12: 688434.

18. Ashton H. Benzodiazepines: how they work and how to withdraw (The Ashton Manual). Newcastle University, 2002. http://www.benzo.org.uk/manual/bzcha01.htm (accessed 26 July 2023).

Psychological aspects of tapering gabapentinoids

The psychological aspects of the discontinuation process from gabapentinoids demonstrate substantial overlap with the issues experienced in discontinuing other dependence-forming medications (see the relevant sections for antidepressants and benzodiazepines)[1,2] These themes are briefly summarised here. The withdrawal process can involve intense emotions, ranging from despair, anger, anxiety, to emotional lability and suicidal thoughts.[1,3,4] These feelings can often be unrelated (or greatly out of proportion) to events or circumstances.[1,2,5] Such experiences can sometimes be familiar emotions to the patient and other times quite novel – and they can be distressing and confusing.[2,6]

Many people cannot tolerate severe withdrawal symptoms. Severe withdrawal effects can impair social and professional functioning, precipitate relapse of underlying conditions and cause the patient to become fearful of the process of reducing their medication or of ever ceasing it.[2,6] Sometimes severe withdrawal effects will prompt people to return to a full dose of medication, or seek other medications or drugs to manage their symptoms. Occasionally severe withdrawal effects will lead people to be admitted to hospital and in some cases to become suicidal.[2,6]

So although there are specific approaches to coping with withdrawal most people do not do well by 'white-knuckling' through the process. The main tool to manage withdrawal symptoms should be to reduce the dose gradually enough to avoid severe withdrawal symptoms. Although there has been only limited research in the area it is reported clinically that experiencing more severe withdrawal symptoms from early rapid reductions may increase the risk of a protracted withdrawal syndrome in the long term and this may be relevant to gabapentinoids.[2,6]

Coping with withdrawal symptoms

There are some examples of general methods of coping with withdrawal symptoms in the introductory chapters, though there are no studies to our knowledge that have examined gabapentinoid withdrawal in particular. Many patients report that it is useful to be made aware that the symptoms that are experienced during the withdrawal process are of a physiological origin and should not be given an existential weight they do not merit.[7] In peer-led withdrawal communities these symptoms are referred to as 'neuro-emotions', denoting emotions that arise because of withdrawal-associated neurological processes, as distinct from 'endogenous' emotions that relate to events in the person's life.[2] Such symptoms, in their more extreme forms, may attract mental health diagnoses from clinicians unfamiliar with this aspect of withdrawal.[2,8]

Sometimes withdrawal symptoms can be difficult to distinguish from an underlying condition, not just for the clinician but also for the patient.[2] Although timing and associated physical symptoms can be helpful to achieve this distinction the subjective similarity of symptoms to the original condition can be confusing for some.[2] Familiar patterns of thoughts and emotions may be triggered by withdrawal symptoms. In the same way as anxiety triggered by, for example, an excess of caffeine in a given individual may have a presentation that depends on an individual's personality and habits of mind, withdrawal symptoms may interact with an individual's typical responses and then closely resemble an underlying condition. In such cases, the pattern of symptoms over time (waxing and waning and corresponding to dose reductions), and co-incident symptoms that are not typical of the patient's mental health condition are most useful to help identify these states.[2]

Techniques such as distraction, acceptance and peer support have been reported by patients to be helpful.[2] Some patients find that learning to manage and cope with withdrawal symptoms also translates to being able to manage the mental health conditions that first prompted medication prescriptions more capably.[2] Reducing stress in life, to the degree this is possible, may facilitate the process. Activity and exercise may be useful both as distraction and to reduce tension but need to be adjusted to the degree of physiological disturbance caused by the withdrawal process in order to avoid sensory overload, which can sometimes exacerbate symptoms.[2,6] Sleep hygiene might be helpful.[2,6]

References

1. Ishikawa H, Takeshima M, Ishikawa H, Ayabe N, Ohta H, Mishima K. Pregabalin withdrawal in patients without psychiatric disorders taking a regular dose of pregabalin: a case series and literature review. *Neuropsychopharmacol Rep* 2021; 41: 434–9.
2. Framer A. What I have learnt from helping thousands of people taper off psychotropic medications. *Ther Adv Psychopharmacol* 2021; 11: 204512532199127.
3. Mersfelder TL, Nichols WH. Gabapentin: abuse, dependence, and withdrawal. *Ann Pharmacother* 2016; 50: 229–33.
4. Bonnet U, Scherbaum N. How addictive are gabapentin and pregabalin? A systematic review. *Eur Neuropsychopharmacol* 2017; 27: 1185–215.
5. Cosci F, Chouinard G. Acute and persistent withdrawal syndromes following discontinuation of psychotropic medications. *Psychother Psychosom* 2020; 89: 283–306.
6. Inner Compass Initiative. The Withdrawal Project. 2021. https://withdrawal.theinnercompass.org/ (accessed 10 July 2023).
7. Guy A, Davies J, Rizq R. *Guidance for Psychological Therapists: Enabling Conversations with Clients Taking or Withdrawing from Prescribed Psychiatric Drugs*. London: APPG for Prescribed Drug Dependence, 2019.
8. White E, Read J, Julo S. The role of Facebook groups in the management and raising of awareness of antidepressant withdrawal: is social media filling the void left by health services? *Ther Adv Psychopharmacol* 2021; 11: 2045125320981174.

Tapering gabapentinoids in practice

The practical process of tapering gabapentinoids is broadly similar to that outlined previously for benzodiazepines and antidepressants. Readers are encouraged to read those sections. The main principles are briefly presented here.

Decision making for deprescribing

- The indications for deprescribing are:
  - adverse effects,
  - lack of efficacy or loss of efficacy (tolerance),
  - the patient wishes to stop,
  - the condition treated has improved or alternative coping skills have been developed, and
  - rationalising medication (e.g. reducing polypharmacy).
- Patients at higher risk from continued use of gabapentinoids are:
  - those on concomitant use of opioids or benzodiazepines,
  - those diagnosed with COPD, severe or uncontrolled respiratory disease, or at risk of respiratory depression,
  - those who have a substance use disorder or a history of overdose, and
  - women who are pregnant or contemplating pregnancy.[1]
- Deprescribing decisions should be agreed between patient and prescriber. Forced tapers are not recommended.
- Life circumstances (e.g. burden of existing stressors and degree of social support available) should be taken into account when deciding when to commence tapering. A brief period of reflection and/or the mobilising of further resources may be required before commencing a taper.
- A key element of a deprescribing intervention is education regarding the risks, benefits and alternatives to gabapentinoids[2] (see 'When and why to stop gabapentinoids').
- Patients should also be educated about the benefits, risks and alternatives to deprescribing (see 'Overview of gabapentinoid withdrawal effects').
- If deprescribing is declined:[3]
  - patients should be advised of the relevant benefits of stopping,
  - any concerns they have about stopping should be addressed,
  - patients should not be pressurised,
  - if appropriate, readdress discontinuation at future appointments, and
  - continue monitoring for adverse effects.
- Note that some patients may be unable to withdraw completely, and a more suitable goal may be dose reduction or maintenance of the current dose.

Before tapering

- Patients should be warned not to stop gabapentinoids abruptly if they have been used for more than a few weeks. Explain that in some cases this can cause severe problems (e.g. rarely, seizures)[4] and might provoke long-lasting withdrawal symptoms.

- Reassurance may be required for those that have rapidly tapered in the past with intolerable consequences. Explain that if tapering is performed gradually and adjusted to their symptoms, it can be tolerable. Rapid withdrawal should be reserved for cases where the medication is causing severe acute harms.
- Preparation for gabapentinoid tapering may be required: for example, bolstering of existing coping skills or development of new ones.[5] These skills can include intentional relaxation (mindfulness, progressive muscle relaxation[6]), controlled breathing exercises,[7] physical exercise (if tolerated), sleep hygiene, acceptance, distraction techniques, CBT for insomnia and stress reduction.[6,8] There are a wide variety of other coping skills that people might find helpful. Lightening of work load or family duties may be useful, if this is possible.
- A support system should be established.[5] This can involve family and friends (who may require education) or more regular contact with clinical staff. Sometimes the introduction of patients to a supportive peer group in person or online can be vital to the process (although beware of exposure to 'worst-case' scenarios, and sometimes inaccurate information).
- Consider replacement treatment for the original condition. Specific treatments for the conditions for which gabapentinoids were originally prescribed (i.e. pain and anxiety) can be helpful for the process. However, there is also general recognition that gabapentinoids may not have marked long-term efficacy for a number of the conditions that they are used to treat.
- Manage expectations. For people that have used gabapentinoids long term, the withdrawal process can take months, or even longer for those sensitive to the process.[9,10] People who have been on the drugs short term may be able to stop completely in a few weeks.[9]
- Past experience of reducing can help predict symptoms that may arise again on tapering so should be noted and can be helpful for monitoring targeted symptoms (see below).
- Familiarity of the patient and the clinician with the wide variety of withdrawal symptoms ('Overview of gabapentinoid withdrawal effects') may help to mitigate unnecessary anxiety when symptoms arise. It should be impressed on patients that unpleasant withdrawal symptoms do not indicate that the drug is needed but that the taper rate should be slowed.

The process of tapering

- It is thought that a patient-directed taper, adjusted to symptoms, is the most successful approach to cessation.[5,9,10] The key elements of a programme of tapering are:
  - that it is flexible and can be adjusted so that the process is tolerable for the patient;
  - that it involves close monitoring of withdrawal symptoms to facilitate timely adjustments to the rate of taper; and
  - that patients are provided with preparations of medication to enable the process of creating doses which cannot be made with widely available tablet or capsule doses (e.g. liquid formulations or smaller-dose formulations of tablets).

The process of tapering involves four steps (Figure 4.3).

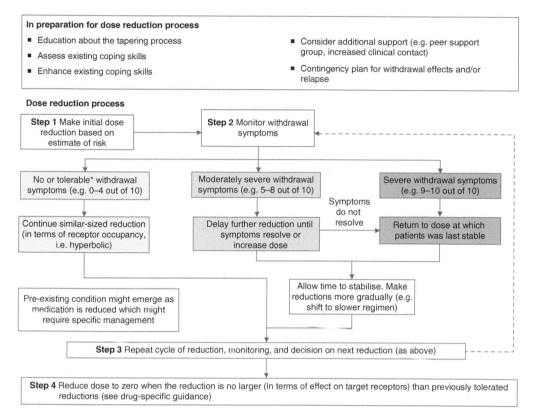

Figure 4.3 An overview of the process of tapering gabapentinoids.
*What constitutes tolerable withdrawal symptoms will vary from person to person.

Step one: estimation of risk of withdrawal and size of the initial dose reduction

Patients may be broadly risk stratified according to what little is known about risk of withdrawal[9] in the suggested approach below. It is better to err on the side of caution when estimating risk category and so the presence of any moderate or high-risk characteristic should assign a patient to that category. Tapers can always be sped up if no difficulties are encountered – but the reverse is not always true.

- **Low-risk** patients could start with approximately 25% (or less) dose reductions from the minimum clinically employed doses (or larger reductions from higher doses) - e.g. the faster regimens given in the drug-specific chapters. This group is characterised by:
  - no evidence of tolerance or inter-dose withdrawal,
  - short-term use (weeks),
  - absent or only mild withdrawal symptoms on stopping or skipping a dose in the past, and
  - no history of multiple episodes of psychiatric medication use and cessation.[11]

■ **Moderate-risk** patients could start with approximately 15% (or less) dose reductions from the minimum clinically employed doses (or larger reductions from higher doses) -e.g. the moderate regimens given in the drug-specific chapters. This group is characterised by:
  ■ some evidence of tolerance or inter-dose withdrawal,
  ■ moderate-length use (months),
  ■ moderate withdrawal symptoms in the past on stopping or skipping a dose, and
  ■ a history of some episodes of psychiatric medication use and cessation.[11]
■ **High-risk** patients could start with 10% (or less) dose reduction from the minimum clinically employed doses (or larger reductions from higher doses) - e.g. the slower regimens given in the drug-specific chapters. This group is characterised by:
  ■ evidence of significant tolerance to the medication or marked experience of inter-dose withdrawal,
  ■ past history of severe withdrawal symptoms on dose reduction or skipping doses,
  ■ long-term use (years),
  ■ older or otherwise physically frail, and
  ■ repeated cycles of psychiatric use and cessation (which is thought to lead to sensitisation, a phenomenon sometimes called kindling).[11]
■ In order to instil confidence in patients in what can be a daunting process, it may be advisable to start with an even smaller dose reduction in order to alleviate patients' fears and promote confidence about the process.
■ None of these regimens should be imposed on the patient but are a starting point to assess how the patient tolerates the process. Some patients may require even slower tapers.[11]
■ If a patient prefers to try a smaller dose reduction than their risk category suggests, this should be supported.

Step two: monitoring of withdrawal symptoms resulting from this initial reduction

■ The most important information to determine the rate of reduction is how the patient experiences the process. Imposed regimens tend to backfire.[11]
■ Although there are various scales used to measure withdrawal symptoms, these can be cumbersome because of the large number of items. Scales may also miss certain individual-specific symptoms and rarely rate the importance of symptoms to the patient. An alternative is to rate a small number of core withdrawal symptoms such as anxiety, insomnia, pain or other prominent symptoms characteristic for the individual out of 10 (0 = no symptoms, 10 = extreme symptoms) or to rate the withdrawal symptoms out of 10 overall. This monitoring often detects a 'wave' pattern of withdrawal symptoms: where symptoms increase, reach a peak, start to resolve and return to or approach baseline (Figure 4.4). See further variations of withdrawal symptoms in Figures 2.11–2.13.

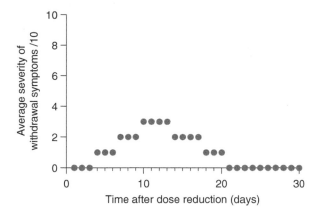

Figure 4.4 Graphical representation of withdrawal symptoms following a dose reduction of a gabapentinoid. These probably constitute mild symptoms. The y-axis shows the average patient-rated severity of withdrawal symptoms. Note the delayed onset of significant symptoms after drug reduction, probably related to drug elimination, followed by a peak and then easing of symptoms, probably related to re-adaptation of the system to a new homeostatic 'set-point'.

Step three: shared decision making for the next dose reduction

The information from withdrawal monitoring can be used to determine the frequency and size of reductions. See further detailed examples in 'Recommendations for stopping antidepressants in clinical practice' but briefly:

- If symptoms take up to 2 weeks to resolve and the severity is mild (e.g. less than 4 out 10) then similar-sized reductions (in terms of receptor occupancy) could be made every 2–4 weeks.
- If symptoms take longer to resolve or their severity is moderate (e.g. 5–8 out of 10) then greater time between reductions will be required and/or smaller reductions made in future.
- If symptoms are severe (e.g. 9 or 10 out 10) then the dose should be increased to the last dose at which the patient was stable, and after stabilisation the rate of reduction should be halved, or slowed even further.

It is important, as already emphasised, that these decisions be reached jointly and that a too rapid rate of taper not be imposed on patients.

Step four: repetition of cycles of reduction and monitoring until cessation

- The steps outlined above in steps 2 and 3 should be repeated. Similar-sized reductions (in terms of effect on target receptors) should produce similar withdrawal reactions, but sometimes these vary over time. Because of this variation, ongoing monitoring of withdrawal symptoms is warranted, with adjustment of the regimen according to the experience of the patient.
  - Reductions should proceed in a hyperbolic pattern to accommodate the nature of the pharmacological effect of the drugs such that reductions in dose become smaller and smaller as the total dose gets smaller.[12,13] Examples of such regimens are displayed in the drug-specific sections of this chapter.

- The taper should be flexible to accommodate periods of stress, increased responsibilities, illness or patient preference.
- The dose should be reduced to zero only when the dose is low enough that the reduction to zero will not cause a larger change (in terms of effect on target receptors) than previous tolerable reductions have caused.

After tapering

Some patients can have ongoing withdrawal symptoms following cessation.[14–16] Sometimes this lasts just for days or weeks but occasionally is extended for months or longer, termed protracted withdrawal syndrome – although it is not known how commonly these syndromes occur for gabapentinoids.[14] There are two main approaches to such problems – either supportive management or small-dose re-instatement.[11] See section on management of protracted withdrawal for further details.

Potential pitfalls

- Physical dependence and the experience of a withdrawal syndrome does not indicate addiction.[17,18] Addiction centres are therefore not suitable for people suffering withdrawal effects from gabapentinoids without abuse or misuse. Sometimes treatment at these centres involves abrupt cessation with other medications added in to 'cover' withdrawal effects, or 12-step approaches inappropriate for medication taken as prescribed.
- Some symptoms can seem bizarre but should not be discounted as many are recognised as withdrawal symptoms (see 'Overview of gabapentinoid withdrawal effects') - e.g. myoclonus, depersonalisation/derealisation, strange tactile sensation, and vertigo.[14,19–21]
- Symptoms of gabapentinoid withdrawal can overlap with the diagnostic criteria for other conditions, leading to misdiagnosis (e.g. functional neurological disorder, medically unexplained symptoms, psychosomatic conditions, chronic fatigue syndrome, anxiety disorders, depression, neurological disorders) and unnecessary testing and medical treatment.[11]
- Withdrawal symptoms are best managed by adjustment of the taper rate, rather than 'white-knuckling' through the process because it is thought that severe withdrawal effects may make a protracted withdrawal syndrome more likely and can sometimes be unbearable.[11]
- Adjunctive medication aimed at treating withdrawal symptoms has not been investigated, but it has shown limited success in tapering other dependence-forming medications[22] and NICE recommends that withdrawal symptoms not be treated with another medication that is associated with dependence or withdrawal symptoms.[9]

References

1. Wise J. Avoid prescribing pregabalin during pregnancy if possible, says UK drug regulator. *BMJ* 2022; 377: o1010.
2. Anderson PA, McLachlan AJ, Shaheed CA, Gnjidic D, Ivers R, Mathieson S. Deprescribing interventions for gabapentinoids in adults: a scoping review. *Br J Clin Pharmacol* 2023; published online May 23. doi:10.1111/bcp.15798.
3. Scenario: Benzodiazepine and z-drug withdrawal. https://cks.nice.org.uk/topics/benzodiazepine-z-drug-withdrawal/management/benzodiazepine-z-drug-withdrawal/ (accessed 7 October 2022).
4. Ishikawa H, Takeshima M, Ishikawa H, Ayabe N, Ohta H, Mishima K. Pregabalin withdrawal in patients without psychiatric disorders taking a regular dose of pregabalin: a case series and literature review. *Neuropsychopharmacol Rep* 2021; 41: 434–9.
5. Cooper RE, Ashman M, Lomani J, Moncrieff J, Guy A. 'Stabilise-reduce, stabilise-reduce': a survey of the common practices of deprescribing services and recommendations for future services. *PLoS One*, 15 March 2023. https://journals.plos.org/plosone/article?id=10.1371/journal.pone.0282988.
6. Guy A, Davies J, Rizq R. *Guidance for Psychological Therapists: Enabling Conversations with Clients Taking or Withdrawing from Prescribed Psychiatric Drugs.* London: APPG for Prescribed Drug Dependence, 2019.
7. Inner Compass Initiative. The Withdrawal Project. 2021. https://withdrawal.theinnercompass.org/ (accessed 19 July 2023).
8. The Withdrawal Project. https://withdrawal.theinnercompass.org/ (accessed 19 July 2023).
9. National Institute for Health and Care Excellence (NICE). Medicines associated with dependence or withdrawal symptoms: safe prescribing and withdrawal management for adults | Guidance | NICE. 2022. https://www.nice.org.uk/guidance/ng215/chapter/Recommendations (accessed 27 June 2022).
10. Somerset CCG. Gabapentinoid suggested tapering regimes. Somerset CCG. www.somersetccg.nhs.uk/wp-content/uploads/2021/05/Tapering-gabapentinoid-1.pdf (accessed 17 June 2023).
11. Framer A. What I have learnt from helping thousands of people taper off psychotropic medications. *Ther Adv Psychopharmacol* 2021; 11: 204512532199127.
12. Horowitz M, Taylor D. Withdrawing from benzodiazepines and z-drugs (in preparation).
13. Delahoy P, Thompson S, Marschner IC. Pregabalin versus gabapentin in partial epilepsy: a meta-analysis of dose-response relationships. *BMC Neurol* 2010; 10: 104.
14. Deng H, Benhamou O-M, Lembke A. Gabapentin dependence and withdrawal requiring an 18 month taper in a patient with alcohol use disorder: a case report. *J Addict Dis* 2021; 39: 575–8.
15. Gabapentin/Lyrica Withdrawal Support. https://www.facebook.com/groups/1438525646474773/ (accessed 17 June 2023).
16. Cosci F, Chouinard G. Acute and persistent withdrawal syndromes following discontinuation of psychotropic medications. *Psychother Psychosom* 2020; 89: 283–306.
17. O'Brien C. Addiction and dependence in DSM-V. *Addiction* 2011; 106: 866–7.
18. Public Health England. Dependence and withdrawal associated with some prescribed medicines: an evidence review. 2019. https://www.gov.uk/government/publications/prescribed-medicines-review-report (accessed 25 May 2021).
19. Mersfelder TL, Nichols WH. Gabapentin: abuse, dependence, and withdrawal. *Ann Pharmacother* 2016; 50: 229–33.
20. Bonnet U, Richter EL, Isbruch K, Scherbaum N. On the addictive power of gabapentinoids: a mini-review. *Psychiatr Danub* 2018; 30: 142–9.
21. Lerner A, Klein M. Dependence, withdrawal and rebound of CNS drugs: an update and regulatory considerations for new drugs development. *Brain Commun* 2019; 1: fcz025.
22. Colorado Consortium for Prescription Drug Abuse Prevention. Benzodiazepine Deprescribing Guidance. Colorado Consortium for Prescription Drug Abuse Prevention. 2022. https://corxconsortium.org/wp-content/uploads/Benzo-Deprescribing.pdf (accessed 16 May 2023).

CHAPTER 4

Management of complications of gabapentinoid discontinuation

Approach to withdrawal akathisia

Akathisia is most commonly seen with long-term antipsychotic exposure and some commentators recommend gabapentinoids to treat this complication.[1] However, akathisia can also be induced by gabapentinoid withdrawal.[2] There is little research in this area but gradual tapering is thought to minimise the risk of this withdrawal effect in other dependence-forming medication,[3] and this may also be true for gabapentinoids. As people can be agitated and quite disordered in their behaviour (pacing, restless, grimacing, etc.) withdrawal akathisia can often misdiagnosed as mania, psychosis or agitated depression, or a variety of physical health conditions by clinicians unfamiliar with this withdrawal effect.[4-6] For some people the condition is so unbearable it can lead to suicide.[7,8] For others it is experienced more as internal restlessness, irritability and tension without manifesting physical signs.[9] Once a patient is in such a state it is difficult to treat and symptoms can be prolonged in some patients.[5] This risk, albeit likely small (though unknown), of too rapid withdrawal is a strong rationale for tapering gradually.

Although there has been little in the way of research on withdrawal akathisia, the most commonly successful approach in clinical practice is re-instatement of the original gabapentinoid at the dose at which the patient had been previously stable.[6] As the response to re-introduction of a gabapentinoid can be somewhat unpredictable when patients are in this state, it is wise to cautiously re-introduce it. It can take some time for symptoms to settle following re-instatement.

If re-instatement is unsuccessful, the drugs most commonly recommended as useful for akathisia are beta-blockers (e.g. propranolol 40–80mg po daily), and $5HT_{2A}$ receptor antagonists (e.g. mirtazapine 15mg po daily and cyproheptadine 8–16mg po daily), although there is a dearth of evidence.[5,6] For example, in one open label trial of patients with neuroleptic-induced akathisia most patients (15/17) treated with cyproheptadine showed marked improvement of their symptoms, which returned when cyproheptadine was ceased.[10] The degree to which this treatment effect is also relevant to gabapentinoid withdrawal-induced akathisia has not been evaluated. The evidence for beta blockers in neuroleptic-induced akathisia is limited, with a Cochrane review finding no evidence of improvement.[11] Anecdotally, some patients with withdrawal akathisia do report an improvement in their symptoms with propranolol.

However, even medications recommended for the treatment of akathisia have been associated with worsening symptoms in some patients.[7] Patient groups advocating for wider awareness of this syndrome, report that antipsychotics, antidepressants and additional benzodiazepines, can sometimes make withdrawal akathisia worse.[7] For example, mirtazapine has been noted to cause akathisia, amongst other movement disorders, in some patients.[12] If re-instatement of the original gabapentinoid is not successful, given the lack of evidence for any specific approach, treatment is largely empirical.[6] Treatment should involve the introduction of one medication at a time for a short period at a low dose as a test of response. Patients should be closely observed to decide whether the drug is helpful, and it should be ceased if it is not, before trialling an additional medication.[5,7]

Aside from re-instatement of the original medication, some patient advocacy groups suggest that another option may be a conservative approach. This essentially means allowing symptoms to resolve over time with minimal intervention, although this can sometimes be difficult for patients to tolerate, especially when symptoms are prolonged.[7] Exercise is widely found to be helpful by patients, who often report that pacing somewhat lessens unpleasant sensations. This is supported by a case study in which the distress caused by a patient's akathisia was relieved by continuously pedalling using a stationary bike.[13] However, in some cases, akathisia will be so unbearable or the patient's consequent suicidality so acute that the use of further medications will be unavoidable. Anti-cholinergics, benzodiazepines, clonidine, and, more rarely, piracetam, buspirone and opioids have all be used in the treatment of akathisia in addition to the agents mentioned above.[6,14]

Management of protracted withdrawal

A wide variety of medications that cause acute withdrawal syndromes, including antidepressants, benzodiazepines, antipsychotics, mood stabilisers, opioids and stimulants[15,16] have also been observed to cause protracted withdrawal syndromes (sometimes called post-acute withdrawal syndromes (PAWS)).[15] This syndrome is often defined as symptoms that persist for more than 6 weeks, but PAWS can persist for months and sometimes years.[15] These protracted withdrawal syndromes are thought to arise because of long-lasting changes to the brain caused by exposure to these drugs.[16,17] There are case studies of patients who have required 18 months to taper off a gabapentinoid[18] suggesting that long-lasting withdrawal symptoms may be possible. Patient-led groups report protracted withdrawal syndrome from gabapentinoids[19,20] – but there has been no study of how commonly this may occur. Clinical experience suggests that more gradual tapering is likely to reduce the risk of protracted withdrawal syndrome,[3] but this has not been evaluated in controlled trials.

Management of protracted withdrawal syndromes from other medication classes normally involves conservative management (no specific intervention) or re-instatement of the original medication,[3] and this may also be applicable to gabapentinoid withdrawal. In general, symptoms of protracted withdrawal from other medication classes improve over time without specific intervention, though this period can be frustratingly lengthy – months and sometimes years.[3,16] A generally healthy lifestyle is thought to be beneficial, although no particular aspect (diet, exercise, relaxation or stress management) has been specifically studied or isolated. A wide variety of supplements are often touted as helpful, but these have not been evaluated in specific studies and patient experience is mixed.[3]

Re-instatement of the original medication is another option. When medications are re-instated soon after withdrawal symptoms onset, quick resolution is almost inevitably the result. When re-instatement is delayed for longer periods than months the results are less predictable, and sometimes delayed, partial or even absent.[3] It is not currently known what determines this relationship. In the case of protracted withdrawal from antidepressants, for example, re-instatement has been observed to produce benefits even years after onset of the syndrome in some people.[23,24] It is not clear if this has relevance for gabapentinoid withdrawal. Some patients report worsening of their symptoms on re-instatement in withdrawal from dependence-forming medications, for

CHAPTER 4

reasons that are poorly understood.[3] One method employed to trial re-instatement whilst mitigating the possibility of a negative outcome is to re-instate a 'test dose' of approximately 5% of usually employed doses, such as 25 mg of pregabalin or 100 mg of gabapentin.[3] If this test dose has positive effects, an increase in dose may be cautiously attempted.[3] If this test re-instatement produces a negative effect then re-instatement could be abandoned (but for some patients symptom resolution can occur after an initial exacerbation).

Addition of other medication is often less successful than re-instatement of the original drug.[27,28] Occasionally, clinicians will trial other medications for pain, neurological or psychological withdrawal symptoms when a patient's level of suffering is untenable, including benzodiazepines, opioids, and anti-epileptic medications, on a case-by-case basis, in the absence of any controlled trials. In such cases, a single medication should be trialled at a time and ceased if not successful to avoid the accumulation of polypharmacy. Sometimes, additional medication can worsen a patient's symptoms (perhaps due to their overall sensitised state), and many of these medications will present issues with dependence and withdrawal themselves.[3]

If patients suffer protracted withdrawal syndromes they may require financial and social support if their ability to work and function is impaired for long periods because the above treatment options were unsuccessful or only partially successful. There is unfortunately limited recognition of protracted withdrawal syndrome by clinicians, making navigating the medical and support systems difficult for these patients, adding to their suffering.[3,22,23] Such patients are often mis-diagnosed as suffering from a mental health condition or a psychosomatic disorder.[3,22,24,25] One of the main requests from patients is that the medical system recognises the difficulties that protracted withdrawal syndromes can cause them and that sufficient support is provided (including completing disability or benefits paperwork where needed).[26]

Some expert clinicians have suggested that this state may be better thought of as a neurological injury.[24] Nevertheless, the vast majority of people eventually recover (albeit some taking years)[26] and one important aspect of treatment is to project optimism for a favourable outcome, as despair in response to slow improvement is common.

Increased sensitivity during withdrawal

Patients can become highly sensitive to psychoactive and neurologically active substances during the process of withdrawal from psychiatric medications,[22,24] and this is also reported for gabapentinoid withdrawal in particular.[26] This phenomenon is thought to be related to an increased sensitivity to stimuli secondary to the de-stabilisation produced by the drug withdrawal process,[3,27,28] though the mechanism is not fully understood. People can respond to a wide variety of substances with activation or other paradoxical effects, including alcohol, neurologically active antibiotics,[29] caffeine, St John's Wort and sometimes even specific foods, supplements and herbs.[3,30] The fluoroquinolone class of antibiotics is particularly notorious for causing problems in benzodiazepine withdrawal[31] probably because this class of antibiotic is thought to interact with the GABA receptor.[32,33] This may be relevant to gabapentinoid withdrawal because of their GABA-mimetic effects.[34]

Where these substances exacerbate withdrawal symptoms it is wise to restrict exposure to them during the withdrawal process, and during the course of protracted withdrawal syndrome.[3] Sensitivities often resolve or improve markedly when the patient recovers from withdrawal.[3] It may not be possible to avoid all implicated medications during the withdrawal process. Decisions will be contingent upon individual circumstances, the risks of exacerbating withdrawal, the risks of the condition to be treated and the alternative treatments available.

References

1. Pfeffer G, Chouinard G, Margolese HC. Gabapentin in the treatment of antipsychotic-induced akathisia in schizophrenia. *Int Clin Psychopharm* 2005; **20**: 179–81.
2. See S, Hendriks E, Hsiung L. Akathisia induced by gabapentin withdrawal. *Ann Pharmacother* 2011; **45**: e31.
3. Framer A. What I have learnt from helping thousands of people taper off psychotropic medications. *Ther Adv Psychopharmacol* 2021; **11**: 204512532199127.
4. Narayan V, Haddad PM. Antidepressant discontinuation manic states: a critical review of the literature and suggested diagnostic criteria. *J Psychopharmacol* 2010; **25**: 306–13.
5. Tachere RO, Modirrousta M. Beyond anxiety and agitation: a clinical approach to akathisia. *Aust Fam Physician* 2017; **46**: 296–8.
6. Lohr JB, Eidt CA, Abdulrazzaq Alfaraj A, Soliman MA. The clinical challenges of akathisia. *CNS Spectr* 2015; **20**(Suppl): 1–14; quiz 15–6.
7. Akathisia Alliance for education and research. Akathisia Alliance for education and research. https://akathisiaalliance.org/about-akathisia/ (accessed 17 September, 2022).
8. Hengartner MP, Schulthess L, Sorensen A, Framer A. Protracted withdrawal syndrome after stopping antidepressants: a descriptive quantitative analysis of consumer narratives from a large internet forum. *Ther Adv Psychopharmacol* 2020; **10**: 2045125320980573.
9. Duma SR, Fung VS. Drug-induced movement disorders. *Aust Prescr* 2019; **42**: 56–61.
10. Weiss D, Aizenberg D, Hermesh H, et al. Cyproheptadine treatment in neuroleptic-induced akathisia. *Br J Psychiatry* 1995; **167**: 483–6.
11. Lima AR, Bacaltchuk J, Barnes TRE, Soares-Weiser K. Central action beta-blockers versus placebo for neuroleptic-induced acute akathisia. *Cochrane Database Syst Rev* 2004; **2004**: CD001946.
12. Rissardo JP, Caprara ALF. Mirtazapine-associated movement disorders: a literature review. *Tzu Chi Med J* 2020; **32**: 318–30.
13. Taubert M, Back I. The Akathisic Cyclist – An unusual symptomatic treatment. 2007. https://orca.cardiff.ac.uk/id/eprint/117286/ (accessed 24 September, 2022).
14. Blaisdell GD. Akathisia: a comprehensive review and treatment summary. *Pharmacopsychiatry* 1994; **27**: 139–46.
15. Cosci F, Chouinard G. Acute and persistent withdrawal syndromes following discontinuation of psychotropic medications. *Psychother Psychosom* 2020; **89**: 283–306.
16. Lerner A, Klein M. Dependence, withdrawal and rebound of CNS drugs: an update and regulatory considerations for new drugs development. *Brain Commun* 2019; **1**: fcz025.
17. Horowitz MA, Taylor D. How to reduce and stop psychiatric medication. *Eur Neuropsychopharmacol* 2021; **55**: 4–7.
18. Deng H, Benhamou O-M, Lembke A. Gabapentin dependence and withdrawal requiring an 18-month taper in a patient with alcohol use disorder: a case report. *J Addict Dis* 2021; **39**: 575–8.
19. Gabapentin/Lyrica Withdrawal Support. https://www.facebook.com/groups/1438525646474773/ (accessed 17 June, 2023).
20. Severe and Protracted Gabapentin Withdrawal Support Group. https://www.facebook.com/groups/1199119827120252 (accessed June 28, 2023).
21. Mersfelder TL, Nichols WH. Gabapentin: abuse, dependence, and withdrawal. *Ann Pharmacother* 2016; **50**: 229–33.
22. Ashton H. Benzodiazepines: how they work and how to withdraw (The Ashton Manual). 2002. http://www.benzo.org.uk/manual/bzcha01.htm (accessed 11 July, 2023).
23. Benzodiazepine tapering strategies and solutions. Benzodiazepine Information Coalition. 2020; published online September 21. https://www.benzoinfo.com/benzodiazepine-tapering-strategies/ (accessed 29 April, 2023).
24. Wright SL. Benzodiazepine withdrawal: clinical aspects. In:. *The Benzodiazepines Crisis* (eds. J Peppin, J Pergolizzi, R Raffa, S Wright). Oxford: Oxford University Press, 2020: 117–48.
25. Guy A, Brown M, Lewis S, Horowitz MA. The 'patient voice' – patients who experience antidepressant withdrawal symptoms are often dismissed, or mis-diagnosed with relapse, or onset of a new medical condition. *Ther Adv Psychopharmacol* 2020; **10**: 204512532096718.
26. Huff C, Finlayson AJR, Foster DE, Martin PR. Enduring neurological sequelae of benzodiazepine use: an Internet survey. *Ther Adv Psychopharmacol* 2023; **13**: 20451253221145560.
27. Otis HG, King JH. Unanticipated psychotropic medication reactions. *J Ment Health Couns* 2006; **28**: 218–40.
28. Smith SW, Hauben M, Aronson JK. Paradoxical and bidirectional drug effects. *Drug Saf* 2012; **35**: 173–89.
29. Bangert MK, Hasbun R. Neurological and psychiatric adverse effects of antimicrobials. *CNS Drugs* 2019; **33**: 727–53.
30. Parker G. Psychotropic drug intolerance. *J Nerv Ment Dis* 2018; **206**: 223–5.

CHAPTER 4

31. McConnell JG. Benzodiazepine tolerance, dependency, and withdrawal syndromes and interactions with fluoroquinolone antimicrobials. *Br J Gen Pract* 2008; 58: 365–6.

32. Unseld E, Ziegler G, Gemeinhardt A, Janssen U, Klotz U. Possible interaction of fluoroquinolones with the benzodiazepine-GABAA-receptor complex. *Br J Clin Pharmacol* 1990; 30: 63–70.

33. Scavone C, Mascolo A, Ruggiero R, et al. Quinolones-induced musculoskeletal, neurological, and psychiatric ADRs: a pharmacovigilance study based on data from the italian spontaneous reporting system. *Front Pharmacol* 2020; 11. doi:10.3389/fphar.2020.00428.

34. Bonnet U, Richter EL, Isbruch K, Scherbaum N. On the addictive power of gabapentinoids: a mini-review. *Psychiatr Danub* 2018; 30: 142–9.

Tapering Guidance for Specific Gabapentinoids

The following sections include guides to tapering pregabalin and gabapentin. To our knowledge, there has been no neuroimaging performed of gabapentinoid receptor occupancy. However, various clinical effects of gabapentinoids (e.g. anticonvulsant properties)[1] demonstrate a hyperbolic relationship with dose, which can be used to infer the relationship between dose and receptor occupancy. As for other medications, the clinical effect presumably mirrors the hyperbolic relationship at the receptor level (as dictated by the law of mass action).[2] Pharmacologically rational regimens were then calculated from these equations and are presented as 'faster', 'moderate' and 'slower' regimens. An attempt has been made to prioritise the use of widely available formulations and simple manipulations (e.g. tablet splitting) unless such approaches are not feasible for the dose reductions suggested.

There is little research to determine which of the three suggested example taper regimens is most suitable for a particular patient. Withdrawal is thought to be more severe for people who have used gabapentinoids at higher doses, for longer periods and for those who have experienced withdrawal in the past on reducing, stopping or missing a dose.[3] A rough guide to estimating initial reductions is shown in 'Tapering gabapentinoids in practice'. However, the response of the patient to initial reductions is the best guide as to the appropriate pace for a patient and the patient's experience should be prioritised over what an algorithm suggests. This patient-led aspect is a crucial part of our suggested regimens.

These guides include a summary of formulations available in selected countries around the world. Licensed and unlicensed (or 'off-label') options are presented. Overall, the guidance given here is broadly consistent with the UK NICE guidelines on how to stop gabapentinoids safely,[3] but we offer considerably more detail in order to allow implementation of deprescribing in clinical practice. Our regimens are informed by contributions from patient advocacy groups who have wide experience in determining the most appropriate rate and manner of withdrawal.[4,5]

Although there are many uncertainties in the field of deprescribing, the aim of this section is to provide some structure to the process of stopping gabapentinoids, while acknowledging that clinical judgement will have to be exercised to modify the regimens to fit the particular circumstances of individual patients. The key feature of these suggested regimens is that they represent a framework around which deviation can take place according to patient experience. Our aim is not necessarily to encourage deprescribing in all instances but rather to assure it is undertaken in a manner that optimises patient experience and outcome.

References

1. Delahoy P, Thompson S, Marschner IC. Pregabalin versus gabapentin in partial epilepsy: a meta-analysis of dose-response relationships. *BMC Neurol* 2010; 10: 104.
2. Holford N. Pharmacodynamic principles and the time course of delayed and cumulative drug effects. *Transl Clin Pharmacol* 2018; 26: 56–9.
3. National Institute for Social and Care Excellence (NICE). Medicines associated with dependence or withdrawal symptoms: safe prescribing and withdrawal management for adults | Guidance | NICE. 2022. https://www.nice.org.uk/guidance/ng215/chapter/Recommendations (accessed 27 June 2022).
4. Gabapentin/Lyrica withdrawal support. https://www.facebook.com/groups/1438525646474773/ (accessed 17 June 2023).
5. Framer A. What I have learnt from helping thousands of people taper off psychotropic medications. *Ther Adv Psychopharmacol* 2021; 11: 204512532199127.

CHAPTER 4

Gabapentin

Trade names: Neurontin, Gabarone, Gralise, Horizant.

Description: Gabapentin is a GABA analogue that binds to the alpha-2-delta ($\alpha 2\delta$) subunit of voltage-dependent calcium channels in presynaptic cell membranes.[1]

Withdrawal effects: The drug manufacturer warns that withdrawal effects from gabapentin (after short- and long-term treatment) can include anxiety, insomnia, nausea, pain, sweating, headache, convulsions, nervousness, depression, ataxia and dizziness.[1,2] No studies to our knowledge have been conducted to evaluate the incidence, severity and duration of withdrawal symptoms from gabapentin. There are no published studies on protracted withdrawal for gabapentin, but it has been reported.[3,4]

Peak plasma: Following oral administration, peak plasma gabapentin concentrations are observed within 2–3 hours.[1]

Half-life: Gabapentin has an elimination half-life of 5–7 hours. It is eliminated unchanged solely by renal excretion. Gabapentin is recommended to be taken three times a day by its manufacturer.[1,2] Dosing less often (including every-other-day dosing) is not recommended for tapering because the marked changes in plasma levels may precipitate inter-dose withdrawal symptoms.

Receptor occupancy: The relationship between dose of gabapentin and its effect on target receptors is hyperbolic as dictated by the law of mass action.[5] This is also reflected in the relationship between dose and clinical effects,[6] which may be relevant to withdrawal effects. Dose reductions made by linear amounts (e.g. 4,800mg, 3,600mg, 2,400mg, 1,200mg, 0mg) will cause increasingly large reductions in effect, which may cause increasingly severe withdrawal effects (Figure 4.5a). To produce equal-sized reductions in effect on receptor occupancy will require hyperbolically reducing doses (Figure 4.5b),[7] which informs the reductions presented. These dose–effect curves are derived from the relationship between dose and anticonvulsant effects in patients.[6]

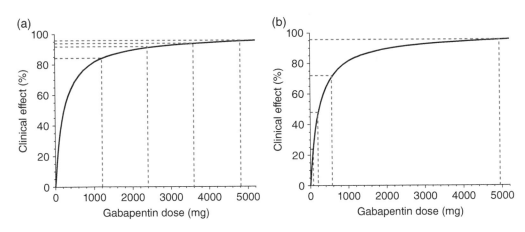

Figure 4.5 (a) Linear reductions of dose cause increasingly large reductions in clinical effect, possibly relevant to withdrawal effects. (b) Equally spaced reductions of effect requires hyperbolic dose reductions. The final dose before stopping will need to be very small so that this step down is not larger (in terms of effect on receptor occupancy) than previously tolerated reductions.

Available formulations: As tablets, capsules, extended-release capsules and liquid.

Tablets

Dosage	UK	Europe	USA	Australia	Canada
100mg	–	–	–	–	✓
300mg	–	–	✓	–	✓
400mg	–	–	–	–	✓
450mg	–	–	✓	–	–
600mg	✓	✓	✓	–	✓
800mg	✓	✓	✓	–	✓
900mg	–	–	✓	–	–

Capsule

Dosage	UK	Europe	USA	Australia	Canada
100mg	✓	✓	✓	✓	–
300mg	✓	✓	✓	–	–
400mg	✓	✓	✓	–	–

Extended- release capsules

Dosage	UK	Europe	USA	Australia	Canada
300mg	–	–	✓	–	–
600mg	–	–	✓	–	–

Liquids

Oral solutions	UK	Europe	USA	Australia	Canada
50mg/mL	✓	–	✓	–	–

Dilutions: In order to make up smaller doses for tapering, dilution of the manufacturer's solution may be required. Adding water to the original solution may have the effect of precipitating gabapentin and so a suspension might be formed.[8] All dilutions need therefore to be shaken thoroughly before use. Gabapentin has limited stability in water[9] and so diluted liquids should be taken immediately after preparation and any remainder discarded.

Dilutions	Solution required	How to prepare solution
Doses ≥ 10mg	50mg/mL	Original solution
Doses < 10mg	5mg/mL	Mix 0.5mL of original solution with 4.5mL of water*

*Other dilutions are possible to produce different concentrations. The above is provided as an example.

Off-label options: Liquid formulations are not universally available. In order to follow some of the suggested regimens, smaller doses are required than can be made using commercially available tablets and capsules. Guidelines for people who cannot swallow tablets[9] suggest that gabapentin capsules can be opened and the contents dissolved in water for administration. Gabapentin is highly soluble in water.[8] The capsule contents may have an unpleasant taste, which could be concealed with juice. For example, water could be added to the contents of a 100mg capsule to make up a 20mL solution (concentration 5mg/mL). The solution should be shaken vigorously before use. It should be consumed immediately, and any unused solution discarded since the drug is rapidly hydrolysed.[9]

Other options to make up small doses include having compounding pharmacies make up suspensions or smaller dose capsules or tablets, including the option of 'tapering strips'.[10]

Worked example: To illustrate how to calculate volumes to make up a given dose using a liquid, a worked example is provided. To make up 10mg of gabapentin using the 50mg/mL solution will require 10/50 = 0.2mL.

Deprescribing notes: There are no established guides to determine the rate of taper for someone stopping gabapentinoids. Withdrawal is thought to be more severe for people who have used gabapentinoids for longer periods, at higher doses, demonstrate evidence of tolerance and for those who have experienced withdrawal in the past on reducing, stopping or missing a dose. The size of the initial reduction should be inversely proportional to the number of risk factors (see 'Tapering gabapentinoids in practice'), with patient preference also taken into account. Sometimes, to start with, an even smaller reduction may be advisable to boost a patient's confidence that they can taper if the process is optimised.

Each reduction should only be made when the withdrawal symptoms from the previous reduction have largely resolved so that subsequent reductions do not lead to cumulative withdrawal symptoms. Withdrawal symptoms should not be too unpleasant: a rate of reduction should be aimed for that produces tolerable withdrawal symptoms that abate within a week or two. Allowing for a sufficient observation period, reductions can therefore be made about every 2–4 weeks, depending on how long it takes withdrawal symptoms to resolve. If withdrawal symptoms are moderately severe or take longer than a couple of weeks to resolve, dose reductions should be postponed until symptoms resolve and then made more gradual by choosing a slower tapering rate. If severe withdrawal symptoms occur, then the patient should return to a higher dose, wait until symptoms resolve and thereafter taper at a slower rate.

Suggested taper schedules for gabapentin: Please note that none of these regimens should be seen as prescriptive – patients should not be compelled to adhere strictly to them. They are given as example regimens and are not 'set and forget' but should be modified in order to ensure that withdrawal symptoms are tolerable throughout a taper. For example, intermediate steps halfway between the doses listed could be added to make a more gradual taper. Ultimately, it is the patient's experience of withdrawal that should guide the rate of taper.

A. A faster taper with up to 10 percentage points of 'clinical effect' between each step – with reductions made every 2–4 weeks*.

Step	CE (%)	AM (mg)	PM (mg)	Night (mg)	Total daily dose (mg)	Form
1	95	1,600	1,600	1,600	4,800	Tablets or capsules
2	89	600	600	600	1,800	Tablets or capsules
3	80	300	300	300	900	Tablets or capsules
4	72	200	200	200	600	Tablets or capsules
5	64	150	100	150	400	Use ¼ or ½ tablets**
6	57	100	100	100	300	Tablets or capsules
			Switch to **50mg/mL solution**			
7	47	70	60	70	200	1.4mL/ 1.2mL/1.4mL
8	40	50	50	50	150	1mL 3 times per day
9	31	35	30	35	100	0.7mL/0.6mL/0.7mL
10	25	25	25	25	75	0.5mL 3 times per day
11	18	20	10	20	50	0.4mL/0.2mL/0.4mL
			Switch to **5mg/mL dilution**			
12	10	10	5	10	25	2mL/1mL/2mL
13	0	0	0	0	0	0

CE = clinical effect

*Patients who have been on the medication for only a few weeks will probably be able to taper more quickly and might follow every second or third step of this regimen and make reductions every few days or so. Normally the duration of the taper should not be longer than the period that the patient has been on the drug for people who have only taken it for a few weeks. For example, if gabapentin is taken for 3 weeks the taper should be less than 3 weeks.

**Alternatively, a liquid formulation of the drug could be used for these doses.

B. A moderate taper with up to 6 percentage points of 'clinical effect' between each step – with reductions made every 2–4 weeks.

Step	CE (%)	AM (mg)	PM (mg)	Night (mg)	Total daily dose (mg)	Form
1	95.5	1,600	1,600	1,600	4,800	Tabs or caps
2	91.3	800	800	800	2,400	Tabs or caps
3	88.8	600	600	600	1,800	Tabs or caps
4	84	400	400	400	1,200	Tabs or caps
5	79.8	300	300	300	900	Tabs or caps
6	76.7	250	250	250	750	Use ½ tabs*
7	72.5	200	200	200	600	Tabs or caps
8	68.7	200	100	200	500	Tabs or caps
9	63.7	150	100	150	400	Use ½ or ¼ tabs*
10	60.6	100	100	150	350	Use ½ or ¼ tabs*
11	56.8	100	100	100	300	Tabs or caps
Switch to **50mg/mL solution**						
12	52.3	80	70	100	250	1.6mL/1.4mL/2mL
13	46.7	70	60	70	200	1.4mL/1.2mL/1.4mL
See further steps in the right-hand column						

Step	CE (%)	AM (mg)	PM (mg)	Night (mg)	Total daily dose (mg)	Form
14	43.4	60	55	60	175	1.2mL/1.1mL/1.2mL
15	39.7	50	50	50	150	1mL 3 times per day
16	35.4	45	35	45	125	0.9mL/0.7mL/0.9mL
17	30.5	35	30	35	100	0.7mL/0.6mL/0.7mL
18	26	30	20	30	80	0.6mL/0.4mL/0.6mL
19	22.2	20	20	25	65	0.4mL/0.4mL/0.5mL
20	18	20	10	20	50	0.4mL/0.2mL/0.4mL
21	13.3	10	10	15	35	0.2mL/0.2mL/0.3mL
Switch to **5mg/mL dilution**						
22	9.9	10	5	10	25	2mL/1mL/2mL
23	6.2	5	5	5	15	1mL 3 times per day
24	2.1	2	1	2	5	0.4mL/0.2mL/0.4mL
25	0	0	0	0	0	

CE = clinical effect, tabs = tablets, caps = capsules
*Alternatively, a liquid formulation of the drug could be used for these doses.

C. A slower taper with up to 3 percentage points of 'clinical effect' between each step – with reductions made every 2–4 weeks.

Step	CE (%)	AM (mg)	PM (mg)	Night (mg)	Total daily dose (mg)	Form
1	95.5	1,600	1,600	1,600	4,800	Tabs or caps
2	93.4	1,100	1,000	1,100	3,200	Tabs or caps
3	91.3	800	800	800	2,400	Tabs or caps
4	88.8	600	600	600	1,800	Tabs or caps
5	87.5	500	500	600	1,600	Tabs or caps
6	86	500	400	500	1,400	Tabs or caps
7	84	400	400	400	1,200	Tabs or caps
8	81.4	300	300	400	1,000	Tabs or caps
9	79.8	300	300	300	900	Tabs or caps
10	77.8	300	200	300	800	Tabs or caps
11	75.4	200	200	300	700	Tabs or caps
12	72.5	200	200	200	600	Tabs or caps
13	70.7	200	150	200	550	Use ½ or ¼ tabs*
14	68.7	150	150	200	500	Use ½ or ¼ tabs*
15	66.4	150	150	150	450	Use ½ or ¼ tabs*
			Switch to **50mg/mL solution**			
16	65.1	150	125	150	425	3mL/2.5mL/3mL
17	63.7	125	125	150	400	2.5mL/2.5mL/3mL
18	62.2	125	125	125	375	2.5mL 3 times per day
19	60.6	120	110	120	350	2.4mL/2.2mL/2.4mL

See further steps in the right-hand column

Step	CE (%)	AM (mg)	PM (mg)	Night (mg)	Total daily dose (mg)	Form
20	58.8	110	105	110	325	2.2mL/2.1mL/2.2mL
21	56.8	100	100	100	300	2mL 3 times per day
22	54.7	100	75	100	275	2mL/1.5mL/2mL
23	52.3	90	70	90	250	1.8mL/1.4mL/1.8mL
24	50.2	80	70	80	230	1.6mL/1.4mL/1.6mL
25	48	70	70	70	210	1.4mL 3 times per day
26	45.5	65	60	65	190	1.3mL/1.2mL/1.3mL
27	43.4	60	55	60	175	1.2mL/1.1mL/1.2mL
28	41.3	55	50	55	160	1.1mL/1mL/1.1mL
29	38.9	50	45	50	145	1mL/0.9mL/1mL
30	36.3	45	40	45	130	0.9mL/0.8mL/0.9mL
31	34.5	40	40	40	120	0.8mL 3 times per day
32	32.6	40	30	40	110	0.8mL/0.6mL/0.8mL
33	30.5	35	30	35	100	0.7mL/0.6mL/0.7mL
34	28.3	30	30	30	90	0.6mL 3 times per day
35	25	25	25	30	80	0.5mL/0.5mL/0.6mL
36	23.5	25	20	25	70	0.5mL/0.4mL/0.5mL
37	21.4	21	20	21	62	0.42mL/0.4mL/0.42mL
38	19.2	18	18	18	54	0.36mL 3 times per day
39	16.8	15	15	16	46	0.3mL/0.3mL/0.32mL

(Continued)

(Continued)

Step	CE (%)	AM (mg)	PM (mg)	Night (mg)	Total daily dose (mg)	Form
40	14.3	12	11	15	38	0.24mL/0.22mL/0.3mL
41	12	10	10	11	31	0.2mL/0.2mL/0.22mL
Switch to 5mg/mL dilution						
42	9.5	8	8	8	24	1.6mL 3 times per day
43	7.3	6	6	6	18	1.2mL 3 times per day
See further steps in the right-hand column						

Step	CE (%)	AM (mg)	PM (mg)	Night (mg)	Total daily dose (mg)	Form
44	5	4	4	4	12	0.8mL 3 times per day
45	2.6	2	2	2	6	0.4mL 3 times per day
46	1.3	1	1	1	3	0.2mL 3 times per day
47	0	0	0	0	0	

CE = clinical effect

*Alternatively, a liquid formulation of the drug could be used for these doses.

D. **An even slower taper** Some patients will be unable to taper at the slowest rates shown here and will need to taper by even smaller decrements, thus lengthening the overall period of the taper. Such a regimen could be constructed by placing intermediate steps in regimen C. For example, 800mg, 700mg, 600mg could be modified to 800mg, 750mg, 700mg, 650mg, 600mg and so on. Further intermediate steps could also be added.

Micro-tapering: The tables above show how to make reductions at intervals of 2–4 weeks. An alternative approach is called 'micro-tapering' whereby very small dose reductions are made every day, as explained in 'Other considerations in tapering gabapentinoids'. Micro-tapering rates can be calculated from the above by dividing the change in dose for each step by 14 or 28 days. For example, for the moderate regimen a reduction of 150mg to 125mg over 14 days is equivalent to a reduction of approximately 1.8mg per day, or 0.6mg reduction per dose (when dosed three times per day). In order to make such small reductions a liquid version of the drug will be needed. By the end of the taper this rate will reduce to reductions of 0.4mg per day. This rate can be adjusted if withdrawal symptoms become too unpleasant.

References

1. SmPC. Gabapentin – Summary of Product Characteristics (SmPC). 2019. https://www.medicines.org.uk/emc/product/2362/smpc#gref (accessed 21 June 2023).
2. FDA. Gabapentin – Highlights of Prescribing Information. 2006. https://www.accessdata.fda.gov/drugsatfda_docs/label/2017/020235s064_020882s047_021129s046lbl.pdf (accessed 30 September 2023).
3. Severe and Protracted Gabapentin Withdrawal Support Group. https://www.facebook.com/groups/1199119827120252 (accessed 28 June 2023).
4. Gabapentin/Lyrica Withdrawal Support. https://www.facebook.com/groups/1438525646474773/ (accessed 17 June 2023).
5. Holford N. Pharmacodynamic principles and the time course of delayed and cumulative drug effects. *Transl Clin* 2018; 26: 56–9.
6. Delahoy P, Thompson S, Marschner IC. Pregabalin versus gabapentin in partial epilepsy: a meta-analysis of dose-response relationships. *BMC Neurol* 2010; 10: 104.
7. Horowitz MA, Taylor D. How to reduce and stop psychiatric medication. *Eur Neuropsychopharmacol* 2021; 55: 4–7.
8. FDA. Neurontin (gabapentin) oral solution label. FDA. https://www.accessdata.fda.gov/drugsatfda_docs/label/2010/021129s029lbl.pdf (accessed 28 June 2023).
9. Smyth J. The NEWT guidelines for administration of medication to patients with enteral feeding tubes or swallowing difficulties. 2011. https://www.newtguidelines.com/index.html (accessed 5 July 2023).
10. Framer A. What I have learnt from helping thousands of people taper off antidepressants and other psychotropic medications. *Ther Adv Psychopharmacol* 2021; 11: 204512532199127.

CHAPTER 4

Pregabalin

Trade names: Lyrica, Lyrica CR, Alzain, Axalid.

Description: Pregabalin is a GABA analogue that binds to the alpha-2-delta ($\alpha2\delta$) subunit of voltage-dependent calcium channels in presynaptic cell membranes.[1]

Withdrawal effects: The drug manufacturer warns that withdrawal effects from pregabalin (after short- and long-term treatment) can include insomnia, headache, nausea, anxiety, diarrhoea, flu syndrome, convulsions, nervousness, depression, pain, hyperhidrosis and dizziness.[1] No studies to our knowledge have been conducted to evaluate the incidence, severity and duration of withdrawal symptoms from pregabalin. There are no published data on whether a protracted withdrawal syndrome is seen with pregabalin, but it has been reported.[2]

Peak plasma: For instant-release pregabalin time to peak plasma is 1 hour[1] and for the controlled release it is 8–12 hours. Food delays absorption with larger amounts of food proportionately delaying the time to peak plasma.[3]

Half-life: Pregabalin has an elimination half-life of 6.3 hours, although controlled release formulations have a longer duration of action owing to delayed disintegration and absorption.[1,3] Pregabalin instant-release is recommended by its manufacturer to be taken two to three times a day, while the controlled release version can be taken once a day.[1,3] Dosing less often (including every-other-day dosing) is not recommended for tapering because the changes in plasma levels may precipitate inter-dose withdrawal symptoms.

Receptor occupancy: The relationship between dose of pregabalin and its effect on target receptors is hyperbolic as dictated by the law of mass action.[4] This is also reflected in the relationship between dose and clinical effects,[5] which may be relevant to withdrawal effects. Dose reductions made by linear amounts (e.g. 600mg, 450mg, 300mg, 150mg, 0mg) will cause increasingly large reductions in effect which may cause increasingly severe withdrawal effects (Figure 4.6a). To produce equal-sized reductions in effect on receptor occupancy will require hyperbolically reducing doses (Figure 4.6b),[6] which informs the reductions presented. These dose–effect curves are derived from the relationship between dose and anticonvulsant effects in patients.[5]

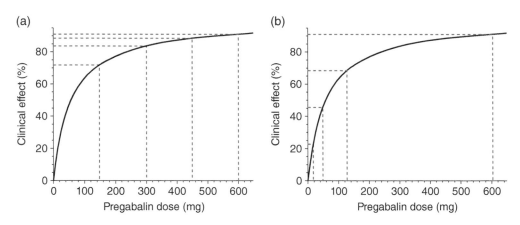

Figure 4.6 (a) Linear reductions of dose cause increasingly large reductions in pharmacological effect, and this is probably relevant to withdrawal effects. (b) Equally spaced reductions of effect requires hyperbolic dose reductions. The final dose before stopping will need to be very small so that this step down is not larger (in terms of effect on receptor occupancy) than previously tolerated reductions.

Available formulations: As tablets, controlled release tables, capsules and liquid.

Tablets

Dosage	UK	Europe	USA	Australia	Canada
25mg	✓	–	–	–	–
50mg	✓	–	–	–	–
75mg	✓	–	–	–	–
100mg	✓	–	–	–	–
150mg	✓	–	–	–	–
200mg	✓	–	–	–	–
225mg	✓	–	–	–	–
300mg	✓	–	–	–	–

Controlled-release tablets

Dosage	UK	Europe	USA	Australia	Canada
82.5mg	–	–	✓	–	
165mg	–	–	✓	–	–
330mg	–	–	✓	–	–

Capsules

Dosage	UK	Europe	USA	Australia	Canada
25mg	✓	✓	✓	✓	✓
50mg	✓	✓	✓	–	✓
75mg	✓	✓	✓	✓	✓
100mg	✓	✓	✓	–	–
150mg	✓	✓	✓	✓	✓
200mg	✓	✓	✓	–	–
225mg	✓	✓	✓	–	✓
300mg	✓	✓	✓	✓	✓

Liquids

Oral solutions	UK	Europe	USA	Australia	Canada
20mg/mL*	✓	✓	✓	–	–

*In order to make up small volumes with this solution, a small syringe (e.g. 1mL) may be required. In order to use this syringe, the bung supplied with the drug to fit the manufacturer's syringe may need to be removed.

CHAPTER 4

Dilutions: In order to make up smaller doses for tapering, dilution of the manufacturer's solution may be required. Adding water to the original solution may have the effect of precipitating pregabalin and so a suspension might be formed.[7] All dilutions need therefore to be shaken thoroughly before use. Drug stability, however, cannot be assured, and so dilutions should be taken immediately after preparation (and any remainder should be discarded).

Dilutions	Solution required	How to prepare solution
Doses ≥ 4mg	20mg/mL	Original solution
Doses < 4mg	2mg/mL	Mix 0.5mL of original solution with 4.5mL of water*

*Other dilutions are possible to produce different concentrations. The above is provided as an example.

Off-label options: Liquid formulations are not universally available. In order to follow some of the regimens suggested, smaller doses than can be made using commercially available tablets and capsules are required. Guidelines for people who cannot swallow tablets[8] suggest that pregabalin capsules can be opened and the contents dissolved in water for administration. Pregabalin, as already mentioned, is highly soluble in water.[7] The capsule contents may have an unpleasant taste,[8] which could be concealed with juice. For example, water could be added to the contents of a 25mg capsule to make up a 25mL solution (concentration 1mg/mL). The mixture should be shaken vigorously before use. Any cloudiness is probably due to insoluble tablet excipients. As its stability cannot be assured it should be consumed immediately and any unused mixture discarded.

Other options to make up small doses include having compounding pharmacies make up suspensions, solutions or smaller dose capsules or tablets, including the option of 'tapering strips'.[9]

Worked example: To illustrate how to calculate volumes to make up a given dose using a liquid, a worked example is provided. To make up 4mg of pregabalin using the 20mg/mL solution will require 4/20 = 0.2mL.

Deprescribing notes: There are no established guides to determine the rate of taper for stopping gabapentinoids. Withdrawal is thought to be more severe for people who have used gabapentinoids for longer periods, at higher doses, demonstrate evidence of tolerance and for those who have experienced withdrawal in the past on reducing, stopping or missing a dose.[10,11] The size of the initial reduction should be inversely proportional to the number of risk factors (see 'Tapering gabapentinoids in practice'), with patient preference also taken into account. Sometimes, to start with, an even smaller reduction may be advisable to boost a patient's confidence that they can taper if the process is optimised.

Each reduction should only be made when the withdrawal symptoms from the previous reduction have largely resolved so that subsequent reductions do not lead to cumulative withdrawal symptoms. Withdrawal symptoms should not be too unpleasant: a rate of reduction should be aimed for that produces tolerable withdrawal symptoms that abate within a week or two. Allowing for a sufficient observation period, reductions can therefore be made about every 2–4 weeks, depending on how long it takes withdrawal symptoms to resolve. If withdrawal symptoms are moderately severe or take longer than a couple of weeks to resolve, dose reductions should be postponed until symptoms resolve and then made more gradual by choosing a slower tapering rate. If severe withdrawal symptoms occur, then the patient should return to a higher dose, wait until symptoms resolve and thereafter taper at a slower rate.

Suggested taper schedules for pregabalin: Please note that none of these regimens should be seen as prescriptive – patients should not be compelled to adhere strictly to them. They are given as example regimens and are not 'set and forget' but should be modified in order to ensure that withdrawal symptoms are tolerable throughout a taper. For example, intermediate steps halfway in between the doses listed could be added to make a more gradual taper. Ultimately, it is the patient's experience of withdrawal that should guide the rate of taper.

A. **A faster taper** with up to 10 percentage points of 'clinical effect' between each step – with reductions made every 2–4 weeks*.

Step	CE (%)	AM (mg)	PM (mg)	Total daily dose (mg)	Form
1	91	300	300	600	Tablets or capsules
2	83	150	150	300	Tablets or capsules
3	79	100	125	225	Tablets or capsules
4	72	75	75	150	Tablets or capsules
5	63	50	50	100	Tablets or capsules
6	56	37.5	37.5	75	Use ½ tablets**
7	46	25	25	50	Tablets or capsules
8	39	18.75	18.75	37.5	Use ¾ tablets**
9	30	12.5	12.5	25	Use ½ tablets**
Switch to pregabalin **20mg/mL solution**					
10	24	9	9	18	0.45mL AM and PM
11	17	6	6	12	0.3mL AM and PM
12	9	3	3	6	0.15mL AM and PM
13	0	0	0	0	

CE = clinical effect

*Patients who have been on the medication for only a few weeks will probably be able to taper more quickly and might follow every second or third step of this regimen and make reductions every few days or so. Normally the duration of the taper should not be longer than the period that the patient has been on the drug for people who have only taken it for a few weeks. For example, if pregabalin is taken for 3 weeks the taper should be less than 3 weeks.

**Alternatively, a liquid formulation of the drug could be used for these doses.

B. **A moderate taper** with up to 5 percentage points of 'clinical effect' between each step – with reductions made every 2-4 weeks.

Step	CE (%)	AM (mg)	PM (mg)	Total daily dose (mg)	Form	Step	CE (%)	AM (mg)	PM (mg)	Total daily dose (mg)	Form
1	91	300	300	600	Tabs or caps	Switch to pregabalin **20mg/mL solution**					
2	86.3	175	200	375	Tabs or caps	16	42.5	22	22	44	1.1mL AM and PM
3	82.2	125	150	275	Tabs or caps	17	38.9	19	19	38	0.95mL AM and PM
4	79	100	125	225	Tabs or caps	18	34.9	16	16	32	0.8mL AM and PM
5	74.6	75	100	175	Tabs or caps	19	30.4	13	13	26	0.65mL AM and PM
6	71.5	75	75	150	Tabs or caps	20	26.9	11	11	22	0.55mL AM and PM
7	69.7	62.5	75	137.5	Use ½ tablets*	21	23.2	9	9	18	0.45mL AM and PM
8	67.7	50	75	125	Tabs or caps	22	19	7	7	14	0.35mL AM and PM
9	65.3	50	62.5	112.5	Use ½ tablets*	23	14.4	5	5	10	0.25mL AM and PM
10	62.6	50	50	100	Tabs or caps	24	11.8	4	4	8	0.2mL AM and PM
11	59.5	37.5	50	87.5	Use ½ tablets*	Switch to pregabalin **2mg/mL dilution****					
12	55.7	37.5	37.5	75	Use ½ tablets*	25	9.1	3	3	6	1.5mL AM and PM
13	51.2	25	37.5	62.5	Use ½ tablets*	26	6.3	2	2	4	1mL AM and PM
14	48.5	25	31.25	56.25	Use ¼ tablets*	27	3.2	1	1	2	0.5mL AM and PM
15	45.6	25	25	50	Tabs or caps	28	0	0	0	0	0
See further steps in the right-hand column											

CE = clinical effect, tabs = tablets, caps = capsules
*Alternatively, a liquid formulation of the drug could be used for these doses.
**Prepared as above

C. **A slower taper** with up to 3 percentage points of 'clinical effect' between each step – with reductions made every 2–4 weeks.

Step	CE (%)	AM (mg)	PM (mg)	Total daily dose (mg)	Form	Step	CE (%)	AM (mg)	PM (mg)	Total daily dose (mg)	Form
1	91	300	300	600	Tabs or caps	25	46.6	26	26	52	1.3mL AM and PM
2	88.8	225	250	475	Tabs or caps	26	44.6	24	24	48	1.2mL AM and PM
3	87	200	200	400	Tabs or caps	27	42.5	22	22	44	1.1mL AM and PM
4	85.4	175	175	350	Tabs or caps	28	40.1	20	20	40	1mL AM and PM
5	83.4	150	150	300	Tabs or caps	29	38.3	18.5	18.5	37	0.93mL AM and PM
6	82.2	125	150	275	Tabs or caps	30	36.3	17	17	34	0.85mL AM and PM
7	80.7	125	125	250	Tabs or caps	31	34.2	15.5	15.5	31	0.78mL AM and PM
8	79	100	125	225	Tabs or caps	32	31.9	14	14	28	0.7mL AM and PM
9	77	100	100	200	Tabs or caps	33	30.4	13	13	26	0.65mL AM and PM
10	74.6	75	100	175	Tabs or caps	34	28.7	12	12	24	0.6mL AM and PM
11	73.1	75	87.5	162.5	Use ½ tablets*	35	26.9	11	11	22	0.55mL AM and PM
12	71.5	75	75	150	Tabs or caps	36	25.1	10	10	20	0.5mL AM and PM
13	69.7	62.5	75	137.5	Use ½ tablets*	37	23.2	9	9	18	0.45mL AM and PM
14	67.7	62.5	62.5	125	Use ½ tablets*	38	21.2	8	8	16	0.4mL AM and PM
15	65.3	50	62.5	112.5	Use ½ tablets*	39	19	7	7	14	0.35mL AM and PM
16	62.6	50	50	100	Tabs or caps	40	16.7	6	6	12	0.3mL AM and PM
17	61.1	43.75	50	93.75	Use ¾ tablets*	41	14.4	5	5	10	0.25mL AM and PM
18	59.5	43.75	43.75	87.5	Use ¾ tablets*	42	11.8	4	4	8	0.2mL AM and PM
19	57.7	37.5	43.75	81.25	Use ½ and ¾ tablets*		Switch to pregabalin **2mg/mL dilution**				
20	55.7	37.5	37.5	75	Use ½ tablets*	43	9.8	3.2	3.2	6.4	1.6mL AM and PM
21	53.5	31.25	37.5	68.75	Use ½ and ¼ tablets*	44	7.7	2.5	2.5	5	1.25mL AM and PM
	Switch to pregabalin **20mg/mL solution**					45	5.5	1.74	1.74	3.48	0.87mL AM and PM
22	51.8	32	32	64	1.6mL AM and PM	46	3.2	1	1	2	0.5mL AM and PM
23	50.1	30	30	60	1.5mL AM and PM	47	1.6	0.5	0.5	1	0.25mL AM and PM
24	48.4	28	28	56	1.4mL AM and PM	48	0	0	0	0	
	See further steps in the right-hand column										

CE = clinical effect, tabs = tablets, caps = capsules
*Alternatively, a liquid formulation of the drug could be used for these doses.

CHAPTER 4

D. **An even slower taper** Some patients will be unable to taper at the slowest rates shown here and will need to taper by even smaller decrements, thus lengthening the overall period of the taper. Such a regimen could be constructed by placing intermediate steps in regimen C. For example, 300mg, 275mg, 250mg could be modified to 300mg, 287.5mg, 275mg, 262.5mg, 250mg and so on. Further intermediate steps could also be added.

Micro-tapering: The tables above show how to make reductions at intervals of 2–4 weeks. An alternative approach is called 'micro-tapering' whereby very small dose reductions are made every day, as explained in 'Other considerations in tapering gabapentinoids'. Micro-tapering rates can be calculated from the above by dividing the change in dose for each step by 14 or 28 days. For example, for the moderate regimen a reduction of 150mg to 137.5mg over 14 days is equivalent to a reduction of 0.9mg per day, or 0.45mg reduction per dose (when dosed twice a day). In order to make such small reductions a liquid version of the drug will be needed. By the end of the taper this rate will reduce to reductions of 0.14mg a day. This rate can be adjusted if withdrawal symptoms become too unpleasant.

References

1. Pregabalin 150mg capsules, hard – Summary of Product Characteristics (SmPC) – (emc). https://www.medicines.org.uk/emc/product/7132/smpc (accessed 17 June 2023).
2. Gabapentin/Lyrica Withdrawal Support. https://www.facebook.com/groups/1438525646474773/ (accessed 17 June 2023).
3. FDA. Lyrica CR: Highlights of Prescribing Information. FDA. www.accessdata.fda.gov/drugsatfda_docs/label/2017/209501s000lbl.pdf (accessed 17 June 2023).
4. Holford N. Pharmacodynamic principles and the time course of delayed and cumulative drug effects. *Transl Clin* 2018; 26: 56–9.
5. Delahoy P, Thompson S, Marschner IC. Pregabalin versus gabapentin in partial epilepsy: a meta-analysis of dose–response relationships. *BMC Neurol* 2010; 10: 104.
6. Horowitz MA, Taylor D. Tapering of SSRI treatment to mitigate withdrawal symptoms. *The Lancet Psychiatry* 2019; 6: 538–46.
7. PubChem. Pregabalin. PubChem. https://pubchem.ncbi.nlm.nih.gov/compound/Pregabalin (accessed 17 June 2023).
8. Colchester Medicines Information. MOC guidelines for tablet crushing in patients with swallowing difficulties. Colchester Hospital University, 2018.
9. Groot PC, van Os J. Successful use of tapering strips for hyperbolic reduction of antidepressant dose: a cohort study. *Ther Adv Psychopharmacol* 2021; 11: 20451253211039330.
10. Framer A. What I have learnt from helping thousands of people taper off psychotropic medications. *Ther Adv Psychopharmacol* 2021; 11: 204512532199127.
11. National Institute for Health and Care Excellence (NICE). Medicines associated with dependence or withdrawal symptoms: safe prescribing and withdrawal management for adults | Guidance | NICE. 2022. https://www.nice.org.uk/guidance/ng215/chapter/Recommendations (accessed 27 June 2022).

Index

The Maudsley® Deprescribing Guidelines: Antidepressants, Benzodiazepines, Gabapentinoids and Z-drugs,
First Edition. Mark Horowitz and David Taylor.
© 2024 John Wiley & Sons Ltd. Published 2024 by John Wiley & Sons Ltd.